Thieme

Mohs Micrographic Surgery: From Layers to Reconstruction

Christopher B. Harmon, MD, FAAD, FACMS
Dermatologic Surgeon
Surgical Dermatology Group;
Director
ACGME Fellowship in Micrographic Surgery and Dermatologic Oncology
Birmingham, Alabama, USA

Stanislav N. Tolkachjov, MD, FAAD, FACMS
Dermatologic Surgeon and Dallas-Fort Worth Area Director
Mohs Micrographic & Reconstructive Surgery
Epiphany Dermatology;
Clinical Assistant Professor
University of Texas Southwestern Medical Center;
Clinical Associate Professor
Texas A&M College of Medicine;
Core Faculty
Division of Dermatology
Baylor University Medical Center
Dallas, Texas, USA

813 illustrations

Thieme
Stuttgart • New York • Delhi • Rio de Janeiro

Library of Congress Cataloging-in-Publication Data
is available from the publisher.

Important Note: Medicine is an ever-changing science undergoing continual development. Research and clinical experience are continually expanding our knowledge, in particular our knowledge of proper treatment and drug therapy. Insofar as this book mentions any dosage or application, readers may rest assured that the authors, editors, and publishers have made every effort to ensure that such references are in accordance with **the state of knowledge at the time of production of the book.**

Nevertheless, this does not involve, imply, or express any guarantee or responsibility on the part of the publishers with respect to any dosage instructions and forms of application stated in the book. **Every user is requested to examine carefully** the manufacturer's leaflets accompanying each drug and to check, if necessary in consultation with a physician or specialist, whether the dosage schedules mentioned therein or the contraindications stated by the manufacturer differ from the statements made in the present book. Such examination is particularly important with drugs that are either rarely used or have been newly released on the market. Every dosage schedule or every form of application used is entirely at the user's risk and responsibility. The authors and publishers request every user to report to the publishers any discrepancies or inaccuracies noticed.

Some of the product names, patents, and registered designs referred to in this book are in fact registered trademarks or proprietary names, even though specific reference to this fact is not always made in the text. Therefore, the appearance of a name without a designation as proprietary is not to be construed as a representation by the publisher that it is in the public domain.

Thieme addresses people of all gender identities equally. We encourage our authors to use gender-neutral or gender-equal expressions wherever the context allows.

Georg Thieme Verlag KG
Rüdigerstrasse 14, 70469 Stuttgart, Germany
+49 [0]711 8931 421, customerservice@thieme.de

Cover design: © Thieme
Cover image source: © Thieme
Typesetting by DiTech Process Solutions Pvt. Ltd., India

MIX
Papier aus verantwortungsvollen Quellen
FSC® C089473
FSC
www.fsc.org

Printed in Germany by Beltz Grafische Betriebe 5 4 3 2 1

DOI: 10.1055/b000000239

ISBN 978-3-13-242017-5

Also available as an e-book:
eISBN (PDF): 978-3-13-242018-2
eISBN (epub): 978-3-13-258252-1

To begin with, I am grateful to my uncle, Dr. John Yarbrough, for his influence to pursue surgical dermatology as a career path over cardiovascular surgery and other surgical subspecialties. "Unc" (as he was affectionately referred to) gave me an appreciation for the art and relational aspect of medicine that supersedes the science of medicine. More than anyone I've known, John had a skill for connecting with patients and compassionately providing care. In his words, "With the frailty of one human being helping another human being ... we practice medicine." He was indeed inclined to treat rather than not treat. Another favorite quote that he borrowed from Dr. John Voorhees was, "I'm not much on diagnosis, but I'm hell on treatment."

As a lifelong learner, I have had the opportunity to continue to learn from the 25 plus Mohs surgery fellows we have trained over a 20-year period. As they now practice in locations from South Carolina to California, our continued collaboration fosters the sharing of ideas, evolving new surgical concepts, best business practices, and most importantly continued friendship and collegiality. Thank you all for the "rebound mentorship" ... keep up the good work.

This text is the result of experience gained from over 80,000 surgical cases in the past 22 years referred to our practice (Surgical Dermatology Group) from the dermatologists and other physicians practicing in Alabama and surrounding states. Your growing friendship over the years is cherished. The vote of confidence you place by entrusting your skin cancer patients to our care is our life blood. We value the great care you provide for your patients and thank you for the opportunity to participate in their care.

I could not have succeeded with undertakings such as this textbook, or the opening of new office locations, and the high volume of surgical cases we perform without our "Surgical Dermatology Group" team members. From physicians to mid-levels and executive team members, to the Ambulatory Surgery Center RNs, CRNAs, our histotechnicians and medical assistants, as well as surgery schedulers, receptionists, and back-office support staff ... thank you all for doing what you do with humility and a commitment to excellence.

For my parents ... thank you for providing a home life that encourages progress and an unending pursuit of excellence. This foundation of love, approval, and support has culminated in this writing and in any successes I have experienced. Ultimately, I dedicate this work to my wife Sandy and our two daughters, Mary Elizabeth and Haley, for supporting my various career endeavors like the undertaking of a textbook which intrudes evenings and weekends. They are the joy of my life and the reason I do what I do ... whether on the tennis court, the mission field, or over prayer time at the dinner table.

Christopher B. Harmon, MD, FAAD, FACMS

To the Almighty God, through Whom all things are possible and Whose will be done. You give us strength when we have none. You lift us up when we are at our depths. You use our hands and the talents You have given us to do Your healing. Your Son made the ultimate sacrifice, so we can forever be with You.

To my selfless and loving wife, Holly. You have stood beside me on the journey from when medicine was just a dream. You have accomplished so much yet stepped back to allow me to chase my dreams. You have been a pillar for our family and a beautiful example of enduring love. You're an incredibly strong individual yet an altruistic best friend. I love you for you.

To my children, Alexander and Ekaterina. Many of the long hours spent on this project I took from you. Every moment spent with you fuels and recharges my soul. There's nothing more precious than watching you grow up loving each other, your family, and the world around you. Your spirit of empathy, honesty, idealism, love, enthusiasm, humor, fun, and care are examples I bring to treat my patients daily. May our bonds continue to grow and may you grow up to be a shining light and a helping hand to the world around you. You are and will always be our greatest achievement.

To my mother and Brian. You brought me from Russia at a young age. We survived on little to nothing, but you taught me the value of hard work, education, and sacrifice. You gave up your dreams for a better life for me. I love you.

Stanislav N. Tolkachjov, MD, FAAD, FACMS

Contents

Videos

Video 1.1: Curettage following sharp debulking.

Video 1.2: Sharp debulking—eyelid.

Video 1.3: Excising the first stage during Mohs surgery.

Video 1.4: Forceps-free atraumatic Mohs initial stage.

Video 1.5: Basic first-stage tissue processing.

Video 1.6: Subsequent Mohs stages.

Video 1.7: Sampling the hinge point on subsequent Mohs stages.

Video 1.8: Deep layer epidermal tag technique.

Video 1.9: Deep layer postage stamp technique.

Video 1.10: Gridding for deep only layers.

Video 1.11: Initial and subsequent stages.

Video 3.1: Shave and sand technique.

Video 3.2: Bilobed flap.

Video 3.3: Forehead flap.

Video 3.4: Conchal bowl full-thickness skin graft.

Video 3.5: Nasolabial flap.

Video 7.1: Helical rim advancement.

Video 7.2: Flip flop flap.

Video 8.1: Repair of a large cutaneous lateral upper lip defect with a crescentic advancement flap. (Courtesy of Stanislav N. Tolkachjov, MD.)

Foreword

I believe that this book is an indispensable addition to educational resources vital to developing and maintaining the skill set essential to the practice of Mohs surgery, from layers to reconstruction. Experience of 30 years as a Mohs and reconstructive surgeon has given me a strong appreciation for the importance of building upon the foundation that we all acquire through our training. Throughout these years, teaching and participating in the education of other physicians has been a big part of my professional activities. Whether educating residents as the Program Director at the Mayo Clinic and later as clinical staff of the University of Pittsburgh, or directing our Micrographic Surgery and Dermatologic Oncology fellowships, the educational resources have always been critical components in providing young physicians a proper foundation. But continuing education for the more experienced practitioner is no less vital to the quality of care provided to patients with skin cancer. Our patients benefit most from a skin surgeon with a solid academic education and who continues to seek new, improved approaches and who assimilates creative nuances in the reconstruction of wounds. After serving as the Program Chair for the annual meeting of the Mohs College in 1999, it became even more evident to me that ongoing education is valuable for all skin surgeons. Since 1999, I have been privileged to serve as Section Editor of the "Reconstruction Conundrums" feature in *Dermatologic Surgery*, which provides new and creative approaches to common and not-so-common cutaneous defects. Through these experiences, I have found that the bottom line in optimizing care for patients with skin cancer through education is to understand that young surgeons yearn for thoughtful, well-reasoned structure for their reconstructive armamentarium and more seasoned operators continue to seek new and creative techniques to handle common and rare reconstructive challenges.

This handbook caters to all.

Dr. Chris Harmon and Dr. Stan Tolkachjov are the perfect team to accomplish the arduous task of formulating a comprehensive book of reconstructions. For the two of them, I know it was a labor of love. Chris, with his quarter century of experience in a high-volume skin cancer practice and whose mastery of Mohs surgery and the aesthetics of reconstruction, underpinned by an exceptionally strong background in cosmetic surgery, is ideally suited for this task. He has been involved for many years in the education of young surgeons through his fellowship training program and through continuous involvement in the educational programs at the most prominent national meetings on dermatology. He has a calm, thoughtful approach to life in general, but particularly in the realm of reconstruction that will be manifest in this textbook.

Stan, on the other hand, is the perfect complement to Chris with his youthful enthusiasm. But don't be fooled by his youth. Stan is years beyond his age in the understanding of reconstructive surgery and of the importance of a structural yet creative resource for the practicing skin cancer surgeon. He has an intimate understanding of what is essential to a young surgeon's development. Together, Chris and Stan are the perfect duo for engineering this important vessel of knowledge.

This textbook is important to skin surgeons because it organizes the specific knowledge needed for competent execution of cancer removal followed by the reconstruction of the defects … and it does so succinctly, with the busy practitioner in mind. It's easy-to-follow format features algorithmic organization complemented by instructive photographs, videos, and illustrations. In short, readers will benefit from the experienced ingenuity of the premiere group of experts who Chris and Stan have assembled to author chapters and who have written about a subject they are passionate about. Their passion is evident in these chapters and will inspire and guide both the younger surgeons and the experienced practitioners who read this book. The chapters herein represent hundreds of hours of preparation and tens of thousands of hours of experience. This collective effort is masterfully organized and condensed for those who choose to spend a few hours absorbing its contents. On behalf of patients with skin cancer across the world and for their sake, I hope that this book becomes a major resource for many, many skin cancer surgeons.

David G. Brodland, MD
Zitelli & Brodland Skin Cancer Center;
Assistant Professor
Departments of Dermatology, Otolaryngology and Plastic Surgery,
University of Pittsburgh
Pittsburgh, Pennsylvania, USA

Preface

As we submit this manuscript to our publisher, we are in the midst of the COVID-19 pandemic. However, for a longer period of time we have been experiencing a skin cancer epidemic globally and in the US. This is primarily because the oldest of the "baby boomers" are now aging beyond 65. Over the next 20 years, as this bolus of population continues to have birthdays into their 80s and 90s, we will see the incidence of skin cancer rise above the current one in five Americans. This context provides the backdrop for what compels us to publish this book ... to share knowledge with our peers today and future generations of dermatologists, Mohs surgeons, and reconstructionists. We are grateful to be working in the field of dermatology, specializing in the removal of skin cancers with the highest curative rates available. The technique of Mohs surgery, developed by Dr. Fred Mohs in the 1950s, has improved over the years, especially with the advent of fresh frozen technique as refined by Stegman and Tromovitch in the 1980s, as noted in their seminal article "Microscopically Controlled Excision of Cutaneous Tumors: Chemosurgery, Fresh Tissue Technique." Today, micrographic surgery allows us to yield a very high cure rate in the patients we serve. Our approach with Mohs surgery is to eradicate each tumor with the least number of stages while providing the best comfort for our patients and sparing the greatest amount of adjacent healthy tissue. Our goal for reconstruction is a systematic approach for each defect in order to achieve the most functional and aesthetically pleasing results for our patients and their referring physicians.

In this textbook, we have brought together the most reputable and experienced group of Mohs and reconstructive surgeons in the field with an overarching theme of creating the systematic approach to subunit reconstruction and a step-by-step description of reconstructive techniques. Each author was chosen for his/her expertise in the field as well as the specific section or anatomic location. For complete understanding of Mohs surgery, we have included chapters on the Mohs technique, how the process is adapted in difficult anatomic locations, preoperative/postoperative considerations, flap and reconstructive mechanics, and "combination reconstructions" stretching over multiple subunits. It is well illustrated and easily implemented in the daily practice.

This book is a complete, yet succinct, guide to Mohs micrographic surgery and reconstruction with the practicing Mohs and facial reconstructive surgeon in mind.

Christopher B. Harmon, MD, FAAD, FACMS
Stanislav N. Tolkachjov, MD, FAAD, FACMS

Acknowledgments

For me personally, this project is a privileged collaboration with mentors and colleagues who represent many of the best surgeons within our specialty. As a dermatology resident at Mayo Clinic in Rochester, Minnesota, both Dr. Randy Roenigk and Dr. Dave Brodland provided mentorship and training that set a trajectory for my career. It is indeed a privilege to have them both contributing to this textbook. Following residency, I had a 3-year Air Force commitment which took me to Keesler Air Force Base in Biloxi, Mississippi, where I continued to do Mohs surgery with another mentor, Dr. Rick Mora. During those 3 years I also had an opportunity to spend several 1-week rotations in Pittsburg working with Dr. John Zitelli and again Dr. Dave Brodland ... further learning surgical techniques before entering a Mohs fellowship.

Following my service in the Air Force, I moved to Birmingham, Alabama, to do a Mohs College sponsored fellowship with Dr. Gary Monheit. I then practiced with Dr. Monheit as a partner for the next 12 years. To this day, much of what we do in our current practice mirrors the surgery, scheduling, workflow, and business acumen I learned during my years with him ... for this I am indebted.

Lastly, Dr. Stan Tolkachjov, a former fellow and practice partner, unequivocally gets credit for being the impetus behind this textbook. His encouragement to undertake the project and his desire to be a hands-on contributing editor were the spark I needed to get this meaningful work underway. The collaborative nature of the text gave me an opportunity to partner with both more senior mentors as described above, and younger contemporaries. Stan and I both feel very fortunate to pull together such an austere group of surgeons and authors. To Stan and the other authors—I am grateful for your contributions and proud of the collaborative work represented here.

Christopher B. Harmon, MD, FAAD, FACMS

I acknowledge the hard work of former and current medical assistants, nurses, histotechnicians, former fellows, and other colleagues in spending time and effort in taking photographs and videos, helping in surgery, obtaining patient consents, and most importantly, taking excellent care of patients. I acknowledge Elizabeth Bryant for help in coordinating these efforts early in the book's inception.

I acknowledge the guidance in fellowship of Dr. Christopher Harmon in learning Mohs surgery and reconstructive techniques and confidence to perform any reconstruction. We believe in being excited about the biggest and most difficult tumors to help patients and improve upon each surgery with an open mind and heart of service. I would also like to thank him for partnering with me on this book.

I greatly appreciate the work of Preston McDonald and Chelsea Decker for help in editing the videos and the funding assistance of Gherghe Pusta and Epiphany Dermatology for video editing.

Lastly, I want to thank my patients for kindly allowing us to use their photographs and images to teach generations of surgeons and improve patient care for others. I also thank my referring providers for entrusting us with their patients. Without our patients and referring providers, this dream would not be possible.

Stanislav N. Tolkachjov, MD, FAAD, FACMS

Contributors

Ashwin Agarwal, MD
Department of Dermatology
Perelman School of Medicine
University of Pennsylvania
Philadelphia, Pennsylvania, USA

David G. Brodland, MD
Zitelli & Brodland Skin Cancer Center;
Assistant Professor
Departments of Dermatology, Otolaryngology and Plastic Surgery,
University of Pittsburgh
Pittsburgh, Pennsylvania, USA

Jonathan Cappel, MD
Surgical Dermatology Group
Birmingham, Alabama, USA

Jason R. Castillo, MD
Micrographic Surgery and Dermatologic Oncology Fellow
Mayo Clinic
Rochester, Minnesota, USA

Gabriela M. Espinoza, MD
Associate Professor
Program Director
Ophthalmology, Plastic and Reconstructive Surgery
Saint Louis University
St. Louis, Missouri, USA

Jeremy R. Etzkorn, MD
Assistant Professor of Dermatology
Hospital of the University of Pennsylvania
Philadelphia, Pennsylvania, USA

Victoria Godinez-Puig, MD, FAAD, FACMS
VitalSkin
Chicago, Illinois, USA

Nicholas Golda, MD
Associate Professor of Dermatology
Dermatology Medical Director
Micrographic Surgery and Dermatologic Oncology Program Director
University of Missouri School of Medicine
Columbia, Missouri, USA

Jennifer L. Hanson, MD, FAAD
Vitalogy Skincare
Georgetown, Texas, USA

Christopher B. Harmon, MD, FAAD, FACMS
Dermatologic Surgeon
Surgical Dermatology Group;
Director
ACGME Fellowship in Micrographic Surgery and Dermatologic Oncology
Birmingham, Alabama, USA

H. William Higgins II, MD, MBE
Assistant Professor of Dermatology
Penn Dermatology Oncology Center
University of Pennsylvania
Philadelphia, Pennsylvania, USA

Thomas Hocker, MD
Advanced Dermatologic Surgery, P.A.
ADS Ambulatory Surgery Center
Overland Park, Kansas, USA

Nicole Howe, MD
Novem Dermatology
Lutz, Florida, USA

George Hruza, MD, MBA, FAAD
Adjunct Professor of Dermatology
St. Louis University
St. Louis, Missouri, USA;
Laser & Dermatologic Surgery Center
Chesterfield, Missouri, USA

Irèn Kossintseva, MD, FRCPC, FAAD, FACMS
Associate Professor
Dermatologic Surgery Centre
Department of Dermatology and Skin Sciences
University of British Columbia
Vancouver, British Columbia, Canada

Aleksandar L. Krunic, MD, PhD, FAAD, FACMS, FEADV, FESMS
Adjunct Associate Professor of Dermatology
Rush University Medical Center;
Director of Dermatologic Surgery
Cook County Hospital Health System;
Health Clinician
Northwestern University Feinberg School of Medicine;
Chicago, Illinois, USA

Christopher J. Miller, MD
Director of Dermatologic Surgery
Hospital of the University of Pennsylvania
Philadelphia, Pennsylvania, USA

Molly Powers, MD
Henry Ford Medical Center
Novi, Michigan, USA

Randall Proctor, Jr, MD, MBA, FACMS
Eastern Dermatology & Pathology, PA
Greenville, North Carolina, USA

Nicola A. Quatrano, MD
SkinCare Physicians
Chestnut Hill, Massachusetts, USA

Randall K. Roenigk, MD
Professor of Dermatology
Director of the Micrographic Surgery and Dermatologic Oncology Fellowship
Mayo Clinic
Rochester, Minnesota, USA

Thomas E. Rohrer, MD
Dermatologic Surgeon
SkinCare Physicians
Chestnut Hill, Massachusetts, USA

Thuzar Shin, MD, FAAD, FACMS
Hospital of the University of Pennsylvania
Philadelphia, Pennsylvania, USA

Joseph F. Sobanko, MD
Mohs Surgery & Reconstruction
Laser Surgery & Cosmetic Dermatology
Director of Dermatologic Surgery Education
Associate Professor, Dermatology
Hospital of the University of Pennsylvania
Perelman Center for Advanced Medicine
Division of Dermatologic Surgery and Cutaneous Oncology
Philadelphia, Pennsylvania, USA

Evan Stiegel, MD, FAAD, FACMS
Wilson Dermatology
An Affiliate of The Skin Surgery Center
Wilson, North Carolina, USA

Stanislav N. Tolkachjov, MD, FAAD, FACMS
Dermatologic Surgeon and Dallas-Fort Worth Area Director
Mohs Micrographic & Reconstructive Surgery
Epiphany Dermatology;
Clinical Assistant Professor
University of Texas Southwestern Medical Center;
Clinical Associate Professor
Texas A&M College of Medicine;
Core Faculty
Division of Dermatology
Baylor University Medical Center
Dallas, Texas, USA

John Zitelli, MD
Adjunct Associate Professor
Departments of Dermatology, Otolaryngology, and Plastic Surgery
University of Pittsburgh Medical Center
Pittsburgh, Pennsylvania, USA

David Zloty, MD, FRCP
Clinical Professor
Faculty of Medicine
Department of Dermatology and Skin Science
University of British Columbia
Vancouver, British Columbia, Canada

1 Mohs Micrographic Surgery

Abstract
The two major goals of Mohs micrographic surgery (MMS) are to provide the highest possible cure rate for the treatment of cutaneous malignancies while also ensuring that the malignancy is removed in the most conservative or tissue-sparing manner possible. While these two tenets of this procedure seem straightforward, there is a considerable amount of attention to detail and process quality that is required to provide the service patients expect from MMS. In this chapter, we outline processes and techniques that will lead to successful, reproducible execution of the MMS.

Keywords: Mohs surgery, micrographic surgery, skin cancer treatment, tissue sparing, complete circumferential peripheral and deep margin assessment, initial Mohs stages/layers, subsequent Mohs stages/layers, process improvement

Capsule Summary and Pearls

- Mohs micrographic surgery (MMS) provides the highest cure rates in the most tissue-conserving manner for most skin cancers.
- Success of the procedure relies on proper tumor selection and careful execution of the technique.
- When excising a Mohs surgical specimen, several refinements in technique can ease tissue processing, accurate tumor mapping, and ultimately reconstruction of the resultant defect.
- Awareness of the surgical and tissue processing issues that may lead to artifacts on the tissue specimen can assist the surgeon in avoiding false positive readings.

1.1 Before the First Stage

Nicholas Golda and George Hruza

1.1.1 Tumor Selection

Mohs micrographic surgery (MMS) is best suited for the treatment of malignancies that grow in a contiguous manner, meaning that they grow in a manner where the entirety of the tumor is part of a singular mass with no part being physically separated from the primary site of growth. Properly trained providers most commonly use MMS for the treatment of all subtypes of basal cell carcinoma (BCC) and cutaneous squamous cell carcinoma (cSCC), but the procedure is also commonly used for nearly all cutaneous adnexal malignancies—dermatofibrosarcoma protuberans (DFSP), cutaneous leiomyosarcoma, extramammary Paget's disease (EMPD), atypical fibroxanthoma (AFX), melanoma in situ (MMIS), and, in some cases, for invasive melanoma, Merkel cell carcinoma (MCC), and other far less common cutaneous malignancies.[1] The unifying feature of all malignancies treated successfully with MMS is that these tumors are contiguous, thereby allowing the surgeon to detect the totality of the microscopic, often subclinical, extent of the tumor while properly carrying out the procedure.[1]

Selection of the most appropriate treatment is very important for producing the best results for the patient. While MMS may be utilized for nearly all forms of cutaneous malignancy, it is important to be discerning with respect to which malignancies are treated with the procedure as there are several other alternatives for the treatment of skin cancer beyond MMS, each with its own merits and drawbacks. MMS, while not a more aggressive or arduous procedure for the patient when compared with a standard excision, is a labor-intensive procedure for the physician and the MMS team, often consisting of several individuals in addition to the physician including nurses and histotechnicians. Acknowledging this, MMS is often reserved for malignancies with any of the following features:

- Malignancies in which there is risk of disfigurement or functional loss, such as those on the head and neck, hands, feet, and genitalia.
- Malignancies that have recurred or have been incompletely treated with other treatment modalities.
- Malignancies in immunosuppressed patients, particularly for cSCC in chronic lymphocytic leukemia (CLL) and solid organ transplant patients.
- Large malignancies in any body site.
- Malignancies in patients in whom the tumor border is poorly defined, often due to severe background actinic damage or subclinical tumor growth that may occur, for example, in infiltrating tumors.
- Malignancies exhibiting aggressive growth features clinically and histologically.
- Malignancies in sites where healing is challenging and a maximally conservative technique will reduce the burden of wound healing for the patient, such as in previously irradiated fields and on the legs in patients with peripheral vascular disease or diabetes.

In an effort to create a decision aid for determining which malignancies are appropriate for treatment with MMS, the American Academy of Dermatology convened a task force to develop MMS Appropriate Use Criteria (AUC). The AUC is a publicly available guideline intended to assist physicians with medical decision-making. As a decision aid, it is not intended to replace the judgment of a treating physician in consultation with their patients. Further, it is not intended to establish a standard of care for the treatment of skin cancer as not all tumors deemed appropriate by this system must be treated with MMS, and, conversely, there are situations where the system may deem MMS inappropriate for a particular tumor, while the treating physician, taking into account additional clinical information not accounted for in the AUC, may make the decision to treat with MMS. It should also be noted that the AUC criteria are in constant evolution and are influenced not only by considerations of what is best for the patient but also by economic forces in the health care system at large.

When selecting the most appropriate treatment for skin cancer, it is important to also recognize that a skin biopsy, particularly because of its superficial nature, can misrepresent the true nature of a skin cancer. It has been shown that while carrying out definitive treatment for skin cancer, the skin biopsy underrepresented the aggressive nature of a skin cancer in up to 33% of cases, while tumors were revealed to be less aggressive than the biopsy in 17% of cases.[2] Further, tumors that are not amenable to completion of treatment under local anesthesia will be challenging to complete in the outpatient setting with MMS, but MMS can be used in many of these cases as a component of multidisciplinary care for particularly advanced skin cancers such as those invading bone, foramina of the skull, or the orbit. Therefore, the clinician's judgment, taking into sum all patient factors including clinical and possible radiologic examination, pathologic correlation with that examination, and a discussion with the patient about their goals for treatment, is still the best tool for selecting a plan for skin cancer management.

1.1.2 Documentation of Site

Cure rates are higher when the procedure is done in the correct location. It seems obvious, but in patients with small lesions or significant background actinic damage, or when anatomically inaccurate verbiage is used to describe the original biopsy site, it can, at times, be difficult to identify the correct site for surgery. Further, patients are often unable to accurately recall the correct site of a biopsy, with one study showing the rate of misidentification of the biopsy site by patients at 16.6%.[3] It is therefore important to have a clearly defined process for identifying the correct site for surgery. Utilizing photography from the time of biopsy is a best practice for avoiding wrong site surgery.[3] Photographs at the time of a skin biopsy should have the planned biopsy site clearly marked and should be taken from far enough away to include anatomic landmarks that can facilitate localizing the site when surgery is eventually carried out. One HIPAA (Health Insurance Portability and Accountability Act of 1996) compliant and relatively simple way to accomplish biopsy site photography is to take a picture of the marked biopsy site with the patient's mobile phone and ask them to bring their phone with them to their surgical visit if the biopsy reveals a malignancy requiring further treatment.[4,5]

In addition to utilizing photography, or when no photograph of the biopsy site is available, providers can use their clinical judgment to identify the biopsy site with confirmation by the patient using a mirror or a photograph on a tablet. Family who are present with the patient, particularly those who have assisted the patient with wound care for the biopsy site, can also be a resource for confirming the correct location for surgery.

If the correct site cannot be confirmed, the surgeon is left with a few options. First, the procedure can be cancelled with the patient returning to the referring provider for site confirmation or monitoring. Alternatively, a frozen section biopsy can be obtained from the most likely candidate location with definitive treatment being done on the same day if the biopsy confirms a skin malignancy. A frozen section biopsy can be carried out by obtaining a biopsy by any technique the surgeon feels will not adversely affect the subsequent definitive procedure if the biopsy is positive and will yield a cosmetically appropriate wound if the site is found to be free of cancer. The biopsy specimen is then processed by vertical sectioning (rather than the tangential sectioning typical of MMS) through the center of the biopsy specimen, stained, and interpreted to confirm the presence or absence of malignancy.[6]

Occasionally, there is an obvious biopsy site or obvious residual tumor with adjacent skin that is clinically suspicious for being involved by skin cancer but not definitely involved. In these cases, we have developed the practice of outlining the definite tumor or biopsy site with a solid line and outlining the area that is suspicious, but not certainly involved, with a dotted line. When confirming the site with the patient, we will explain that we will only start with the area marked with the solid line, but that we are suspicious that their cancer may be larger in the area of the dotted line. This helps manage our patients' expectations by letting them know that we are doing everything we can to be conservative, but that their cancer may be larger than they thought previously (▶ Fig. 1.1).

Once the correct surgical site has been marked and confirmed, photography and clinical examination can be used to document the site that will be operated upon as well as the native presurgical state of the patient's

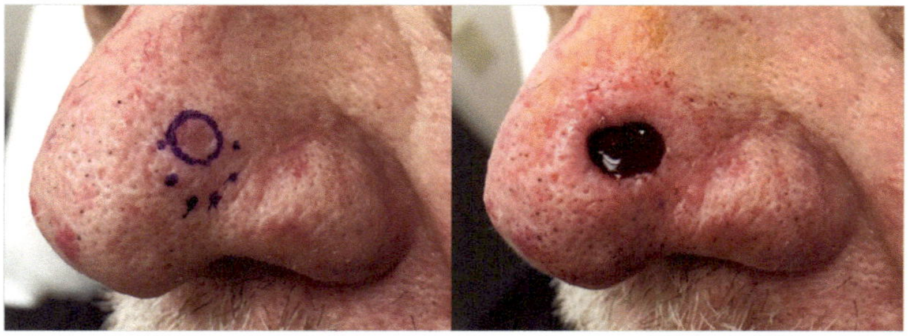

Fig. 1.1 Initial marking of a tumor showing the area that is certainly involved with a *solid line* and the area that is suspicious for involvement with a *dotted line*. Illustrating where you are concerned the tumor may extent prior to starting surgery can help patients prepare mentally for a defect that is larger than they may anticipate.

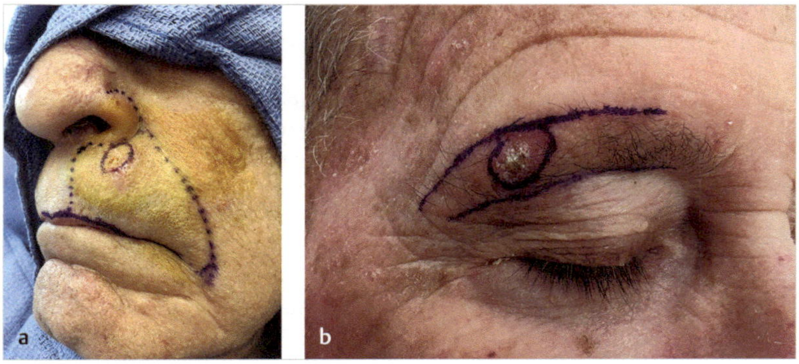

Fig. 1.2 (a,b) Marking anatomic boundaries preoperatively can be helpful in identifying these boundaries following MMS during reconstruction planning. These boundaries are often distorted by edema following tumor removal.

anatomy. Photographic documentation and discussion of the patient's presurgical state can assist with eventual reconstruction planning as well as protect the treating physician from being implicated as the cause of any asymmetries, deformities, or palsies that the patient has prior to the planned surgical procedure. Additionally, during this time, it can also be helpful to mark relevant anatomic boundaries prior to the instillation of anesthesia if these boundaries will be helpful during reconstruction planning. A common example where this is helpful is marking the white roll of the lip as the edema from surgery and injected anesthesia can make this landmark more challenging to visualize reliably, especially in older patients with a less well-defined vermilion border (▶ Fig. 1.2a, b).

1.1.3 Time-Out

A critical practice for the safe and accurate execution of a surgical procedure is the surgical "time-out." This can be carried out in a number of ways, but essentially, the physician who will be doing the procedure must confirm that the correct procedure is being done on the correct site for the correct patient. Many Mohs surgeons do formal time-outs at the outset of the MMS and less formal time-outs with subsequent stages. The time-out for a subsequent stage can be particularly important if patients are being moved to different rooms throughout the day to ensure that the correct Mohs map is being referenced and the correct instruments are being used.

1.2 Procedures before the First Stage

Nicholas Golda and George Hruza

1.2.1 Curettage

Curettage is a common procedure in dermatology often used as a definitive treatment for superficial skin cancers in noncosmetically sensitive areas. At the outset of MMS, curettage is done to grossly define the breadth and depth of the skin cancer, but the procedure is carried out differently from curettage done in the course of malignant destruction. Prior to MMS, curettage is carried out more gently in a manner to avoid unnecessarily disrupting the surrounding epidermis in skin that is clinically uninvolved by skin cancer. This is often accomplished with reusable dermal curettes, which are typically less sharp and therefore more specific for tumor than single-use disposable curettes, which tend to be overly sharp for this purpose. Generally, working from the center of a lesion out to the periphery, the tumor shells out relatively easily providing firmer tactile feedback to the surgeon when normal dermis is encountered both peripherally and at the deep margin. Once this rigid feedback is encountered at all margins, and no soft skin cancer remains to be removed, curettage is stopped and the operative site is cleansed with gauze to remove any fragments of skin cancer that may have been freed by curettage but remain on or near the surgical site. This gauze is then discarded in order to avoid reintroducing these fragments of skin cancer to the operative field and increasing the risk of a false-positive histologic margin due to a displaced tumor fragment (▶ Video 1.1).

There are several benefits to curettage prior to the first layer of MMS:

- Site confirmation as tumor in a correctly identified surgical site will typically readily curette away.
- Removal of the bulk of the malignancy gives the surgeon a better concept of the gross breadth and depth of the tumor.[7] Curettage can confirm the surgeon's clinical impression of the size of a malignancy, but it can also inform the surgeon that the malignancy is either larger or smaller than originally thought, thereby sparing the patient unnecessary subsequent layers or allowing for a more conservative procedure, respectively.
- "Floaters" and other artifactual tumor on the Mohs margins can be reduced by curettage. By removing the gross tumor, tumor fragments are less likely to be displaced into the peripheral or deep margin during tissue processing, thereby reducing the chance of false-positive tumor at the margin and making histologic interpretation less challenging.
  - False-positive tumor displacement into the deep margins during relaxing cuts or specimen division is referred to as a "push-through" error (▶ Fig. 1.3a).
  - Residual tumor in the center of the specimen that hinges into the deep margin following specimen division thereby causing a false positive on the deep margin is referred to as a "fall over" error (▶ Fig. 1.3b).
- Tissue relaxing for the purposes of tissue processing is facilitated by removal of the central bulk of the tumor by curettage.

There are also pitfalls to the curettage process:

- Fibrous, infiltrative, incompletely excised, and recurrent malignancies will not curette well, so curettage is unreliable in these settings for defining the gross extent of the tumor.
- Curettage in areas where skin is particularly weak or thin and prone to tearing, such as an aged eyelid affected significantly by solar elastosis, may inadvertently remove normal, uninvolved tissue and introduce skin tears that can make tissue orientation and subsequent reconstruction more challenging.
- If care is not taken with the procedure or if overly sharp disposable curettes are used, then the process of curettage may damage surrounding uninvolved epidermis and make the Mohs excision larger than necessary to achieve a cure.

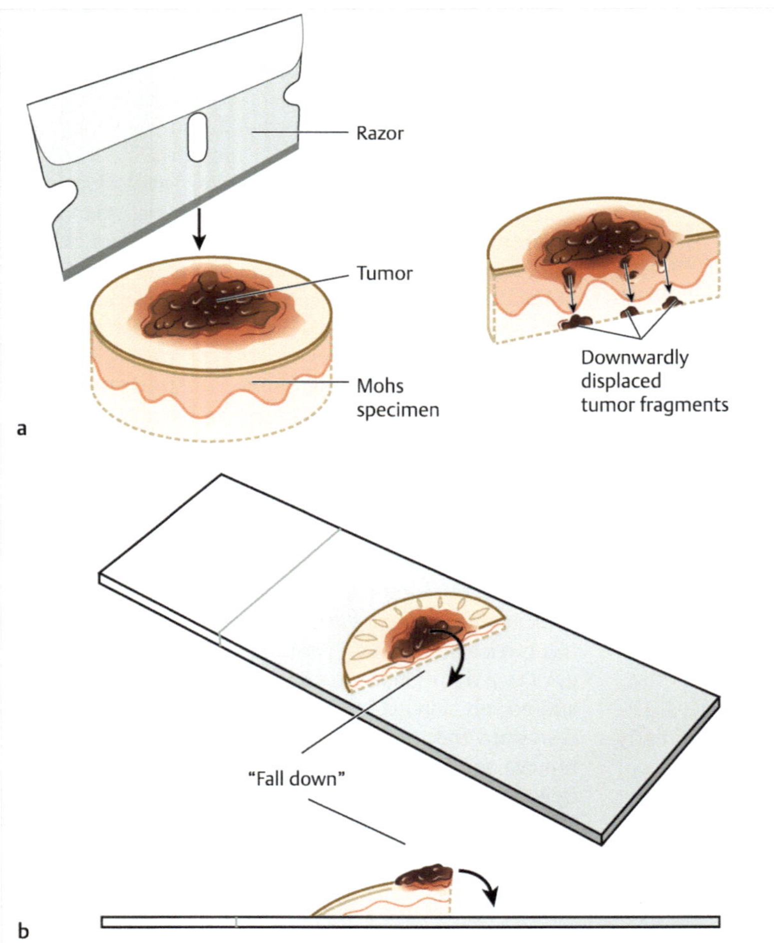

Fig. 1.3 (a,b) Curettage can assist in reducing the risk of histologic errors later in the procedure, particularly push-through artifact where gross tumor is pushed into the deep margin during processing and fall over artifact where gross tumor falls into the deep margin from the center of the tumor in divided specimens.

1.2.2 Sharp Debulking

The intent of sharp debulking of a tumor prior to excision can be manifold. The most typical use of sharp debulking is to remove the gross bulk of an exophytic tumor, thereby facilitating subsequent curettage and/or tissue processing. The surgeon may also want to obtain the center section of a tumor for histologic analysis, so this can be compared with the margins while attempting to clear the tumor. This technique can be particularly helpful for less common malignancies or malignancies where the histology is atypical or somehow in question (a "know your enemy" biopsy). Analysis of the center of a tumor may also be helpful for identifying high-risk features of the malignancy that may not have been evident on the initial diagnostic biopsy and may not be manifest on the margins of the Mohs specimens. This additional information may assist with obtaining more complete tumor staging, such as in cases of cSCC, and may provide important information for future management of the patient. Processing of the debulking specimen can either be done with horizontal frozen section processing and interpretation by the Mohs surgeon or by submitting the specimen for frozen or permanent section analysis by a dermatopathologist. In either case, a pathology report should be produced to document the findings of such biopsies.

The benefits of sharp debulking prior to the first layer of MMS are similar to those seen with curettage. Namely, removing the tumor bulk will reduce the chance of malignant tissue becoming dislodged from the tumor mass during excision and tissue processing and ending up on the examined histologic margins of the MMS specimen. When tumor cells become dislodged in this manner, it can increase false-positive interpretations or make histologic interpretation more challenging as the surgeon works to determine if the tumor is at the margin. Typically the deep margin in these cases, where specimen division or relaxing cuts push malignant tissue into the margin, is a true or false positive.

The primary pitfall of taking a debulking specimen is that the surgeon is at risk for inadvertently taking too wide or too deep a debulk, thereby making the final Mohs excision larger than necessary. This risk can be minimized through careful technique (▶ Video 1.2).

1.3 The First Stage

Nicholas Golda and George Hruza

1.3.1 Essentials of the First Stage

Recall that the two principal goals of MMS are oncologic cure and maximal tissue conservation, in that order. With that said, the goal with each stage of MMS should be to conservatively remove the malignancy in its entirety. Clinical examination by the Mohs surgeon to identify the clinically obvious extent of the tumor is the best tool for determining the size of the first stage. This examination can be augmented as previously discussed by the use of curettage prior to the first stage. It is important to reiterate that while the surgeon may have suspicion that the tumor may be larger than it appears, only the clinically obvious extent of the tumor should be removed with the first stage with the surgeon using histology of the MMS margins to either confirm or refute the initial clinical suspicion. Using this technique may result in an additional stage being necessary, but it also allows for maximal tissue conservation.

The first stage consists of complete removal of the entire gross tumor as well as a 1- to 2-mm margin of clinically normal skin immediately around and deep to the tumor (▶ Video 1.3). For very large or aggressive tumors, a larger initial margin may be useful to reduce the number of stages needed for tumor clearance. This rim of clinically normal tissue is needed to prove negative margins as well as to allow for monitoring of tissue processing quality by the surgeon, as will be discussed later. If care is taken while excising Mohs stages to make the tissue specimen easier for the surgeon or the histotechnician to process, the histologic section will be processed faster, and will be of higher quality and easier to interpret. Following is an outline of the first stage with suggestions for facilitating tissue processing and optimizing quality.

The first stage begins with a very superficial incision or score around the tumor at a 90-degree angle relative to the skin surface. This incision defines the margin of the specimen that will be processed. To aid in subsequent tissue processing, the border of the Mohs layer should consist of smooth, rounded, convex contours. Sharp corners, concave shapes, and start-stop chatter (rifling layers) are more challenging to relax and flatten into the proper plane for tissue processing. These imperfections in the Mohs excision can create areas where the epidermis is missing, thus making that section of the specimen uninterpretable and necessitating additional stages of surgery that may have been avoidable. Further, start-stop chatter can also cause the introduction of false tissue scores that can make tumor localization challenging (▶ Fig. 1.4).

The initial incision for the Mohs excision is made superficially because the goal is to leave the specimen in perfect orientation relative to the site on the patient where it is being removed so tissue orienting marks can be precisely placed on the specimen and patient. These orienting marks can be made by different techniques and in different patterns based on surgeon preference and tumor size and shape (▶ Fig. 1.5). The key when placing orienting marks is to ensure that, if tumor is present, the surgeon will be able to precisely localize the residual tumor on the patient based on these marks. Therefore, the marks are placed prior to incising through the full thickness of the dermis in order to ensure that the mark on the specimen side corresponds exactly to the mark on the patient side. Orienting marks are most commonly

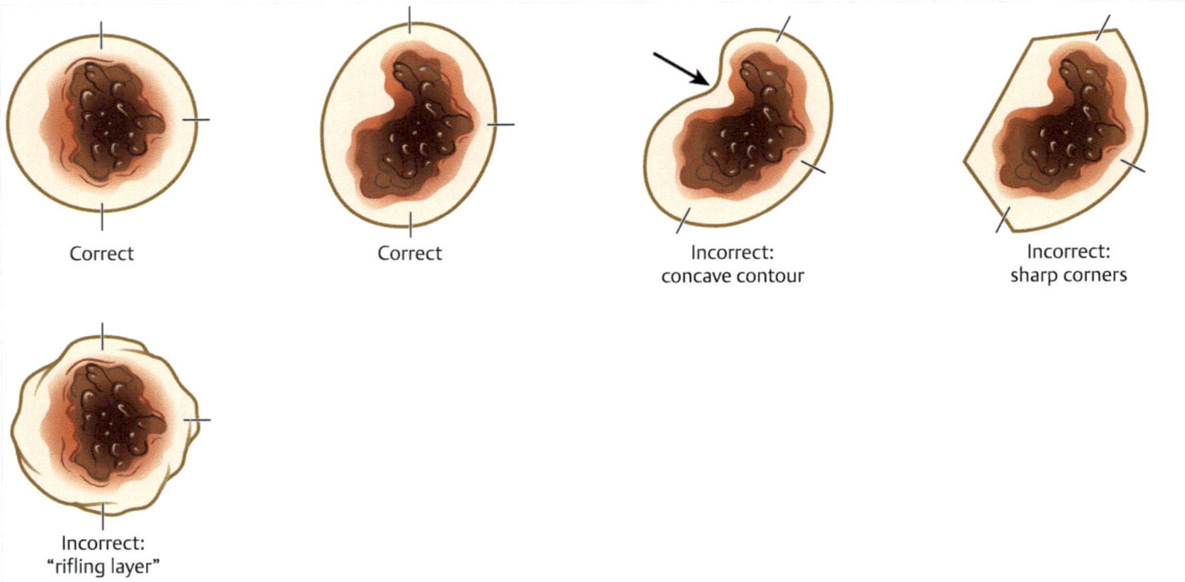

Fig. 1.4 A proper first stage of the MMS consists of a smooth incision immediately around the gross tumor with convex edges and inwardly beveled walls to facilitate tissue processing. Sharp corners, concave shapes, and start-stop chatter are to be avoided.

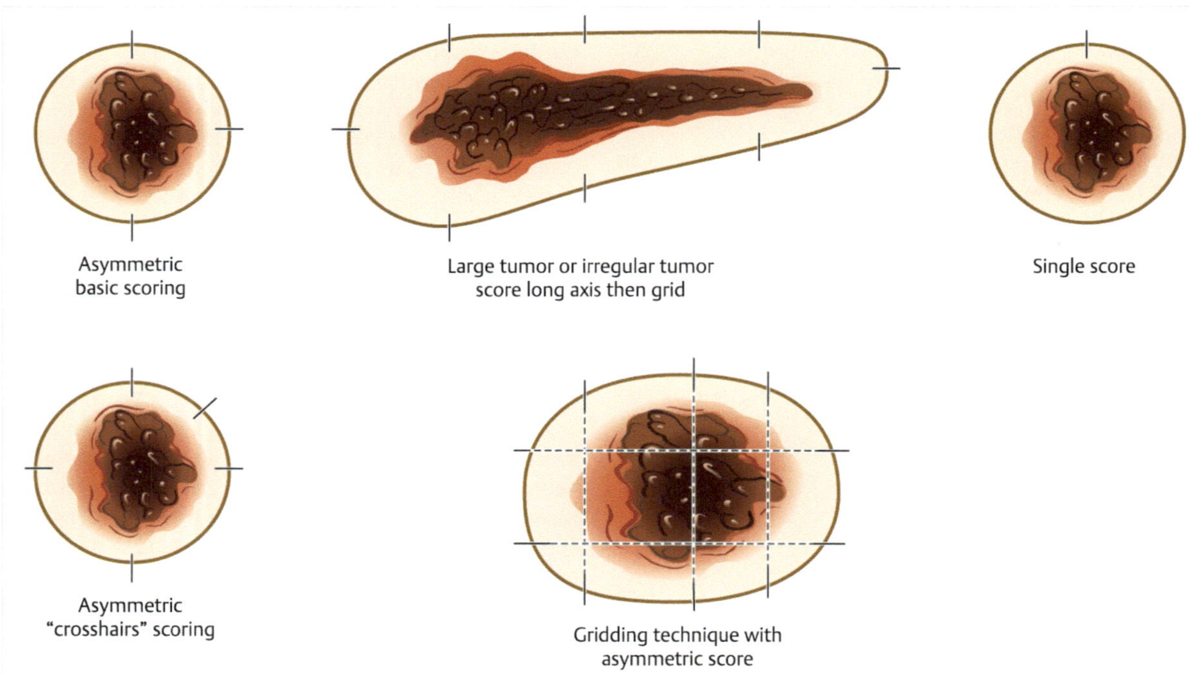

Fig. 1.5 Common patterns for placing tissue orientation marks.

made by making a shallow nick with the scalpel in the tissue. This nick should be deep and large enough to be readily found if a subsequent stage is required, but not so large and deep as to interfere with reconstruction. The pattern of tissue nicks is highly variable among surgeons. The surgeon must select the technique they feel will allow them the greatest ability to locate and selectively excise residual tumor using histologic maps. One key is that, regardless of what technique is used, the orienting marks should be asymmetric. By making the marks asymmetric, the surgeon can reorient the specimen to the patient if any tissue handling error occurs during tissue processing, such as a dropped specimen or a mislabeled map, because the specimen will only "fit" on the patient's defect one way much like an asymmetric shaped peg will only fit into its corresponding hole in the correct orientation.

Surgeons use several techniques to make orienting marks. Some use gentian violet in order to avoid tissue scores, but gentian violet has a tendency to lose its sharpness on the skin ("bleed") and can be washed away by surgical preps and blood between stages, thus negatively affecting precision of tumor location. More commonly, surgeons use orienting nicks in the tissue as discussed earlier. Common asymmetric patterns include a single score in one location and three scores in a 12, 3, and 6 o'clock position or similar asymmetric orientation. Alternatively, many providers will place four scores in a symmetric crosshairs orientation, though this does require more care to maintain orientation as the symmetry of the scores does not allow reorientation if there is a tissue handling error during tissue transfer, grossing, or processing. When tissue nicks are placed, it is helpful to place them in line with the most likely vector of closure, so the nicks will be excised with standing cones and not confound epidermal approximation during wound closure. Larger tumors are best scored with a "gridding" technique that allows the highest possible resolution for residual tumor in the deep margin within the larger field of these tumors. In this technique, scores are placed such that the tissue can be divided into graph paper–like squares during tissue processing. Another method of marking very large tumors is the use of skin staples around the defect margins matching staples in the specimen excised. Staples can also be useful for orienting deep margin tumor resection without a skin edge with the staples used to outline the margins of the specimen excised (▶ Fig. 1.6).

When placing scores, the surgeon must balance resolution of tumor location during tissue analysis with the fallibility introduced by placing several orienting scores in the specimen. The ability of the surgeon to precisely identify, on the patient, where residual tumor remains for selective re-excision in a subsequent stage is improved if the tumor is near an orienting score. Therefore, the more scores a surgeon places in the specimen, the greater their ability to precisely locate the residual tumor on the patient. Scores, however, introduce potential error into the MMS because each score produces an area where epidermis may be incompletely laid down into the sectioning plane. If the score results in failure to visualize focal residual tumor on a margin because of incomplete epidermal lay-down, then cure rates can be negatively affected. The decision for how many scores are necessary to accomplish the goals of MMS is therefore left to the surgeon to determine based on confidence in individual practice laboratory techniques and ability to localize tumor within a specimen with more or less scores.

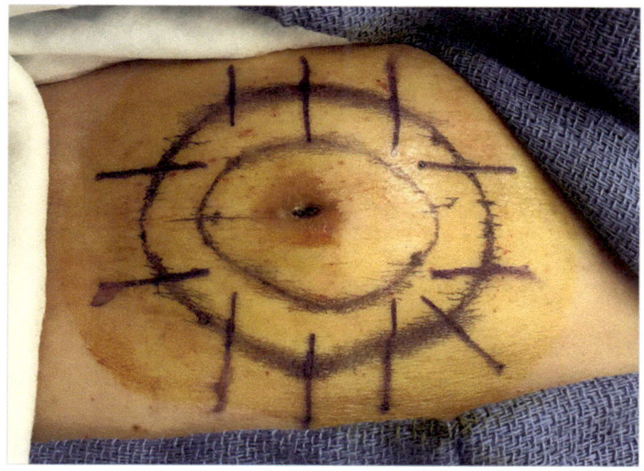

Fig. 1.6 Large tumors, such as the dermatofibrosarcoma protuberans pictured, are best oriented with marks placed in a grid pattern so residual tumor at deep margins can be easily resolved and accurately removed. Large tumors such as these are best marked redundantly with gentian violet and tissue scores.

Next, a beveled incision is used to incise into the skin, and into deeper tissues, if necessary, to the desired depth of the excision below the grossly evident depth of the malignancy. This beveled incision is accomplished by taking several passes around the specimen within the superficial initial incision, at approximately a 45-degree angle in most cases, until the correct depth is reached. Excising the tissue with a bevel eases the process of laying the epidermal edge flat into the same plane as the deep margin during tissue processing as the epidermal edge travels a smaller distance and encounters less torsional resistance when the tissue is beveled relative to a 90-degree excision (▶ Fig. 1.7). The amount of bevel needed varies based on the anatomic site of the tumor (as the dermis is more or less rigid in different sites) and the depth of the tumor (shallow, dermis-only layers need a greater degree of beveling as do tumors that are deeper than they are wide).[8] It is common, for example, on distal nasal and nasal alar lesions to take a transdermal layer in an effort to facilitate a better outcome with a skin graft or second intention healing, but such transdermal layers typically need more extreme beveling in order to facilitate high-quality tissue processing due to the stiffness of the

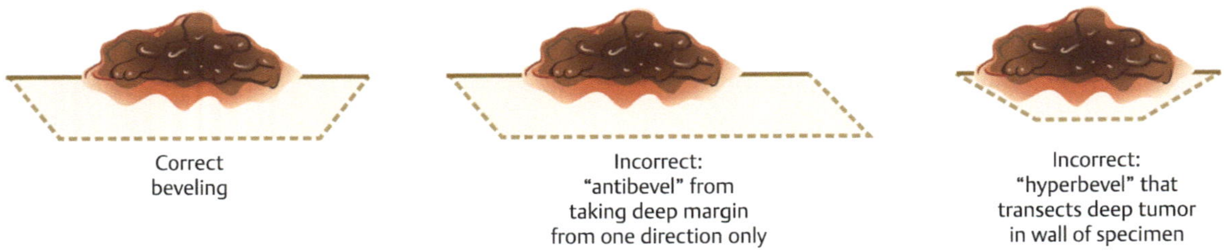

Fig. 1.7 Demonstration of appropriate bevels. Having too little bevel can cause difficulty with tissue processing, while too much bevel may inadvertently transect the tumor within the wall of the specimen.

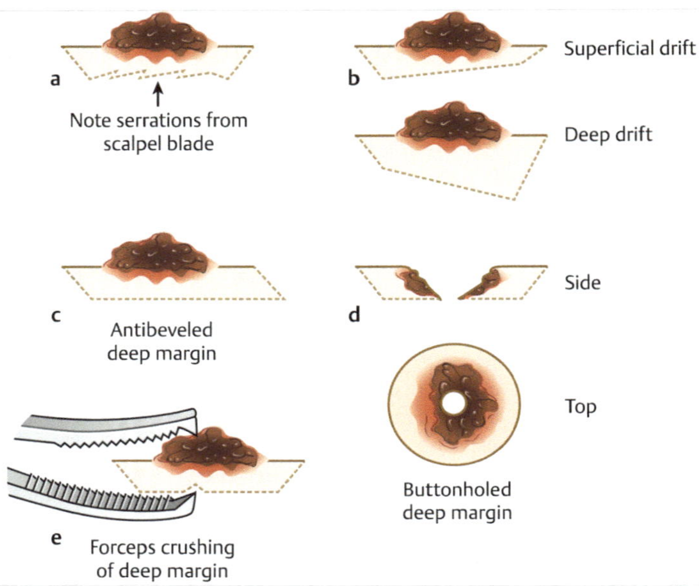

Fig. 1.8 Pitfalls with the deep margin on an initial Mohs stage. **(a)** A jagged deep margin. **(b)** Drifting superficially or deep within the deep plane. **(c)** Antibeveled deep margin. **(d)** A buttonholed deep margin. **(e)** Grasping the deep margin too firmly with toothed forceps producing a hole in the deep margin.

dermis (▶ Video 1.4). This has been referred to as the partial-thickness layer technique.[8,9]

Finally, once the beveled incision at the periphery of the specimen is complete, the specimen is removed from the patient by making a flat incision across the deep margin of the specimen at a depth just below the deepest extent of the tumor. In some cases, this depth may be intradermal. In others, it may be deeper at any level down to and including periosteum. Errors that can be made during incision of the deep margin include the following (▶ Fig. 1.8a–e):

- Making an incision that is not flat: A jagged deep marginal incision will increase the likelihood of dropout areas, leading to the possibility of false negatives.
- Making an incision that drifts more superficially or more deeply across the deep margin:
  - Shallow drift: Risks more stages by inadvertently incising into the deep margin of the tumor.
  - Deep drift: Unnecessary tissue waste, volume loss, and possible damage to deeper structures such as nerves or vessels.
- Creating an antibevel that interferes with tissue relaxing by incising the entirety of a deep margin across the specimen from one direction.
- Incomplete or buttonholed deep margin:
  - Creates an area of uninterpretable deep margin "dropout" by incising into the curetted deep margin of the specimen or creating extra notches mimicking those planned for orientation.
- Grasping the tissue too firmly with toothed forceps while removing the specimen can create triangular impressions in the deep margin that impair assessment of the complete deep margin:
  - Toothed forceps may also transfer malignant tissue from the tumor to the deep margin if care is not used to only use one side of the forceps on the tumor side and the other on the deep side while grasping the tissue.

1.3.2 Incomplete Excision and Recurrence

The process of taking a first Mohs stage from a site that has been previously excised or is recurrent following a prior excisional procedure presents unique challenges. An incompletely excised tumor is one where an excision has been attempted and the pathology revealed persistent malignancy at a lateral or deep margin. Having information about whether the residual tumor is present at lateral or deep margins, or having the slides from the original excisional specimen available for review, can be helpful when planning subsequent MMS. The issue created by an incompletely excised or recurrent tumor is that the malignancy may no longer be contiguous and/or may be obscured by scar clinically and histologically. This is why cure rates for MMS are highest when MMS is the first treatment selected for a tumor.[10,11] In our practice, we will typically execute a "mapping layer" in the cases of incomplete excision as the first stage of MMS (▶ Fig. 1.9). A mapping layer essentially consists of a narrow re- excision of the entirety of the scar from the prior procedure to include tissue below the deep margin of the prior procedure. This complete re-excision of the deep margin below the prior scar is essential to prove negative deep margins with MMS. The deep margin of a prior excision can be identified both clinically and histologically by visualizing scar rather than normal subcutaneous fat on the deep margin. In cases of recurrence and incomplete excision, it is only possible to prove clear margins by complete histologic assessment of the prior surgical margins. This requires careful re-excision of the prior procedure and understandably causes additional tissue loss and occasionally large defects that may have been avoided if MMS was used for primary treatment of the malignancy.

1.4 Tissue Processing

Nicholas Golda and George Hruza

1.4.1 Tissue Transfer

Once the MMS specimen has been excised, it is placed on a transfer medium for transport to the grossing table. The medium used is variable among Mohs practices and may consist of cardstock or paper with or without anatomic drawings drawn or preprinted, filter paper, nonadherent pads, or saline-soaked gauze. Further, some practices use Petri dishes to house tissue and the aforementioned transfer medium to transport tissue to the laboratory for processing. Regardless of the transfer medium selected by an individual surgeon, some things are consistent between practices:

- Most media have a mechanism for identifying the location of orienting marks, or at least the 12 o'clock position, on the excised tissue. This can be accomplished with detailed drawn maps on preprinted cards or a simple ink mark on a nonadherent pad or gauze (▶ Fig. 1.10).
- There must be a mechanism for identifying the patient and site or accession number to avoid confusing specimens with one another in the lab (▶ Fig. 1.10).
- Once processing is complete, a mechanism must be used to track which frozen tissue specimen corresponds with which patient in case further sections are required. Some surgeons use color-coded slide labels and optimal cutting temperature (OCT) medium, while others label by order within the cryostat.

1.4.2 Relaxing Incisions and Dividing

The goal of relaxing incisions is to bring the entirety of the epidermal margin into the same plane as the deep margin of the specimen. Understanding that the epidermal edge must move into the same plane as the deep margin by rotating about a pivot or "hinge" point prior to tissue freezing is one of the critical elements of tangential sectioning of MMS[12,13] (▶ Fig. 1.11). If the entirety of the epidermal edge of a specimen is not moved into this plane, then it cannot be examined microscopically and the opportunity for missing a positive margin and recurrence of malignancy is increased.[14]

Practices may use any of the following options for relaxing the tissue or a combination of these, as we do in our practice. The first step to allowing the epidermal edge to move into the proper plane is debulking and curettage as discussed previously. Removal of the central mass of malignant tissue allows the epidermal edge to fall into

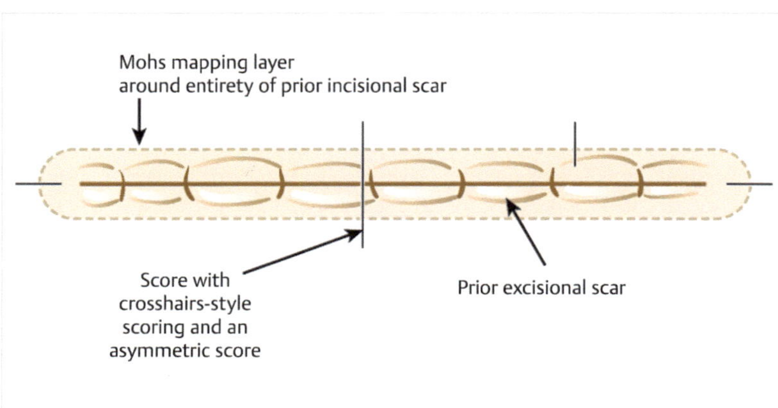

Fig. 1.9 Mohs mapping for a previously excised tumor (Mohs for a prior incomplete excision).

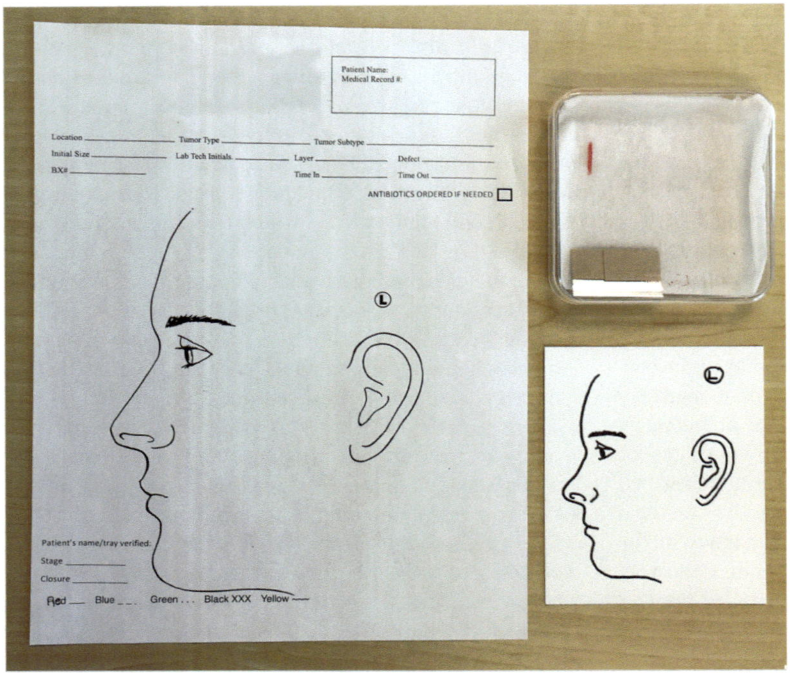

Fig. 1.10 Sample map and labeled petri dish for tissue transport to the lab.

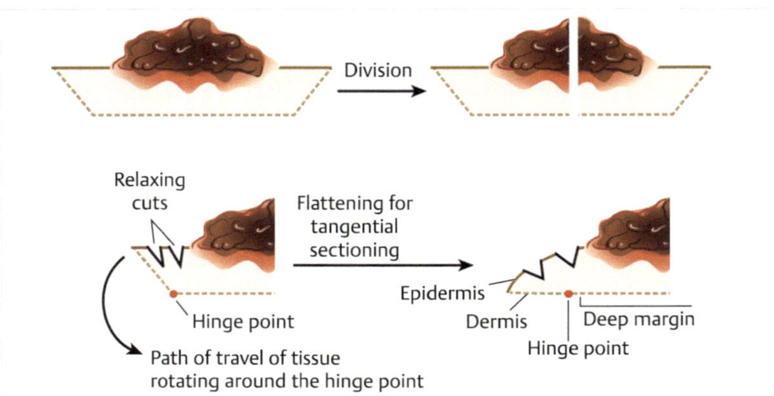

Fig. 1.11 Illustration of tissue being rotated around the "hinge point" in order to produce tangential sectioning.

the proper plane more easily and also reduces the opportunity for malignant tissue transfer to the margins during processing with resultant false positives. Next, radial and circumferential relaxing incisions can be made in the tissue. For both types of relaxing incisions, it is important to avoid incising completely through a specimen into the dermal face or deep margin of the specimen as this can result in "push-through" artifact, where tumoral cells are pushed by the blade into the margin of the specimen, thereby making histologic interpretation more difficult and possibly causing false positives. Radial incisions are incisions in the tissue oriented perpendicular to the wound edge pointing toward the center of the specimen. Radial incisions should not incise all the way to the epidermal margin of the specimen in order to avoid introducing false tissue scores at the margin. Circumferential incisions course parallel to the wound edge within the specimen. These allow the epidermal edge to move into the deep margin via an accordionlike motion

Based on surgeon preference, MMS specimens can be divided before freezing and sectioning or can be processed as a single piece.[15,16] There are merits and drawbacks to both approaches. There is obvious time efficiency gained in the lab when a specimen is processed as a single piece, provided the histotechnician is facile with getting the entire epidermal margin properly relaxed into the deep plane. If getting the entirety of the epidermis is challenging for the Mohs histotechnician resulting in lost time or recuts, then the efficiency of a single piece may be lost. A divided specimen is always required if the excised tumor is too large to fit on a microscope slide. Mohs surgeons may also choose to divide specimens to further increase the ease of getting the epidermis properly laid down as the division serves as an additional relaxing procedure for the specimen. There are some potential pitfalls that can occur at this stage of tissue processing:

- A divided specimen may result in "push-through" artifact where tumor is pushed down into the deep margin by the blade when it is being divided resulting in false-positive deep margins.
- Tumoral tissue from the superficial part of the specimen may roll or fall down onto the plane of the deep margin potentially causing a false positive on the deep margin.
- The deep margin in divided specimens may be incompletely laid down into the plane of section, thus not allowing histologic assessment of the entirety of the deep margin.
- Excessive downward pressure on the specimen while freezing the tissue into the planar orientation for tangential sectioning may inappropriately press tumoral tissue closer to the deep margin and predispose to false positives.
- Excessive facing into the frozen tissue block due to suboptimal epidermal relaxation can inadvertently cut into the gross tumor when it may not have been present in the true margin if the specimen had been sectioned more conservatively.
  - The surgeon can often visualize that a block has been cut too deeply by observing that superficial structures of the skin are present in the central, or deep, portion of the tumor. Additionally, the peripheral epidermal edges will begin to show tangential sectioning with a honeycombed network of rete ridges being visible in sections cut too deeply into the tissue block.

1.4.3 Tissue Inking

Permanent tissue dyes are used to color code the tissue specimen so that the anatomic orientation of the tissue specimen is known (▶ Video 1.5). This inking is consistent with a simultaneously created tissue map that shows a drawing of the specimen with all orienting marks, often set in the context of nearby anatomic structures. When tissue inking is completed, the specimen should correspond to the Mohs map in only one orientation so that the surgeon will be able to accurately map any residual tumor based on the ink visible on the histologic slides.[8] Several techniques can be carried out to ensure inking assists maximally in tissue orientation and tumor identification (▶ Fig. 1.12):

- Ink should be applied sparingly to avoid excess ink running into and falsely marking more than one margin or tissue nick.
- Inking should, whenever possible, follow a predetermined convention for all cases, for example, blue indicates the superior part of the tumor, red the inferior part, and green the lateral asymmetric score. On the other hand, one mnemonic used is: green to the grass, blue to the sky, red to the right. The editors use a blue ink to indicate the 6 o'clock position and red ink to indicate the 3 o'clock position, which allows proper orientation even without inking the 9 or the 12 o'clock positions.
- Inking should be done in a manner that reinforces asymmetry of the tissue specimen to avoid mapping errors.
- Attempt to avoid using the same color in two different sections of the same specimen to avoid confusion during tumor mapping.
- In divided specimens, particularly large specimens with several pieces, ink the deep margin where the division occurred in a manner to identify the specimen on the map and not allow different specimens in the same map to be confused with one another.
- In deep margin-only specimens, the sides of the specimen, or nicks in the sides of the specimen, may be inked in a manner to illustrate their orientation relative to the patient anatomically.
- Some advocate inking on cardstock and retaining this cardstock until the end of the surgical day in case there are questions about inking that can be answered by referencing the saved inked and oriented transfer cardstock.[8]

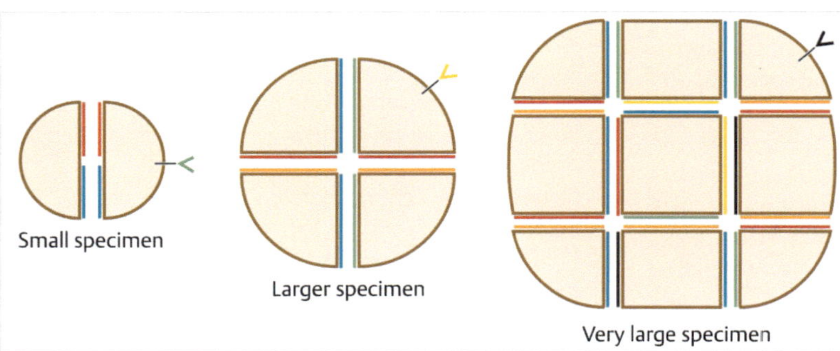

Fig. 1.12 Potential tissue inking patterns for simple and complex tumors.

1.5 Histologic Interpretation/ Mapping

Nicholas Golda and George Hruza

A significant part of MMS training includes the proper interpretation of tangentially processed frozen section histology for a variety of common and uncommon skin malignancies. Histologic interpretation not only requires the ability to recognize subtle changes consistent with the trailing edge of skin cancer at the margins of a Mohs excision, but also requires the ability to assess each tissue specimen for quality of histologic processing and staining as deficiencies in these areas can result in a decreased ability of the Mohs surgeon to recognize the presence of malignancy at a margin. Training for this is cumulative through dermatology residency training where trainees are exposed to both dermatopathology and MMS and, in many cases, through fellowship training in micrographic surgery and dermatologic oncology where the trainee has the opportunity to have rigorous training in the procedure including laboratory technique, treatment of rare or advanced tumors, as well as advanced reconstructive techniques. Of note, not all providers who perform MMS have undergone a formal MMS fellowship or even a dermatology residency.

An important first step in interpretation is awareness of the tumor that is being excised. While common malignancies are more easily recognized after years of training and work in practice, less common variants of skin cancer can be more challenging. In these cases, it is often helpful to review the original diagnostic biopsy slides or to take a frozen section biopsy for vertical sectioning from the center of the malignancy on the day of surgery.

1.5.1 Initial Slide Quality Review

Prior to rendering a histologic interpretation of the specimen, the surgeon first completes an initial quality review of the slide. Errors in slide preparation and interpretation have been shown to account for a large proportion of recurrences following MMS.[14,17,18] The labeling of the slide, often with an accession number or other identifying information, should be confirmed with the labeling of the Mohs map on which the surgeon will document findings.

Next, the surgeon may visually inspect the specimen to confirm that there are no features that would indicate that it is not the correct specimen for the patient to whom or the site to which it is attributed. Examples of ways to detect potential errors in this way include the following: size of specimen does not match what was excised from the identified patient (too large or small), anatomic area does not match what was excised from the identified patient (i.e., a specimen with mucosa or conjunctiva from a specimen identified as having come from the scalp), and so on.

Next, the surgeon will examine the slide microscopically to ensure that it has been prepared properly. The following laboratory issues can interfere with histologic interpretation and should be addressed by the surgeon with the laboratory staff:

- Coverslipping errors can produce air bubbles. This can be addressed by placing coverslipping medium directly on the slide in sufficient but not excessive quantity and placing the coverslip slowly from one end.
- Insufficient xylene or xylene substitute clearing can result in brown discoloration requiring removal of the coverslip and reclearing.
- Poor staining can make tumor more difficult to distinguish from normal structures in the specimen. This can be the result of an error in the staining protocol, old staining reagents, or a mechanical error in an automated stainer.
- Specimens cut too thick are easier to transfer from the cryostat to the slide but make staining too dark and interpretation challenging. We have observed the upper limit for interpretable thickness in our practice to be approximately 8 µm.

Next, the surgeon should assess the slide to ensure the specimen is complete. If any marginal tissue, from either the epidermal edge or the deep margin is missing, then the specimen cannot be interpreted with certainty, and the surgeon should consider acting to ensure a complete specimen is obtained and interpreted. This may require either re-embedding and/or recutting deeper sections into the specimen, "rocking" the specimen in a direction to get the necessary missing edge to lay down for an extra cut, or taking additional tissue from the patient to ensure complete marginal analysis. Factors that may contribute to missing tissue at the margin may include the following:

- Missing epidermis:
  - Curettage of epidermis prior to taking Mohs stage.
  - Loose epidermis in areas of scar that slides/shears off the specimen during processing.
  - Incomplete epidermal relaxation into the plane of section during tissue grossing.
  - Incomplete epidermal "lay-down" immediately adjacent to orienting scores.
  - Specimen edges that are concave, jagged, or otherwise not smooth.
  - Folding of the epidermal edge, especially if a dull or incompletely cleaned blade is used in a cryostat at the point where the blade first encounters the embedded tissue.
  - Chatter artifact from a defective or dull cryostat blade.
  - Chatter artifact from thick hair in the specimen deflecting the path of the cryostat blade. This can be relieved by manually plucking hair present in the specimen in anatomic sites where the tissue is otherwise delicate such as eyelid and nasal mucosa.

- Missing tissue in the deep margin:
  - Incomplete freezing of fat, which requires longer freeze times to be preserved on the specimen.
  - Toothed forceps trauma to the deep tissue causing triangular defects in the deep margin.
  - Insufficient relaxation of tissue can cause the central portion of the deep margin to lift when epidermis is being laid down, thereby raising it out of the plane of section.
  - Failure of surgeon to remove the deep margin as a flat plane when taking the stage.
  - Chatter artifact from a defective or dull cryostat blade.
  - Deep margin continuity is most readily assessed in specimens that are not divided and are processed as a single piece, though this is not always possible.

1.5.2 Histologic Interpretation

Once the surgeon has completed a quality review of the slides and determined they are appropriate for making a histologic determination about the margins of the excised specimen, the surgeon may then proceed with slide interpretation. The fact that the surgeon also renders the histologic assessment is a feature unique to MMS and is, in fact, a required part of MMS. The high standards for specimen orientation and ability to precisely identify the location of residual tumor in a specimen margin that are typical for MMS require that the surgeon and pathologist be the same individual. Furthermore, Mohs surgeons are well trained in the assessment and histologic mapping of frozen section tissue processed by tangential sectioning for both common and rare malignancies of the skin. The recognition of obvious as well as subtle residual malignancy in a specimen margin is well addressed in entire textbooks and atlases dedicated to this topic and is beyond the scope of this chapter. What is important to note in this work are the potential opportunities for error at this stage of the procedure beyond a lack of training or ability to recognize persistent malignancy in a margin, and how a surgeon may avoid these errors.

First, the surgeon should be alert for factors that may obscure tumor present in the margin. During tissue processing, the epidermis may fold slightly over onto the specimen, thereby obscuring the margin with a double thickness of tissue. While the section may be thin enough to make an interpretation through this folded tissue, it is more challenging and does increase the risk that subtle malignancy, such as focal superficial BCC or SCC in situ, may be missed.[14] Inflammation is another factor that may mask tumor in a margin. Inflammation, typically manifesting as dense lymphocytic aggregates in the specimen, can occur for a variety of reasons: in response to a recent biopsy, as a reaction to nearby malignancy (peritumoral inflammation), rosacea in sebaceous facial tissue, or due to other primary inflammatory processes or leukemia cutis in the skin unrelated to skin cancer.[13] In addition, certain sites such as the conchal bowl deep to the cartilage have inflammation at baseline, and while pursuing deep tumors, lymph nodes mimicking as peritumoral inflammation may be encountered. While dense inflammation may make interpretation more challenging by obscuring small foci of invasive malignancy, it can also be helpful in many cases by drawing the surgeon's attention for closer inspection, thereby making the detection of small foci of malignancy, in some cases, easier. Dense inflammation and histologic evidence of fibrosis has been shown to herald residual SCC with one study showing residual SCC on a subsequent layer in 1.9% of cases where another MMS stage was taken due to these histologic findings.[19] Due to this, surgeons may consider taking an additional stage when these findings are visualized histologically. A similar correlation between dense inflammation and residual BCC has not been shown,[20] although stromal tissue may lead some surgeons to take an additional layer.

Tumoral tissue may also be artifactually present on the MMS histologic slides due to circumstances that occur during excision and tissue processing. If a surgeon is not comfortable recognizing artifactual tumor, false-positive histologic interpretations may occur, leading to unnecessary additional surgery for the patient. In addition to having the ability to recognize artifact if it occurs on pathology specimens, it is important to improve processes earlier in the procedure in order to minimize the occurrence of artifactual tumor. Some artifacts are simple to identify. These are commonly referred to as floaters. The use of the word floater is a misnomer in MMS, as the term originates from extraneous tissue from a prior specimen that would float off in a water bath and end up on another specimen during paraffin-based permanent section processing.[21] In MMS, these are more appropriately referred to as displaced tumoral tissue, though, however imprecise, the term floater is part of common parlance. These tumor fragments often manifest as tumoral tissue completely separated and physically removed from the primary specimen on the slide. Occasionally, tumor fragments can come to rest on the specimen itself. This can occur in two scenarios: the tumor fragment comes to rest on top of the tissue specimen or the fragment comes to rest in a gap or defect in the specimen. When it lies on top of the section, it can be easily identified as a floater because the tumoral tissue will be in a different plane than the tissue section and will not be in focus under the microscope when the true specimen is in focus. When the tumoral fragment lies in a defect in the tissue section, identification as a false positive can be more challenging and may rely on the surgeon's judgment that the tumor fragment does not correspond with the surrounding tissue architecturally. Further, a tumor fragment may come to rest on the deep margin of a divided specimen (▶ Fig. 1.13). This may cause a false-positive interpretation of a deep margin if this goes

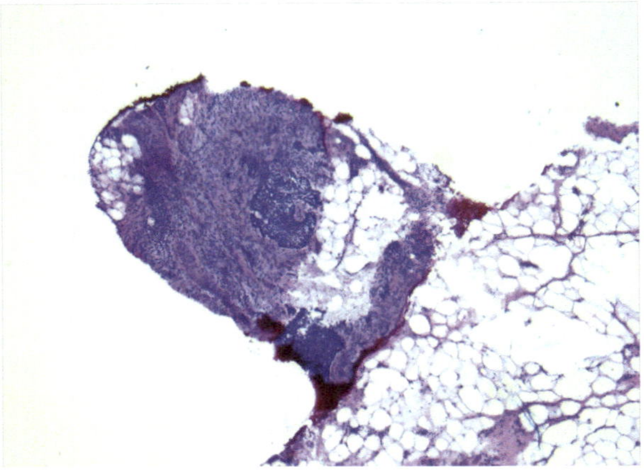

Fig. 1.13 Tumor "floater" at the deep margin of a Mohs specimen.

unrecognized as a floater. Often these tumor fragments can be differentiated from a true positive by the fact that displaced tumor will often be completely surrounded by tissue marking ink and may also not be architecturally consistent with the nearby true deep margin of the specimen. When there is doubt, the surgeon should err on the side of excising a thin layer of additional tissue to confirm that the margins are free of tumor as oncologic cure is the most important motivating factor for performing MMS.

While ensuring complete removal of the malignancy is a primary goal of MMS, tissue conservation is also a critical element of the procedure. One means of being maximally conservative is to be knowledgeable of the histologic appearance of all of the normal structures of the skin that can occur in different anatomic areas as well as of the benign tumors of this skin that may be present incidentally during Mohs histology. One must not take the inappropriate course of surgically removing any abnormality noted in the skin due to an inability to distinguish malignant from benign neoplasms.[22]

Structures in the skin that may mimic malignancy include the following:

- **Salivary glands:** When performing surgery on the lip or on the cheek, especially the area immediately anterior and inferior to the ear, salivary glands can be present on Mohs specimens. These structures can be differentiated form BCC by their well-organized epithelium of serous (dark) and mucous (foamy and pink) cuboid and columnar epithelial cells with ducts.
- **Hair follicles and sebaceous glands:** In some sections, particularly sections that tangentially glance an edge of a hair follicle or sebaceous gland, hair follicles and sebaceous glands may be concerning for malignancy. This can often be resolved by examining deeper sections of a tissue block to see the area of concern evolve histologically into a normal follicle or gland.
- **Conjunctival epithelium:** The conjunctival epithelium is a nonkeratinized stratified squamous epithelium with goblet cells. It can be challenging to process and is vulnerable to incomplete marginal lay-down during issue grossing. Further, care should be used to avoid confusing goblet cells with pagetoid cells particularly when Mohs is being carried out for sebaceous carcinoma of the eyelid. Transitional epithelium in the urethra can pose similar difficulty.
- **Follicular basaloid proliferation (benign follicular proliferation or benign follicular hamartoma):** Interconnecting strands of basaloid cells resembling infundibulocystic BCC, but this benign neoplasm exhibits a normal perifollicular stroma versus the myxoid stroma of BCC as well as a more normal- appearing cytology.[23]
- **Benign adnexal neoplasms:** Commonly encountered benign adnexal neoplasms that may be confusing for malignancy include trichoepithelioma, trichoblastoma, tumor of the follicular infundibulum, syringoma, etc.[23]
- **Calcinosis cutis:** Calcinosis will often appear as a clearly identified floater; however, small calcium deposits may mimic BCC or sheets of cSCC.

When performing histologic interpretation of MMS tissue specimens, the surgeon should use care to not neglect other malignancies that may be encountered on the specimens. It is not uncommon to encounter an incidental new malignancy while treating a patient. For example, one may encounter an incidental BCC while using MMS to treat a cSCC and vice versa. It is appropriate to recognize and treat this additional tumor during that same patient encounter for MMS. In addition, nearby and clinically evident tumors that may fall in a potential reconstruction, such as a flap, should also be treated.

Finally, it is ideal for the Mohs surgeon to examine the tissue specimens not only for the presence or absence of malignancy, but also for the presence of factors that may contribute to the patient's care such as finding and documenting features that may upstage a patient's SCC from a Brigham and Women's Hospital (BWH) T2a to a T2b tumor stage[24] and documenting the presence of lymphocytic infiltration consistent with lymphoproliferative disease, such as CLL, and initiating a diagnostic workup if these features are identified.[25]

1.5.3 Tissue Mapping

MMS is effective because the surgeon and the pathologist are the same person. As discussed previously, because the surgeon is completely aware of the orientation of a tissue specimen as it is removed from the patient, has control of all of the laboratory processes between excision and histologic interpretation, and performs the histologic interpretation, the surgeon is able to accurately pinpoint the exact location of any residual malignancy on the patient and selectively re-excise it. Histologic mapping is the tool that allows documentation of residual malignancy in relation to the patient's anatomy and the orienting marks the surgeon has placed on the patient and specimen.

Mohs surgeons employ a variety of different media for mapping tumors ranging from straightforward drawings of the specimen and orienting marks to predrawn maps showing the excised specimen and orienting marks in relation to a standardized anatomic drawing, to intraoperative photographs of the patient with the orienting marks and mapping superimposed either physically with hand drawings or digitally with photo editing software.[26] Some additionally use a standardized anatomic numbering system to localize tumors to very specific locations.[27] This technique can be useful in conducting retrospective research where precise anatomic location of the tumor is essential. Regardless of the actual map used, the process of transferring the information the surgeon observes on the histologic specimens to the map is similar. First, as a point of quality assurance, the surgeon must confirm that the map and the histologic specimen are from the same site on the same patient. This is commonly accomplished by the use of accession numbers or other unique identifying information that is present on both the map and the microscope slides. This can further be confirmed by the surgeon by examining the gross size of the histologic specimen and the histologic appearance of the specimen to confirm that the specimen and map agree. For example, when a map from a large tumor accompanied by slides with a small specimen do not agree, it should serve as a cue for the surgeon to explore the possibility of a laboratory error. As a further example, the histologic appearance of scalp, nasal skin, eyelid, back, and so on is somewhat unique, so the surgeon should also be concerned about a tissue transfer or laboratory error if a map from one anatomic area is accompanied by slides that are evidently from another anatomic area upon histologic examination. Finally, the surgeon will examine the inking of the specimen and the placement of any asymmetric scores to ensure that the inking and orientation of the tissue and the illustration of the inking and orientation of the specimen on the map agree and that the tissue specimen has not, for example, been rotated 180 degrees relative to its original anatomic orientation. This step is important in order to avoid inadvertently mapping tumor to the wrong site on the specimen, thereby leading to the unnecessary excision of normal skin and, worse, the failure to excise residual malignant tissue.

Once these quality checks are done, the surgeon proceeds with histologic interpretation of the specimen. During this stage, one of the most obvious issues that can lead to a recurrence following MMS is failing to recognize tumor at the margin of the specimen. The risk for this is greatest in cases of unusual or particularly insidious tumors where recognition of the tumor at its periphery, where the histologic evidence of residual tumor can be subtle, may be challenging. Beyond this, there are errors that can be made in mapping residual tumor that may account for tumor recurrences. Imprecise mapping may lead to selective re-excision of the incorrect site, or re-excision of an inadequate breadth or depth of the correct site. Selective re-excision of the incorrect site is particularly challenging because the result will be a histologically tumor-free margin on the subsequent layer and false reassurance that the tumor was properly treated.

When mapping a tumor, it is important for the surgeon to keep in mind that the tumor being mapped is a three-dimensional (3D) figure with an edge, a wall, a "hinge point" where the wall transitions to the base, and a deep margin. Often there is histologic evidence that aids the surgeon in accounting for tumor in the wall of a specimen and tumor in the hinge point or base. The most obvious form of this evidence comes in the form of hair follicles, which are sectioned vertically in the wall and horizontally in the base. Careful attention to the precise 3D location of the residual tumor when mapping is important. This is particularly true for residual tumors that reside in the hinge point, where resampling an edge without extending through the hinge into the deep margin will produce a false-negative margin on a subsequent stage. Proper tumoral mapping should include the tumor type and subtype and anatomic depth. The notation of scar tissue, when observed, is a federal payer requirement and may aid the surgeon in resolving if the true deep or lateral margin has been reached and histologically assessed in a recurrent or incompletely excised tumor.

The surgeon may also wish to note histologic abnormalities that are not malignancies in order to document that these were observed and deemed to not be a positive margin. Such structures may include benign adnexal neoplasms, hair follicles or sebaceous glands that do not appear absolutely typical, intradermal melanocytic nevi, and seborrheic keratoses. Noting actinic keratoses may be helpful in that the surgeon has noted in the medical record the presence of background actinic damage that did not require excision by the Mohs technique but may require subsequent superficial treatment and in order to avoid confusion with a recurrent tumor at a later date. Noting normal structures that were involved by the tumor is also helpful such as when the lacrimal canaliculi, parotid or other salivary glands, or other normal structures are involved in the Mohs excision. Knowing the lacrimal canaliculus was damaged, for example, is important if one wishes to surgically attempt to restore function of this structure. In our practice, we note these nonmalignant structures in a color other than the red we use for noting the presence of malignancy in order to avoid confusion about whether an area requires selective re-excision or not. Cartilage, which may be seen on ear or nose layers, may also be illustrated on the map to show the sides of the cartilage where a tumor may be present.

The histologic map is a tool to aid the surgeon in precisely locating the site on the patient involved by residual tumor. The more precisely that tumor and nonmalignant structures are labeled, the more likely the surgeon will be to produce a cure for the patient. Further, the map is an important part of the medical record illustrating the observations the surgeon makes histologically and the decision-making regarding structures that will require re-excision because they were determined to be malignant and those that will be left behind because they were determined to be benign or more appropriately treated by other means such as in the case of actinic keratosis. A surgeon may wish to make written comments on the map as well to add clarity to decisions that are made based on histology and to guide selective re-excision of residual tumor such as tumor present on the deep tissue cuts examined that may clear on the true surgical margin cuts.

1.6 Subsequent Layers

Nicholas Golda and George Hruza

The rate of recurrence increases in MMS, requiring multiple stages to completely remove a malignancy.[18] The rationale behind this is manifold. Tumors requiring multiple stages are more likely to be more biologically aggressive, the ability for the surgeon to reorient may diminish with additional layers, and there are more opportunities for an error such as inaccurate mapping or inaccurate marginal resampling.

With respect to subsequent layers, as the number of subsequent layers needed to treat a particular tumor increases, the ability of the Mohs surgeon to maintain precise resolution of where the next stage needs to be taken from becomes more challenging. Being purposeful in the planning and execution of subsequent layers is important. While the surgeon should attempt to completely remove all residual tumor with each subsequent layer, the goal remains to also be conservative, so the surgeon should also excise the subsequent layer in a manner that will allow easy reorientation to the site if yet another stage is required.

When preparing to take a subsequent layer, a moment should be taken to reorient to the histologic map and the patient. The surgeon should confirm that the correct maps for the correct patient and tumor are present. Attention should be paid to the location of anatomic landmarks and orienting marks with confirmation that these correspond to what is present on the map.

Once these are confirmed, the surgeon proceeds with excision of the subsequent layer. One may wish to employ a technique known as "flanking," where a small amount of tissue in each dimension around the tumor (both sides and deep) is included with the selective re-excision. This small additional amount of tissue is often inconsequential to the planning of a repair and provides a measure of insurance to the surgeon if the location of the residual tumor is not exact or if the tissue edges at the tips are incompletely laid down during tissue processing. This technique also aids in situations where the residual tumor is near the hinge point, as a small fringe of the deep margin can be included in the layer to provide histologic evidence that the proper depth was re-excised to prove negative margins (▶ Video 1.6, ▶ Video 1.7).

The extent of the subsequent layer can be indicated on the patient in various ways. The most common of these is the placement of tissue scores in the skin at either side of a selective re-excision where the curvature of the edges fades back into the rounded contour of the original rounded MMS stage. Care should be taken to terminate these layers at pre-existing scores or to somehow make these terminal scores discernible from those in place already from earlier layers. Alternatively, some surgeons may elect to square off subsequent layers at their terminal points, while still others will use unique geometric shapes for subsequent layers to reduce potential confusion about the location of a subsequent layer. There may be debate about which of these techniques is superior. However, the most important factor should be which technique consistently allows a surgeon the greatest confidence in accurate reorientation if yet another layer should be needed.

Just as with first layers, surgeons may also wish to place tissue-orienting marks or scores on subsequent layers. The benefits and drawbacks of tissue scores for first stages persist in subsequent stages, so the surgeon must determine what is best for the clinical situation at hand. Many surgeons choose to place midpoint scores in subsequent layers in order to increase the resolution of the location of residual tumor. Additionally, if a surgeon determines that more than one distinct tissue specimen should be excised during a single subsequent layer, these specimens can be differentiated from one another by the placement of a midpoint score in one specimen and no score in the other. Careful attention must be paid to inking of multiple tissue specimens in one layer that may be placed on one histologic slide (one block) or separate slides (separate blocks of the same stage).

1.6.1 Subsequent Layers When Malignancy is Present Only in the Deep Tissue

At times, the surgeon may need to re-excise residual tumor that is present only in the deep margin of the specimen. There are several approaches to maintaining tissue orientation when the more fragile deep tissue, consisting often of fat and possibly muscle, requires re-excision. The challenge that arises from deep margin–only specimens is how to maintain tissue orientation such that any residual tumor that persists on the deep tissue only subsequent layer can be accurately mapped and properly re-excised. Because deep tissue–only layers lack a dermal component in most cases, traditional orientation utilizing dermal scores or marks is not possible. Following are some techniques that have been described for addressing this issue:

- **Dermal tag technique:** In this technique, the necessary deep tissue is removed as well as a nearby thin margin of dermis. The location of this dermal tag is marked by a tissue score. When tissue processing is done, the dermis is laid down as per normal Mohs tissue processing and any residual tumor in the deep margin can be mapped using this dermal tag as a reference point (▶ Video 1.8).
- **Rhombus or "postage stamp" technique:** This technique is best suited for large tumors where there is a large field of deep tissue and the surgeon must use the previously described gridding technique to accurately locate residual tumor on a deep margin. Once the appropriate zone or zones in the grid that requires re-excision are identified, the surgeon excises the entirety of that polygon of involved tissue and inks the flat sides with different colors to correspond with the map. This allows precise location of any residual deep tumor relative to the uniquely inked margins (▶ Video 1.9, ▶ Video 1.10).
- **Entire depth resampling:** If a smaller lesion has involvement of any part of the deep margin, the surgeon may determine that it is most appropriate to resample the entirety of the deep margin to ensure that the margin is completely sampled and rechecked for residual malignancy. Orientation in these cases can be accomplished by placing scores in the deep tissue–only re-excision that corresponds to the original tissue scores placed for the preceding layer. These scores can then be inked and located during histologic analysis, allowing precise mapping of residual malignancy if present. Taking the entire depth of the previous stage may also be helpful in reconstruction (such as removing excess tissue on the nose or back for a primary repair) or even change the reconstructive plan (such as taking a deeper layer on the nasal ala necessitating a flap or even a multiple-stage reconstruction as opposed to a full-thickness skin graft).
- **Staples for tissue orientation:** Placing staples within the defect at the edges of the excised specimen helps localize the area being excised and placing matching staples into the specimen helps orient the specimen relative to the defect. The number of staples in the defect should be counted to ensure that no staples are left behind at the conclusion of the case.

Regardless of which technique is used, the critical element of deep-only layers is the same as that for all subsequent layers: complete removal of the malignancy. Often re-excision of additional deep tissue is not impactful from a reconstructive or functional standpoint, so resampling the zone that has been determined to have residual malignancy as well as a flank of additional tissue around this zone is appropriate to ensure complete re-examination of the margin and reducing the risk of a false-negative MMS layer. ▶ Video 1.11 illustrates the process of taking an initial stage as well as mapping and removing a subsequent stage.

1.7 Nonstandard Situations

Nicholas Golda and George Hruza

There are anatomic situations where the previously described techniques for tissue excision, processing, and mapping do not hold or special attention to difficult-to-process tissue or to the 3D aspects of the excised tissue is required. These most often present in the form of through-and-through defects of the more anatomically complex areas of the face such as the ear, nose, lip, and the eyelid.

First, in a through-and-through defect, the traditional orientation of "deep" and "superficial" is lost as there is epidermis, mucosa, or conjunctiva that requires analysis on the entire circumference of the tissue being processed. Additionally, the "deep" part of these excisions lies at the center between these two epithelial layers and may contain rigid tissue such as cartilage or tarsal plate. If the surgeon determines it is reasonable to do so, initial and subsequent layers in these settings should be excised in a manner that facilitates ease of tissue processing. It stands to reason that the easier a given piece of tissue is to process with complete representation of all epithelial and deep margins intact, the easier it will be to interpret and accurately identify and map residual tumor. Tissue specimens that are harder to process will result in more challenging interpretations and a greater possibility of incomplete treatment or unnecessary additional stages of MMS. The best approach for easing histologic processing is to take MMS stages that require through-and-through resections at the same level or to the same depth internally versus externally such that the specimen can essentially be placed flat on a microscope slide with both epithelial layers and the deep margin in full contact with the slide immediately following excision from the patient and any division of the specimen that may be necessary.

A further challenge in these situations is accurate tissue orientation and mapping. This is especially true for wedge-style Mohs stages on the ear where the skin on both sides of the auricular cartilage is similar in histologic appearance (unlike eyelid, nose, and lip where tissue differs histologically inside vs. out). Cases such as these require excellent communication between the surgeon and laboratory staff, careful mapping, and thoughtful placement of orienting scores.

1.8 Mohs Layers in Special Sites

Thomas Hocker

The primary objective of MMS at *any* site is complete tumor extirpation; therefore, it is sometimes necessary to sacrifice cosmetically or functionally important anatomic structures. However, it is important to understand the unique anatomic aspects that exist in these "special sites" so that unnecessary morbidity can be avoided. Thorough discussion of the complex anatomy of these sites has been eloquently described elsewhere and will not be the focus of our discussion. Instead, we will try to highlight some practical surgical pearls and pitfalls.

1.8.1 Eyelid

Eyelid anatomy is perhaps the most complex of any site Mohs surgeons operate (▸ Fig. 1.14, ▸ Fig. 1.15). For a full discussion of relevant anatomy, we recommend the excellent review article by Patel and Itani.[28]

Anatomic Keys

- Eyelid skin is the thinnest anywhere on the body (< 1 mm), with essentially **no subcutaneous fat** between it and the underlying orbicularis oculi muscle.
- Eyelid is divided primarily into **anterior and posterior lamellae**; although usually not discussed as such, a "middle lamella" also exists at portions of the eyelid (see ▸ Fig. 1.14):
  - Anterior lamella: **skin** and **orbicularis oculi** muscle.
    - Orbicularis oculi is a muscle of facial expression → hence, innervated by branches of facial nerve (cranial nerve [CN] 7). Orbicularis oculi muscle is a **sphincterlike** muscle divided into two main concentric subunits. (1) Orbital— outermost ring of muscle, under voluntary control, and responsible for **forced lid closure**; overlying skin is easily undermined above the muscle allowing for great mobility. (2) Palpebral—inner ring of muscle, under voluntary and involuntary control, responsible for **blinking and winking**, and contiguous with lateral canthal tendon (attaches laterally to Whitnall's tubercle) and medial canthal tendon (MCT; a bifurcated structure that envelops the lacrimal canaliculi at the medial portion of the orbit). Palpebral orbicularis oculi is further subdivided into a peripheral **preseptal** and a central **pretarsal** portion. Preseptal orbicularis oculi: skin is loosely attached and mobile; deep to this layer lies the "middle lamella" consisting of the orbital septum, orbital fat pads, and the lid retractor muscles/aponeuroses (levator palpebrae superioris and Muller's muscle superiorly, and capsulopalpebral fascia inferiorly). Pretarsal orbicularis oculi: overlying skin is tightly adherent to posterior lamella.
  - "Middle lamella": Deep to the preseptal portion of the orbicularis oculi muscle lies (in order from superficial to deep) **orbital septum**, **orbital fat pads**, and the **lid retractors** (levator palpebrae superioris, Muller's muscle, inferior tarsal muscle, and capsulopalpebral fascia):
    - Levator palpebrae superioris: the **major eyelid elevator**, innervated by oculomotor nerve (CN3), attached to the tarsal plate via its aponeurosis, and is compromised in Horner's syndrome (miosis, ptosis and anhidrosis).
    - Sympathetic innervation: Muller's muscle and inferior tarsal muscle.
    - *Pearl*: If a laceration to the preseptal portion of the eyelid results in a large amount of herniating fat, then you know that the orbital septum has been compromised.
  - Posterior lamella: **conjunctiva** and **tarsal plate:**
    - Tarsal plate: fibrous tissue, comprises the structural support of the lid, and houses Meibomian glands → provides oily secretions that prevent tear evaporation.
- Lacrimal canaliculi are located deep to superficial wing of the MCT:
  - Lacrimal drainage system is protected anteriorly by MCT.
- Lacrimal gland is located at the superolateral aspect of the upper eyelid.
- Vascular supply of the eyelid is extremely rich!
  - Numerous anastomoses exist between branches of the internal and external carotid systems:
    - Notably, at the MCT, branches of the facial artery (external carotid) anastamose with the ophthalmic artery (internal carotid).
  - *Pearl*: The rich vascular supply of the eyelid makes for an excellent wound bed for skin grafts; flaps are also well vascularized and robust in this location.
- Lymphatic drainage (important for understanding regional metastatic disease):
  - **Lateral two-thirds** of upper eyelid and lateral one-third of the lower eyelid → **preauricular** nodes.
  - **Medial one-third** of upper eyelid and medial two-thirds of the lower → **submandibular** nodes.

Mohs Pearls

- **Chlorhexidine prep is contraindicated** near the eye due to the risk of keratitis; povidone–iodine is recommended.
- Chalazion clamps assist in hemostasis and facilitate Mohs excisions (especially of the lid margin).
- Eye shields: use during MMS is controversial:
  - Questionable benefit for periocular surgery.
    - Used by up to 75% of Mohs surgeons, but only used consistently 10% of the time by those who use them.[29]
    - Roughly one-third of Mohs surgeons have, at some point, had a patient who experienced corneal abrasions due to eye shield use; usually self-resolves in 2 to 3 days with conservative pain-relief measures ± topical antibiotics (erythromycin ointment or quinolone drops).
  - Plastic (polymethyl methacrylate) eye shields are recommended over stainless steel eye shields for all

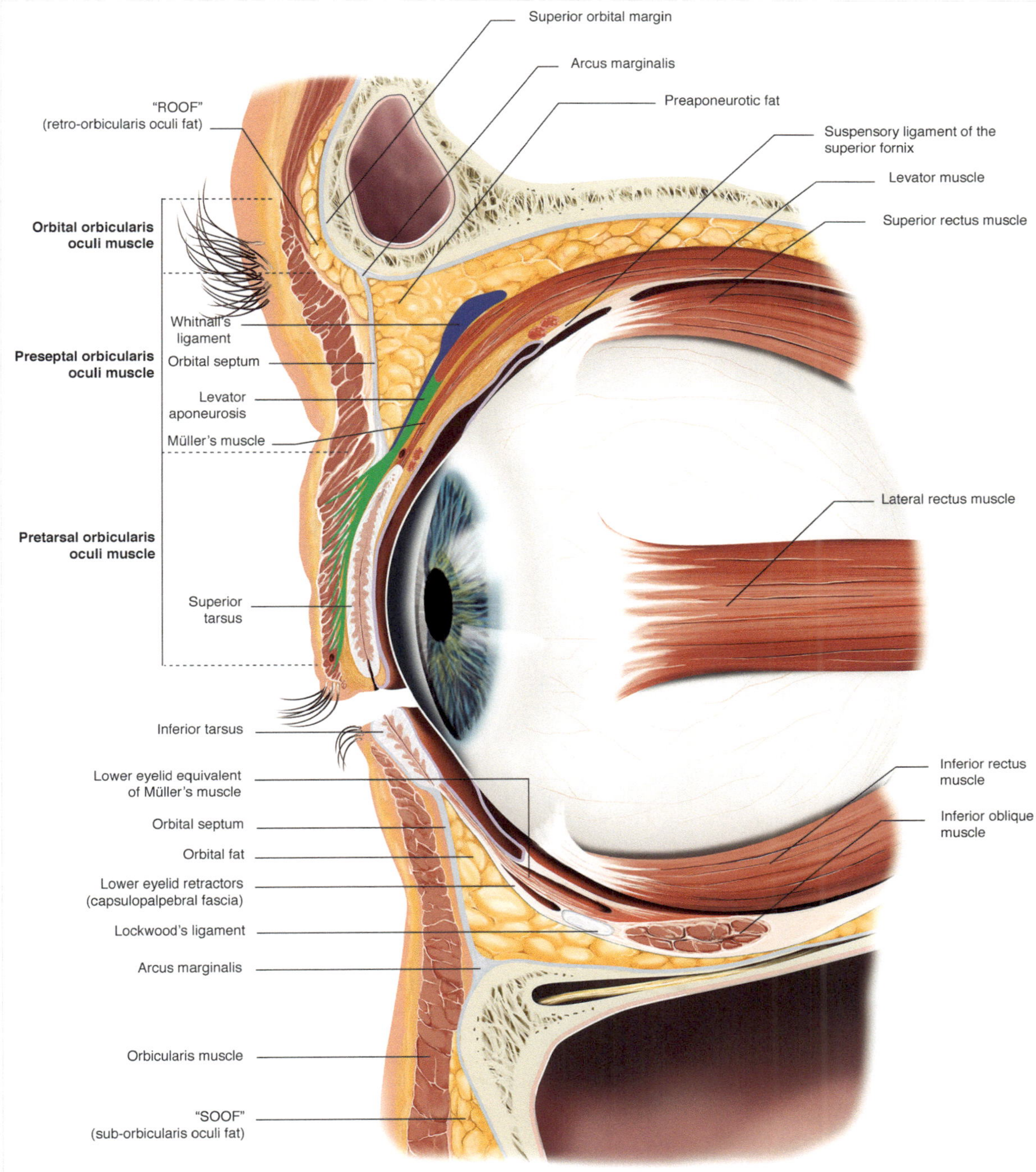

Fig. 1.14 Eyelid anatomy: sagittal section. Reproduced from Leatherbarrow B. Oculoplastic Surgery. 3rd Edition. New York: Thieme; 2019.

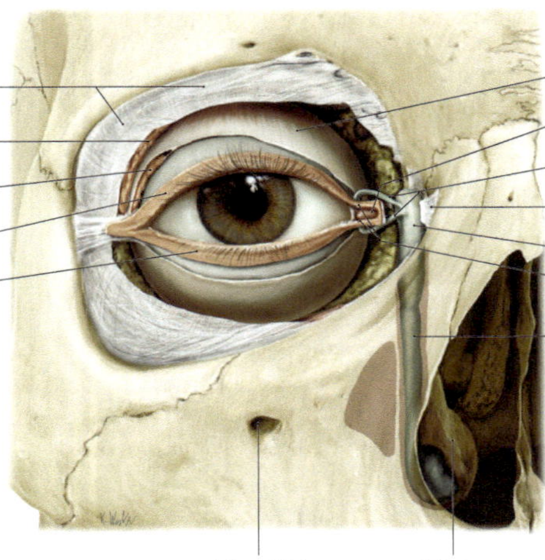

Fig. 1.15 Basic eyelid anatomy: frontal view. Reproduced from Schuenke M, Schulte E, Schumacher U. THIEME Atlas of Anatomy: Head, Neck, and Neuroanatomy. Illustrations by Voll M and Wesker K. © Thieme 2020.

nonlaser procedures[30]; cannot use with laser procedures due to risk of thermal-induced corneal damage:
  - Lower risk of sharp edges and burs than stainless steel → decreased risk of corneal abrasion.
  - Less likely to conduct energy from electrosurgical units.
  - Cheaper.
- Must ensure the shields are properly fitted and have a smooth, intact surface → otherwise, risk of corneal abrasion.
- Technique:
  - Apply proparacaine topically to anesthetize eye.
  - Inspect eye shield for scratches, burs, sharp edges, or debris.
  - Apply lubricant (methylcellulose-based lubricants are preferred over Lacri-Lube or antibiotic ointments).
  - Insert eye shield: (1) Tell the patient to look up and then retract the lower lid. (2) Insert inferior edge of the eye shield posterior to the lower eyelid, all the way down to the fornix. (3) Tell the patient to look down and retract the upper eyelid (superior edge of the eye shield will fall into place).

- Tissue distortion can become problematic with high volumes of local anesthetic → use minimal required amount of anesthetic.
- Breach of orbital septum → risk of retrobulbar hematoma.
- Having an assistant **pull the skin taut during Mohs** excision is key, since periocular skin is thin and loose. One way of doing this on the eyelid margin is having an assistant keep traction, gently but firmly, with one forceps while the surgeon uses another forceps to grip the other side while taking a layer. The editors prefer to grip the eyelid margin with the forceps on behalf of the assistant first, which is a critical step with risk of causing injury, and subsequently allow the assistant to take over the forceps and keep tension.
- Using a no. **11-blade or 15c blade** is helpful for incisions on the floppy portions of eyelid (skin overlying the orbital portion of the orbicularis oculi):
  - These sharper blades are also helpful along the free margin of the lid, which is an area where it is difficult to achieve great side-to-side tension from your assistant.
- Mohs layers on the eyelid often do not need to be angled at 45 degrees, since the skin is so lax. Even vertical Mohs excisions can typically be laid down with ease. The lid margin is often relaxed with small vertical incisions on the superficial portion due to the thickness of sebaceous tissue.
- Given the thin and floppy nature of the eyelid skin, it is often more difficult to take narrow subsequent Mohs stages compared to other thicker-skinned sites. Vertical incisions using a no. 11 blade or 15c blade are helpful in this regard.
- To ensure high-quality Mohs slides, extra attention is required when inking and laying down Mohs layers on eyelid skin.
  - Loose, redundant skin can lead to folding artifact.
  - Lid margin and conjunctival layers may be confusing to lay-down for your histotechnician, since conjunctiva may be mistaken for missing epidermis → it is helpful to bring them into the room during the Mohs layer to show them the *in vivo* orientation of the true margin.
  - *Editor's note*: To this extent, when a layer must be taken on the bulbar conjunctiva, it is also important to make sure the edges are not folded as this tissue is extremely thin. Typically, experienced Mohs surgeons comfortable with eyelid layers can continue to take layers from the lid margin down to the palpebral and bulbar conjunctiva if needed. However, one must understand and review the unique nuances of conjunctival frozen section histology. Practically, taking a conjunctival layer, once over the sclera, allows for one

chance at margin evaluation, if the histotechnician and surgeon are able to properly orient and embed the tissue for evaluation. If positivity is noted once the limbus is approached, other therapeutic options will be considered by a cornea surgeon such as excision with cryotherapy, plaque radiotherapy, or orbital exenteration.

It is important to note that once the palpebral conjunctiva layers are exhausted and the tumor extends on the bulbar conjunctiva, further surgery may risk severe eye damage and even loss of an eye. Therefore, if a severe tumor is suspected, all possible risks, alternative treatments, and outcomes, including exenteration, should be discussed with the patient in detail prior to surgery to obtain informed consent, and such surgery should be done by or in conjunction with a cornea or oculoplastic surgeon.

In Dr. Tolkachjov's experience, taking such layers in a multidisciplinary setting and in conjunction with a cornea surgeon and anesthesia would be ideal, if a Mohs surgeon has privileges at an "eye" hospital or can supervise and guide a cornea surgeon (with the help of an intraoperative microscope) making the incisions and using blunt and sharp scissors dissection while keeping the conjunctiva taut to remove conjunctival tissue from the limbus over to the canthus if tumor involvement is suspected. Clinically, SCC (conjunctival intraepithelial neoplasia or ocular surface squamous neoplasia) spreading over the conjunctiva may mimic a pterygium or a pinguecula, a yellowish, raised thickening of the bulbar conjunctiva on the sclera, close to the edge of the cornea. While pingueculae are not cancerous, rapid changes or severe overgrowth may signal a possible SCC formation.

- Frozen section histopathology:
  - Excess ink can obscure true skin edge margins and impair precise tissue lay-down → carefully laying out the specimen on a piece of cardboard and applying only pinpoint amounts of tissue ink helps minimize this problem. As discussed earlier, folding artifact is common if tissue is not properly laid down prior to sectioning.
  - Conjunctival tissue appears different than skin histologically. Conjunctival mucosa has a very thin layer of epithelium, and usually, an underlying lymphoplasmacytic bandlike infiltrate in the superficial dermis.
  - Familiarity of conjunctival histopathology, especially when transitioning from palpebral conjunctiva to bulbar conjunctiva, is necessary as vasculature and glands of the bulbar conjunctiva may often resemble glandular SCC.

1.8.2 Lip

The lip is a fairly simple, highly mobile anatomic structure comprising a sphincteric muscle (orbicularis oris), hair-bearing cutaneous lip skin, and mucosa.

Anatomic Keys

- Similar to orbicularis oculi, the orbicularis oris muscle is a sphincteric muscle of facial expression that is innervated by CN7.
  - However, orbicularis oris has no bony attachments → lip has greater laxity/mobility → easier to rearrange tissue during reconstruction.
  - Like the eyelid, the orbicularis oris muscle fibers attach directly to the overlying skin and mucosa, with essentially no intervening subcutaneous fat.
- Vascular supply is extensive:
  - Anastomosing arcades provided by labial arteries, which run deep to the orbicularis oris muscle.
- Motor innervation of lip:
  - Orbicularis oris is innervated by the buccal branch of CN7.
  - Lip depressors are innervated by the marginal mandibular branch of CN7:
    - *Major danger area is where the nerve courses over the mandible.*[31] Typically occurs 3 cm anterior to the masseteric tuberosity (approximately one-fourth of the distance between the masseteric tuberosity and the mental midline; ▶ Fig. 1.16).
- Sensory innervation of lip:
- Upper lip is innervated by the **infraorbital nerve** (branch of V2).
- Lower lip and chin are innervated by the **mental nerve** (branch of V3).

Mohs Pearls

- Nerve blocks of the infraorbital nerve (upper lip) and mental nerve (lower lip) are highly effective and can minimize anesthetic-related tissue distortion.
- The vermilion border becomes blanched and distorted after local anesthesia injection:
  - Prior to anesthesia injection, **mark the vermilion border** with a skin marker while it is easily seen before distortion with local anesthetic.
  - During your initial Mohs layer, make superficial scalpel hash marks along the previously marked vermilion border, since skin marker often washes off throughout the course of the day.
- In addition to the vermilion border, the location of the nasolabial folds and apical triangle are important landmarks in reconstructive approaches. Use a marking pen to delineate these landmarks prior to distorting the tissue with local anesthesia.
- The **lip is a free margin** and thus can be difficult to stabilize during Mohs excision. We recommend the following methods to achieve adequate tension and stabilization during excision:
  - Tell the patient, "please do not talk during this part, you don't want me to have a moving target!"
  - Standard four-point lateral surface tension often works well for the cutaneous lip.

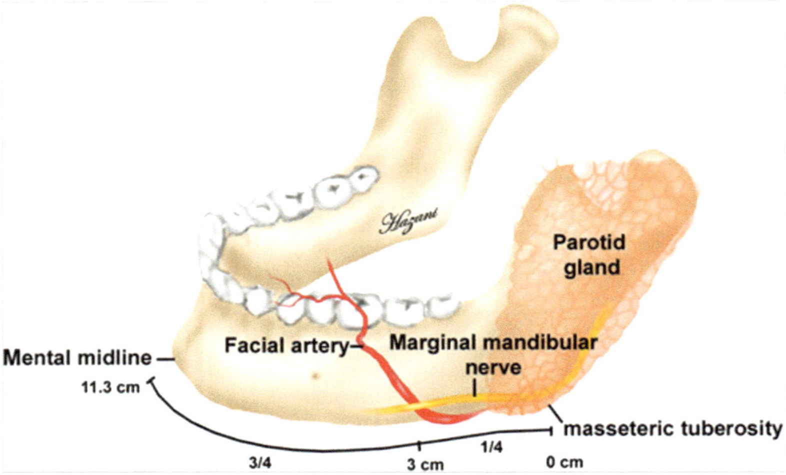

Fig. 1.16 Anatomic landmarks that can be used to predict the location of the marginal mandibular nerve. Reproduced with permission from Hazani R, Chowdhry S, Mowlavi A, Wilhelmi BJ. Bony Anatomic Landmarks to Avoid Injury to the Marginal Mandibular Nerve. Aesthet Surg J 2011;31 (3):286–289.

- If greater tension is needed, or you are operating closer to the vermilion border, the following methods are helpful:
  - Place rolled-up gauze inside the mouth between the teeth and the inner surface of the lips and then apply surface tension. The roll of dry gauze serves as a more stable “backstop” than slippery wet teeth do; the bulkiness of the gauze also serves to evert the lip.
  - “Pinch-pull method”: the assistant uses index fingers and thumbs of both hands to pinch inside and outside the lips on both sides of the surgical site; then they stretch and evert the lip. Pinching or grasping with gauze provides better traction and grip. This method has the added benefit of hemostasis via occlusion of the labial arteries.

- Consider **sharp**/scalpel **debulking** of tumor rather than curettage, as it offers many benefits and few downsides:
  - Sharp debulking helps lay down/process the tissue more easily and minimizes the chance of deep tumor positivity.
  - Very little is sacrificed by employing sharp debulking because defect depth is not important on the lip (unless through and through):
    - Most lip Mohs defects are closed primarily or with flaps.
    - Grafts are not generally a good reconstructive option for the mobile lip.
- Superficial tumors on the upper and lower lips can sometimes be curetted lightly and cleared with a thin conservative thickness Mohs layer (CTL) and allowed to heal by second intention with good cosmesis.[8]
- Orbicularis muscle fibers insert directly into overlying skin with minimal or no intervening fat → difficult to establish subdermal undermining plane during reconstruction:
  - Because of the muscle fiber insertion into the skin, primary closures have a tendency to heal with inversion due to the band of scar tissue in the muscle, which retracts/inverts the skin surface → it is critical to achieve hypereversion via buried vertical mattress sutures as well as epidermal vertical mattress sutures.

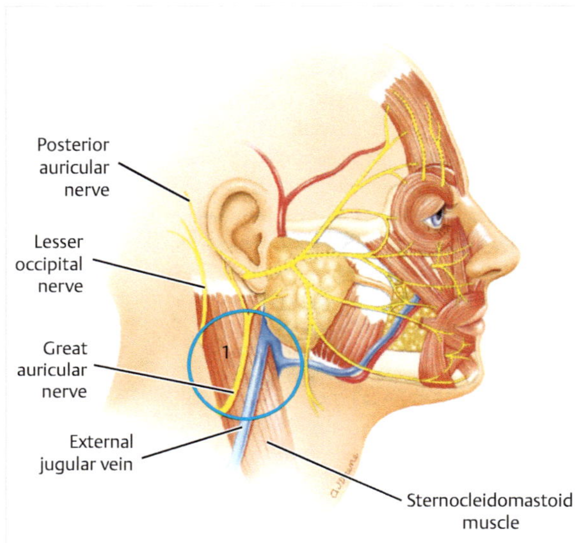

Fig. 1.17 Key periauricular anatomy. Reproduced from Janis J. Essentials of Plastic Surgery. 3rd Edition. New York: Thieme; 2022.

1.8.3 Ear

The ear is a highly convoluted 3D structure whose shape is dictated by the underlying cartilaginous scaffolding. The key periauricular anatomy is shown in ▶ Fig. 1.17. The ear is in close proximity to the main trunk of CN7, the parotid gland, and numerous named sensory nerves. The primary considerations during MMS are to (1) minimize damage to critical neighboring motor and sensory nerves and (2) preserve hearing by protecting the patency of the external auditory canal (EAC).

Anatomic Keys

- Skin on the ear differs based on location:
  - Anterior surface: very thin (1 mm or less), no subcutaneous fat, **difficult to undermine** off of deep tissues, and relatively **immobile.**
  - Posterior surface: thicker skin with **increased mobility** and subcutaneous fat, and **easy to undermine and mobilize** for reconstructions.
- Vascular supply is provided by branches off two vertically oriented vessels:
  - Superficial temporal artery (STA): supplies anterior ear through horizontally oriented unnamed branches, is a terminal branch of external carotid system that originates in parotid by the mandible, and courses 1.5 cm anterior to tragus.
  - Posterior auricular artery (PAA): supplies posterior ear and courses upward within the postauricular sulcus.
- EAC length = 2.5 cm from conchal bowl to tympanic membrane:
  - Lateral one-third of EAC = cartilage (conchal bowl).
  - Medial two-thirds of EAC = bone (temporal bone).
- Important structures to consider:
  - Main trunk of CN7 and STA are both located 1 to 1.5 cm anterior and deep to the tragus.
  - EAC: only 7 to 8 mm in diameter → **even slight EAC stenosis can lead to hearing loss!**

Mohs Pearls

- For all areas of the ear, skin grafts are a valuable reconstructive option → **attempt to preserve the perichondrium** whenever feasible.
- Palpate all ear lesions!
  - If the lesion is mobile over the cartilage → tumor less likely to be invading into cartilage → make a strong attempt to preserve perichondrium on the initial Mohs stage.
  - If the lesion is **immobile** over the cartilage → **cartilage likely involved.**
- Conchal bowl is a difficult area to take standard beveled Mohs layers, due to its concave nature:
  - Angled scalpel blades can be helpful.
  - If a standard no. 15 blade is used, start by using the very tip of the blade to thinly incise a circle around the lesion. Then begin your Mohs layer from the lateral aspect of the ear and use a shaving motion to pass under the lesion all the way through to the opposite (medial aspect).
  - Have your assistant place their fingers on the posterior ear and push up on the underside of the conchal bowl to flip it outward/make it less concave.
- Scissors are helpful for dissecting in the potential space between the skin and perichondrium.

1.8.4 Nose

The nose is one of the most common sites for skin cancer due to its anterior projection and thus direct exposure to sunlight. This is unfortunate, since the nose is perhaps the single most important facial structure from a cosmetic standpoint, due to its centrofacial location and 3D symmetry of multiple convoluted cosmetic subunits. Because of these factors, there are multiple books dedicated solely to nasal aesthetics and reconstruction. Refer to ▶ Fig. 1.18 showing the cartilaginous nasal structure.

Anatomic Keys

- The nose is divided into distinct cosmetic subunits: root, dorsum, sidewall, tip, soft triangle, and ala.
- Skin on the different subunits varies in texture, mobility, and risk of tension-related distortion.
- Skin texture:
  - **Sebaceous, thick skin**: ala, tip, and root:
    - Skin grafts often are conspicuous at these sites.
  - **Shiny, thin skin**: dorsum, sidewall, dorsum, soft triangles, and columella:
    - Skin grafts are a good option in terms of cosmetic match for these sites.
- Mobility:
  - **High mobility**: dorsum, sidewall, and root:

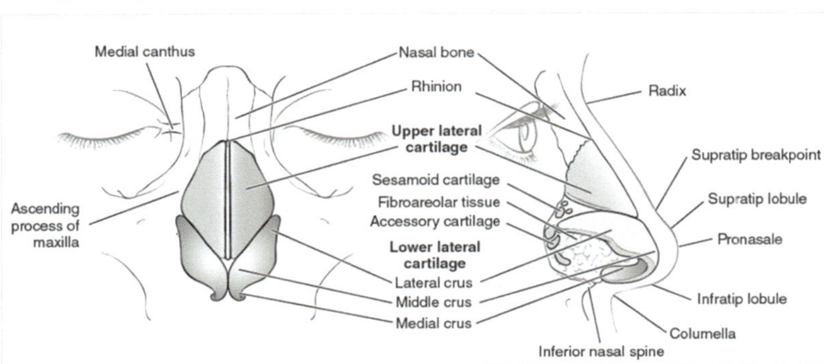

Fig. 1.18 Cartilaginous nasal structure. Reproduced from Janis J. Essentials of Plastic Surgery. 2nd Edition. New York: Thieme; 2014.

    - This greater mobility is partly related to the presence of subcutaneous fat layer separating skin from underlying muscles of facial expression.
  - **Low mobility**: ala, columella, tip, and soft triangle:
    - Undermining in these areas is very challenging and unrewarding in terms of gained mobility.
- Three zones of cartilage provide the nose with its shape:
  - Septal cartilage:
    - Responsible for degree of anterior nasal projection.
    - Anchored to bone → **rigid**.
    - Medial boundary of internal and external nasal valves.
  - Upper lateral cartilages (paired):
    - Provides structural support to nasal sidewall.
    - Anchored to bone → semi-rigid (but is still subject to distortion by compressive forces).
    - Lateral boundary of internal nasal valve (susceptible to compressive forces).
  - Lower lateral cartilages (paired):
    - Contributes to nasal tip projection, alar crease prominence, and provides support to external nasal valve.
    - NOT anchored to bone → **very mobile** and **easily distorted** by compressive forces.
- Risk of positional distortion is determined by the presence or absence of rigid underlying bone, which resists compression; the lower alar cartilages are insufficiently rigid to resist great compressive forces:
  - **Low risk of distortion**: dorsum, sidewalls, and nasal root.
  - **High risk of distortion**: ala, nasal tip, and soft triangle.
- Nasal valves allow for proper airflow and may be compromised by closure-related tension on portions of the nose NOT braced by underlying bone:
  - External valve: allows passage of air through distal nostril:
    - *Pearl*: Test structural integrity by occluding opposite nostril and having the patient forcibly inspire → if nostril collapses, then structural support is required.
  - Internal valve: the major contributor to airflow resistance; is located superior to external nasal valve.
    - Borders: inferior portion of upper lateral cartilage, nasal septum cartilage, and turbinate.
    - Increased risk of valve dysfunction: deviated septum and compression of inferior portion of upper lateral cartilage.
- Vasculature: nasal skin has ample blood supply via branches of the internal (dorsal nasal artery, a branch off the ophthalmic artery) and external (facial/angular arteries) carotid systems:
  - **Medial canthus is location of anastomosis** between angular artery (external carotid) and dorsal nasal artery (internal carotid).
  - **Vessels are located superficial to nasal musculature** → undermining in submuscular plane is a relatively bloodless plane and preserves major vessels.

Mohs Pearls

- More so than at other sites, it is important to minimize not only breadth of tissue removal during Mohs, but also depth:
  - Minimizing depth of defects allows for greater reconstructive options and also decreases risk of iatrogenic nasal valve incompetence.
  - The distal third of the nose leads itself to clearing tumors with conservative thickness layers, and these defects heal nicely by second intent. In some cases, the defect and surrounding sebaceous skin, or even rhinophyma, can be treated with wire brush dermabrasion in the same operative session as tumor clearance with a CTL.[8,9]
  - Because nasal cartilages are responsible for nasal contour, excision of cartilage during MMS often necessitates cartilage replacement in order to restore normal contour.
- **Greater degree of beveling** is often required for proper lay-down of thick, sebaceous nasal skin.
- Nasal skin is the most common site for subclinical **"basaloid follicular proliferations"** (BFPs) or "funny-looking basaloid follicular structures" → awareness of nasal BFPs/"funny follicles" helps minimize risk of overly aggressive resections.
- Shape and **rigidity of the alar bulb is due to fibrofatty tissue, not cartilage:**
  - Even if no cartilage has been resected during Mohs excision, the external nasal valve may become compromised → if so, must re-create structural support via cartilage struts or similarly rigid tissue.
    - *Pearl*: Folded paramedian forehead flaps and Spear's flaps (cheek interpolation flap) often possess enough intrinsic rigidity to obviate the need for cartilage struts, but you must assess on a case-by-case basis.

1.8.5 Periosteum/Bone

Performing Mohs layers near the bone is technically challenging for both the surgeon and histotechnician. Challenges include maintaining layer contiguity, mapping, tissue lay-down, and sectioning. Periosteum is extremely thin, loose tissue that is prone to folding.

Mohs Pearls

- When tumors penetrate near periosteum on your initial Mohs layer, it is often difficult to accurately correlate the precise location of the tumor seen on the Mohs slides with the in vivo location where further resection is required. As such, it is common to resect periosteum broadly around the suspected area of positivity, or even to remove the entire depth of the prior Mohs defect (complete removal of the periosteum in the operative site). Tumors that approach the periosteum are highly infiltrative, by definition, and thus have an increased risk of recurrence. It is therefore critical to ensure that whatever approach you take results in a high degree of confidence that you have fully extirpated the tumor. Given the difficulty with precise localization when only the deep margin is positive, the author usually leans toward removing the periosteum from the entire depth of the surgical site.

- When removing periosteum, it is worth remembering that **periosteum often retracts beneath the skin edges.**
  - To avoid an incomplete layer due to periosteum retraction, it is **helpful to excise a small margin of skin** (2–3 mm) peripheral to the prior Mohs defect all the way down to bone, and then dissect the periosteum off the bone.
  - In addition, including a thin rim of peripheral skin allows the surgeon to place hash marks for mapping, and provides a better area for gripping the tissue during periosteum removal.
- **Periosteum is delicate tissue and easily perforated** with sharp tips. To avoid perforation, one should use a periosteal elevator with the curved edge facing downward. The periosteum can then be gradually freed from the bone with multiple small pushing actions.
  - If scissors or a scalpel is used instead (not recommended), it is critical that the sharp tip be pointed downward toward bone in order to avoid perforation.
- Transfer the tissue carefully to a small piece of moistened cardboard, which will adhere to your specimen and make it easier to maintain orientation and ink:
  - Caution: do not apply too much ink, which can obscure the tissue edges and make it harder for your histotechnician to process accurately:
    - It is often preferable to have your histotechnician do the inking while being present in the room during the layer.
- It is difficult for your histotechnician to evenly cut a specimen that contains both skin and periosteum, due to their vastly different thicknesses and structural properties → it is commonly necessary to separate the periosteum in order to provide quality frozen section slides.
- Instruct your histotechnician to cut thin sections and avoid deeply freezing (can lead to brittle tissue and fracturing).
- If deep tumor remains positive in your periosteum Mohs layer → consider referral to ENT or neurosurgery for possible bone (outer table of the calvarium) resection—the outer table of the calvarium can be burred down with a dermatome or in the office setting with a coarse diamond fraise or a dermabrading hand engine. While this technique does not allow microscopic examination of the margins, it does provide an extra measure of tumor removal below missing or torn areas of periosteum—this technique also increases the vascularity of exposed cranium for second intent healing or split-thickness grafting.

1.8.6 Nail

MMS is extremely valuable in the treatment of nail unit malignancies, as it can offer high cure rates and digital sparing.

Anatomic Keys

- Nail unit: the nail plate overlies the matrix, nail bed, proximal and lateral nail folds, hyponychium, and neurovascular structures.
- The major **neurovascular structures** run along the **lateral and medial aspects** of the digits and are easily anesthetized with nerve blocks.
  - A large study of 1,111 patients undergoing digital nerve blocks for hand surgery compared use of plain lidocaine (without epinephrine) to lidocaine with epinephrine → no complications were observed when lidocaine with epinephrine was used → data support the use of lidocaine with epinephrine for digital blocks (exercise caution if the patient has a vasoocclusive disorder).[32]
  - Combining bupivacaine with the lidocaine with epinephrine may provide prolonged anesthesia and decrease postoperative pain.[33]
- The two most commonly used digital nerve blocks are the following:
  - Proximal digital block:
    - Injection site: lateral and medial portions of the proximal digit, near the MCP/MTP.
    - Slow onset (15–20 minutes).
    - Risk of damage to major neurovascular bundles.
    - Does not provide hemostasis.
  - Distal digital blocks ("wing blocks"):
    - **Faster** in onset, **safer**, and provide **hemostasis**, compared to proximal digital blocks; more painful if a prior proximal digital is not done.
    - Injection site: 5 mm proximal and lateral to the lateral edges of the proximal nail fold.

Mohs Pearls

- Ensure a bloodless field:
  - The assistant can pinch the radial and ulnar aspects of the digit to occlude blood flow.
  - Tourniquet can be made from gauze or penrose drain or glove.
- Understanding of the nail deformity allows you to make an educated guess as to where the tumor lies:

- Matrix lesions → pigment or thickening within the nail plate proper.
- Nail bed → normal-appearing nail plate will be elevated off of the nail bed.

- The 3D shape of the distal bone and the convolutions of the nail folds make it challenging to maintain a uniform, uninterrupted Mohs layer. Trying to ensure completeness of the deep margin can be particularly problematic, as there is little subcutaneous tissue separating the nail unit from the underlying bone.
  - Often, your best chance of obtaining a high-quality Mohs specimen is during your initial Mohs stage.
  - If the deep margin is positive on your first Mohs stage, you will likely need to use similar techniques and tools as described earlier for periosteum Mohs layers.
- Due to the complex 3D structure of the nail unit, be sure to bring your histotechnician into the room to show them how the specimen appeared in vivo, so they can be more confident about what represents the "true margin" during tissue relaxation and processing.

1.8.7 Anogenital Region

Tissue conservation in the anogenital region is critical for preservation of function and cosmesis of this highly sensitive area. Anogenital skin presents unique challenges due to its thin nature, laxity, and its transition zones from squamatized epidermis to the mucosal epithelium of the gastrointestinal and genitourinary tracts. EMPD and SCCs of the anogenital area are not infrequent indications for MMS, due to the desire for maximal tissue sparing.

Mohs Pearls

- Scrotum/vulva/penis: The thin and highly redundant nature of genital skin presents unique challenges:
  - Your assistant will need to fully stretch out the redundant skin so that your incisions yield sharp margins.
  - Due to the thinness of the skin and the importance of underlying fascial and soft-tissue structures, it is critical to avoid unnecessarily deep incisions.
  - The surgeon should aim to incise only the epidermis and dermis with their scalpel during the initial Mohs excision. To ensure a contiguous deep tissue margin and prevent perforation of the underlying structures, iris scissors are preferred for elevation and removal of the Mohs layer after the lesion has been circumferentially incised with a scalpel.
  - Hash marks may be extremely difficult to identify on both the Mohs specimen and the patient's skin surrounding the Mohs site. It is often useful to suture a single interrupted stitch at each of the hash marks on the patient. It is also critical to pay close attention to the location of the hashes on the Mohs specimen before inking it and/or giving it to your lab.
- Perianal region: many of the same challenges and approaches that were discussed for genital skin apply to the perianal region. Fortunately, there are fewer deep structures of concern, and therefore, less emphasis is placed on achieving super-thin Mohs excisions.

References

[1] Tolkachjov SN, Brodland DG, Coldiron BM, et al. Understanding Mohs micrographic surgery: a review and practical guide for the nondermatologist. Mayo Clin Proc. 2017; 92(8):1261–1271

[2] Stiegel E, Lam C, Schowalter M, Somani AK, Lucas J, Poblete-Lopez C. Correlation between original biopsy pathology and Mohs intraoperative pathology. Dermatol Surg. 2018; 44(2):193–197

[3] McGinness JL, Goldstein G. The value of preoperative biopsy-site photography for identifying cutaneous lesions. Dermatol Surg. 2010; 36 (2):194–197

[4] Lichtman MK, Countryman NB. Cell phone-assisted identification of surgery site. Dermatol Surg. 2013; 39(3, Pt 1):491–492

[5] Highsmith JT, Weinstein DA, Highsmith MJ, Etzkorn JR , Jr. BIOPSY 1-2-3 in dermatologic surgery: improving smartphone use to avoid wrong-site surgery. Technol Innov. 2016; 18(2–3):203–206

[6] Starling J , III, Coldiron BM. Outcome of 6 years of protocol use for preventing wrong site office surgery. J Am Acad Dermatol. 2011; 65 (4):807–810

[7] Dika E, Fanti PA, Ismaili A, et al. Basal cell carcinoma margin delineation: is curettage useful? A surgical and histological study. J Dermatolog Treat. 2013; 24(3):238–242

[8] Tolkachjov SN, Cappel JA, Bryant EA, Harmon CB. How We do it: utility of conservative thickness layers in Mohs micrographic surgery in selected patients. Dermatol Surg. 2018; 44(9): 1227–1229

[9] Tolkachjov SN, Cappel JA, Bryant EA, Harmon CB. Conservative thickness layers in Mohs micrographic surgery. Int J Dermatol. 2018; 57 (9):1128–1134

[10] Rowe DE, Carroll RJ, Day CL , Jr. Long-term recurrence rates in previously untreated (primary) basal cell carcinoma: implications for patient follow-up. J Dermatol Surg Oncol. 1989; 15(3):315–328

[11] Rowe DE, Carroll RJ, Day CL , Jr. Mohs surgery is the treatment of choice for recurrent (previously treated) basal cell carcinoma. J Dermatol Surg Oncol. 1989; 15(4):424–431

[12] Li JY, Silapunt S, Migden MR, McGinness JL, Nguyen TH. Mohs mapping fidelity: optimizing orientation, accuracy, and tissue identification in Mohs surgery. Dermatol Surg. 2018; 44(1):1–9

[13] Lee E, Wolverton JE, Somani AKA. A simple, effective analogy to elucidate the Mohs micrographic surgery procedure: the peanut butter cup. JAMA Dermatol. 2017; 153(8):743–744

[14] Hruza GJ. Mohs micrographic surgery local recurrences. J Dermatol Surg Oncol. 1994; 20(9):573–577

[15] Godsey T, Jacobson R, Gloster H , Jr. Large elliptical specimens and the single section method. Dermatol Surg. 2017; 43(9):1189–1191

[16] Randle HW, Zitelli J, Brodland DG, Roenigk RK. Histologic preparation for Mohs micrographic surgery. The single section method. J Dermatol Surg Oncol. 1993; 19(6):522–524

[17] Zabielinski M, Leithauser L, Godsey T, Gloster HM , Jr. Laboratory errors leading to nonmelanoma skin cancer recurrence after Mohs micrographic surgery. Dermatol Surg. 2015; 41(8):913–916

[18] Campbell T, Armstrong AW, Schupp CW, Barr K, Eisen DB. Surgeon error and slide quality during Mohs micrographic surgery: is there a relationship with tumor recurrence? J Am Acad Dermatol. 2013; 69 (1):105–111

[19] Macdonald J, Sneath JR, Cowan B, Zloty D. Tumor detection after inflammation or fibrosis on Mohs levels. Dermatol Surg. 2013; 39 (1, Pt 1):64–66

[20] Katz KH, Helm KF, Billingsley EM, Maloney ME. Dense inflammation does not mask residual primary basal cell carcinoma during Mohs micrographic surgery. J Am Acad Dermatol. 2001; 45(2):231–238

[21] Gephardt GN, Zarbo RJ. Extraneous tissue in surgical pathology: a College of American Pathologists Q-Probes study of 275 laboratories. Arch Pathol Lab Med. 1996; 120(11):1009–1014

[22] Launhardt A, Golda N, North J. Atypical adnexal tumors adjacent to basal cell carcinoma: a difficult problem in patients with Brooke-Spiegler syndrome undergoing Mohs surgery. Dermatol Surg. 2014; 40(3):354–357

[23] Stanoszek LM, Wang GY, Harms PW. Histologic mimics of basal cell carcinoma. Arch Pathol Lab Med. 2017; 141(11):1490–1502

[24] Karia PS, Jambusaria-Pahlajani A, Harrington DP, Murphy GF, Qureshi AA, Schmults CD. Evaluation of American Joint Committee on Cancer, International Union Against Cancer, and Brigham and Women's Hospital tumor staging for cutaneous squamous cell carcinoma. J Clin Oncol. 2014; 32(4):327–334

[25] Padgett JK, Parlette HL, III, English JC, III. A diagnosis of chronic lymphocytic leukemia prompted by cutaneous lymphocytic infiltrates present in Mohs micrographic surgery frozen sections. Dermatol Surg. 2003; 29(7):769–771

[26] Alcalay J. Mohs mapping in the cloud: an innovative method for mapping tissue in Mohs surgery. J Drugs Dermatol. 2015; 14(10): 1127–1130

[27] Tolkachjov SN. Utilization of topographical Mohs micrographic surgery maps for rapid review of clinicopathologic characteristics of nonmelanoma skin cancers of the ear. Dermatol Surg. 2018; 44 (1):25–30

[28] Patel SY, Itani K. Review of eyelid reconstruction techniques after Mohs surgery. Semin Plast Surg. 2018; 32(2):95–102

[29] Ogle CA, Shim EK, Godwin JA. Use of eye shields and eye lubricants among oculoplastic and Mohs surgeons: a survey. J Drugs Dermatol. 2009; 8(9):855–860

[30] Shih S, Khachemoune A. Use of eye shields for mohs micrographic surgery of the eyelids and periorbital area. Dermatol Surg. 2019; 45 (2): 210–215

[31] Condie D, Tolkachjov SN. Facial nerve injury and repair: a practical review for cutaneous surgery. Dermatol Surg. 2019; 45(3):340–357

[32] Chowdhry S, Seidenstricker L, Cooney DS, Hazani R, Wilhelmi BJ. Do not use epinephrine in digital blocks: myth or truth? Part II. A retrospective review of 1111 cases. Plast Reconstr Surg. 2010; 126 (6):2031–2034

[33] Vinycomb TI, Sahhar LJ. Comparison of local anesthetics for digital nerve blocks: a systematic review. J Hand Surg Am. 2014; 39(4): 744–751.e5

2 Facial Subunit Reconstructive Principles and General Considerations

Christopher J. Miller, Joseph F. Sobanko, Nicole Howe, Thuzar Shin, Jeremy R. Etzkorn, and H. William Higgins II

Abstract
Adhering to fundamental principles of surgical reconstruction and understanding tissue biomechanics are the keys to reliable reconstruction outcomes after Mohs micrographic surgery. Disregarding these fundamental principles leads to inconsistent outcomes or noticeable scars. This chapter will review guiding principles for facial reconstruction.

Keywords: reconstruction, design principles, tissue biomechanics, systematic wound assessment, flap, facial reconstruction

Capsule Summary and Pearls

This chapter will review fundamental principles of facial reconstruction design, tissue biomechanics, anatomy, and selection of reconstruction options.

- Fundamental principles of reconstructive design:
  - To preserve and restore free margins and contour.
  - To hide scars in cosmetic subunit junctions and relaxed skin tension lines.
  - To optimize skin color and texture match.
- Fundamental principles of tissue biomechanics:
  - Reconstructions to repair central facial defects favor tissue movement from lateral to medial locations.
  - Reconstructions to repair lateral facial defects favor tissue movement from inferior to superior locations.
  - Linear closures and sliding flaps have the greatest tension at the primary defect.
  - Transposition and interpolation flaps transfer the greatest tension away from the primary defect to the tissue donor site.
  - Ideal undermining planes vary with the anatomic location of the face and affect blood supply to flaps.
- Fundamental principles of anatomy:
  - Blood supply to the face comes from both the external and internal carotid systems. Incorporating vessels into flap pedicles can improve blood supply and flap survival.
  - The superficial musculoaponeurotic system (SMAS) protects the branches of the facial nerve.
- Fundamental principles to assess facial wounds and to select an ideal reconstruction:
  - Define the missing anatomic layers in a defect and replace them with similar tissue whenever possible.
  - Preserving free margins and contour is the top priority. Hiding scars in cosmetic subunit junction lines and relaxed skin tension lines and matching color and texture are secondary priorities.
  - If wound edges can be approximated without tension or distortion of anatomy, linear closure or sliding flaps are usually possible.
  - If approximating wound edges has high tension or distorts anatomy, transposition and interpolation flaps or skin grafts may be necessary.

2.1 Design Principles of Facial Reconstruction

2.1.1 Overview

We observe faces as we do highways: we disregard the expected; we notice the unexpected. Just as we ignore the characteristics of the highway until painted lines are altered or we encounter bumps or holes, we do not pay attention to facial scars unless they surprise us with unexpected lines or contours. The surgeon's job is to leave scars that blend into the background and restore the expected contours of the face. In descending order of importance, the fundamental principles of reconstructive design are to preserve and restore free margins and contour, to hide scars in cosmetic subunit junctions and relaxed skin tension lines (RSTLs), and to optimize color and texture match with imported tissue.

2.1.2 Free Margins

The eyelids, distal nose, lips, and helical rim are "free margins" because they are unsupported on one side. These structures define our appearance, as demonstrated by the prominence of free margins in a facial sketch (▶ Fig. 2.1). Preserving and restoring the free margins of

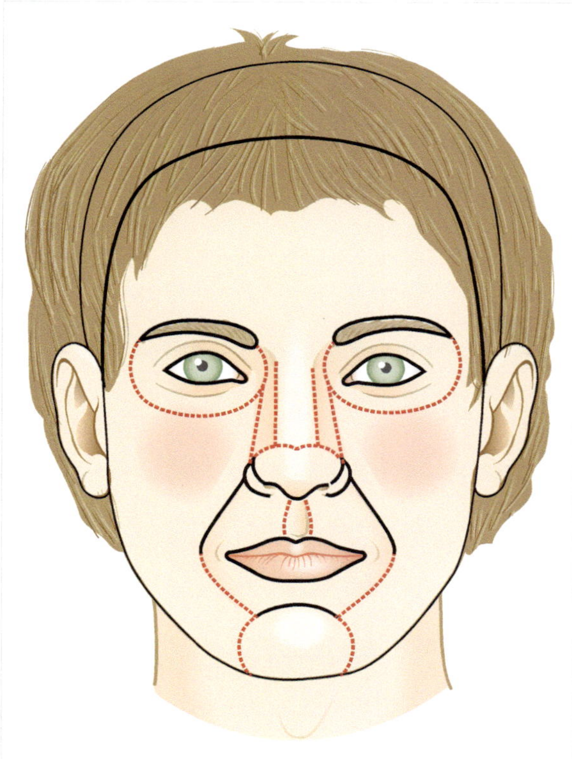

Fig. 2.1 Cosmetic subunits and free margins of the face.

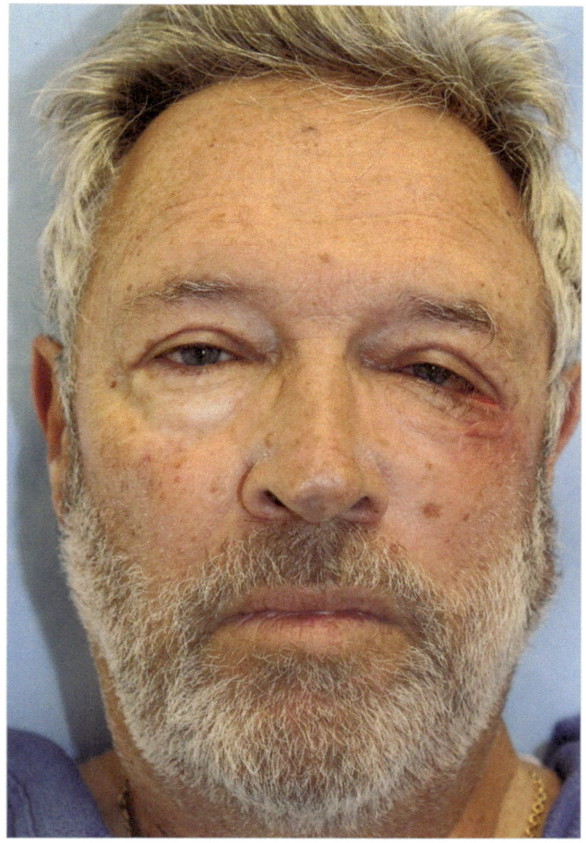

Fig. 2.2 Patient with lateral ectropion of the left eye due to contracted scar tissue from prior repair. Malposition of the free margin causes conspicuous changes in appearance.

the eyelids, the distal nose, the lips, and helical rim is a top priority during reconstructive surgery. Tension from reconstructive surgery or subsequent contraction from resulting scars can change the position of these delicate structures and create noticeable changes in contour and symmetry (▶ Fig. 2.2). Strategies to preserve free margin position include orienting tension vectors parallel to free margins, transferring tension to tissue reservoirs remote from free margins,[1] and tacking tissue to immobile deep structures so that dermal sutures near free margins are tension free.

2.1.3 Contour

Contour determines how light reflects off our faces. Concavities (alar groove, medial canthus, philtrum) cast shadows; convexities (zygoma, tip of nose) reflect shiny light; and planar surfaces (cheek, forehead) reflect a subtle, even light. Unnatural contours on the face are noticeable because they interrupt the expected play of light. Too much volume (e.g., thick forehead flap on the nasal tip), too little volume (e.g., a skin graft in a deep defect), or failure to recreate natural contours (e.g., flaps that ablate the alar groove) will draw attention to these aberrations in facial contour (▶ Fig. 2.3a–c). A top priority of reconstructive surgery is to recreate natural contours by filling wounds with tissue of similar surface area and thickness.

2.1.4 Cosmetic Subunit Junction Lines

Cosmetic subunit junction lines create natural shadows and reflections at transition zones between facial structures (▶ Fig. 2.1).[2,3] In complex cosmetic subunits such as the nose, further subdivisions are evident between the tip, dorsum, sidewalls, alae, and soft triangles.[4] For example, the alar groove separates the ala and nasal sidewall. Around the mouth, the vermilion cutaneous junction divides the shiny red vermilion from the hair-bearing skin of the cutaneous lip. The nasolabial fold separates the lip from the cheek. Intentionally placing scars in cosmetic subunit boundaries camouflages them within natural shadows and reflections (▶ Fig. 2.4). Wounds near the boundaries of cosmetic subunits may be expanded to hide scars in the junction lines (▶ Fig. 2.5, ▶ Fig. 2.6).

2.1.5 Relaxed Skin Tension Lines

RSTLs correspond to the wrinkles that form with animation of the underlying muscles of facial expression. RSTLs run perpendicular to the direction of the underlying muscle fibers. For example, contraction of the vertically

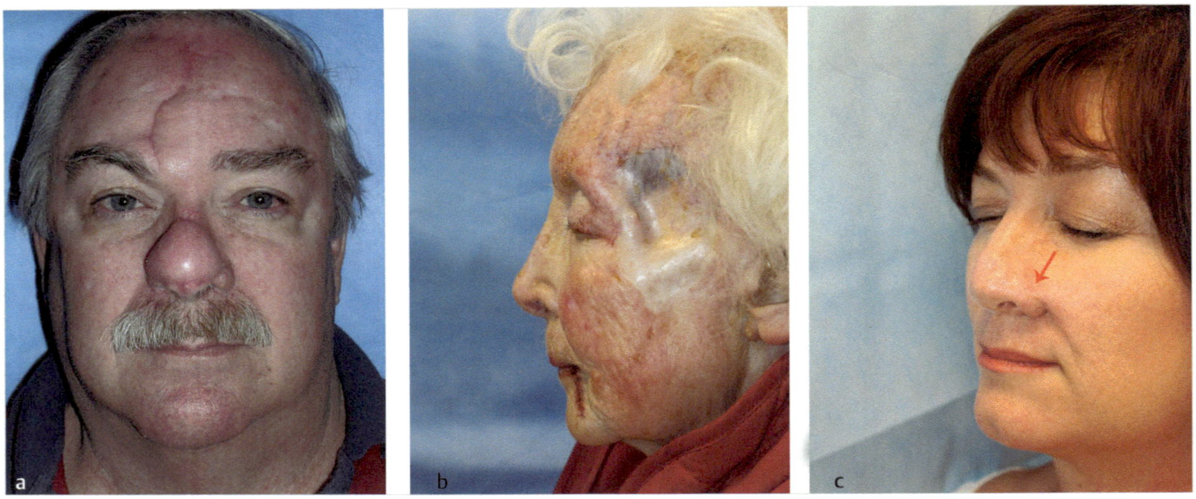

Fig. 2.3 **(a)** Unnatural light reflections draw attention to this bulky paramedian forehead flap. **(b)** This split-thickness skin graft is noticeable for both its white color and depressed contour. **(c)** A cheek advancement flap blunts the natural concavities of the nasofacial sulcus and alar groove.

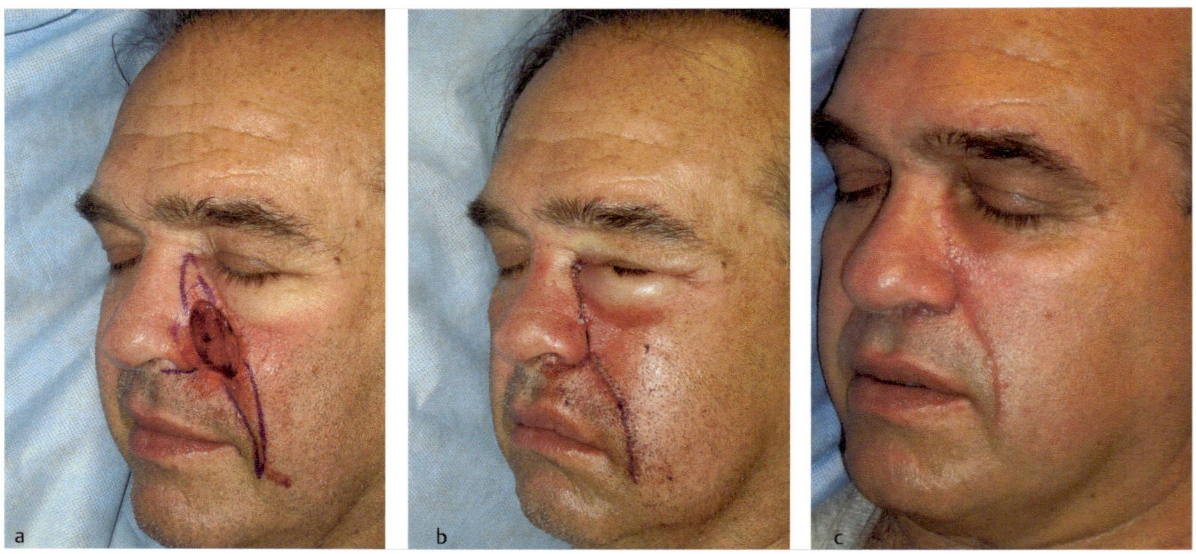

Fig. 2.4 **(a)** This defect resides along the cosmetic subunit junction lines that separate the cheek from the nose and mouth. **(b)** Appearance immediately after a linear repair that falls within the nasofacial sulcus and nasolabial fold. **(c)** Weeks after surgery, the pink scar is less conspicuous because it falls in the cosmetic subunit junction lines where a viewer expects to see lines or shadows.

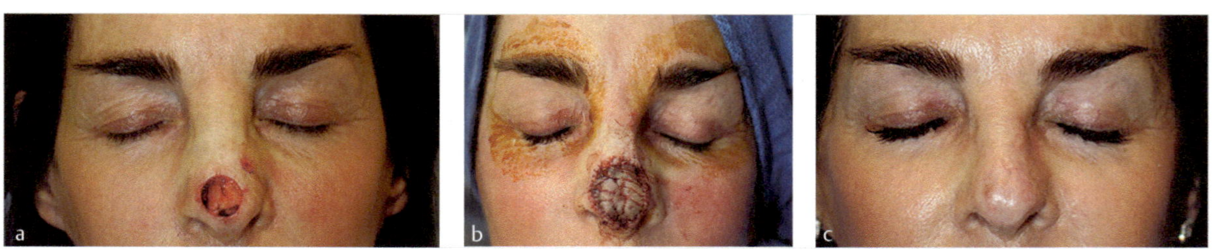

Fig. 2.5 **(a)** Tension from a local flap for this nasal tip defect risked distortion of the free margins. **(b)** The defect was expanded to the boundaries of the nasal tip subunit and repaired with a full-thickness skin graft. **(c)** The scars along the cosmetic subunit boundaries are inconspicuous and the free margins and contour are restored.

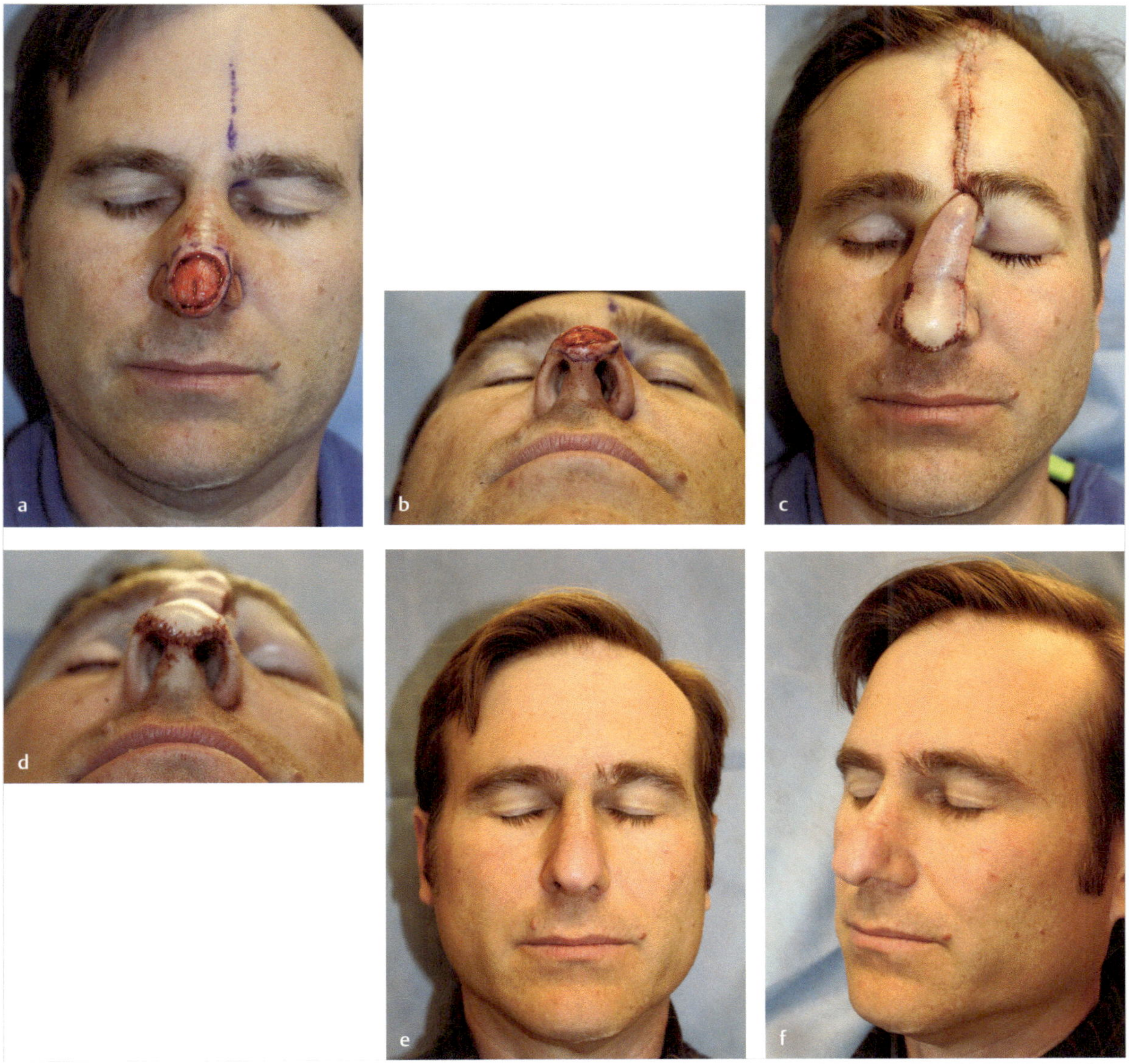

Fig. 2.6 (a,b) The defect was expanded to the purple markings so that the edges of the paramedian forehead flap conformed to the boundaries of the nasal tip subunit: frontal view. **(c,d)** Paramedian forehead flap repair. **(e,f)** Months after surgery, the scars at the cosmetic subunit junction lines are hard to notice.

oriented frontalis muscle fibers creates horizontal rhytids on the forehead and contractions of the circumferential orbicularis oculi and orbicularis oris muscles form rhytids that radiate perpendicularly from the free margins of eyelids and lips, respectively (▶ Fig. 2.7). As we age, these lines become more visible even without animation of facial muscles. Scars are less noticeable and have less tension when they align with RSTLs. However, placing scars in RSTLs should not violate higher priority reconstruction principles. For example, if a horizontal closure on the forehead would cause asymmetric lift of the eyebrow, it is better to perform a vertical closure that crosses RSTLs but preserves brow position.

2.1.6 Color and Texture

Mismatches in color and texture can make scars noticeable, a common outcome with skin grafts (▶ Fig. 2.3b, ▶ Fig. 2.8). Linear closures and local flaps are preferred, because they recruit adjacent skin of similar color and texture. Mismatches in the density of hair and sebaceous glands can still occur with local flaps (▶ Fig. 2.9), especially if terminal hairs are transposed to areas normally containing vellus hairs. Replacement of specialty skin, such as the vermilion lip or eyelid margin, may not be possible. When it is impossible to avoid color and texture mismatches, conforming to higher priority reconstruction

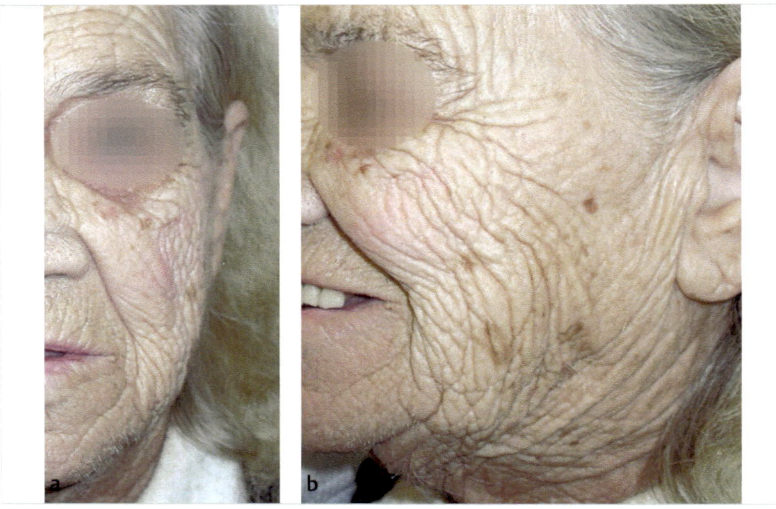

Fig. 2.7 (a, b) Periorbital and perioral lines.

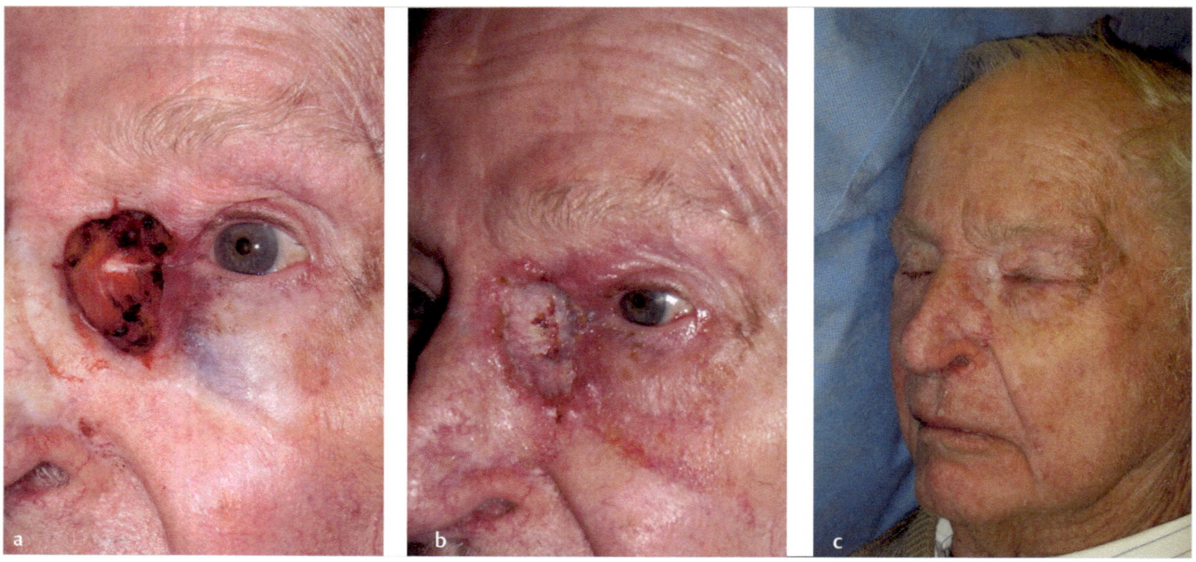

Fig. 2.8 (a) Large defect of the left medial canthus. (b) Healing skin graft. (c) While there is good anatomical position of the eyelids, there is noticeable mismatch in color of the graft in comparison to the surrounding skin.

principles (free margins, contour, cosmetic subunit junction lines, RSTLs) often makes these differences acceptable (▶ Fig. 2.9).

2.2 Principles of Tissue Biomechanics

2.2.1 Overview

Surgical reconstruction moves tissue from one area to another along preferred vectors on the face. Basic principles guide tissue movement, and understanding the preferred vectors for tissue movement can make the difference between a high- and a low-tension reconstruction. The location of the defect and tension vectors relative to the primary defect will dictate reconstruction design. Undermining in an efficient tissue plane can also facilitate skin movement.

2.2.2 Preferred Vectors to Move Facial Tissue

The direction in which a skin flap slides toward the defect is called the primary tissue motion, and the countermovement of the surrounding tissue to meet the flap is considered secondary tissue motion. Facial skin moves along preferred vectors (▶ Fig. 2.10).

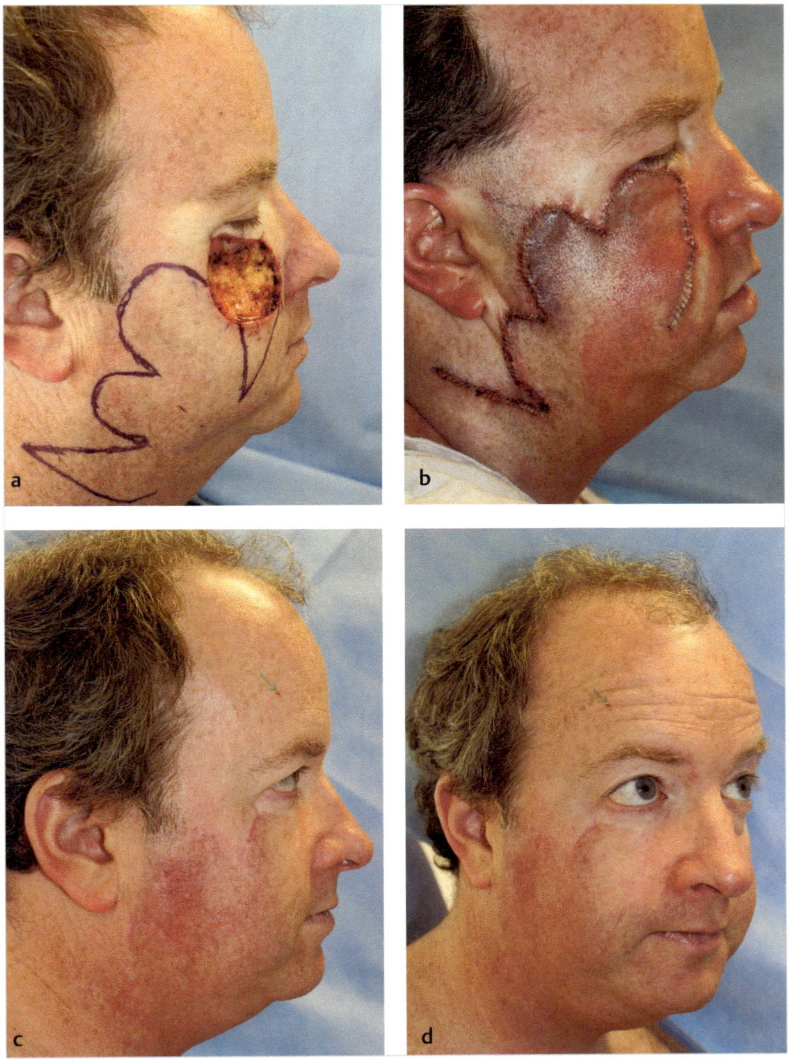

Fig. 2.9 (a) Large Mohs defect on the right infraorbital cheek. (b) Trilobed flap sutured in place. (c,d) Well-healed flap with excellent restoration of contour and no pull on the ipsilateral lower lid. While incision lines are fine, note that the flap is more conspicuous given terminal hair follicles were transposed to an area of normally vellus hair–bearing skin.

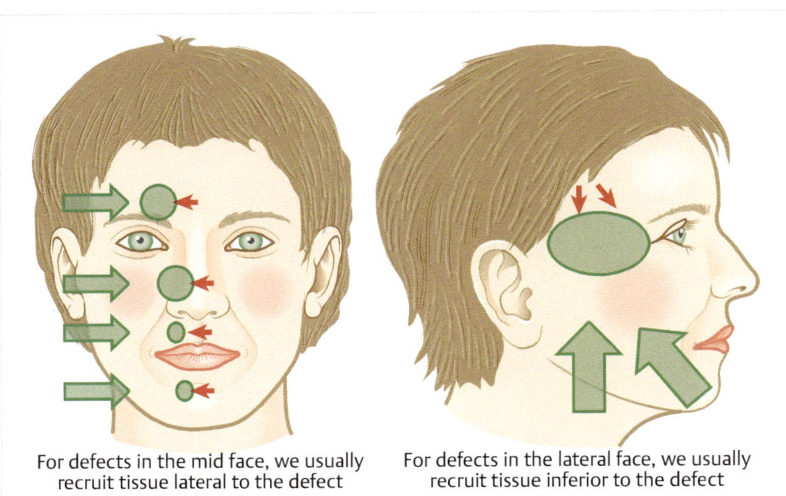

Fig. 2.10 Preferred vectors along which skin flaps move on the lateral and central face.

To repair defects of the central face (mid-forehead, glabella, nose, lips, chin), the primary tissue motion occurs along a medial or superomedial vector that recruits skin from the lateral cheek or jowl toward the midline. The horizontal/medial vector parallels the free margins of the eyelids, distal nose, and lips, and helps preserve their position.

To repair defects of the lateral face (lateral forehead, temples, lateral cheek), the primary tissue motion occurs along a superior or superolateral vector that moves skin from the neck and jowl to more superior locations on the face. The superior vector has minimal impact on the contours of the central face. In general, facial reconstructions are most successful when the primary tissue motion follows these vectors.

2.2.3 How Different Reconstructions Affect Location of Tension Relative to the Primary Defect

Primary closures and sliding flaps (i.e., advancement and rotation) recruit skin immediately adjacent to the wound and maintain greatest tension at the primary defect. When tension at the primary defect is too great for direct closure or if tension will distort anatomy, then transposition (e.g., rhombic, bilobed, and trilobed flaps) and interpolation flaps (e.g., paramedian forehead flap and nasolabial interpolation flap) or grafts may be necessary. These flaps transfer tension to a remote donor site so that tissue can be inset at the primary defect with minimal tension. Whether tension is at the primary defect or a remote donor site, all of these reconstruction options work best when the main tension falls along preferred vectors (lateral to medial in the midface and inferior to superior on the lateral face; ▶ Fig. 2.10).

2.2.4 Tissue Planes for Undermining and Elevating Flaps

Most local reconstructions of the face require undermining to mobilize tissue. Undermining releases either the skin edges or flap from underlying attachments to gain mobility.

The ideal surgical plane for facial undermining varies based on the location (▶ Table 2.1). If the surgeon is working in an efficient surgical plane, flap elevation and undermining should occur with ease and minimal bleeding. Undue resistance or excessive bleeding while lifting tissue usually signifies an inefficient anatomic plane (e.g., most commonly splitting the subcutaneous fat, rather than working at the junction of the fat and fascia).

On the lateral face, the ideal plane to elevate flaps or undermine tissue is at the junction of the subcutaneous fat and fascia of the superficial musculoaponeurotic system (SMAS) (▶ Fig. 2.11). This plane preserves the branches of the facial nerve, which lie deep to the SMAS. On the central face, excising deep to the muscles of facial expression/SMAS poses minimal risk for motor deficits. The most common surgical plane on the nose and central forehead is deep to the SMAS (▶ Fig. 2.12). For smaller procedures in the central face, the surgeon may choose a surgical plane superficial to the SMAS, such as a small horizontal closure on the forehead or narrow linear closure on the cutaneous lip.

The vascular supply to a flap varies according to the anatomic plane and extent of undermining. Flaps elevated too superficially (e.g., immediately subdermal) may not have adequate blood supply.[5,6] To optimize blood supply, local flaps should contain at least the epidermis, dermis, and the tight columnar cells of subcutaneous fat immediately adherent to the dermis. Undermining deep to muscle or fascia improves flap blood supply but may increase morbidity, depending on the anatomic location of the surgery. For example, in the central face (e.g., nose and central forehead) and scalp, undermining deep to the muscles of facial expression or galea, respectively, is desirable in most cases. By contrast, on the lateral face, temple, and posterior triangle of the neck, undermining deep to the SMAS and investing fascia of the neck, respectively, can damage underlying motor nerves.

Undermining too widely can threaten a flap's blood supply or increase the risk for postoperative bleeding and hematoma.[7,8] In general, the surgeon should undermine

Table 2.1 Ideal surgical plane for facial undermining based on location

Anatomic location	Preferred anatomic plane	Comments/critical structures to consider
Lateral face and neck	Junction of the subcutaneous fat and superficial musculoaponeurotic system (SMAS)	The motor branches from the facial nerve always lie deep to the most superficial layer of SMAS.[a] Excision at the junction of the subcutaneous fat and SMAS will always protect the motor nerves.
Central one-third of the face and scalp	At the junction of subcutaneous fat and SMAS or deep to the muscles of the SMAS (central face) or galea (on scalp)	Because the branches of the facial nerve have arborized before reaching the central one-third of the face, excision deep to the SMAS is less likely to cause motor deficits (e.g., excision of midline and paramedian frontalis muscle does not leave motor deficit on the forehead). On the midline nose, forehead, and scalp, undermining deep to the SMAS is frequently desirable.

[a]In areas where the muscles of facial expression are layered, for example, lip depressors and elevators, the motor nerves innervate the deepest muscles from their superficial surface.
Abbreviation: SMAS, superficial musculoaponeurotic system.

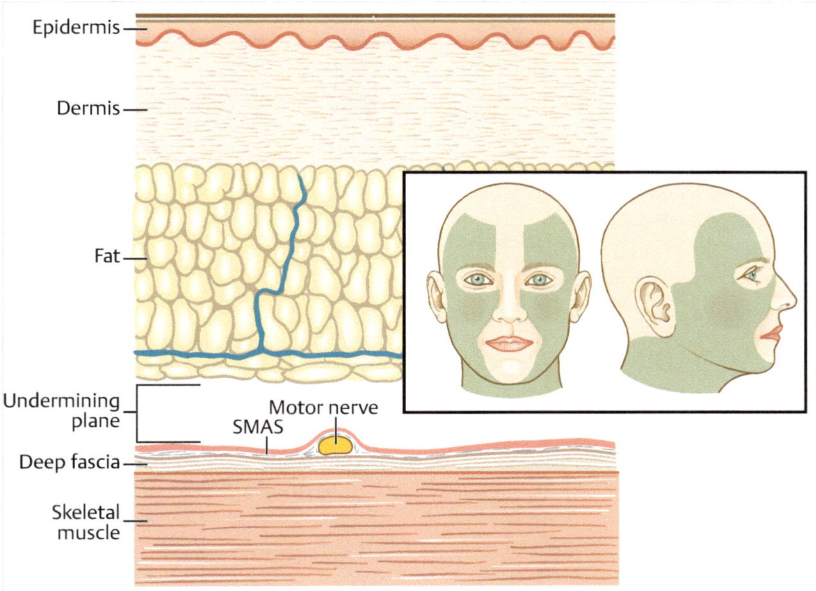

Fig. 2.11 The ideal plane for undermining on the lateral face is between the subcutaneous fat and fascia of the superficial musculoaponeurotic system. SMAS, superficial musculoaponeurotic system.

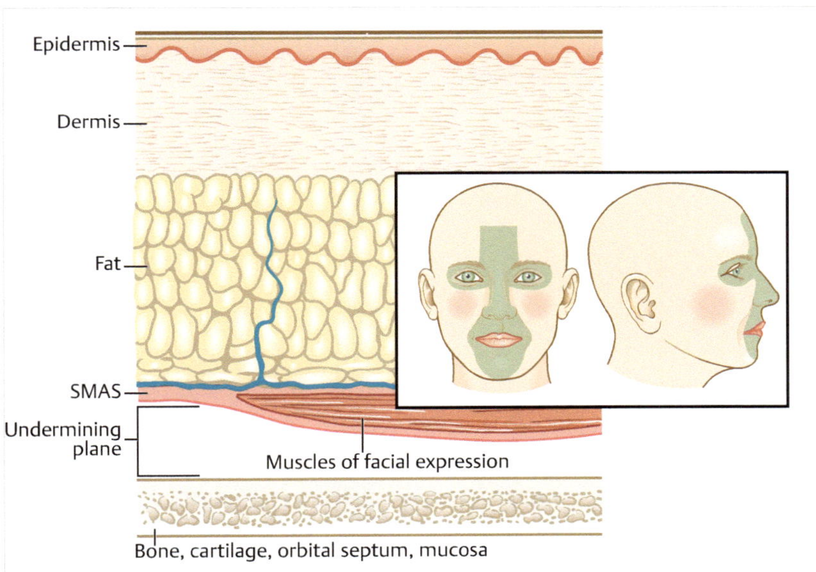

Fig. 2.12 The ideal plane for undermining on the central face is deep to the superficial musculoaponeurotic system and muscles. This minimizes risks of motor defects. SMAS, superficial musculoaponeurotic system.

just enough to move the flap into place. Frequent assessment of skin edge mobility helps avoid unnecessarily wide undermining. When the skin edges comfortably stretch to their desired target, additional undermining is rarely helpful or necessary.

2.3 Key Principles of Anatomy

2.3.1 Overview

A comprehensive discussion of facial anatomy is beyond the scope of this introductory chapter. A few guiding principles of facial anatomy are especially important for reconstruction. Understanding the blood supply of axial flaps helps ensure survival, as does a precise grasp of the depth of motor nerves in relation to facial musculature and the SMAS.

2.3.2 Blood Supply to the Face

Blood supply to the face comes from both the external and internal carotid systems. The external carotid artery and its branches supply blood to the lateral forehead, temple, cheek, ear, distal and lateral nose, and lips. The internal carotid artery and its branches supply blood to the mid-forehead, upper eyelid, and central nose. Linear closures, sliding flaps, and transposition flaps typically have a random-pattern blood supply from the subdermal plexus, so the proper plane of undermining (at least under the subdermal fat) is the most important factor for flap survival. By contrast, axial flaps contain named arteries in their pedicles (e.g., supratrochlear artery in the paramedian forehead flap and labial artery in the Abbé lip switch flap). Precise knowledge of anatomy is necessary to include the artery in the flap pedicle.

2.3.3 Superficial Musculoaponeurotic System

The SMAS is a term to describe the muscles of facial expression and fascia that envelope the face and protect the facial nerve branches. The SMAS is continuous with the platysma inferiorly and the galea aponeurotica and superficial temporal fascia superiorly.[9] The branches of the facial nerve are most vulnerable after they emerge from the parotid gland, because they are covered by only a thin layer of fascia until they innervate the central facial muscles from their lateral undersurface. The temporal and marginal mandibular branches are most vulnerable. Working in the tissue plane immediately superficial to the SMAS protects the facial nerve branches and is the most common plane to elevate tissue on the temple and the mandible.

2.4 Systematic Approach to Assessing Facial Wounds and Choosing Reconstruction

2.4.1 Overview

A systematic approach to assessing surgical defects helps conform to fundamental principles of surgical design and tissue biomechanics. Replacing "like with like" is a principle of reconstruction (e.g., if cartilage is missing, replace the cartilage).

2.4.2 Define What Is Missing

The first step to reconstructing facial defects is to define the missing anatomic layers. Reconstruction under local anesthesia is generally limited to soft-tissue defects that can range from superficial defects with loss of the superficial dermis to deep defects with loss of skin, muscle, and cartilage. In general, reconstructions should replace "like with like." For example, full-thickness skin grafts may be ideal for shallow defects with missing epidermis and dermis, but they rarely restore contour for defects involving cartilage or muscle. If defects include cartilage on the nose and ear, a free cartilage graft is usually necessary to prevent contraction of an overlying flap or graft.

In addition to replacing missing anatomic layers, donor sites ideally have skin of similar color, thickness, and density of hair and sebaceous glands. Flaps that contain hair will be conspicuous if they replace normally hairless skin (▶ Fig. 2.9). Cheek flaps with a generous layer of subcutaneous fat will look distended if they replace normally taut lip or nasal skin.

2.4.3 Prioritize Principles for Reconstruction Design

After examining the missing anatomic layers on the wound, consider the following questions to take inventory of the major principles of reconstruction. Does the wound involve a free margin? Could tension from the reconstruction push or pull on a free margin? What surface area and thickness of tissue do I need to restore contour, and will tension from the reconstruction change facial contour? Can I design a reconstruction that hides scars in cosmetic subunit junction lines or RSTLs? Can I cover the wound with skin of similar color and texture? Is terminal hair-bearing skin being moved into a normally vellus hair-bearing area?

2.4.4 Choose among Reconstruction Options

Assessing wound tension by pushing the edges of the defect centripetally (i.e., toward the center of the wound) determines if the wound edges can be approximated and demonstrates the impact of different tension vectors on adjacent free margins and contour. Observation of this simple test can help the surgeon choose the ideal reconstruction. If the wound edges can be pushed together, then reconstructions that maintain tension at the primary defect—linear closures and advancement and rotation flaps—are usually possible. If the wound edges cannot be pushed together because of excessive tension or if doing so would distort free margins and contour, then reconstructions that transfer tension to remote tissue reservoirs—transposition flaps and interpolation flaps—are ideal. If local tissue reservoirs have too much tension for a transposition flap, a staged interpolation flap, skin graft, or second intention healing may be necessary.

2.5 Reconstruction Options for Facial Reconstruction

2.5.1 Overview

This section will review fundamental principles of different reconstruction options on the face, including second intention healing, linear closure, grafts, and flaps.

2.5.2 Second Intention Healing

Second intention healing has two predictable outcomes: (1) the scar will have a shiny texture and (2) the scar will contract. Therefore, ideal wounds for second intention healing are located in areas where the skin normally has a shiny texture and where scar contraction will not cause anatomic distortion. Areas on the face where second intention scars have reasonable texture match include the scalp, upper forehead, ear, and nasal dorsum or proximal sidewall. By contrast, scars from second intention healing may contrast against the sebaceous skin of the nasal tip and ala or the hair-bearing skin of the cheek and lip. Scars from second intention healing may also hide in or recreate concave contours, such as the alar groove and medial canthus.[10] However, this strategy must be employed judiciously, since scar contraction may blunt the concavity.

Contraction of second intention wounds can change the position of nearby free margins and cause webbing of adjacent, loose skin, such as the ectropion of the eyelid. The likelihood of anatomic distortion and webbing of the scars is greater for deep wounds spanning the concave junction between cosmetic subunits. The ideal defect to minimize distortion from second intention healing is shallow and has surrounding stiff skin. Patients should expect evolving color and volume of the second intention scar. Scars that are initially pink and hypertrophic usually mature to a hypo- or hyperpigmented color with flatter contour.

2.5.3 Linear Closure

Linear closure is the side-to-side approximation of the edges of a fusiform wound. Tension lies along a single vector running perpendicular to the long axis of the fusiform wound and is greatest at the center of the wound. To avoid standing cones and to maintain normal contour, the ideal angles at the apices of a fusiform excision are greater than 30 degrees, which requires a length-to-width ratio of 3:1 or greater. In some anatomic locations, such as the nasal tip/columella, helical rim, or malar cheek, standing cones may need to be elongated to reduce tension and to maintain contour.

Primary linear closure is the most common reconstruction on the face. On the central face, primary linear closures are usually oriented with a vertical long axis so that the tension vector of the wound parallels the free margins of the face. Vertically oriented closures of the central face can still distort free margin position. When the curved lines of a fusiform excision are joined to form a straight line, the long axis of the fusiform excision elongates and can push up or down on adjacent free margins.[11] Linear closures can also compress the soft tissue of free margins, creating a fat lip or a bulky alar margin. On the lateral face, primary closures are usually oriented with a horizontal or diagonal long axis so that the primary tissue motion follows a vector from inferior to superior. The scars from primary closures on the lateral face often fall within RSTLs.

2.5.4 Skin Grafts

Skin grafts lack an intrinsic blood supply, so their survival depends on inosculation with the blood vessels of the wound bed. Grafts will not survive on devascularized wounds, such as forehead or scalp defects that lack periosteum or nasal tip defects without perichondrium. Full-thickness skin grafts (epidermis plus full-thickness of dermis) usually have better color and texture match because they retain hair follicles and eccrine glands. Split-thickness skin grafts (epidermis plus partial-thickness dermis) can cover larger wounds, but they usually have worse color and texture because they lack adnexal structures.

Skin grafts have sufficient volume to restore contour only for shallow wounds. Skin grafts covering deep wounds will result in depressed contour or a skeletonized appearance (▶ Fig. 2.3b). Full-thickness wounds of the alar margin, soft triangle, and columella may require composite grafts, which contain both skin and cartilage. Composite grafts have an especially high risk for failure, due to their high metabolic demand. As a result, composite grafting is usually limited to wounds less than a centimeter in diameter. The root of the helix is a common donor site for composite grafts.

Donor skin should match, as closely as possible, the color and texture of removed skin at the defect. Skin grafts usually are less conspicuous when they replace thin, nonsebaceous skin. By contrast, grafts are usually readily apparent on sebaceous or hair-bearing skin.

2.5.5 Sliding Flaps

Sliding flaps move adjacent skin directly into the defect, and the greatest tension lies at the primary defect. Examples include advancement flaps, V-Y island pedicle advancement flaps, and rotation flaps.

Advancement Flaps

Advancement flaps are useful for wounds that could be closed with a fusiform excision, except one of the standing cones would encroach on a free margin (e.g., eyelid, lip, distal nose, and helical rim) or cosmetic subunit junction (e.g., eyebrow, vermilion cutaneous junction, and alar groove; ▶ Fig. 2.13). Like fusiform closures, advancement flaps maintain tension along a single vector, but they displace one or both of the standing cones to preserve a free margin or hide the scar in a cosmetic subunit junction line or RSTL.

Common locations for advancement flaps are near free margins on the face, such as the upper and lower cutaneous lip, the nasal sidewall, the infraorbital cheek and lower eyelid, the forehead and temple, the preauricular cheek, and the helical rim. Advancement flaps are also useful for small paramedian nasal tip defects (e.g., East-West flap).[12] For defects of the midline face, the primary tissue motion of advancement flaps is usually lateral to medial so the tension vector parallels the free margins of

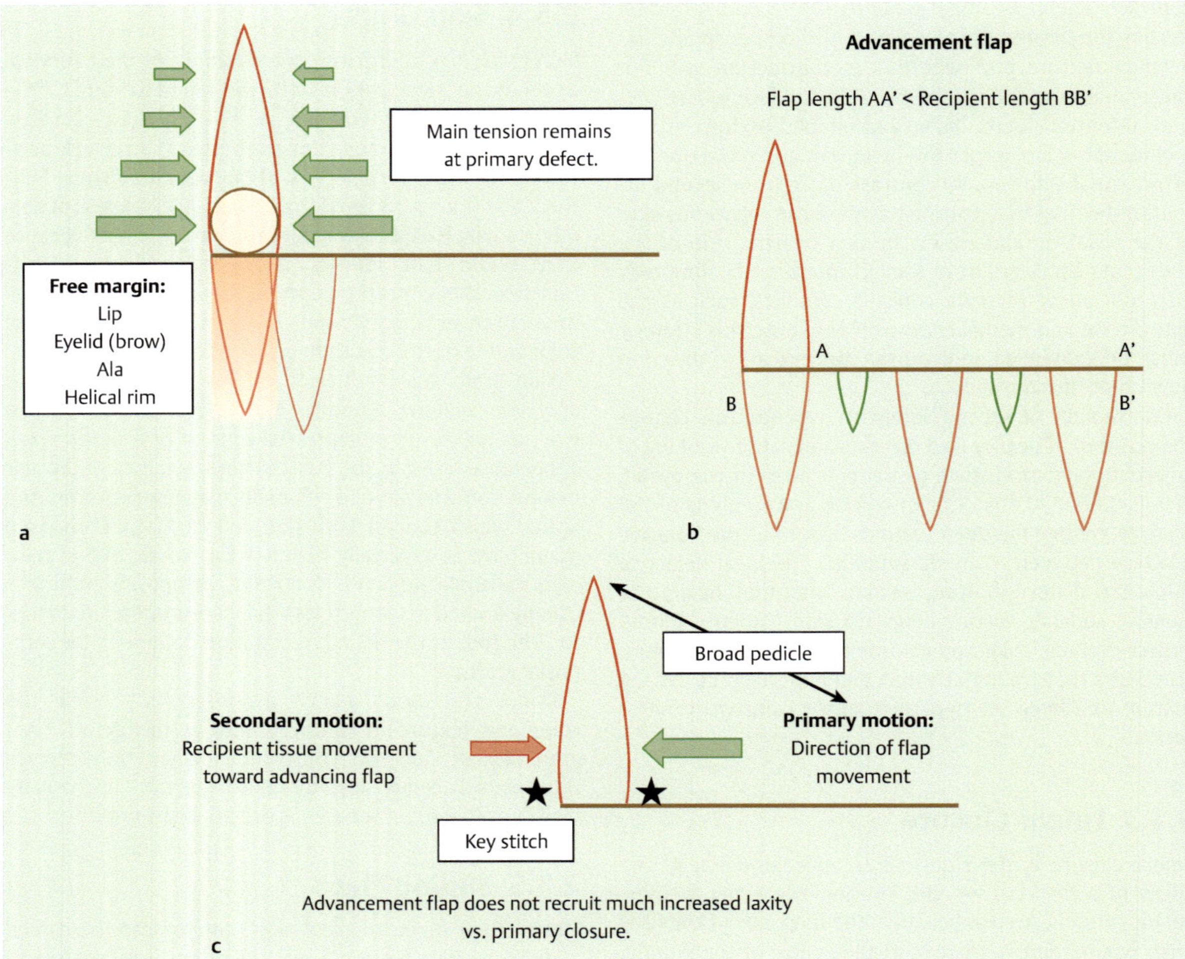

Fig. 2.13 (a–c) Key principles of an advancement flap.

the eyelids, nose, and lips. For defects of the lateral face, the primary motion is usually inferior to superior.

V-Y Island Pedicle Advancement Flaps

V-Y island pedicle advancement flaps differ from the other sliding flaps (i.e., advancement and rotation) in that their entire blood supply comes from the flap's undersurface. A triangular shaped flap is designed with its base at the edge of the defect. Incisions are made through the dermis of the two side limbs, creating the "island" that gives the flap its name. A key suture advances the leading edge of the flap toward the defect. The secondary defect at the trailing edge of the flap is closed primarily, resulting in a suture line that resembles a "Y."

V-Y island pedicle advancement flaps on the face are most commonly used to repair defects of the lateral upper cutaneous lip (▶ Fig. 2.14), nasal sidewall and alar groove, cheek, and brow.

Rotation Flaps

The hallmark of a rotation flap is the arciform incision used to mobilize the surrounding skin (▶ Fig. 2.15). Rotating the flap into the primary defect creates a secondary defect along the arciform incision. In contrast to the single tension vector of advancement flaps, rotation flaps distribute tension across multiple vectors along both the primary and secondary defects.

A simple test to choose between a rotation and an advancement flap is to push the wound edges together (▶ Fig. 2.16). If there is a clearly preferred tension vector at the primary wound but the standing cone of a linear closure would impinge on adjacent free margins, then an advancement flap will work. If there is no clearly dominant tension vector, but the wound edges nearly approximate by pushing in multiple directions, then a rotation flap may be ideal to distribute tension across multiple vectors at the primary defect. The scalp is a classic

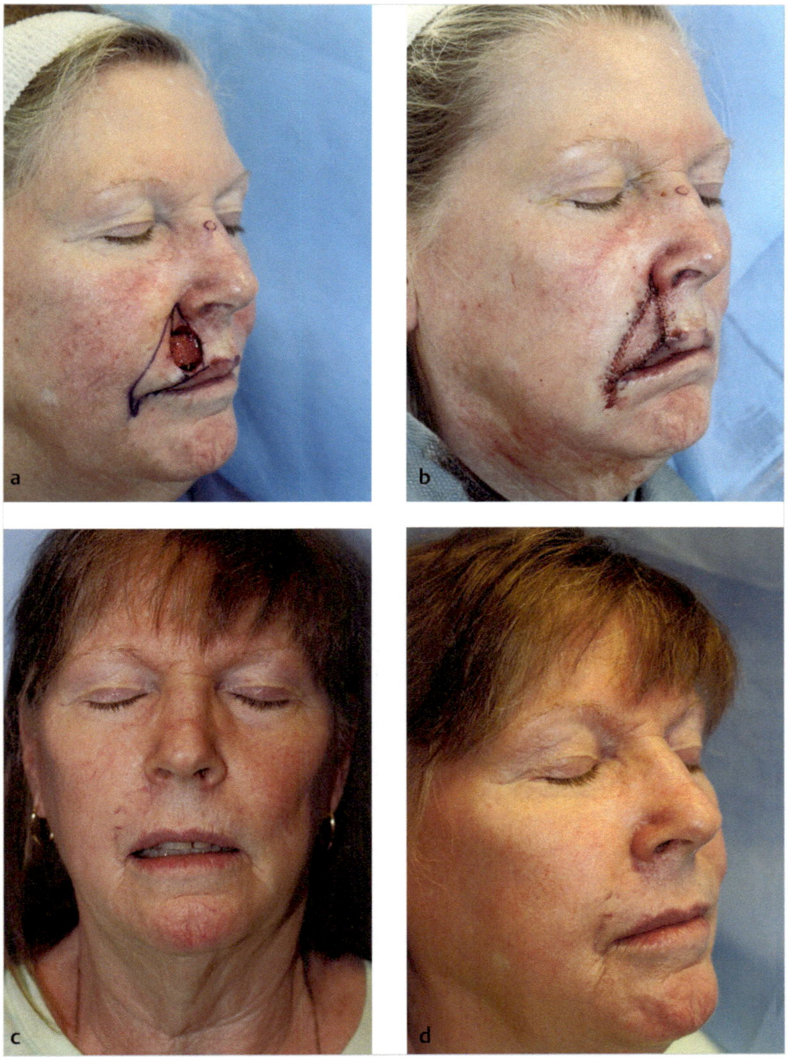

Fig. 2.14 **(a)** Mohs defect on the upper cutaneous lip. **(b)** V-Y advancement flap sutured in place. **(c,d)** Patient at follow-up with well-concealed incision lines along the nasolabial fold and vermilion border.

location for rotation flaps because wounds at this location often do not have a preferred tension vector.

Rotation flaps on the face are most commonly used to repair medial cheek defects that recruit skin from the lateral cheek and neck, lateral forehead defects that recruit from the temple, and nasal tip defects that recruit skin from the nasal sidewall and glabella.[13,14]

Transposition Flaps

If linear closure or use of sliding flaps would result in excessive tension or distortion of free margins (e.g., eyelids, distal nose, and lips), then a transposition flap may be useful to transfer tension to a more generous tissue reservoir. Three common transposition flaps include the rhombic or banner (single-lobed), bilobed, and trilobed flaps (▶ Fig. 2.17). As opposed to sliding flaps, which have the greatest tension at the primary defect, transposition flaps displace the greatest tension to the final donor site (i.e., secondary defect of a rhombic flap, tertiary defect of a bilobed flap, and quaternary defect of a trilobed flap). Closing the terminal donor site allows rotation of the flap into the primary defect with minimal tension. Adding lobes to transposition flaps recruits tissue from reservoirs increasingly remote from the primary defect and displaces tension to more favorable vectors.

Because they transfer key tension vectors away from the primary defect, transposition flaps are especially useful to repair facial defects near the free margins of the nose, eyelids, and lips.

Interpolation Flaps

Interpolation flaps transfer skin from remote reservoirs with a pedicle that bridges an isthmus of skin between the primary defect and the donor site. The flap pedicle remains intact until the ingrowth of blood vessels from the recipient site provides sufficient nourishment to the

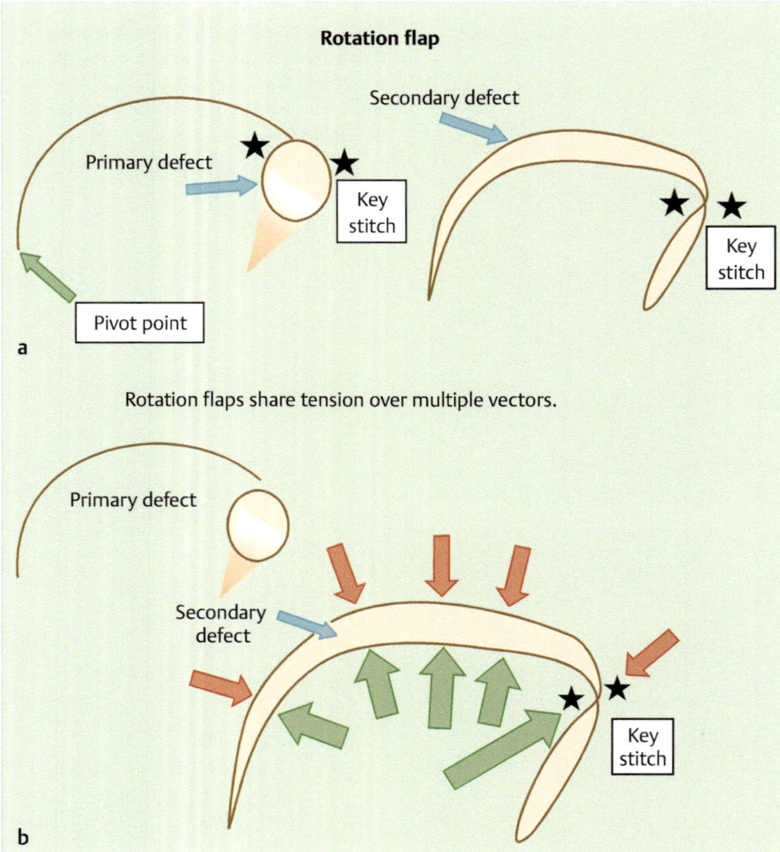

Fig. 2.15 (a, b) Key principles of a rotation flap.

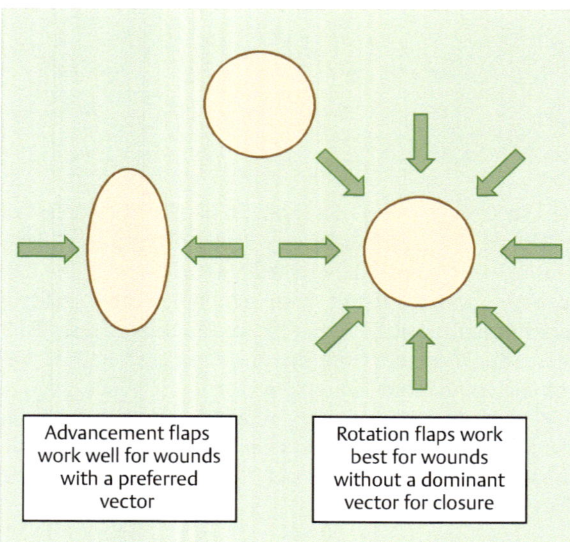

Fig. 2.16 Simple test for choosing between advancement and rotation flaps. Advancement flaps work well for wounds with preferred vectors. Rotation flaps work well for wounds without a dominant vector for closure.

transferred skin. The ingrowth of new vessels is usually reliable after approximately 3 weeks, at which time the pedicle can be divided during a second surgical procedure.

Interpolation flaps are ideal for defects at or near free margins of the face. The paramedian forehead flap[15] (▶ Fig. 2.6) and nasolabial interpolation flap repair distal nasal defects,[16] the retroauricular interpolation flap repairs helical rim defects,[17,18]; the Abbé flap repairs large defects of the lip margin[19]; and the Hughes and Cutler–Beard flaps repair defects of the eyelid margin.[20,21] All of these flaps transfer tension away from the primary defect and help preserve and restore free margins.

2.6 Conclusion

Fundamental principles of design and tissue biomechanics are the cornerstones of successful facial reconstruction. A systematic approach to assessing wounds can help choose reconstructions that adhere to these key principles.

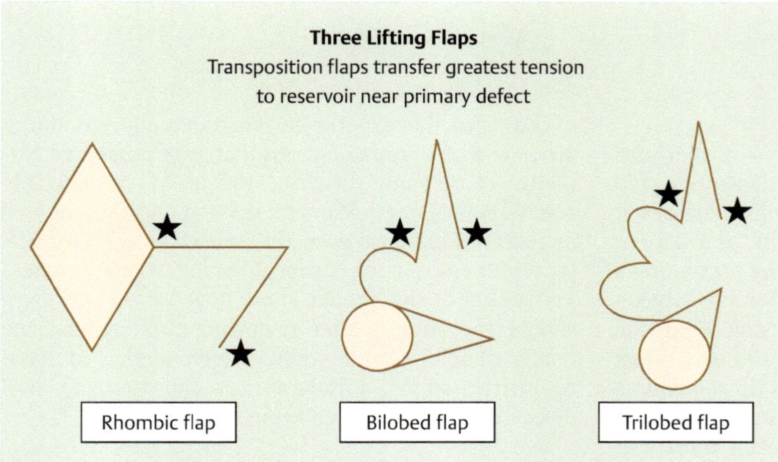

Fig. 2.17 Three common transposition flaps (rhombic, bilobed, and trilobed), all of which transfer greatest tension to reservoir near the primary defect. Stars represent closure of the key stitch.

References

[1] Miller CJ. Design principles for transposition flaps: the rhombic (single-lobed), bilobed, and trilobed flaps. Dermatol Surg. 2014; 40 Suppl 9:S43–S52

[2] Burget G. Discussion: reconstruction of the nasal soft triangle subunit. Plast Reconstr Surg. 2013; 131(5):1051–1054

[3] Burget GC. Aesthetic reconstruction of the tip of the nose. Dermatol Surg. 1995; 21(5):419–429

[4] Burget GC, Menick FJ. The subunit principle in nasal reconstruction. Plast Reconstr Surg. 1985; 76(2):239–247

[5] Pearl RM, Johnson D. The vascular supply to the skin: an anatomical and physiological reappraisal: part II. Ann Plast Surg. 1983; 11 (3):196–205

[6] Pearl RM, Johnson D. The vascular supply to the skin: an anatomical and physiological reappraisal: part I. Ann Plast Surg. 1983; 11(2): 99–105

[7] Cutting C. Critical closing and perfusion pressures in flap survival. Ann Plast Surg. 1982; 9(6):524

[8] Cutting C, Ballantyne D, Shaw W, Converse JM. Critical closing pressure, local perfusion pressure, and the failing skin flap. Ann Plast Surg. 1982; 8(6):504–509

[9] Ghassemi A, Prescher A, Riediger D, Axer H. Anatomy of the SMAS revisited. Aesthetic Plast Surg. 2003; 27(4):258–264

[10] Zitelli JA. Wound healing by secondary intention. A cosmetic appraisal. J Am Acad Dermatol. 1983; 9(3):407–415

[11] Etzkorn JR, Sobanko JF, Miller CJ. Free margin distortion with fusiform closures: the apical angle relationship. Dermatol Surg. 2014; 40 (12):1428–1432

[12] Geist DE, Maloney ME. The "east-west" advancement flap for nasal defects: reexamined and extended. Dermatol Surg. 2012; 38(9): 1529–1534

[13] Rigg BM. The dorsal nasal flap. Plast Reconstr Surg. 1973; 52(4): 361–364

[14] Zimbler MS, Thomas JR. The dorsal nasal flap revisited: aesthetic refinements in nasal reconstruction. Arch Facial Plast Surg. 2000; 2 (4):285–286

[15] Brodland DG. Paramedian forehead flap reconstruction for nasal defects. Dermatol Surg. 2005; 31(8, Pt 2):1046–1052

[16] Fader DJ, Baker SR, Johnson TM. The staged cheek-to-nose interpolation flap for reconstruction of the nasal alar rim/lobule. J Am Acad Dermatol. 1997; 37(4):614–619

[17] Nguyen TH. Staged cheek-to-nose and auricular interpolation flaps. Dermatol Surg. 2005; 31(8, Pt 2):1034–1045

[18] Johnson TM, Fader DJ. The staged retroauricular to auricular direct pedicle (interpolation) flap for helical ear reconstruction. J Am Acad Dermatol. 1997; 37(6):975–978

[19] Millard DR , Jr, McLaughlin CA. Abbe flap on mucosal pedicle. Ann Plast Surg. 1979; 3(6):544–548

[20] McNab AA, Martin P, Benger R, O'Donnell B, Kourt G. A prospective randomized study comparing division of the pedicle of modified hughes flaps at two or four weeks. Ophthal Plast Reconstr Surg. 2001; 17(5):317–319

[21] Fischer T, Noever G, Langer M, Kammer E. Experience in upper eyelid reconstruction with the Cutler-Beard technique. Ann Plast Surg. 2001; 47(3):338–342

3 Nose

Evan Stiegel and John Zitelli

Abstract

Mastering nasal reconstruction requires a thorough understanding of nasal anatomy, flap dynamics, and proficiency with repair options depending on defect location, skin type and nasal topography, and patient expectations. Herein, the authors begin by presenting a review of nasal anatomy, a prerequisite for any surgeon endeavoring to master nasal reconstruction. Next, the authors review repair options according to each nasal cosmetic subunit, starting with the nasal tip and ending with the nasal sidewall. While innumerable repair options exist for each particular nasal defect, those that are presented are the result of the senior author's trove of reconstructive experience, which has allowed him to arrive at a set of repair options that, when executed correctly, consistently produce the most reproducible results. Finally, the authors review complications as well as revisions, because even the best reconstructive surgeon will encounter occasional complications despite a perfect effort and should know how to manage these should they occur. After reviewing this chapter, the reader should have a sound understanding of nasal reconstruction and a framework to approach any nasal defect he or she should encounter.

Keywords: nasal reconstruction, flap, graft, nose

Capsule Summary and Pearls

- Superficial defects on any nasal location can have an excellent aesthetic outcome when allowed to heal by second intention, especially when augmented by the use of the "shave and sand" technique.
- Deeper defects on concave areas like the alar crease and nasal root/inner canthus can also achieve good results when left to heal.
- While full-thickness skin grafts are a remarkably versatile option for range of defects on the nose, defect size, depth, neighboring skin quality, and patient preference dictate when their use is most appropriate. The conchal bowl provides the best match for wounds of the lower third of the nose, whereas postauricular skin is favored for wounds on the upper two-thirds.
- Primary closure is an outstanding option for small to medium midline wounds on the nasal tip and dorsum, though several modifications of the classic fusiform closure must be employed to attain an optimal result.
- Local transposition flaps are the most reliable repair options for full-thickness defects on the nose not amenable to primary closure.
- The bilobed transposition flap is the preeminent flap choice for small to medium full-thickness defects on the lower third of the nose, especially the tip, whereas the rhombic flap is preferred for the upper two-thirds.
- The forehead flap is the ideal choice for larger defects of the nasal tip and ala, especially when used in conjunction with cartilage grafts in the cases where functional integrity of the nose is compromised.
- For full-thickness perforating defects, all three nasal layers including skin, cartilaginous or fibrofatty structural support, and nasal lining must be repaired in order to thwart damaging aesthetic and functional repercussions.
- Before and during repair, nasal valve competency should be assessed and restored as needed.
- In order to decrease risk of pincushioning, wide undermining to promote formation of a platelike scar, aggressive flap defatting, and use of buried vertical mattress sutures to pull deep tissues back to suture line are required.
- At the time of surgery, patients should be informed of their need to return in 3 months for potential dermabrasion in order to correct any visible incision lines or contour asymmetry.

3.1 Introduction

Repairing the nose poses one of the greatest challenges for the reconstructive surgeon. The combination of the nose's complex topography, unique sebaceous texture, minimal laxity, and freely mobile free margins requires a mastery of the skills necessary to repair this complex structure. The nose plays a pivotal role aesthetically as the centerpiece of the face while also having a significant role in respiration. Thus, a poor reconstructive effort may have both cosmetic and functional repercussions for the patient. Approaching nasal defects algorithmically based on size, skin type, and location can assist in selecting the most appropriate repair option for a given patient. However, because noses drastically differ among patients, one should simply not apply a "cookie cutter" approach to nasal reconstruction. The surgeon must therefore address each nasal defect individually when selecting the optimal repair option for a particular patient.

While innumerable methods to repair a particular defect on each nasal subunit have been published, in our experience, there are a limited a number of reliable repair options for each subunit that routinely achieve high-quality results. Herein, following a review of nasal anatomy, we discuss the various repair options that we believe consistently provide superb results for patients.

3.2 Anatomy

Possessing a thorough understanding of nasal anatomy is essential to achieve operative success and avoid complications. The unique nasal topography, an elegant synthesis of convexities, concavities, inflections, and grooves, allows its division into aesthetic subunits. These aesthetic subunits include the tip, dorsum, sidewalls, alar lobules, and soft triangles.[1] It has been advocated that superior results are achieved when skin within an aesthetic subunit is repaired with like skin possessing similar texture and color. However, many flaps on the nose that do not adhere to the subunit principle will still accomplish highly aesthetic results. A quintessential example is the bilobed flap, which uses lax donor skin from the upper sidewall to repair defects on the tip. Furthermore, many, especially in plastic surgery literature, advocate resurfacing an entire subunit even at the expense of enlarging a defect. While the authors will often employ this technique for larger staged flaps, excellent outcomes can still be attained without sacrificing more skin. Similarly, while the borders of aesthetic subunits are theoretically an ideal place for scar placement, scars placed elsewhere with the intention of preventing distortion should be a preferred goal.

The nose can be thought of as a three-layered structure consisting of skin, cartilage or fibrofatty tissue, and a mucosal lining. The nasal lining consists of a thin layer of vascular mucosa that is tightly adherent to overlying cartilage and bone. Failure to repair the mucosal portion of a full-thickness perforating nasal defect can have grim complications including flap contraction, nasal distortion, and airway obstruction.

The majority of the nasal "skeleton" consists of cartilage with a small bony base comprising the most proximal aspect (▶ Fig. 3.1). This bony base is formed by two symmetric nasal bones, which correspond with the nasal bridge. The nasal bones are bordered superiorly by the skull's frontal bone at an intersection point termed the nasion (corresponding to the nasal root on the skin's surface) and are bordered laterally by the frontal processes of the maxilla. After extending anteriorly and inferiorly, the nasal bone attaches to the septal cartilage, which continues to extend in an anterior and inferior direction to form the spine of the nose. The upper lateral cartilage projects laterally from the nasal septum to form the overlying nasal sidewall. Inferiorly, the lower nose is reinforced bilaterally by the lower lateral cartilages. Each lower lateral cartilage possesses both a lateral crus, which supports the nasal tip and medial ala, and a medial crus, which supports the nasal columella. Importantly, while the bulk of the nasal ala is not supported directly by cartilage, the rigid quality of its unique fibrofatty tissue allows it to resist collapse upon inspiration. The nasalis muscle extends superiorly and medially from the maxilla and is responsible for flaring the nostrils. Its incorporation into various flaps on the nose allows for excellent flap viability.

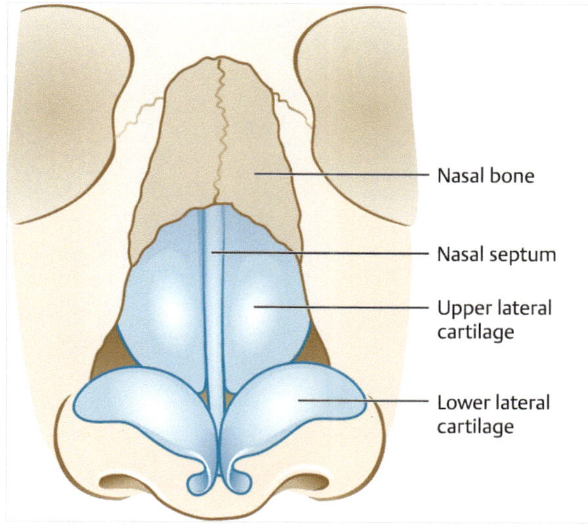

Fig. 3.1 Cartilage and bony "skeleton" of the nose.

When executing a nasal flap or graft, an understanding of the zones of skin thickness is critical when selecting ideal donor skin (▶ Fig. 3.2). The skin on the upper half of the nose (zone I) is thin, shiny, nonsebaceous, and relatively lax. On the tip, supratip, ala, and lower sidewall, skin tends to be significantly thicker, more sebaceous, and rigid (zone II). Moving caudally down the nose, starting at the infratip and continuing onto the soft triangles and columella, the skin transitions back to being thin and nonsebaceous (zone III), similar to that of the upper nose. While it is important to understand the zones of the nose conceptually, the size of each zone on a particular patient may vary. Likewise, the degree of sebaceous composition and size of the various nasal cartilages account for the heterogeneity of nasal shapes and sizes that exist among patients.

The nose has a rich vascular system, owing to a blood supply that comes from branches of both the external and internal carotid artery systems with extensive anastomoses (▶ Fig. 3.3). At the level of the lateral lip, the facial artery (external carotid system) gives off its two terminal branches: the superior labial artery and the angular artery. After coursing medially along the upper lip, the superior labial artery gives off septal branches to

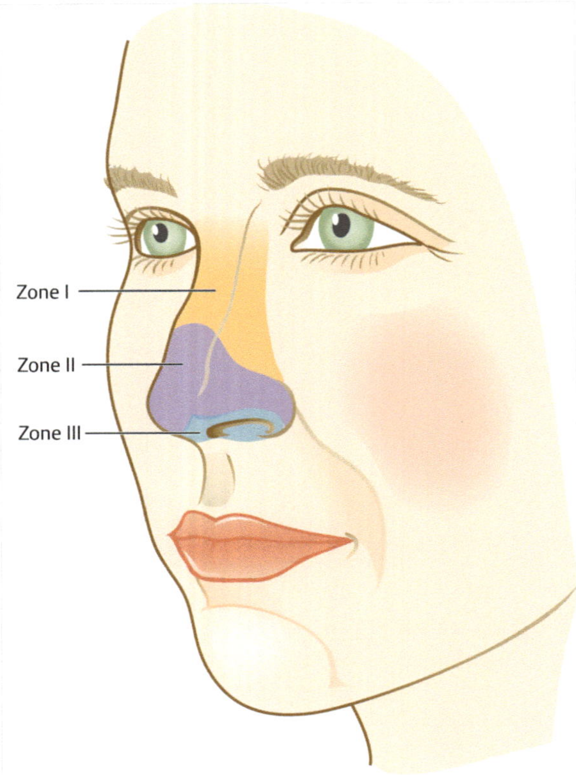

Fig. 3.2 Zones of the nose used to describe areas of the nose with similar skin thickness and sebaceous quality.

supply the anterior portion of the nasal septum and ultimately a branch that supplies the columella. In its upward course, the angular artery gives off the lateral nasal artery and provides blood supply to the lateral portion of the lower one-third of the nose. The external nasal branch of the anterior ethmoidal artery is a branch of the ophthalmic artery (internal carotid system) and provides part of the blood supply to the nasal tip. The dorsal nasal artery branches off the ophthalmic artery and pierces through the orbital septum superior to the medial canthal ligament supplying a large portion of the upper sidewall and dorsum. The nose's extensive vascular network allows for excellent viability of both flaps and grafts.

The sensory input to the nose stems from the ophthalmic (V1) and maxillary (V2) branches of the trigeminal nerve. The ophthalmic nerve gives off the supratrochlear, infratrochlear, and external nasal nerves, which supply the skin of the root, upper sidewall, dorsum, and tip. The infraorbital branch of the maxillary nerve gives sensory supply to the caudal nasal sidewall and nasal alae. The nose contains no major motor nerves; however, transection of some of the aforementioned sensory nerve branches may result in anesthesia that is likely to resolve over the course of a year. Nerve blocks are infrequently used on the nose.

A review of nasal anatomy would be incomplete without mention of the internal nasal valve. The valve is the narrowest part of the nasal airway and the area of greatest resistance. It is formed by the caudal border of the upper lateral cartilage, the nasal septum, the nasal sidewall, and the inferior turbinate. Because the nasal sidewall is the most mobile border, cancer extirpation or repairs involving the sidewall adjacent to the alar groove can risk collapse of the valve, resulting in impaired airflow during inspiration. Therefore, it is essential to assess patency of the valve prior to repair to determine whether correction is necessary. In the remainder of this chapter, we will review our approach to nasal reconstruction, describing various repair options for each nasal subunit.

3.3 Nasal Tip

Due to the immobility of the thick sebaceous nasal tip skin, even minimal tissue movement can lead to distortion. Therefore, a precise reconstructive plan is vital. Second intention healing, primary closure, flaps, and grafts are all reconstructive options for the nasal tip, depending on the nature of the defect.

3.3.1 Second Intention Healing

In patients with highly sebaceous skin, superficial defects anywhere on the nose are amenable to healing by second intention (▶ Fig. 3.4).[2] Aesthetic results when utilizing alternative reconstructive approaches can be unpredictable, as healed surgical incisions are particularly prone to postoperative scar depression on highly sebaceous skin.

While many defects can heal by second intention with no additional intervention, a "shave and sand" technique can often be employed to enhance results (▶ Video 3.1). This technique can be performed immediately postoperatively or delayed and is particularly useful for superficial defects with abrupt edges. Using a scalpel blade placed horizontally on the skin immediately adjacent to the defect, light pressure is applied removing thin shavings skin in order to blend the transition between the defect and its surrounding skin. To further camouflage the surgical site, coarse 80-grit sterile aluminum oxide sandpaper is then rubbed over the whole subunit until fine pinpoint bleeding is observed. We describe this technique to patients by comparing it to sanding a scratch on wood furniture. While this method typically yields excellent cosmetic results in those with highly sebaceous skin, very rarely patients may develop increased pore size and/or hypopigmentation. In the editors' experience, a manual dermabrasion apparatus may also be used with a diamond fraise for younger or nonsebaceous skin and a wire brush for thick sebaceous and rhinophymatous skin. In patients with nonsebaceous skin, surgical repair consistently yields superior results and is our favored approach, unless a defect is exceptionally thin.

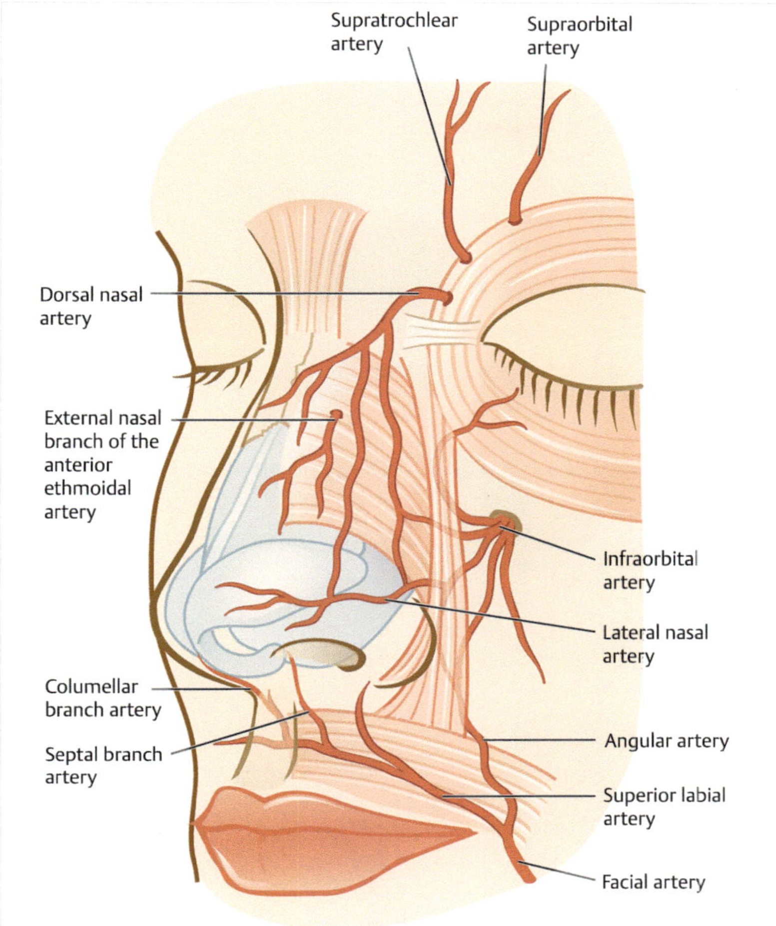

Fig. 3.3 Arterial supply of the nose.

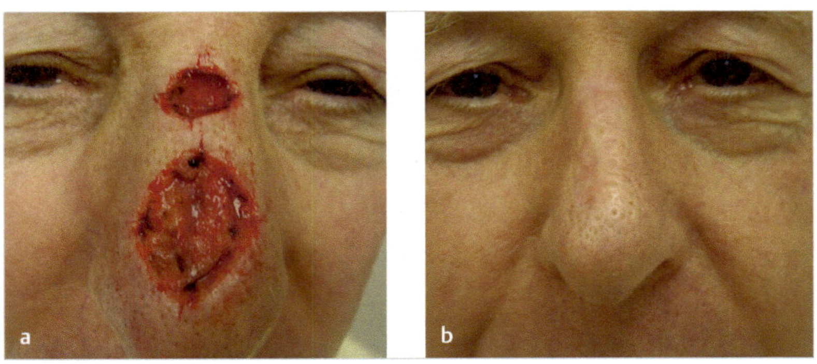

Fig. 3.4 **(a)** Superficial defects on the nose of a 68-year-old man with a sebaceous nose. **(b)** Results at 3 months when wounds were allowed to heal by second intention.

3.3.2 Primary Closure

Primary repair on the nasal tip should be reserved for small to medium-sized midline defects (▶ Fig. 3.5).

Design

There are several important points in designing and executing a successful fusiform closure on the nose.[3] When designing the repair, at least a 5:1 length-to-width ratio is employed with the apices ending above the bony hump of the nasal dorsum (where the nasal bone connects to cartilage) and below the inferior margin of the nasal tip about the infratip or columella. Using standard 3:1 length-to-width ratio design may increase closure tensions and result in prominent standing cutaneous deformities, significantly distorting the nasal profile.

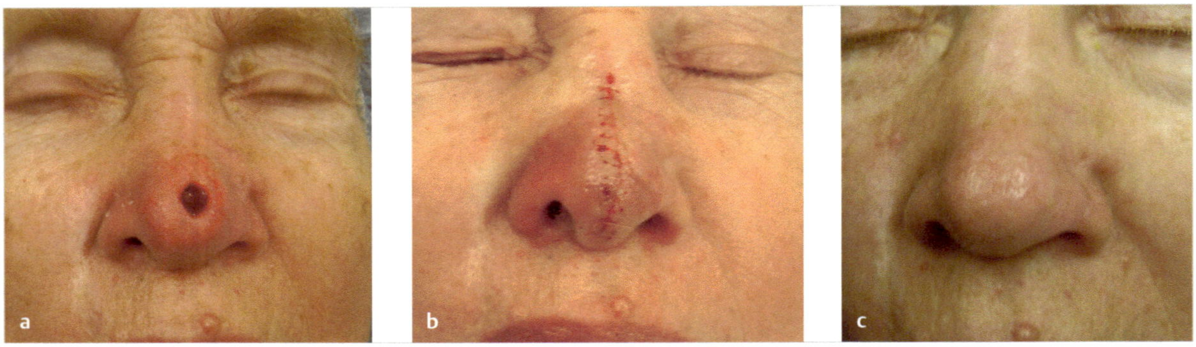

Fig. 3.5 **(a)** Defect on the midline nasal tip of a 74-year-old woman. **(b)** Fusiform repair utilizing a 5:1 length-to-width ratio. **(c)** Results at 3-month follow-up.

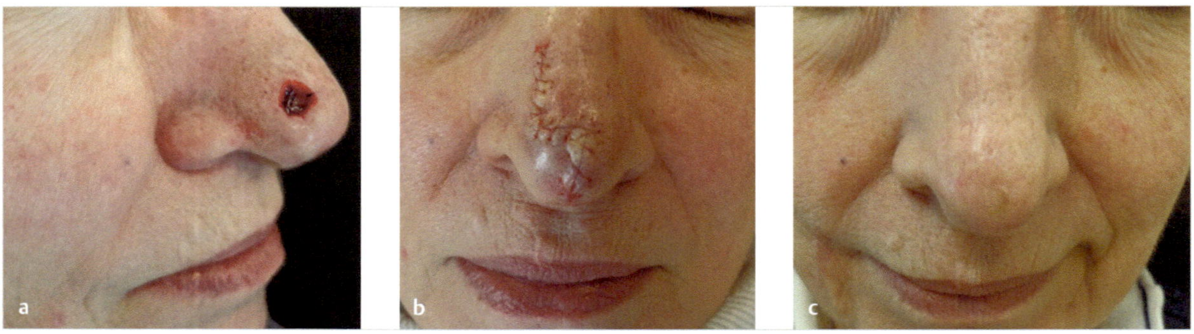

Fig. 3.6 **(a)** Defect on the lateral nasal tip in a 71-year-old woman. **(b)** Repair with a Burow's advancement flap. **(c)** Results at 3-month follow-up.

Execution

After widely anesthetizing the area, the ellipse including the defect is incised to the level of the perichondrium and periosteum. Undermining in a submuscular plane, often as wide as the nasofacial sulcus for larger defects, is necessary to recruit sufficient skin laxity for closure under minimal tension. Hemostasis is then performed. For a nose with prominent telangiectasia, there is often a desire to cauterize superficial vessels to allow for a bloodless field. However, doing so may result in epidermal necrosis with scarring. Rather, this bleeding should be anticipated by allowing ample time for the epinephrine in the anesthesia to work. The defect is then closed using 5–0 polyglactin 910 buried vertical mattress sutures.[4] When suturing on the nose, entry points on the wound edge should be in the deep reticular dermis, as more superficial bites can leave persistent nodules. Also, underlying muscle should be included in each bite in order to prevent a depressed scar.

For defects that are slightly off-center, the inferior triangle can be displaced medially, creating a Burow's advancement flap, sometimes called the "East-West" flap on the nose[5] (▶ Fig. 3.6). This variation should only be used on individuals with a wide infratip and columella; otherwise, closing the inferior triangle may distort the nares.

If size of a nasal tip defect precludes complete fusiform closure, a superiorly based Burow's graft can achieve an excellent aesthetic result (▶ Fig. 3.7). Burow's grafts have the advantage of providing adjacent skin for superb color and texture match.

3.3.3 Bilobed Flap

Our workhorse repair option for defects under 1.5 cm on the nasal tip is the bilobed flap (▶ Video 3.2).[6] What makes the bilobed flap the ideal option for nasal tip repair is its ability to deftly recruit laxity from upper nose to close defects where the immediate adjacent skin lacks sufficient mobility to use single transposition or other local flaps. In addition, it has an inherent Z-plasty-like motion, which provides a lengthening effect that creates a downward force, preserving the position of the free alar margin.

Design

Proper design of the bilobed flap is crucial for its success (▶ Fig. 3.8a). For tip defects, the flap is most commonly

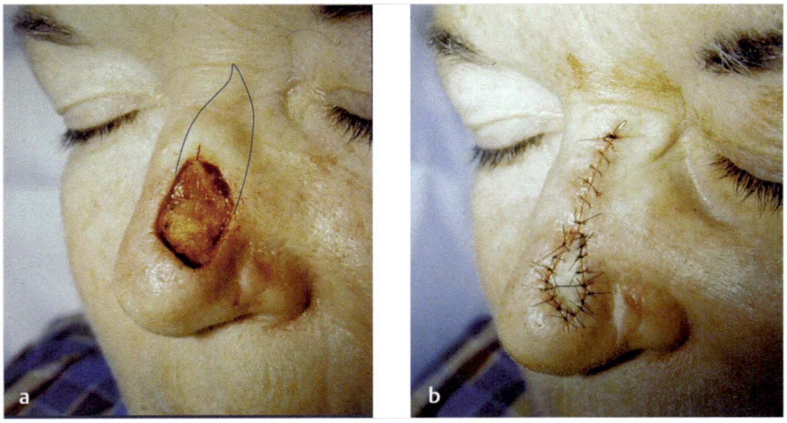

Fig. 3.7 **(a)** Defect on a 66-year-old woman with Burow's graft designed. **(b)** Repair with Burow's graft.

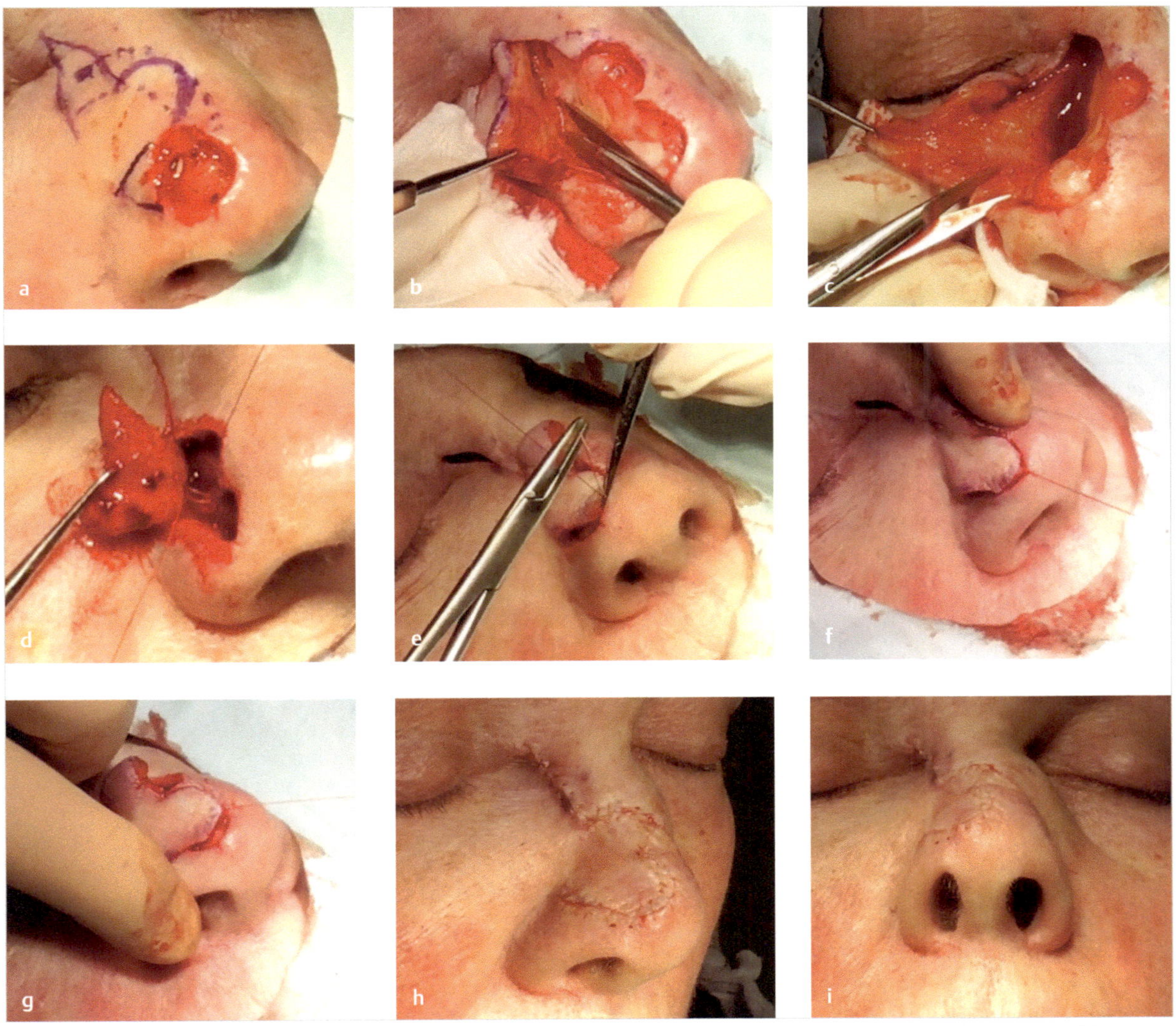

Fig. 3.8 **(a)** Proper design of the bilobed flap for defect on in a 58-year-old woman. **(b)** Severing unnamed ligament to allow for flap release. **(c)** Trimming tissue at pivot point of flap. **(d)** Nasal valve "stenting" suture to base of flap. **(e)** Correct placement of "key" suture. **(f)** Improper low placement of key suture causing "bulldozing" of ipsilateral ala and elevation of contralateral ala. **(g)** Improper high placement of key suture causing ipsilateral alar elevation. **(h)** Lateral view of completed flap. **(i)** Worm's eye view of demonstrating no alar distortion.

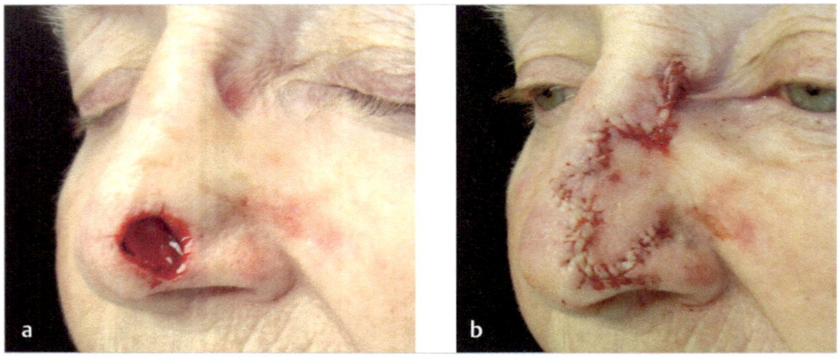

Fig. 3.9 Trilobed flap. If a bilobed flap were chosen in this case, the secondary lobe could not have designed vertically. Adding a tertiary lobe allows its orientation perpendicular to the ala. **(a)** Post-Mohs defect in an 84-year-old woman. **(b)** Completed flap.

laterally based. The dog-ear is drawn to be approximately 1.5 times the diameter of the defect and its superior arm drawn horizontally, permitting the secondary lobe of the flap to be drawn vertically along the length of the nose. Designing the secondary lobe vertically effectively places closure tension perpendicular to the ala, preventing its displacement when suturing in the flap. Our endeavor is to match the size of the primary and secondary flap lobes to that of the defect. Designing flap lobes that are too small may cause secondary movement upon flap closure that could result in alar displacement, while lobes too large may result in pincushioning. For defects that are more distal on the nasal tip, the Burow's triangle needs to be drawn with its apex oriented more vertically, avoiding its placement through the ala. When doing so, we will often add a third lobe, creating a trilobed flap (▶ Fig. 3.9), in order to place the quaternary defect perpendicular to the alar free margin as discussed previously.

Execution

The flap is first incised to the level of the perichondrium, and the defect is deepened to the level of the cartilage if necessary. Next, the flap is widely undermined, using skin hooks intermittently to assess if the flap will cover the defect without significant tension. Like primary closure described earlier, undermining is often carried out as wide as the nasofacial sulcus. We have found that severing an unnamed ligament, which exists at the lateral junction of the nasal bone and upper lateral cartilage, provides substantial flap movement allowing it to easily fall into place (▶ Fig. 3.8b). The primary lobe, especially the leading edge of the flap, should then be thinned and defatted as necessary to match the level of the skeletonized defect. We have also found that trimming tissue at the point of rotation minimizes the chance of a persistent dog-ear (▶ Fig. 3.8c). Hemostasis is then performed with care not to cauterize vessels of the superficial skin edge.

Like other transposition flaps, the distal defect is closed first, which is the tertiary defect in the case of the bilobed flap. Because the bilobed flap often traverses the alar crease, which overlies the internal valve, a tacking suture is often placed, allowing the nasal valve to remain patent (▶ Fig. 3.8d). Next, we place what we believe is the "key" stitch. This stitch is the one that aligns the primary lobe of the flap into the defect. In addition to correct design, proper placement of this stitch is essential to preserve nasal symmetry and prevent distortion (▶ Fig. 3.8e). If placed too low, a "bulldozing" effect of the ipsilateral ala can occur (▶ Fig. 3.8f), while if placed too high, displacement of the contralateral side may occur (▶ Fig. 3.8g). The remainder of the flap is then anchored into place, the secondary lobe is trimmed, and a fast gut suture is run along the scar to finely approximate the epidermis (▶ Fig. 3.8h, i). Prior to starting the repair, we inform patients of the potential for visible incision lines, which may inevitably occur on a sebaceous nose despite immaculate suture technique, and routinely have them return to assess the need for dermabrasion in 3 months.

3.3.4 Dorsal Nasal (Rieger's) Flap

The dorsal nasal flap is a rotation flap widely used for midline defects less than 2.5 cm on the nasal tip and supratip (▶ Fig. 3.10).[7] We use this flap infrequently due to some of its limitations; we use it only in circumstances where a defect may be too large for a bilobed flap and when the patient prefers a one-staged flap. The pivotal restraint encountered with this flap is amplified compared to that faced with other rotation flaps due to the thick sebaceous quality of the nasal skin. Therefore, increased closure tension is frequently encountered, which can often lead to conspicuous scarring and distortion. Another significant limitation is that the flap rotates thick glabellar skin into the medial canthus, often requiring subsequent revision.

Design and Execution

The flap is first designed with a Burow's triangle angled superiorly in the direction of the base of the flap. Importantly, the leading edge is extended past the defect to overcome the inherent rotational shortening that accompanies this flap. The arc is drawn in the alar sulcus, upward along the nasofacial sulcus, continued onto the medial canthus, and then terminated on the glabella. The arc should be completed superiorly on the glabella in order to facilitate closure of the secondary defect, and a

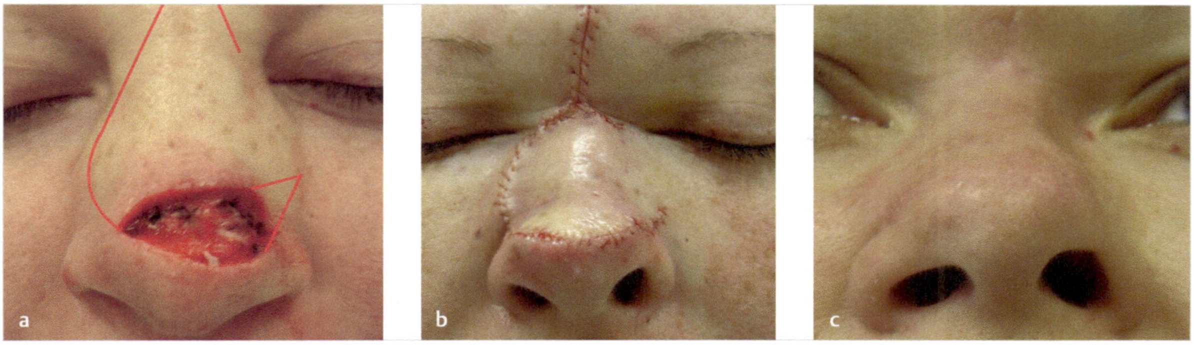

Fig. 3.10 **(a)** Design of dorsal nasal flap for defect in a 42-year-old woman. **(b)** Completed flap. **(c)** Results at 3 months showing depressed right ala. Picture included to demonstrate inconsistent results of the dorsal nasal flap despite proper design and technique.

generous back cut is designed downward no more inferior than the contralateral medial canthal tendon to enable ample rotation.

After anesthesia is achieved, the flap is incised and then undermined above the perichondrium and periosteum past the nasofacial sulcus. Hemostasis is achieved in preparation for flap inset. The glabellar donor site is closed first, and the remainder of the flap closed in a layered fashion, paying careful attention to avoid nasal tip elevation. The glabellar standing cutaneous deformity is amputated, and the remaining skin in this area that is rotated into the medial canthus should be thinned to overcome the skin thickness mismatch of these two areas.

3.3.5 Forehead Flap

For large (typically > 2 cm) or complex nasal tip or alar defects not amenable to repair with local flaps, we often employ a forehead flap (FHF) to restore the subunit with a staged approach (▶ Video 3.3, ▶ Fig. 3.11).[8,9] Its reliability, ease of transfer, capacity to provide bulk when lost, and excellent color and textural match make the FHF unsurpassed in its ability to repair such defects. Relative contraindications of the FHF include patients with poor mental status who may be at risk pulling the flap's pedicle, patients who do not understand the multiple steps required of the procedure, and patients who are at risk for not returning for a second stage. Anatomic contraindications include patients with additional skin cancers or scarring on the forehead donor site or patients who do not possess adequate forehead height to generate sufficient flap length, although if other options are limited, the flap can be curved laterally, like a hockey stick, or hair-bearing scalp can be used with a plan to do hair removal.

Preoperative Planning

First and foremost, informed consent should be obtained, discussing with patients the multiple stages that are required and the prospect of having a "tube" connecting their forehead to their nose for a 3-week period. We will also show patients representative cases in our atlas to facilitate their understanding of the multiple stages requisite of this flap. Proper planning of the FHF is a prerequisite for the flap's success. The height of the forehead is first assessed to determine if extension of the flap onto hair-bearing skin or if extension of the flap below the orbital rim is necessary to achieve adequate length. Next, attention is paid to the nose, evaluating for any loss of lining or structural integrity as well as airway patency. If any of these elements are compromised, they will need to be addressed prior to raising the FHF. There are several approaches to addressing loss of nasal mucosa[10] including lining flaps, hinge flaps, or a folded FHF. For loss of structural integrity or reduced airway patency, cartilage grafts may need to be harvested. The authors prefer use of conchal bowl cartilage due to its strength, ease of harvesting, and large reservoir available. For defects that encompass greater than 50% of the nasal tip or ala, we will typically employ the subunit principle and resurface the entire subunit. Not until all of the aforementioned factors are addressed should the surgeon start the FHF.

Design

While the traditional paramedian FHF has classically been described as an axial pattern flap based on the supratrochlear artery, our center has demonstrated that it is really a random pattern flap and that a paramidline approach provides equivalent clinical outcomes.[11] As such, the authors and the editors do not use a Doppler preoperatively as the flap's robust blood supply is a result of the dense anastomosing network of blood vessels throughout the central forehead, rather than the singular supratrochlear artery.

First, a template is crafted out of foil from a suture packet to match the defect exactly (▶ Fig. 3.11d). One should ensure that the template reflects the three-dimensional nature of the defect. A template too large may result in pincushioning, whereas one too small may result in secondary tissue movement in order to close the wound. The template should also not be created until any extranasal portions of the defect are addressed and after any cartilage grafts are placed to ensure it reflects the true nature of the operative defect. Second, the template is then transferred to the upper forehead and transposed 180 degrees medially to account for its rotation during interpolation. Next, the pedicle is designed on the ipsilateral side of the nasal defect and drawn with the planned medial incision starting at the midpoint of the glabella and the lateral incision near the edge of the medial eyebrow, allowing for a pedicle width of 1.2 cm. Both planned incisions are carried upward vertically to reach the flap template. Prior to making any incisions, however, appropriate pedicle length should be evaluated by using a gauze strip held at the flap's base and pivoted onto the nose (▶ Fig. 3.11e).

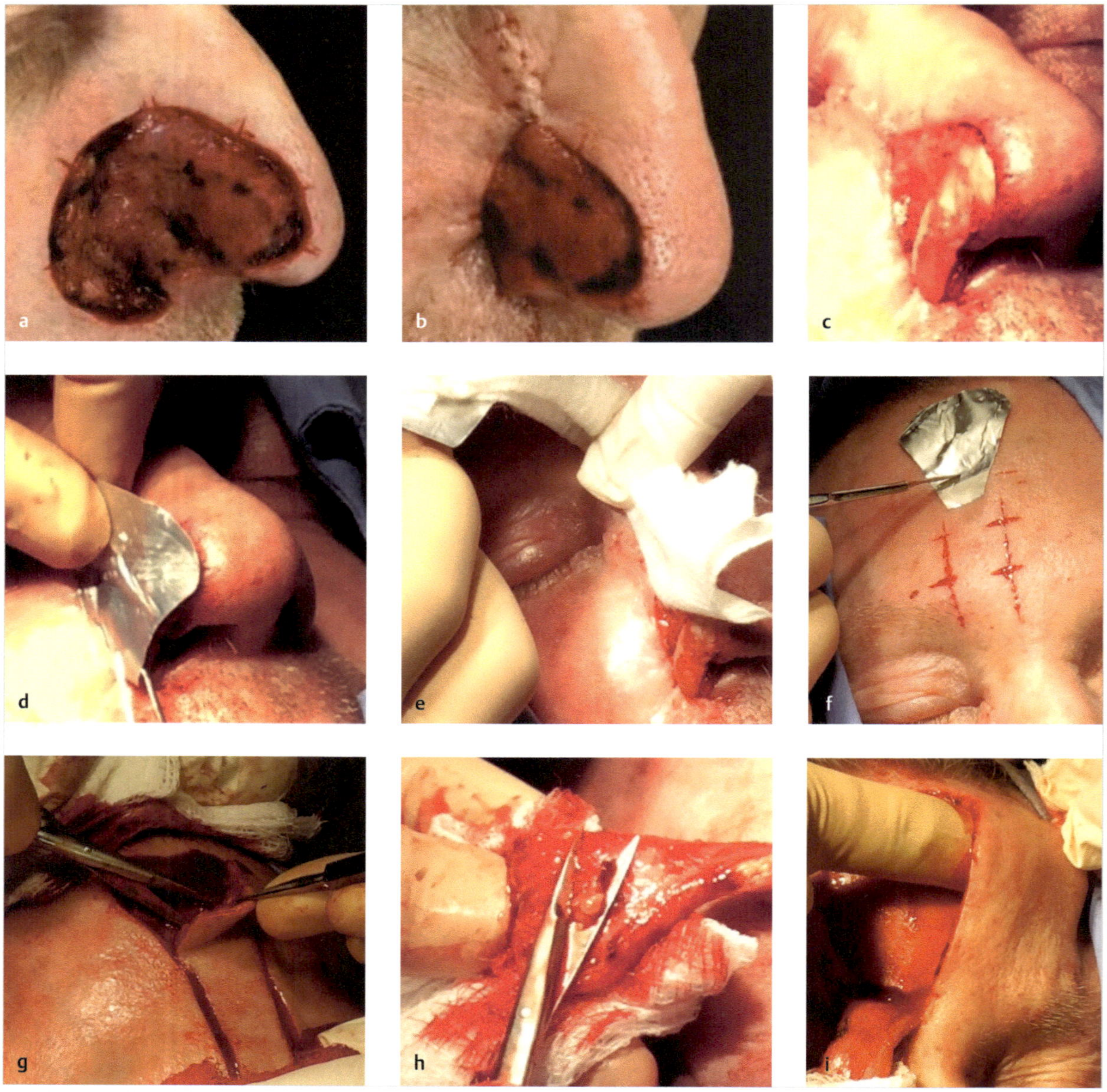

Fig. 3.11 **(a)** Defect in a 45-year-old man encompassing cheek, lip, and nasal cosmetic subunits. **(b)** Remaining nasal defect following advancement of the cheek. **(c)** Cartilage graft harvested from the conchal bowl sutured in place to provide structural integrity to lost nasal ala. **(d)** Template crafted from suture packet foil. **(e)** Gauze strip used to ensure adequate pedicle length prior to making any incisions. **(f)** Paramidline location of flap pedicle incised. Superficial nicks are made for accurate realignment during closure of the forehead donor site. **(g)** Distal flap elevated in superficial subcutaneous plane. **(h)** Aggressive thinning of distal flap. **(i)** Blunt digital undermining to allow for closure of the forehead donor site.

(Continued)

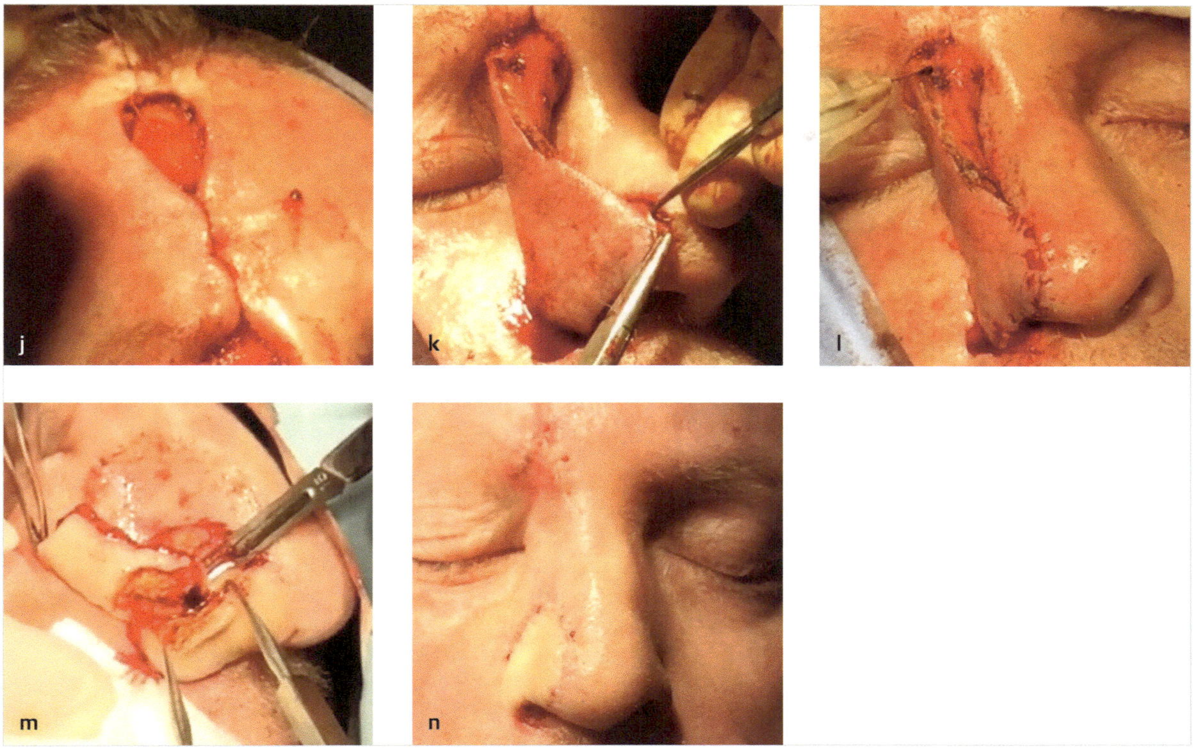

Fig. 3.11 *(continued)* **(j)** Layered repair of the forehead. Superior portion was too tight to close and was allowed to heal by second intention. **(k)** Flap sewn into place using 5–0 Vicryl. **(l)** Completed flap. Vigorous electrodessication of the pedicle's edge is performed to minimize postoperative bleeding. **(m)** At takedown, flap is debulked of granulation and subcutaneous tissue to match surrounding nasal skin. **(n)** Final results after takedown.

Execution

As the FHF is an arduous procedure for patients, a small dose of an oral benzodiazepine is offered for anxiolysis. We believe the minor antihypertensive effect of oral benzodiazepines also minimizes bleeding throughout the surgery. We use supraorbital nerve blocks to provide long-lasting anesthesia as well as small aliquots of numbing medication around the pedicle and donor site areas for the epinephrine effect. After allowing sufficient time for epinephrine to work, the flap and donor site are scored with the scalpel. Superficial nicks are made in the patient's horizontal forehead lines so these lines can be readjoined at the time of donor site closure (▶ Fig. 3.11f). Failure to do so can result in noticeable asymmetry upon healing of the flap. The templated area is then elevated in a superficial subcutaneous plane (▶ Fig. 3.11g). Incisions for the pedicle are then carried through subcutaneous fat, muscle, and fascia to the level of periosteum and the flap is subsequently raised (▶ Fig. 3.11h). We consistently carry incisions beyond the supraorbital ridge toward the nasal root to increase flap reach and allow inset of the pedicle within the favorable glabellar and corrugator skin tension lines. The distal flap can be thinned aggressively as needed (▶ Fig. 3.11i), allowed for by the robust vascular supply of this flap. Diligent hemostasis is then achieved as postoperative bleeding with FHFs is quite common; however, care should be taken to avoid the deeper structures of the pedicle. Direct electrodessication of the pedicle's skin edge is acceptable as this area will be transected with the flap takedown. The editors frequently run a locking suture (6–0 nylon) along the edge of the pedicle to further reduce bleeding from the transected edges of the connecting pedicle.

Attention is then paid to the closure of the forehead donor site. A cursory job closing the forehead can lead to an obvious scar that in many cases can overshadow an excellent result on the nose. To assist in its closure, the forehead is bluntly undermined widely in the avascular subfascial plane (▶ Fig. 3.11j) and then closed in a layered fashion. The galea and deep fascia of the frontalis muscle are closed first in order to prevent a depressed scar, and the dermis is closed subsequently (▶ Fig. 3.11k). Care is taken to reapproximate the nicks previously made when incising the flap to maintain the patient's natural forehead lines. For larger nasal reconstructions, closing the cephalic portion of the forehead may not be possible. While other surgeons employ additional flaps or grafts to close this defect, we prefer to manage this area by second intention healing. Additional procedures introduce increased costs and morbidity and are unlikely to have superior aesthetic results to second intention in this particular area.

Next, attention is paid to the nasal defect. The nasal wound margins are conservatively undermined to allow for wound edge eversion and formation of platelike scar to minimize pincushioning upon healing. The flap is sutured into place in a layered fashion up to the superior portion of the defect to avoid impinging the vascular pedicle.

Wound Care and Second Stage

Prior to bandaging the flap, the pedicle should be inspected again for bleeding and hemostasis achieved as the epinephrine effect has often started to wear off by this time. The pedicle is first covered in Gelfoam powder, wrapped in petrolatum-impregnated gauze, and then a pressure bandage is placed. Opioid and antiemetics are often prescribed to address the common complaint of pain and nausea due to the tightness of the forehead donor site. We typically have the patient return the following day for a bandage change, again redressing the pedicle in a similar fashion. One week later, as we do with most of our repairs, we have the patient return, at which point the bandage is again changed and the wound assessed. A light, flat bandage is placed over the wound at this time.

At 3 weeks postoperatively, the patient returns for flap division and insertion, allowing enough time for the establishment of sufficient collateral circulation. While others have advocated for an additional interim stage for flap refinement or delayed cartilage placement at this time prior to takedown of the flap, we have found that doing so is unnecessary to consistently generate excellent results.

After anesthesia, the pedicle is severed in the middle, before attention to the proximal and distal aspects. At the origin of the pedicle, any granulation tissue is debulked and subcutaneous tissue thinned to an appropriate depth that matches the neighboring glabellar skin. A defect is then created around the pedicle in an inverted **V** shape, and the pedicle is trimmed and inset here in a layered fashion (▶ Fig. 3.11m). At the nasal defect, the superior part of the flap is similarly debulked of granulation and subcutaneous tissue to match the surrounding nasal skin and excess skin is trimmed. A well-placed linear closure can also be used to close the pedicle origin. The flap is then inset in a layered fashion and both wounds are bandaged.

We have the patient return 3 months postoperatively for wound assessment. Additional revisions are performed at this time if the patient desires, which may include thinning or sculpting of the flap and dermabrasion. All of our patients are informed of the possibility of any revisions at the time of the initial surgery.

3.3.6 Prelaminated and Prefolded Forehead Flap

When there is complete nasal tip loss, the senior author has previously described a prelaminated and prefolded FHF as a novel method for repairing this formidable defect. Performed in three to six stages, a three-dimensional nose is formed upside on the distal forehead and ultimately transferred to the nose. The main advantage of this flap is that the difficult work is performed on the forehead precluding intranasal manipulation. This allows for good visibility and is advantageous for the patient with anxiety or oxygen requirements. Additionally, there is a robust vascular supply due to the delayed pedicle formation.

Design and Execution

While the flap is being created, the nasal defect is temporarily covered with a split-thickness skin graft. First, a template from hydrocolloid film (DuoDerm; ConvaTec, Skillman, NJ) is molded to recreate the nose. The paper backing of the DuoDerm is replaced with gauze in order to make the template more pliable. In order to recreate the three-dimensional shape of the nose, the film is folded under itself (▶ Fig. 3.12a) by pushing both thumbs where the nasal airways would be (demarcated with *dotted lines* in the figure). The cartilaginous support should then be demarcated on the template (*solid red* lines in the figure).

The template is flattened out upside down on the distal forehead. The distal flap is incised and lifted, but the pedicle is left. Like a conventional FHF, the distal third is raised below the deep dermis, the middle third below adipose, and proximal third below the periosteum. An entire conchal bowl cartilage is then harvested and fashioned into three separate grafts: two cupped ovals recreate the lower lateral cartilage of the nose, and a long batten rod to support the dorsum, tip, and columella. These grafts are then positioned corresponding to their position on the nasal tip and sewn into place using 4–0 Polyglactin 910. The first two stitches fold the corners of the flap down (▶ Fig. 3.12b). The next two stitches will create the flap's three-dimensional shape (▶ Fig. 3.12c). First, a stitch pierces the proximal three parts of the flap, which will correspond to the lateral-most parts of both the alar groove and the septum. Once this stitch is tied, the three parts are snugged together, and the alar grooves recreated. Next, a similar stitch is placed piercing the same three portions of the flap more distally, further securing the flap's shape. The newly created "nose" is then secured to the underlying forehead fascia, and then covered with petrolatum, petrolatum gauze, Telfa, and thermoplastic cast (Aquaplast PS; WFR, Avondale, PA).

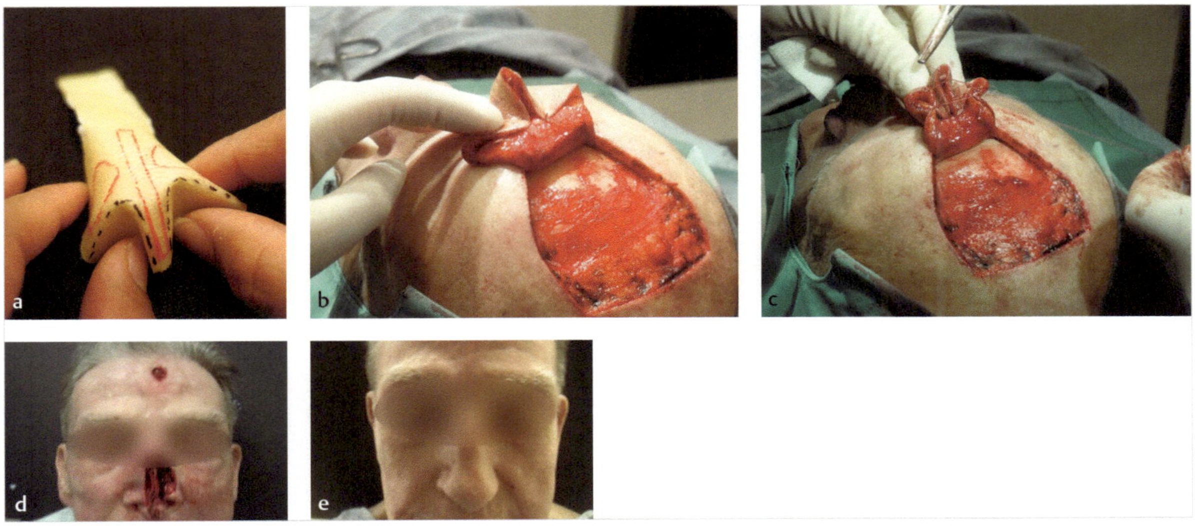

Fig. 3.12 (a) Duoderm folded under itself to recreate the 3-dimensional shape of the nose. (b) First two stitches of flap that fold corners of the flap down. (c) Next two stiches that create flap's 3-dimensional shape. (d) Defect in 62-year-old man. (e) Flap appearance 6 months post-op.

On week 2, the pedicle is delayed by incising it down the brow, but not lifted, leaving the pedicle in place attached to the forehead. Delaying a flap refers to incising it but leaving it in its original position. This tactic has been reported to increase vascularity as a response to stress.[12]

On week 4, the split-thickness graft on the nose is removed and the nasal recipient bed is freshened. The FHF is lifted, transferred to the nose, and sewn into place. The forehead defect is closed.

On weeks 6 and 7, the sectioning of the pedicle is delayed by respectively only sectioning one lateral third of the pedicle at a time. These steps are optional but recommended in order to increase vascular supply of the flap. On week 8, the remaining portion of the pedicle is divided. The flap and residual pedicle are then sewn into place, similarly to a conventional FHF. ▶ Fig. 3.12d and e depict the defect after tumor extirpation and the final result of the flap several months post-op.

3.3.7 Conchal Bowl Full-Thickness Skin Graft

In select settings on the nasal tip and ala, skin grafts can rival the results obtained with flaps (▶ Video 3.4, ▶ Fig. 3.13). We most commonly use skin grafts for small, shallow defects not amenable to second intention healing in our elderly patient population. The conchal bowl is routinely selected as a donor reservoir for the distal nose because of the excellent color and texture color similarity between the two areas. This similarity is owed to the comparable sebaceous gland density and pore size.[13] Furthermore, the donor site reliably yields excellent results when allowed to heal by second intention.

Design and Execution

A template of the nasal tip defect using the foil from a suture packet is shown in ▶ Fig. 3.13b. After anesthesia, the graft is harvested above cartilage. The inclusion of perichondrium in the graft has been shown to lead to less graft contraction and increased retention of epidermal appendages (▶ Fig. 3.13c).[14] To expedite healing of the donor site, multiple perforations are made in the cartilage using punch biopsy tool to promote granulation. If needed, the graft is thinned to match the thickness of the skin surrounding the defect. In acutely convex locations on the nasal tip, the editors find it helpful to circumferentially undermine around the defect to reduce the incidence of pincushioning. This is less important in concave locations such as the alar groove. We use 6–0 fast absorbing gut to sew in the graft. Simple interrupted sutures anchor in the graft at four points such as at the 12, 3, 6, and 9 o'clock positions, and the remaining graft is sutured in a running fashion. While suturing the graft, one should pay careful attention to ensure reapposition of the epidermis and the entire dermis by taking full-thickness bites (▶ Fig. 3.13d). A common error is to take too superficial of bites, only including the epidermis and papillary dermis, because the reticular dermis tends to retract toward the center of the graft. Failure to reappose the epidermis and entire dermis can lead to a depressed wound edge and depressed scar. Following graft inset, a bolster is sewn on to ensure contact between the wound bed and base of the graft in order to enhance graft imbibition. An assistant applies petrolatum to the graft, followed by a nonstick gauze like Telfa, then a folded 2 × 2 gauze on top. The bolster is secured with one or two figure-of-eight stitches using 4–0 silk (▶ Fig. 3.13f). The

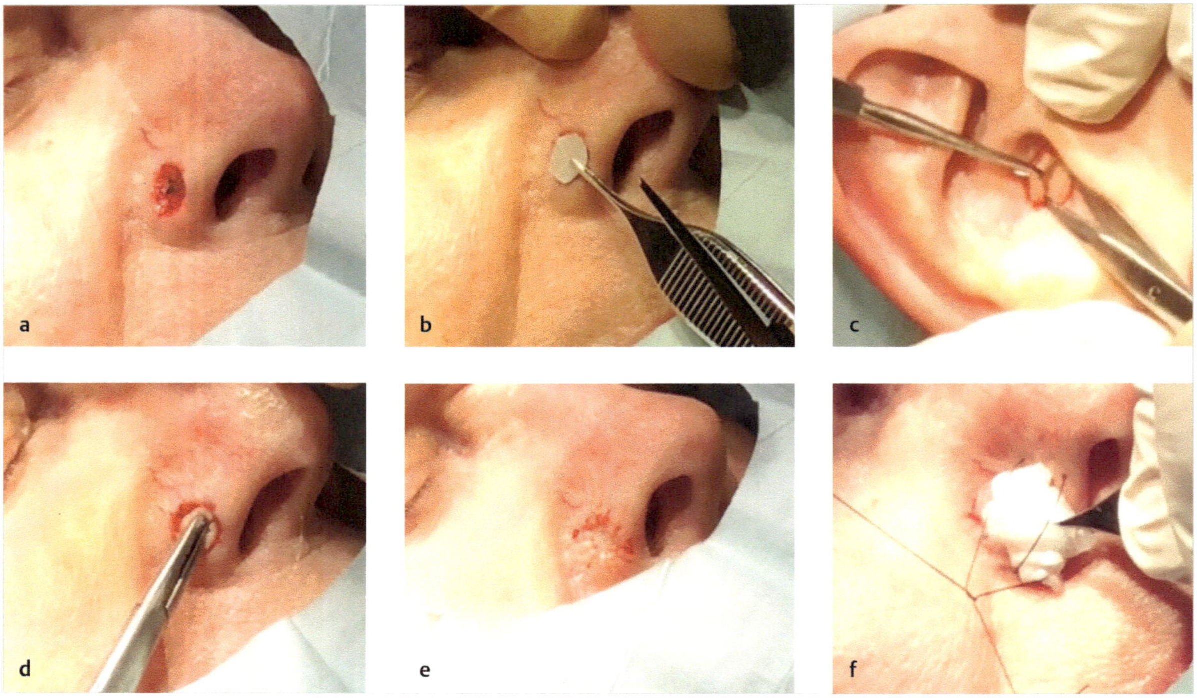

Fig. 3.13 (a) Alar defect in a 65-year-old woman. (b) Foil template matching the size of the defect. (c) Graft harvested directly above cartilage. (d) Full-thickness suture bites are taken, otherwise failure to reappose the epidermis and entire dermis can lead to a depressed wound edge and depressed scar. (e) Graft completely sewn in. (f) Placement of bolster using 4–0 silk suture with a figure-eight knot.

patient returns 1 week later for bandage and bolster removal, at which point graft survival is assessed.

3.4 Nasal Ala

Proximity to a free margin, poor tissue mobility, and the necessity of conserving function of the external nasal valve complicate the repair of alar defects. While the tip and ala share sebaceous and thickness qualities, the ala lacks underlying cartilaginous support relying only on its fibrofatty nature to maintain its patency to allow for airflow. Thus, it is essential that the surgeon evaluate remaining structural integrity following tumor extirpation to determine the need to replace structural support.

3.4.1 Second Intention

Defects that are limited to the concave region of the ala can demonstrate excellent results when allowed to heal by second intention, regardless of wound depth. Even some wounds that straddle the concave and convex areas of the ala can produce good results, as long as the aspect of the wound on the convex alar lobule is at least 4 mm from the alar rim. Wounds near the alar rim allowed to be healed by second intention risk creation of a distracting notch, a complication that is notoriously difficult to revise. Very superficial defects on the alar lobule are an exception. We will often employ the shave and sand technique to contour superficial wounds on the ala. Partial-thickness defects on the ala and the distal third of the nose also respond nicely to recontouring with a wire brush or diamond fraise driven by a hand engine. Especially in men with highly sebaceous skin or rhinophyma, for which the wire brush is best, the shoulders of the defect can be eliminated while the rhinophyma of the entire distal third of the nose is also treated (▶ Fig. 3.14a–c).[15]

3.4.2 Grafts

Wounds of intermediate depth on the ala can often be reconstructed with a full-thickness skin graft (▶ Fig. 3.13). Like the nasal tip, the conchal bowl provides the most optimal donor site. We have found that for smaller wounds, utilization of a graft on the alar lobule often provides superior contour than a flap would if used to repair the same wound. The major limitation of selecting a graft is the resultant skin color discrepancy. In women, this discrepancy can be easily camouflaged with makeup.

Any time structural integrity of the ala may be compromised, a cartilage graft should be considered. Cartilage grafts can be used in conjunction with both flaps and full-thickness skin grafts. The conchal bowl is our preferred donor site, which makes it convenient when harvesting both cartilage and skin from this location when

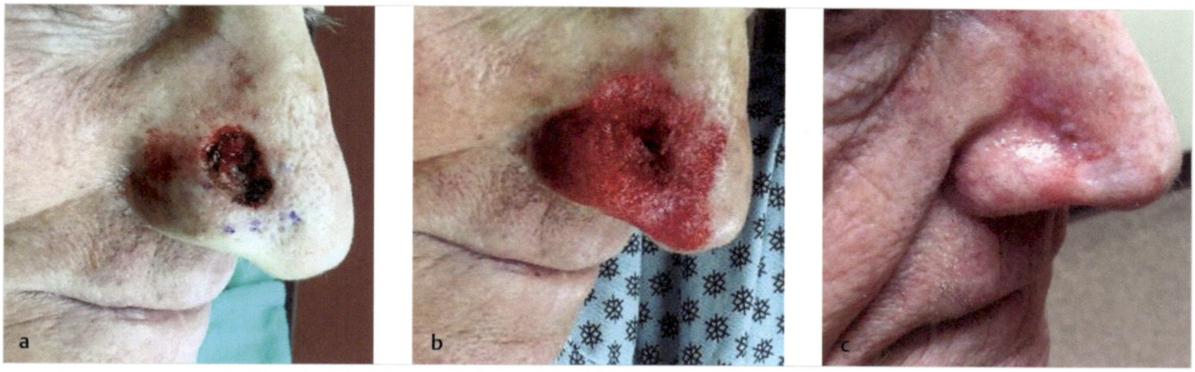

Fig. 3.14 Dermabrasion of the nasal ala subunit as a reconstruction after Mohs surgery. **(a)** Alar defect after Mohs surgery. **(b)** Dermabrasion of the nasal ala subunit to knock down wound edges and blend surrounding skin. **(c)** Two-week follow-up with mild polysporin dermatitis but improved wound edge transition. (These images are provided courtesy of Stanislav N. Tolkachjov, MD.)

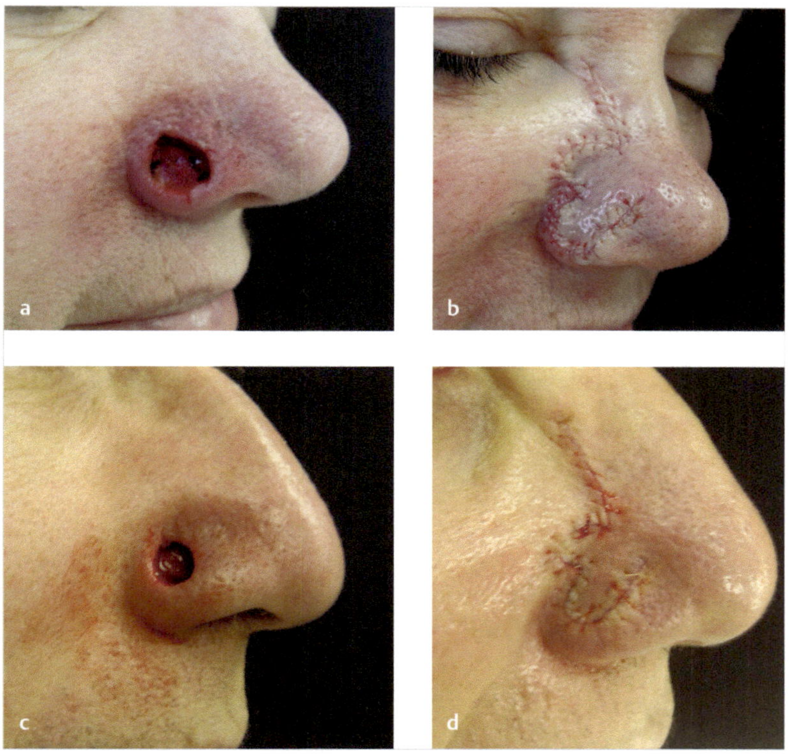

Fig. 3.15 **(a)** Defect in a 38-year-old woman. **(b)** Repair with medial-based bilobed flap. **(c)** Defect in a 51-year-old man. **(d)** Repair with a medial-based bilobed flap.

repairing an alar lobule defect. A strut slightly longer than the inferior aspect of the defect is harvested. The cartilage is thinned as needed, and pockets are created on either site of the defect where the strut is inserted after which it is secured with sutures. If the depth of the defect is greater than the harvested skin graft, chopped up pieces of cartilage can also be placed in the bottom of the defect before the graft is sewn into position. This can help maintain the convex contour of the ala.

3.4.3 Medial-Based Bilobed Flap

Partial- or full-thickness alar defects that measure ≤ 1.5 cm can dependably be repaired with a bilobed flap that is medially based, especially if they are situated at the anterior aspect of the ala (▶ Fig. 3.15). A medially based bilobed flap is designed and executed in the same fashion as its laterally based counterpart, with the exception that when undermining, the plane of undermining should

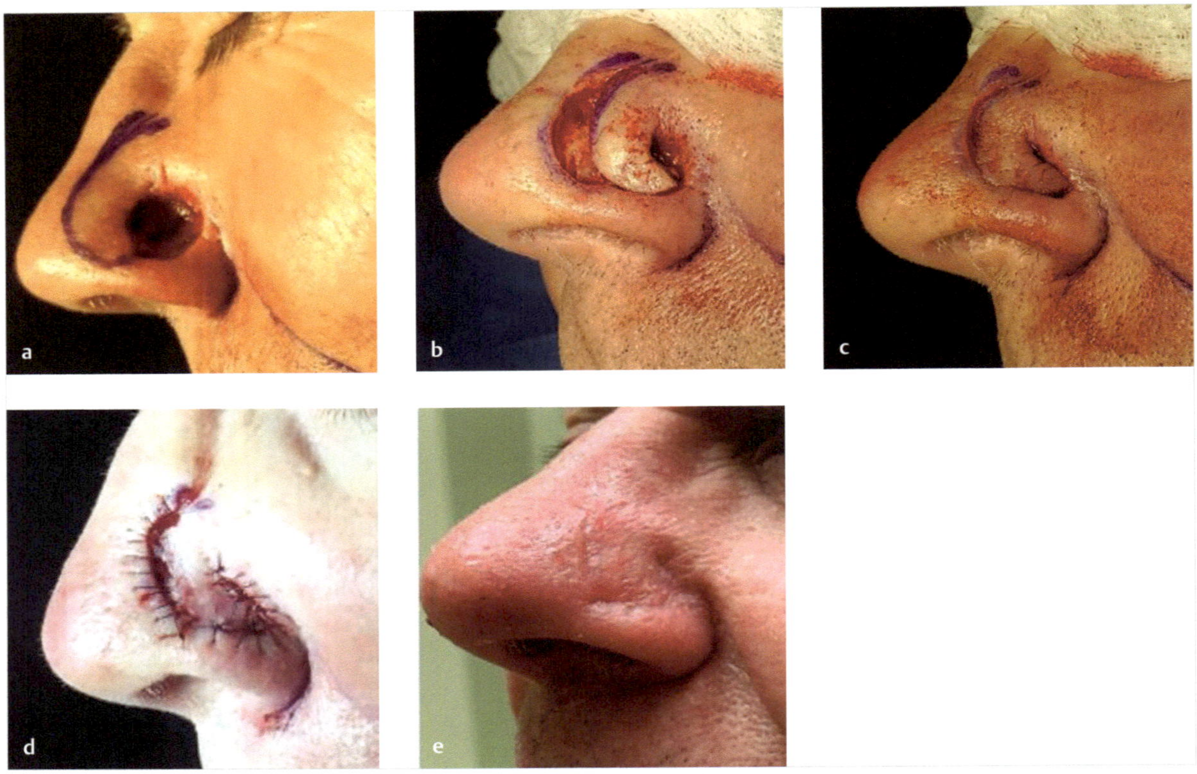

Fig. 3.16 Spiral flap. (a) Defect involving the superior nasal ala and a portion of the nasal alar groove with the flap drawn out. Note the anterior portion of the flap is designed wider than diagram due to the width and vertical height of the defect. (b) Key stitches: the first stitch brings the flap tip to itself and the second stitch aligns the flap to the alar rim portion of the defect. Of note, the editor may often tie the flap base to the nasal valve if concerned for flap collapse or potential internal scar compression. (c) Deep stitches in place. (d) Immediate postoperative appearance. (e) One-month follow-up. Flap outline is still visible at this point but may fade over time or can be improved by dermabrasion. (These images are provided courtesy of Stanislav N. Tolkachjov, MD.)

transition from above cartilage on the nose to a subcutaneous plane on the cheek.

3.4.4 Spiral Flap

Similar-sized defects that are more proximal and may fall on both sides of the alar groove can also be repaired with a spiral flap (▶ Fig. 3.16a, b).[16] This flap is designed from the wound edge at point A and spirals upward so that "B" is the diameter of the defect and "C" is 1.5 times the diameter (▶ Fig. 3.16c). Again, undermining is wide and below the level of the muscle. Using 6–0 polyglactin 910, the tip of the spiral is sutured onto itself. Then the remainder of the flap is advanced forward into the defect in a spiral fashion to close the defect and maintain convexity of the nasal ala.

3.4.5 Cheek-to-Nose Interpolation Flap

Full-thickness defects ≥ 1.5 cm that are confined to the alar lobule can be repaired with the cheek-to-nose interpolation flap (CNIF; ▶ Fig. 3.17). The CNIF can be designed as either a peninsula or an island, but we prefer a peninsula as it theoretically should be better vascularized. While the CNIF is a robust flap that allows for an aesthetic repair, one must keep in mind that it is not quite as well vascularized as the FHF. Like the FHF, the subunit principle is adhered to on a situational basis, depending on the nature of the defect.

Design

First, a template is created to exactly match the defect. The template is placed on the cheek lateral to the melolabial fold and superior to the oral commissure. While the template should be placed inferiorly enough to allow for sufficient pedicle length, it should not be too long where there is a chance of the flap's blood supply being compromised. Importantly, the superior aspect of the template should be placed medially, adjacent to the melolabial fold, to account for the rotation of the flap into the defect. A peninsula is drawn encompassing the flap template with the base situated above the defect. The inferior apex of the peninsula should be drawn acutely enough to allow for closure of the secondary defect without a residual standing cone deformity.

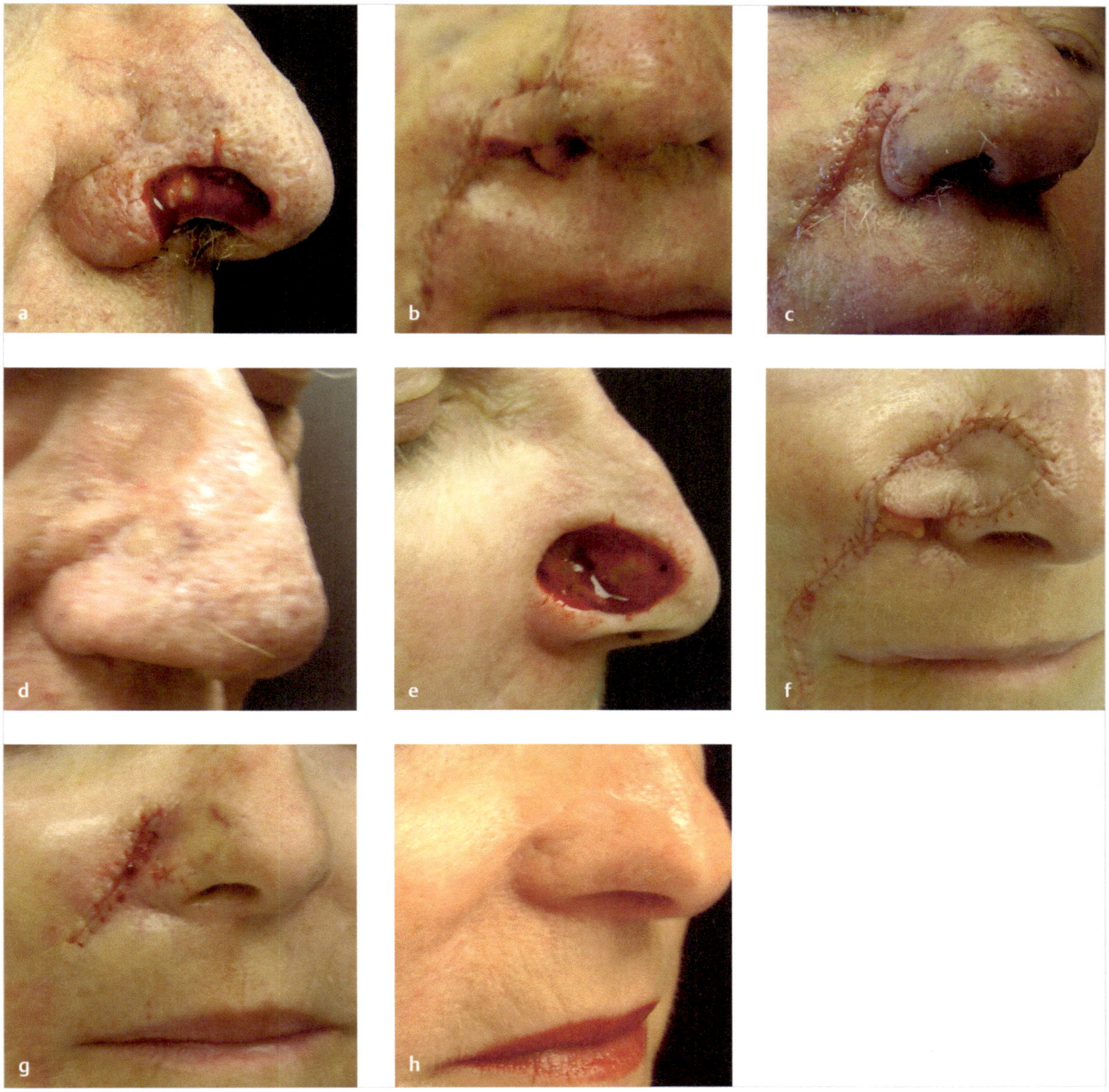

Fig. 3.17 **(a)** Defect in a 79-year-old man. **(b)** Repair with cheek-to-nose interpolation flap. **(c)** Results after takedown of flap at 3 weeks. **(d)** Results at 3 months. **(e)** Defect in a 55-year-old woman. **(f)** Repair with cheek-to-nose interpolation flap. **(g)** Results after takedown of flap at 3 weeks. **(h)** Results at 3 months.

Execution

The flap is incised from the base of the peninsula to the apex. It is important to remove the Burow's triangle inferior to the template until adequate reach of the flap into the defect is ensured. Once incised, the flap is undermined at the superficial subcutis. As undermining is continued proximately, the level of undermining is deepened to the deep subcutis to allow for a well-vascularized base. Once sufficient reach is guaranteed, the Burow's triangle is removed, and the flap is aggressively thinned distally. Hemostasis is achieved, and the flap sewn in in a layered fashion

Second Stage

At approximately 3 weeks, the flap is taken down. First, the pedicle is severed distally. At this time, if following the subunit principle, the remainder of the posterior aspect of the alar lobule can be excised leaving a 1- to 2-mm rim laterally. Subcutis and granulation tissue are removed so the flap can be sewn in flush the surrounding tissue. Attention is then turned to the base of the pedicle, which is severed and removed along with any granulation tissue. Although this site can be closed primarily or in a V-Y fashion, we prefer a primary closure because we feel a V-Y in this area tends to pincushion more readily.

3.4.6 Spear Flap

For defects where there is full-thickness loss of the ala and vestibular lining extending to the lateral alar crease, the Spear flap is an excellent option to recreate the hemicylindrical convexity of the alar rim and the crease of the alar cheek fold (▶ Fig. 3.18).[17] The Spear flap is a reverse nasolabial island pedicle flap that is flipped over and turned upon itself, allowing it to recreate the missing alar skin.

Design

A peninsula is drawn off the lateral edge of the wound with its apex oriented inferiorly. The medial arm of the peninsula is situated in the melolabial fold. The width of the flap should match the width of the defect, and the apex should be acute enough (< 30 degrees) to allow for donor site closure without resultant standing cone deformity. The base of the flap is what will ultimately be sutured to provide nasal lining.

3.4.7 Technique

The medial and lateral arms of the flap are incised down to the subcutis. The apex is undermined proximally to its base in a subcutaneous plane. After aggressive thinning of the flap and undermining of the donor site, the donor site can be closed, allowing for closure of the remainder of the flap under little tension. The flap is then hinged on its subcutaneous base medially, likened to flipping a page of a book. What was originally the *superior/medial* corner of the island is sewn into the *superior/lateral* corner of the nasal lining defect. The original inferior/medial corner of the island is then sewn into the *inferior/medial* corner of the lining defect. The lateral portion of the upper island is then

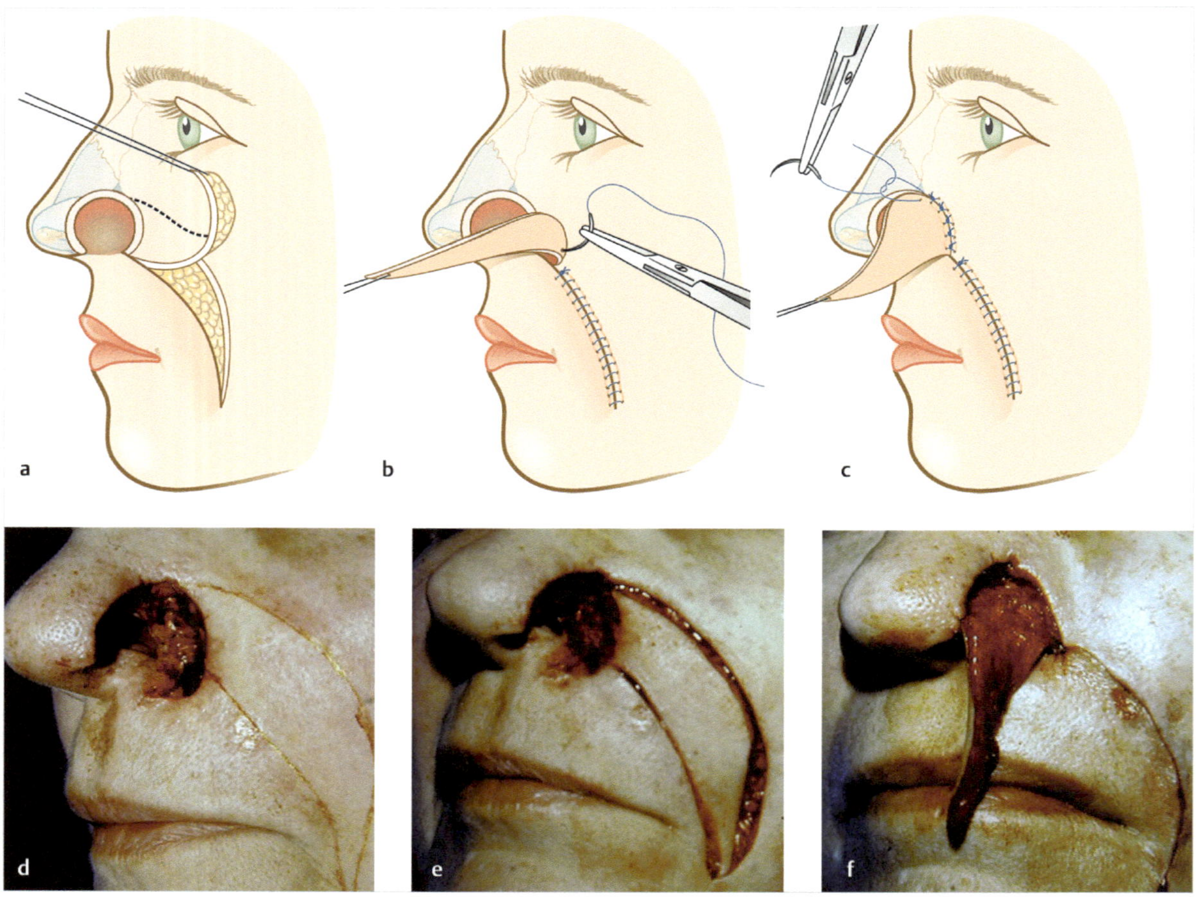

Fig. 3.18 (a–c) Pictorial representation of how a spear flap is executed. **(d)** Defect in a 53-year-old woman with Spear island flap designed. **(e)** Spear island flap incised to subcutaneous plane. **(f)** Flap hinged on its subcutaneous base medially and sewn into mucosal portion of defect.

(Continued)

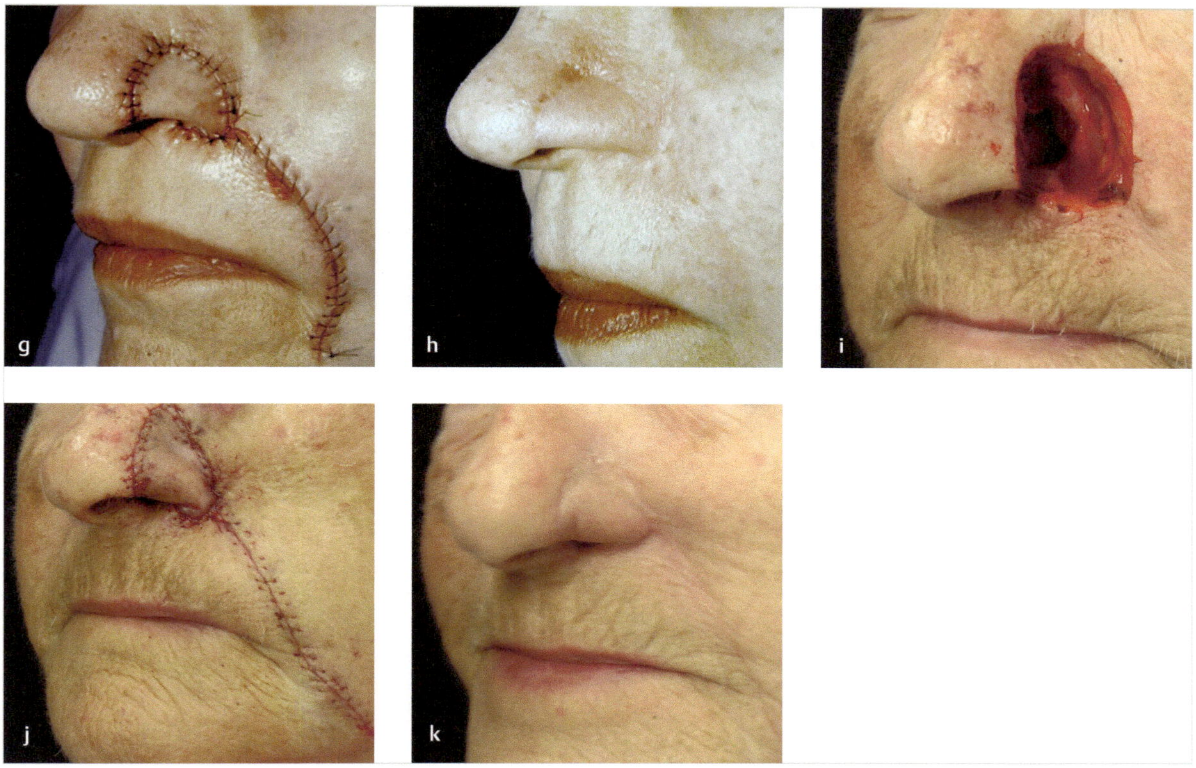

Fig. 3.18 (*Continued*) **(g)** Flap sewn into place. **(h)** Results at 3 months. **(i)** Defect in an 81-year-old woman. **(j)** Repair with Spear flap. **(k)** Results at 3 months.

sutured to the medial nasal lining with the inferior apex hanging down from the inside of the nose. The flap is then folded upon itself to form the external ala. It is important that the flap is folded upon itself at the right point in order to provide symmetry with the contralateral ala. Periosteal sutures can be used at the lateral aspect of the flap to prevent flaring of the newly created ala. The remainder of the flap can then be sewn in using a layered technique.

3.5 Soft Triangle/Columella

The soft triangle is a complex subunit of the nose, suspended between the nasal infratip and alar rim. It is composed of a vestibular lining, a very thin subcutaneous space, and nasal skin that is significantly thinner and less sebaceous than the remainder of the lower third of the nose. Although it is a small structure, loss of the soft triangle will result in an aesthetically noticeable notched appearance.

The columella can be a very difficult structure to repair. Small superficial defects can be allowed to heal by second intention with satisfactory results, while slightly larger columellar defects may be adequately repaired with a full-thickness skin graft. Complete loss of the columella may necessitate a cartilage graft in conjunction with an interpolated flap (forehead or cheek-to-nose) in order restore function and cosmesis.

3.5.1 Turnover Flap

The turnover flap is a simple method to repair defects of the soft triangle or correct notches that occur as a secondary complication of other flaps or grafts in the area (▸ Fig. 3.19).[18] While the turnover flap is an effective choice for repairing defects limited to the soft triangle area, for larger defects it may also be used to provide vestibular lining for surface flaps as well as blood supply for an overlying skin graft.

Design and Execution

The contralateral soft triangle serves as a template in estimating the amount of tissue that is required to be replaced. A triangle-shaped turnover flap is designed at the junction of the inferior nasal tip and the columella with its apex pointing toward the contralateral ala. Ultimately, the inferior arm of the triangle will become the new free margin of the soft triangle.

The flap is incised, and the apex is undermined until it can be turned over so it can reach the alar rim. The portion of the alar rim that will receive the flap's edge (superior

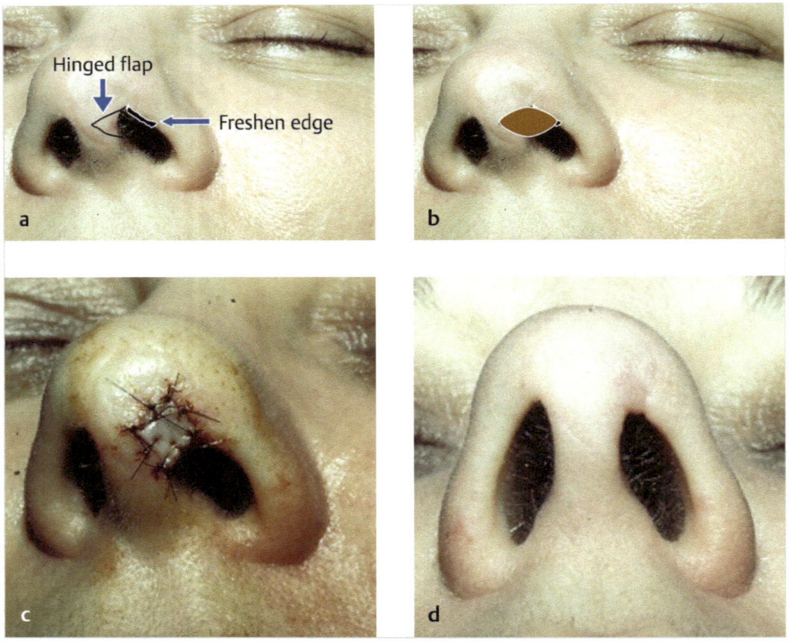

Fig. 3.19 (a) Soft triangle notch in a 39-year-old woman 3 months after a repair with a full-thickness skin graft. A hinge flap is designed. **(b)** Illustration depicting where full-thickness skin graft will be placed. **(c)** Repair with soft triangle turnover hinge flap, covered with a postauricular full-thickness skin graft. **(d)** Results at 3 months.

arm of the initial triangular flap) is freshened with excision of the skin edge to a depth that allows suturing of both the turnover flap and an overlying full-thickness skin graft. After hemostasis is achieved, the superior margin of the flap is sutured to the vestibular margin of the alar rim. The inferior margin of the flap should extend an additional 1 to 2 mm below the contralateral soft triangle to compensate for eventual wound contraction that will occur, and bilateral free margin symmetry can be established. A full-thickness skin graft from the postauricular sulcus is designed to cover both the exposed flap surface and the flap's donor site. The postauricular sulcus is chosen because its thin skin provides a suitable match for the thin smooth skin of the soft triangle. The graft is harvested, sewn in, and immobilized with a tie-over bolster dressing.

3.5.2 Nasal Tip Rotation Flap

Small partial-thickness defects at the junction of the soft triangle, lateral nasal tip, and anterior ala can present a significant reconstructive challenge. A useful repair option for these defects is the nasal tip rotation flap.[19] This flap elegantly hides incision lines at the junction of the nasal tip and dorsum and is able to maintain nasal tip topography with a low risk of alar rim elevation.

Design

A Burow's triangle is drawn paralleling a line connecting the inferior nasal tip to the mid alar rim (▸ Fig. 3.20). For defects that are more inferior placed, the Burow's triangle should be angled more inferiorly toward the nasal infratip/columella. Proper placement of this triangle will prevent notching of the alar rim. When possible, the angle of flap rotation is designed within the cosmetic junction line between the nasal tip and the nasal dorsum. However, the angle of flap rotation may need adjustment depending on the vertical dimension of the defect, nasal laxity, and the patient's particular nasal tip topography. Defects with larger vertical dimensions, thick or inelastic sebaceous tissue, and bulbous nasal tips may necessitate a greater arc of rotation, sometimes beyond the midline, which allows for increased tissue movement. A displaced Burow's triangle is then drawn due to the length discrepancy between the longer outer and shorter inner arcs.

Execution

The flap is incised, and both Burow's triangles are excised. Undermining is carried out widely, mobilizing the entire nasal tip subunit above the lower lateral alar cartilage in order to recruit ample tissue. The displaced Burow's triangle is closed first, followed by securing the leading edge of the flap into the inferoposterior aspect of the defect. The remainder of the flap is sutured in a layered fashion.

3.6 Nasal Dorsum

The nasal dorsum, also sometimes referred to as the "bridge" of the nose, has considerable aesthetic importance. Repair options for the nasal dorsum have been described in detail in other sections. Like other areas of the nose, superficial defects can heal adequately, although employment of the previously described shave and sand technique will often optimize the result. Primary repair can effectively close the majority of small to medium

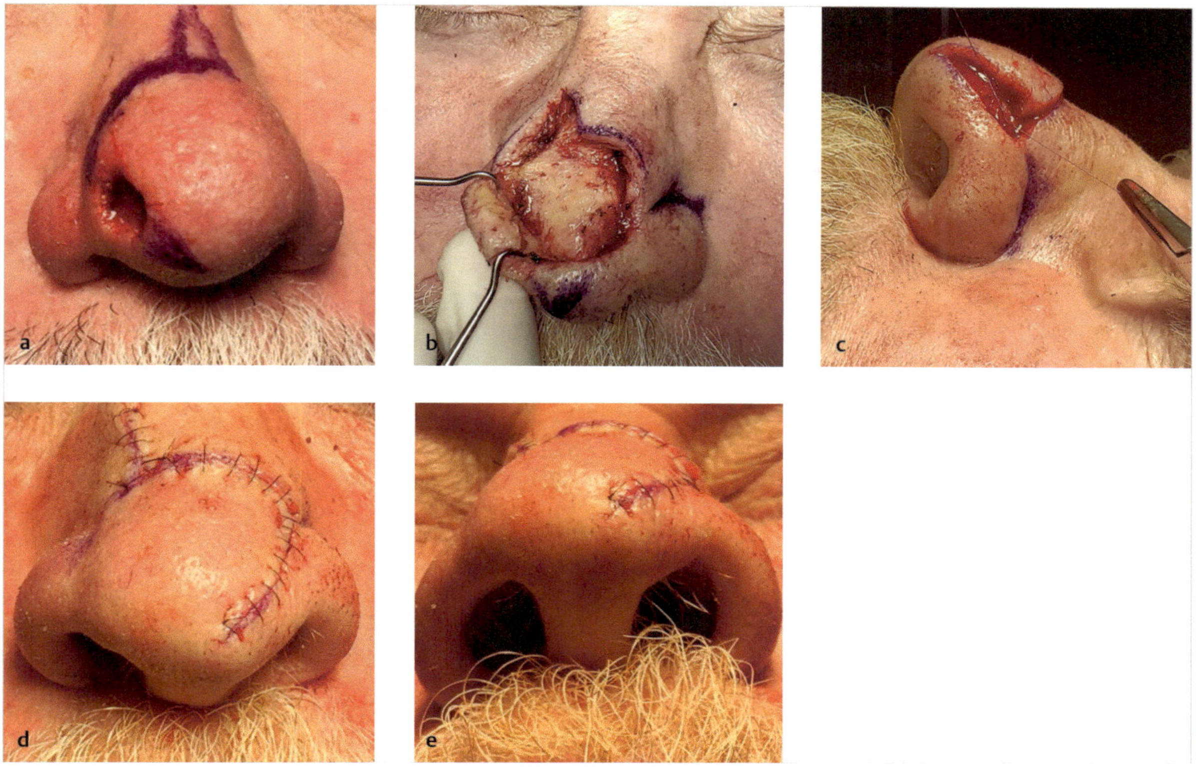

Fig. 3.20 Nasal tip rotation flap. **(a)** Deep lateral nasal tip defect of a bulbous nose illustrating flap design (different patient). **(b)** Flap elevated after complete undermining of the nasal tip above cartilage and the nasal dorsum to allow a platelike internal scar to form. **(c)** Second key stitch (after closure of the secondary defect) demonstrating alignment of the leading flap edge to close the primary defect. **(d)** Immediate postoperative appearance (anterior view). **(e)** Immediate postoperative appearance (worm's eye view). The alar rim lift and slight notching is temporary in these flaps, if properly executed, and typically resolve over several weeks. (These images are provided courtesy of Stanislav N. Tolkachjov, MD.)

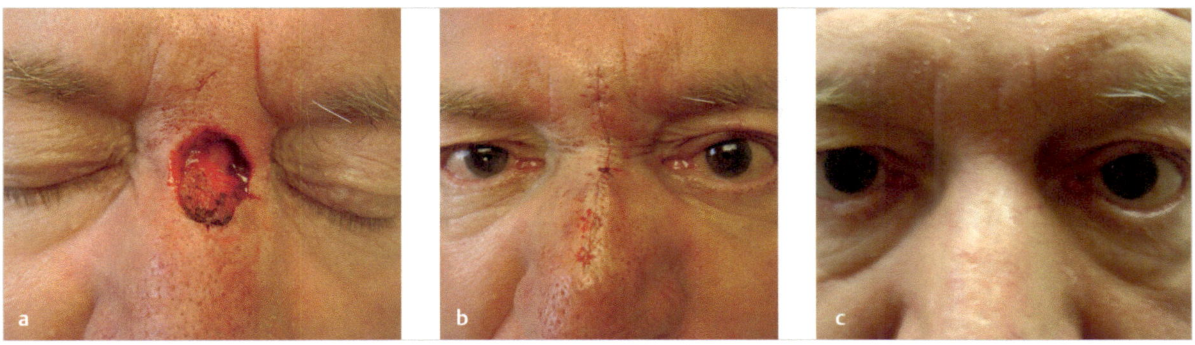

Fig. 3.21 **(a)** Defect on the nasal dorsum/root area. **(b)** Primary closure. **(c)** Results at 3 months.

full-thickness midline defects (▶ Fig. 3.21). Defects where size may seem to initially preclude use of primary closure can often be closed after extensive undermining to recruit lax skin on the bilateral nasal sidewalls, offering the advantage of excellent color and texture match. For defects on the lateral nasal dorsum where primary closure runs the risk of alar retraction, a local flap is preferred. The various options for these defects will be discussed in Chapter 3.8.

Very large defects on the nasal dorsum that cannot be satisfactorily closed using adjacent skin can be closed using a full-thickness skin graft (▶ Fig. 3.22) or an FHF. A postauricular donor site is preferred as it provides an

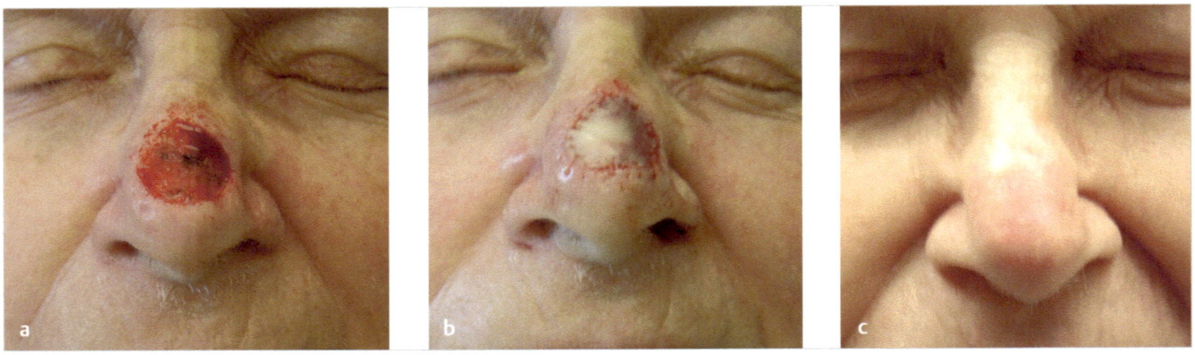

Fig. 3.22 **(a)** Defect on a 69-year-old man. **(b)** Repair with a full-thickness skin graft harvested from the postauricular sulcus. **(c)** Results at 3 months.

excellent match for the thinner skin of the upper two-thirds of the nose. The donor site is closed primarily in the sulcus leaving a nearly imperceptible scar. When defects are too large for a postauricular donor site, the supraclavicular fossa is preferred.

3.7 Nasal Root/Lower Glabella

Due to its concave nature, small to medium-sized defects on the nasal root can heal wonderfully by second intention. For a deeper defect, second intention is still a good option; however, there is often enough laxity for a primary closure. For nonmidline defects, when executing a fusiform repair, the ellipse is oriented obliquely toward the inner canthus.

One situation in our experience where repair with a full-thickness skin graft is preferred over flap is for larger wounds of the nasal root area. Grafts in this area frequently yield excellent results, more so than grafts in other areas. Further, the propensity of flaps to cause webbing, contour deformity, and distortion in this area often makes grafts the better repair choice. Again, a postauricular donor site is preferred.

3.8 Nasal Sidewall

Like the other subunits of the nose, superficial wounds can heal by second intention, often in conjunction with the shave and sand technique. Small, full-thickness wounds can be closed primarily, with the ellipse oriented obliquely, running parallel to a line extending from the nasal tip to the inner canthus. Closing larger wounds on the nasal sidewall in a fusiform fashion runs the risk of ipsilateral alar retraction, and thus should be avoided. Instead, large defects are optimally repaired with the local transposition flap.

3.8.1 Rhombic Transposition Flap

The rhombic flap is our "workhorse" for repairing small to medium-sized defects less than 1.5 cm on the nasal sidewall due to its reliability, efficiency, and cosmetic elegance (▶ Fig. 3.23).[20] In the majority of cases, the laxity of the superior nasal sidewall supports using an inferior base. Small to medium-sized defect on the lower sidewall may necessitate use of a bilobed flap in order to draw from the reservoir of lax skin on the superior sidewall.

Design

Like the bilobed flap, the most crucial design aspect of the rhombic flap is vertical orientation of the donor site. Vertical orientation will prevent pull on the ala when closing the donor site. The donor site is drawn with its apex less than 30 degrees, and its width should equal the vertical diameter of the defect. The Burow's triangle is drawn with its superior arm parallel to the arm of the flap that in not connected to the defect.

Execution

The flap is incised and undermined widely in a submuscular plane. The donor site is closed first, followed by the Burow's triangle. Once the remainder of the flap is secured, the flap is trimmed to fit the size of the defect. While some advocate extending the defect to fit the angulated flap, we favor conserving normal tissue, and find no difference in the ultimate aesthetic appearance as long as excellent suture technique is employed.

3.8.2 Superior-Based Bilobed Flap

For vertically oriented ovoid defects on the lateral nasal dorsum or the anterior nasal sidewall, we occasionally will perform a superior-based bilobed flap.[21] The vertical orientation of the defect may preclude the use of a rhombic flap, as a significantly larger flap must be designed in order to situate the donor site perpendicular to the ala. The particular use of a bilobed flap in this area utilizes lax cheek skin as a reservoir, similar to the single-stage nasolabial flap.

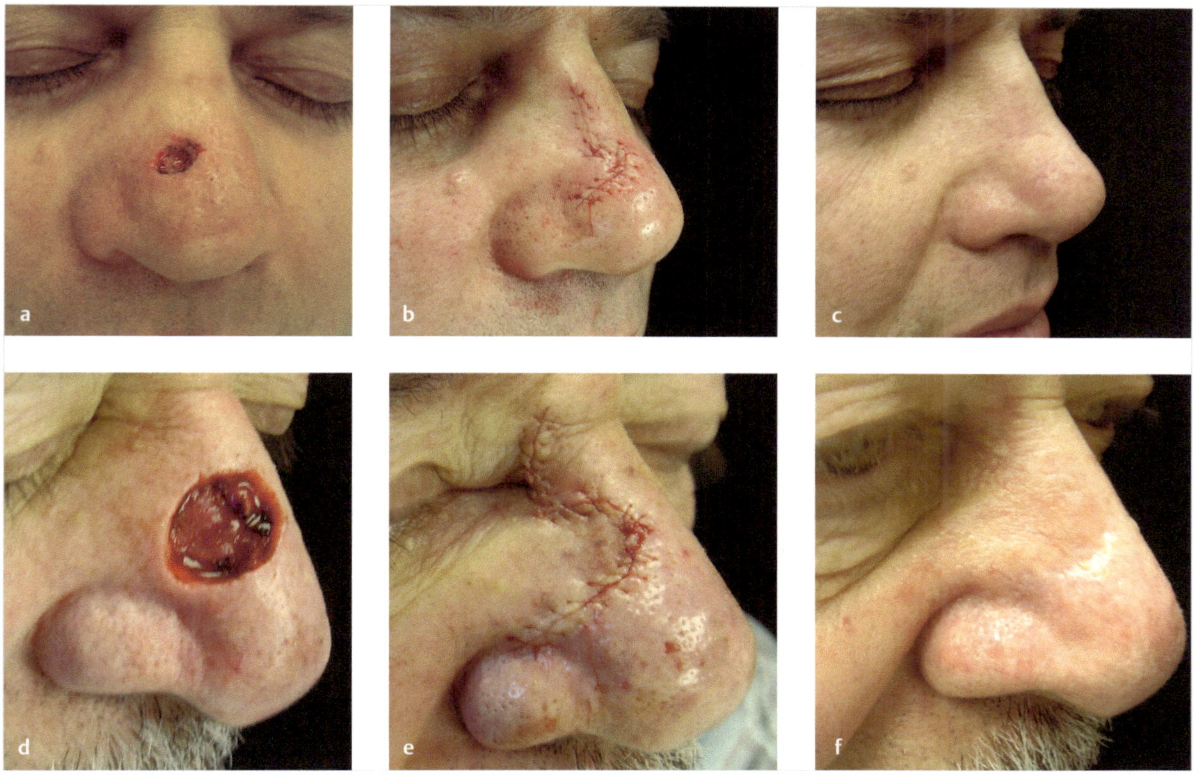

Fig. 3.23 **(a)** Defect in a 39-year-old man. **(b)** Repair with rhombic transposition flap. **(c)** Results at 3 months. **(d)** Defect in a 63-year-old man. **(e)** Repair with rhombic transposition flap. **(f)** Results at 3 months.

3.8.3 Lateral-Based Rotation Flap/ Crescentic Advancement Flap/Cheek-Based Burow's Advancement Flap

For the editors, nasal sidewall defects that are distal but do not cross the alar groove can also be repaired nicely with a lateral-based rotation flap that recruits laxity from the medial cheek. The flap is designed along the alar groove and lengthened out on to the cheek a distance equal to the diameter of the defect superior to the defect. Superior to the defect a Burow's triangle is removed. The key stitch should be placed at the nasal tip crease and close the defect from side to side. The second stitch is placed in the proximal alar groove and starts with a bite in the floor to become a three-point stitch and lifts up the collapsed nasal valve. As the remainder of the donor site is closed, care must be taken to inset the cheek skin edge and prevent blunting of the alar groove.

3.8.4 V-Y Flap

In some patients, the portion of the mid-nasal sidewall that extends into the nasofacial sulcus can do so with a slight convexity or hump. Defects of 1 to 2 cm situated in this location or even more proximal encroaching the medial canthus can be nicely repaired with a V-Y flap that recruits skin from the medial cheek.

Design

The flap is designed as a V extending inferolaterally from the defect. The proximal portion of the flap is the same width as the defect and tapers to a 30-degree angle—staying above the melolabial fold.

Execution

The incision of the flap is extended into the deep subcutaneous tissue. As with any island pedicle flap, the pedicle is lengthened by blunt/sharp dissection downward and turning laterally so as to also undermine the tissue on either side of the donor site. Once hemostasis is achieved, the proximal edge of the flap is advanced in a superior direction onto the nasal sidewall. As it is advanced, it can be rotated to meet the opposite side of the defect in such a way to keep the primary tissue movement vector horizontal and not pull down on the eyelids. The corners of the leading edge of the flap are trimmed to match the shape of the defect. The remainder of the flap and the donor site can be closed with buried vertical

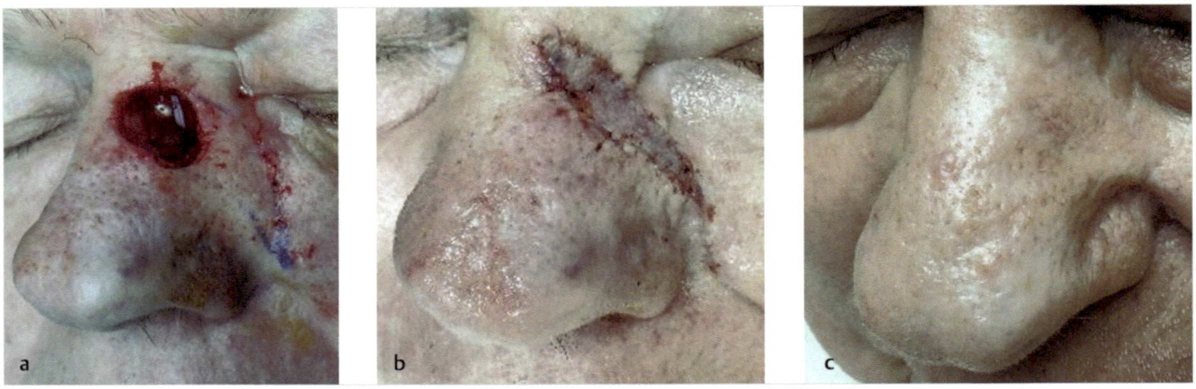

Fig. 3.24 Nasal sidewall V-Y advancement flap. **(a)** Proximal to mid-nasal sidewall defect. **(b)** V-Y advancement flap sewn into place. Notice suturing from flap to base set the flap edge lower than the base in order to account for likely natural pincushioning of this flap even with wide undermining. **(c)** Eight-month follow-up. (These images are provided courtesy of Stanislav N. Tolkachjov, MD.)

mattress sutures and 6–0 fast-absorbing suture on the surface (▶ Fig. 3.24).

3.8.5 Single-Stage Nasolabial Flap

Defects measuring greater than 1.5 cm on the lateral or inferior portion of the lateral sidewall are readily repaired with a nasolabial transposition flap (▶ Video 3.5). The nasolabial flap is a superior-based transposition flap that utilizes lax cheek skin as a donor reservoir. Perforating defects and those that obliterate the alar rim can also be repaired with a nasolabial flap. The flap provides an excellent color and texture match for the missing nasal skin, and the scar is well-hidden within the melolabial fold. Although it is a transposition flap by definition in that the flap is transposed over the lateral ala, the sliding advancement of the cheek allows the nasal portion of the flap to be closed under minimal tension. However, for wounds that are greater than 2.5 cm or patients without abundant cheek laxity, an alternative repair should be chosen. Modifications of the nasolabial flap have simplified the its design and execution, precluding the need for a second stage and minimizing the standing cone deformity and trapdoor phenomenon that classically result from the original design.

Design

The medial arm of the flap starts at the midpoint of the lateral aspect of the defect and descends along the melolabial fold. Importantly, this incision should not transect the apical triangle as this is an important structure that should be preserved. The lateral arm of the flap should extend higher than the point of transposition over the lateral ala, and the width of the flap should match exactly the width of the defect. A Burow's triangle is drawn superiorly above the defect with its apex less than 30 degrees and directed toward the medial canthus (▶ Fig. 3.25a).

Execution

The flap is incised down to subcutis and undermined widely to facilitate formation of a platelike scar. Success of the flap is contingent on placement of four key periosteal sutures (▶ Fig. 3.25b), which maintain contour and relieve tension on the flap. The initial periosteal suture connects that lateral aspect of the cheek wound to the lateral alar crease at the apex of the apical triangle of the lip, reforming the contour of the melolabial fold and relieving tension on closure of the donor site. This suture has been deemed one that "separates the men and women from the boys and girls" as its successful placement deep in the alar crease requires significant technical expertise. The remainder of the donor site can then be closed in a layered fashion. The second periosteal suture is placed in the nasofacial sulcus to prevent tenting that would otherwise occur. The suture is placed from the nasofacial sulcus to a point at the base of the flap approximately 1 cm superior to the alar crease. Like the first key suture, this one also relieves tension on the advancing flap. At this point, the flap should be thinned and defatted. Any fat remaining on the underside of the flap will fibrose and contract and contribute to the trapdoor phenomenon; therefore, "fat is your enemy." The third periosteal suture is placed at the anterior distal aspect of the flap in order to direct closure tension in a horizontal direction and mitigate pulling on the ala that would otherwise occur. The last key periosteal suture is placed connecting the distal aspect of the flap to the alar crease, which has two purposes. First, this suture recreates the alar crease that would otherwise be blunted without its placement. Second, this suture stents open the nasal valve that collapses when there is wounding in this area. Once the periosteal sutures have been placed, the distal aspect of the flap can be amputated, and the remainder of the flap sewn in slightly concave from the adjacent wound edges in a layered fashion. ▶ Fig. 3.25c, d depicts a defect suitable for this flap with immediate postoperative results.

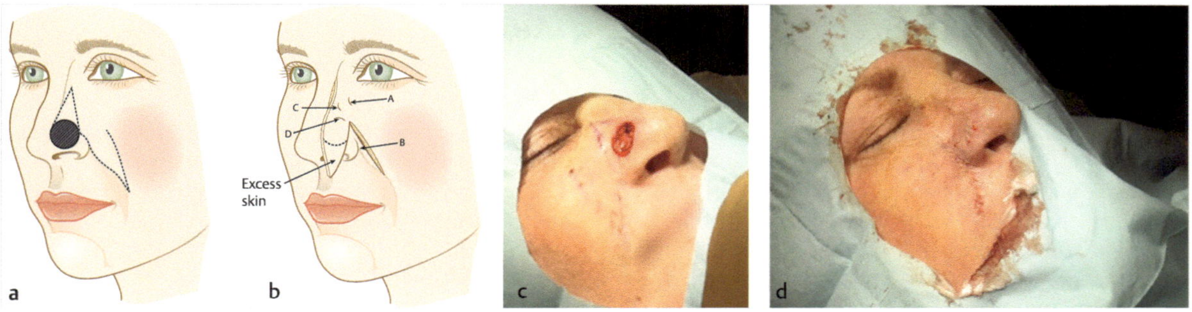

Fig. 3.25 **(a)** Design of the single-stage nasolabial flap. **(b)** Four key periosteal tacking sutures crucial for flap's success. **(c, d)** Pre- and post-op photos of nasolabial flaps.

3.9 Complications and Revisions

While complications are sometimes inevitable, the vast majority can often be avoided with careful planning, execution, and meticulous attention to surgical technique. Pincushioning, a common complication during nasal reco- nstruction, can be prevented if one exactly matches the primary flap lobes and grafts to the size of the defect, performs wide undermining to promote formation of a platelike scar, defats flaps to prevent fat fibrosis, and uses buried vertical mattress sutures to pull deep tissues back to suture line.

In the first few months postoperatively, it is important to suppress the urge to overcorrect any flap irregularities, remembering that it takes a full year for scars to fully mature. For example, flaps have the tendency to retain fluid due to the disruption of lymphatics. Compression of the flap that reduces flap "puffiness" can highlight this phenomenon. Collateral lymphatic channels eventually reform, which can be hastened by instructing patients to perform vigorous scar massage starting 1 month postoperatively. Visible incision lines or contour asymmetry can be corrected with dermabrasion. We typically perform this at a minimum of 3 months postoperatively. As mentioned previously, we always inform the patient of the need for dermabrasion at the time of surgery so that it does not appear later that dermabrasion is suggested as a cover-up for surgical incompetence. Persistent flap fullness may necessitate use of intralesional triamcinolone at a strength of 40 mg/mL. If no improvement is observed with this intervention, the flap may need to be elevated and thinned of scar and subcutaneous tissue.

References

[1] Burget GC, Menick FJ. The subunit principle in nasal reconstruction. Plast Reconstr Surg. 1985; 76(2):239–247
[2] Zitelli JA. Wound healing by secondary intention. A cosmetic appraisal. J Am Acad Dermatol. 1983; 9(3):407–415
[3] Cook J, Zitelli JA. Primary closure for midline defects of the nose: a simple approach for reconstruction. J Am Acad Dermatol. 2000; 43 (3):508–510
[4] Zitelli JA, Moy RL. Buried vertical mattress suture. J Dermatol Surg Oncol. 1989; 15(1):17–19
[5] Goldberg LH, Alam M. Horizontal advancement flap for symmetric reconstruction of small to medium-sized cutaneous defects of the lateral nasal supratip. J Am Acad Dermatol. 2003; 49(4):685–689
[6] Zitelli JA. The bilobed flap for nasal reconstruction. Arch Dermatol. 1989; 125(7):957–959
[7] Rieger RA. A local flap for repair of the nasal tip. Plast Reconstr Surg. 1967; 40(2):147–149
[8] Cook J, Zitell JA. Axial pattern flaps. In: Robinson JK, Hanke CW, Sengelmann RD, Siegel DM, eds. Surgery of the Skin: Procedural Dermatology. Philadelphia, PA: Mosby; 2005:311–343
[9] Brodland DG. Paramedian forehead flap reconstruction for nasal defects. Dermatol Surg. 2005; 31(8, Pt 2):1046–1052
[10] Menick FJ. Aesthetic refinements in use of forehead for nasal reconstruction: the paramedian forehead flap. Clin Plast Surg. 1990; 17 (4):607–622
[11] Stigall LE, Bramlette TB, Zitelli JA, Brodland DG. The paramidline forehead flap: a clinical and microanatomic study. Dermatol Surg. 2016; 42(6):764–771
[12] MCFARLANE RM, HEAGY FC, RADIN S, AUST JC, WERMUTH RE. A study of the delay phenomenon in experimental pedicle flaps. Plast Reconstr Surg. 1965; 35:245–262
[13] Rohrer TE, Dzubow LM. Conchal bowl skin grafting in nasal tip reconstruction: clinical and histologic evaluation. J Am Acad Dermatol. 1995; 33(3):476–481
[14] Portuese W, Stucker F, Grafton W, Shockley W, Gage-White L. Perichondrial cutaneous graft. An alternative in composite skin grafting. Arch Otolaryngol Head Neck Surg. 1989; 115(6):705–709
[15] Tolkachjov SN, Harmon CB. How we do it: dermabrasion as a primary reconstruction option for nasal defects. Dermatol Surg. 2019; 45 (4):627–630
[16] Mahlberg MJ, Leach BC, Cook J. The spiral flap for nasal alar reconstruction: our experience with 63 patients. Dermatol Surg. 2012; 38 (3):373–380
[17] Spear SL, Kroll SS, Romm S. A new twist to the nasolabial flap for reconstruction of lateral alar defects. Plast Reconstr Surg. 1987; 79 (6):915–920
[18] Zitelli JA. Repair of the soft triangle of the nose. J Dermatol Surg Oncol. 1994; 20(12):839–841
[19] Benoit A, Hollmig ST, Leach BC. The nasal tip rotation flap for reconstruction of the lateral nasal tip, anterior ala, and soft triangle: the authors' experience with 55 patients. Dermatol Surg. 2017; 43 (10):1221–1232
[20] Zitelli JA, Fazio MJ. Reconstruction of the nose with local flaps. J Dermatol Surg Oncol. 1991; 17(2):184–189
[21] Kelly-Sell M, Hollmig ST, Cook J. The superiorly based bilobed flap for nasal reconstruction. J Am Acad Dermatol. 2018; 78(2):370–376

4 Forehead and Temple Reconstruction

Joseph F. Sobanko, Ashwin Agarwal, and Christopher J. Miller

Abstract

The forehead and temple are upper facial subunits readily visible to onlookers. Disruption of brow position and symmetry or interruption of the smooth transition from the slightly convex forehead to the mildly concave temple can be distracting. Successful forehead and temple reconstruction accounts for these anatomic relationships. Reconstruction must also strive to preserve motor and sensory function. This chapter reviews the relevant anatomy and proposes a systematic approach to repairing forehead and temple soft-tissue defects.

Keywords: forehead, temple, eyebrow, reconstruction, flap, graft

Capsule Summary and Pearls

- Preservation of the subdermal plexus of vascular anastomoses increases the viability of local flaps.
- The supraorbital nerve is vulnerable to injury at the mid-pupillary line bilaterally at distances of 1 cm and greater above the superior orbital rim. In this region, the surgeon may attempt to undermine superficially above the frontalis muscle with blunt separation of tissue.
- Consider designing midline and paramedian excisions with a vertical orientation in order to avoid supratrochlear nerve (STN) and supraorbital nerve (SON) transection. A vertical incision also allows undermining deep to the frontalis muscle, preservation of the nerves and vessels on the superficial surface of the muscle, and potential perpendicular tension to muscle movement of this area.
- Dissect superficial to the superficial temporal fascia to preserve the temporal branch of the facial nerve.

4.1 Forehead and Temple Anatomy

4.1.1 Boundaries of the Forehead and Temple Subunits

The forehead has a rectangular shape bounded superiorly by the frontal hairline, caudally by the nasal root and eyebrows, and laterally by the bony prominences of the temporal crest. The upper forehead has a shinier texture with thinner dermis and fewer sebaceous glands than the lower forehead.[1] Fibrous connections tether the dermis of the forehead skin to the underlying frontalis muscle and limit mobility.

The temple, on the other hand, has a triangular shape with its base at the zygomatic arch, a medial limb along the orbital rim and temporal crest, and a lateral limb at the temporal hairline. The skin of the temple has dermal thickness and sebaceous gland density similar to the upper forehead, but it is more mobile due to looser connections with the underlying superficial temporal fascia.

4.1.2 Muscles of the Forehead and Temple

The forehead has four underlying muscles of facial expression: the frontalis, procerus, the corrugator supercilii, and superior portions of the orbicularis oculi. The frontalis muscle originates at the anterior portion of the galea aponeurotica of the scalp and inserts into the subcutaneous tissue and skin of the lower forehead and brows. Its fibers also interdigitate with the procerus, corrugator supercilii, and orbicularis oculi muscles. As the galea descends from the scalp, it splits to invest the frontalis muscle with fascia on its superficial and deep surfaces. Contraction of the frontalis muscle raises the eyebrows and produces horizontal rhytides or relaxed skin tension lines (RSTLs). The procerus muscle originates on the nasal bone and inserts on the frontalis muscle. Contraction of the procerus draws down the medial angle of the eyebrows and creates transverse rhytides at the nasal root. The corrugator supercilii muscles have their origins at the medial end of the superciliary arch and insert on the skin of the medial brows. They reside deep to the frontalis muscle. Contraction of the corrugator supercilii muscles pulls the brow inferiorly and medially and creates oblique rhytides between the brow and the glabella. The superior aspects of the orbicularis oculi muscles, which serve to close the eyelids forcefully, lay superficial to the frontalis muscle.

There are no muscles of facial expression specific to the temple. The superficial temporal fascia, which is continuous with the frontalis muscle, lies deep to the subcutaneous fat of the temple and separates the skin from the underlying temporalis muscle. Because of this, contraction of the temporalis during mastication does not create overlying rhytides. Instead, RSTLs on the temple occur from contraction of the adjacent orbicularis oculi and frontalis muscles. Radial rhytides on temple skin are a result of dynamic muscle activity of the orbicularis oculi muscle.

In both the forehead and temple cosmetic units, actinic damage, age, and muscle use contribute to the permanent etching of rhytides, even at rest, consequently providing convenient sites to hide surgical incisions.

4.1.3 Blood Supply to the Forehead and Temple

The internal carotid artery supplies blood to the forehead via the paired supratrochlear and supraorbital arteries. These vessels share numerous anastomoses as they course cephalically in the subcutaneous fat of the forehead. Pushing the forehead skin toward the midline creates vertical and oblique wrinkles corresponding to the path of the underlying arteries in the glabellar region.

The supratrochlear artery is a terminal branch of the ophthalmic artery from the internal carotid arterial system. It exits the orbit by piercing the orbital septum at the superomedial orbital rim within 5 mm to a vertical line drawn at the medial canthus.[2] Its pulse can be palpated at its exit point found approximately 12 mm (range: 10.2–14.5 mm) superior to the medial canthus.[3] It has mean diameter of 0.9 mm.[3] Some surgeons use this landmark and even ultrasound to identify the supratrochlear artery for the formation of the paramedian forehead flap.

After emerging from the septum, the supratrochlear artery travels superficial to the periosteum and corrugator supercilii muscle and deep to the orbicularis oculi and frontalis muscles.[4] It pierces the orbicularis oculi and frontalis muscles to reach the subcutaneous fat between 10 and 25 mm superior to the supraorbital rim.[2,5] On the lower forehead, the artery and its branches travel in the deep subcutaneous fat closer to the frontalis muscle.[2,5] On the upper two-thirds of the forehead, the artery approaches the dermis as it courses cranially past the junction of the sagittal and coronal sutures at the top of the skull.[6] Along its course, the supratrochlear artery has branches that communicate with numerous vessels, including the angular, supraorbital, paracentral, and central arteries.[2]

The surgeon can utilize topographic landmarks to identify the course of the supratrochlear artery. The most prominent glabellar frown line corresponds to the junction of the medial corrugator and procerus muscles, and can be accentuated by pushing the medial brows inferomedially toward the midline.[7] The supratrochlear artery is located anywhere from this glabellar frown line to 6 mm laterally.[7]

The supraorbital artery exits the orbit through a foramen or notch 30 mm lateral to the midline and has a mean diameter of 0.84 mm. It enters the corrugator supercilii muscles and divides into superficial and deep branches, most commonly at the level of the supraorbital rim. The superficial branches travel through the corrugator, orbicularis oculi, and frontalis muscles before becoming superficial to the frontalis. It pierces the frontalis muscle approximately 30 mm above the supraorbital rim and transitions to the subcutaneous fat between 40 and 60 mm above the rim to reach the superior third of the forehead. The supraorbital artery gives an average of two to four superficial branches that supply the frontalis muscle.[8]

The deep branches of the supraorbital artery arise at the level of the supraorbital rim and travel cranially just above the periosteum and within deep layers of the subgaleal fascia to perfuse the pericranium and fascia. Flaps designed in this area and undermined in a subgaleal plane just beneath the frontalis muscle can preserve these deep branches of the supraorbital artery by elevating muscle but leaving down the loose areolar connective tissue atop the periosteum.

Of note, the supraorbital and supratrochlear arteries share many rich anastomoses across the medial and lateral forehead as they travel cranially to the scalp. They form a vascular arcade across the glabellar and nasal regions via connections with the bilateral angular arteries of the central face. Further, a supraorbital plexus approximately 3 mm above the supraorbital rim connects the supraorbital, supratrochlear, and dorsal nasal arteries from the nasal sidewall.[6] Anastomoses also exist between distal deep branches of the supraorbital artery and the superficial temporal artery.

The temple subunit is similarly perfused by an anastomotic vascular network. Temporal skin and superficial temporal fascia are supplied by branches of the zygomatico-orbital, zygomaticotemporal, zygomaticofacial, and transverse facial arteries, all of which originate from the superficial temporal artery of the external carotid system. This network communicates with the deep temporalis fascia via perpendicular penetrating vessels.

Surgery Pearl

Preservation of the subdermal plexus of vascular anastomoses increases the viability of local flaps.

4.2 Preservation of Sensory and Motor Function

4.2.1 Sensory Function

The STN and SON of the ophthalmic division (V1) of the trigeminal sensory nerve (cranial nerve [CN] V) provide sensation to the forehead and frontal scalp. An understanding of the location and course of the SON and STN is important for dermatologic surgeons, as surgery or reconstruction in this area can lead to transection that results in paresthesias, pruritus, or traumatic neuroma formation.[9] Nerve injury leads to anesthesia extending in a column from the point of injury to the frontal scalp, although nerve regrowth and collateral formation may restore sensation months later.

The frontal nerve of CN V1 divides within the orbits into the SON and the STN after passing through the superior orbital fissure. The SON innervates the upper eyelid, forehead, frontoparietal, and vertex scalp, and emerges through a supraorbital notch or foramen on average around 4 mm above the superior orbital rim[9] and approximately

2.6 cm from the midline. A vertical line drawn superiorly from the pupil is one method of mapping the path of the nerve. The SON then divides a few millimeters above the orbital rim into a superficial and a deep branch. The superficial branch courses through the corrugator supercilia before eventually traveling beneath the frontalis muscle. Many smaller branches emerge from this superficial branch and pierce the frontalis muscle in a fanlike distribution at around 2.6 cm above the superior orbital rim to innervate the forehead. The medial branches of this superficial SON branch cross-innervate a shared territory with the STN.[9] Meanwhile, the deep branch of the SON courses more laterally after emerging from the supraorbital rim and remains subgaleal, deep to both the frontalis and the corrugators to innervate the vertex and frontoparietal scalp. Careless undermining below the frontalis muscle can injure this nerve branch and affect sensation to the frontal and vertex scalp. Forehead sensation will remain intact as the superficial branch does not travel below the galea.

Surgery Pearl

The SON is vulnerable to injury at the mid-pupillary line bilaterally at distances of 1 cm and greater above the superior orbital rim. In this region, the surgeon may attempt to undermine superficially above the frontalis muscle with blunt separation of tissue.

The more medially located STN provides sensation to the skin and underlying tissue of the glabella, lower forehead, upper eyelid, and conjunctiva. It exits the orbit through the frontal notch or foramen approximately 4 mm cranial to the superior orbital rim and 18 mm from the midline. The STN then travels cranially approximately 1.6 cm from midline.[10] To avoid transection, a similar anatomic danger zone can be considered in an area spanning 3 cm across the glabellar midline. After emerging from the orbit, the nerve separates into two branches within the retro-orbicularis oculi fat before penetrating the corrugator and branching into multiple smaller endings.

Surgery Pearl

Consider designing midline and paramedian excisions with a vertical orientation in order to avoid STN and SON transection. The vertical incision also allows undermining deep to the frontalis muscle and preservation of the nerves and vessels on the superficial surface of the muscle.

Sensation to the lateral forehead and temple is provided by the zygomaticotemporal, zygomaticofacial, and auriculotemporal nerve branches of the trigeminal nerve. Both the zygomaticotemporal and the zygomaticofacial nerve originate from the zygomatic nerve of the maxillary division (V2) of CN V as they branch at the level of the lateral orbit. The zygomaticotemporal nerve courses through the zygomaticotemporal foramen to enter the temporal fossa and finally emerges approximately 22 mm above the zygomatic arch to innervate the lateral forehead and temple.[11] During its course, it also communicates with the zygomaticofacial and auriculotemporal nerves.

The auriculotemporal nerve contributes to innervation of the posterior temple. It courses over the posterior zygomatic arch, posterior to the temporomandibular joint, and then travels cranially within the temporoparietal fascia anterior to the external auditory canal. For much of its path, the auriculotemporal nerve can be found in proximity to the superficial temporal artery. Moving cephalad, both the auriculotemporal nerve and the superficial temporal artery become superficial to the superficial temporal fascia.[11] The superficial temporal branch is the terminal ending that innervates temple skin, and emerges at a distance from the tragus of approximately 15 mm cranially and 7.5 mm medially.[12]

4.2.2 Motor Function

The temporal branch of facial nerve provides motor function to the frontalis muscle, the upper portion of the orbicularis oculi muscle, corrugator supercilii, and temporoparietalis muscles. In most patients, it is the single innervating branch to the frontalis muscle. Injury to the temporal nerve results in ptosis of the skin of the brow and upper eyelid with noticeable facial asymmetry and potential obstruction of the superior visual field. The facial nerve (CNVII) travels through the temporal bone of the skull before it exits the stylomastoid foramen and delivers the posterior auricular branch behind the ear. It will emerge from the parotid gland approximately 2.5 cm anterior to the tragus. The temporal nerve then runs obliquely 1.5 cm lateral to the lateral orbital rim and deep to the superficial temporal fascia before innervating the lateral undersurface of the frontalis muscles.

Drawing a line from 0.5 cm below the tragus to 1.5 cm above the lateral brow approximates the course of the underlying nerve.[13] In this region, the nerve is most at risk of transection after exiting the parotid gland and traveling just below and over the middle zygomatic arch, where it is protected only by thin overlying superficial temporal fascia through the temple and lateral forehead.[14] Usually the facial nerve branches run between the superficial musculoaponeurotic system (SMAS) and the deep muscular fascia, and are therefore susceptible to injury in areas without overlying muscle. Undermining superficial to the superficial temporal fascia protects the temporal branch of the facial nerve.

Surgery Pearl

Dissect superficial to the superficial temporal fascia to preserve the temporal branch of the facial nerve.

4.3 Achieving Reproducibly Excellent Cosmetic Results

Adhering to key principles optimizes outcomes for forehead and temple reconstruction. Preserving the position and symmetry of the eyelids and brows is paramount. Restoring contour to the normally smooth surfaces of the forehead and temples is equally important. Hiding incisions along the cosmetic subunit boundaries and RSTLs of the hairline, brow, and orbital rim improves cosmesis. However, these incisions must not compromise free margin position or skin contour. Horizontally oriented linear closures on the forehead might align with RSTLs, but they may also cause ipsilateral and asymmetric brow elevation, especially for defects closer to the brow. Following these principles with sound surgical technique minimizes the visibility of forehead and temple scars.

Box 4.1 General Principles of Forehead and Temple Reconstruction

1. Maintain natural position of brow and eyelids.
2. Preserve contour of cosmetic subunits.
3. Align scars with cosmetic subunit boundaries of the hair and brow or in horizontally oriented RSTLs if free margin position can be preserved.
4. Oblique scars, skin grafts, and displaced eyebrows may lead to conspicuous results.
5. Recruitment of skin for flaps of the forehead will be from lateral to medial; for recruitment of skin for the temple, it is often inferior to superior from the cheek.
6. Postoperative staged revisions may be necessary for optimal cosmetic results.

4.4 Evaluating Wounds on the Forehead and Temple

Box 4.2 Prereconstruction Considerations

1. What is the location of the defect within or across cosmetic subunits?
2. What structures are exposed by defect (e.g., subcutaneous tissue, fascia, and periosteum)?
3. Are there special structures and free margins that need to be preserved (e.g., eyebrow)?
4. Are there risk factors for poor healing (e.g., prior radiation, current tobacco use, etc.)?

A systematic approach to evaluating forehead and temple wounds guides selection of the optimal reconstruction. First, determine the missing anatomic structures and decide what structures can be preserved or need replacement. For example, wounds extending to the subcutaneous fat may heal by second intention or allow reconstruction that preserves sensory nerves. If the frontalis muscle has been removed, then wound closure will offer better contour than second intention healing. Additionally, if periosteum is missing, then the wound bed will not support a skin graft.

After taking such anatomic considerations into account, push the wound edges toward each other to see if they approximate. If so, primary linear closure or a sliding flap offers the most reproducible results. Next, observe the effect of various tension vectors on the nearby free margins of the brow and eyelid, and choose a tension vector that preserves their position and contour. On the forehead, particularly for defects near the brow, most reconstructions recruit skin from lateral to medial along a horizontal vector to avoid elevating the brow. On the temple, the preferred tension vector is usually vertical, recruiting skin from inferior to superior. Subsequently, assess opportunities to hide scars in cosmetic subunit junction lines along the brow and hairline or in RSTLs. Consider extending wounds to the edges of the hair or brow to disguise scars. Also, take into account patient history of poor wound healing and donor skin quality (e.g., prior radiation) to predict the impact of closure tension on wound healing. Finally, choose surgical materials appropriate for the wound (Box 4.3 (p. 69)).

Box 4.3 Selection of Intraoperative Materials

1. Forehead wounds that extend through the frontalis and expose periosteum benefit from reapproximation of the frontalis muscle. 2–0 or 3–0 braided suture assists with closure of this layer (PS-4 needle facilitates movement of suture).
2. 4–0 long-acting monofilament suture is used for dermal buried vertical mattress sutures on the forehead and temple.
3. 5–0 monofilament sutures may be used for dermal buried vertical mattress sutures on thin temple skin and when approaching the lateral canthal skin.
4. 5–0 or 6–0 nonabsorbable or fast-absorbing suture may be used for the cuticular layer.

4.5 Reconstruction Options for the Forehead and Temple

This section will review different options for forehead and temple reconstruction.

Box 4.4 Suggested Guidelines for Temple and Forehead Reconstruction

1. Evaluate the depth and location of the wound.
2. Design a closure that preserves symmetry and position of the eyebrows and eyelids.
3. Place incisions in cosmetic junction borders and RSTLs whenever possible.
4. Minimize wound closure tension.

4.5.1 Second Intention

Second intention healing is a helpful approach for partial-thickness defects on the upper forehead and temple for patients who prefer to avoid surgical reconstruction. Second intention healing produces shiny, sometimes hypopigmented, scars. Healed skin may camouflage well in patients with lighter complexions with minimal photodamage. Since the wounds heal by keratinocytes migrating inward with associated centrifugal contraction, larger defects adjacent to free margins such as the eyebrows may not be ideal candidates for granulation. Tissue composition also influences the success of second intention healing. For example, granulation on the lower forehead can produce visibly shiny scars that compare poorly with adjacent sebaceous skin. Second intention healing can preserve skin contour if the defect selected to heal is relatively superficial (e.g., above frontalis muscle). Patients should be counseled that scar erythema can take many months to fade. A common example where a forehead defect is allowed to heal on its own is in patients undergoing forehead flap reconstruction. Second intention healing of the donor site mitigates excessive incisional tension and frequently heals well because of its cephalic position on the forehead (▶ Fig. 4.1).

If a forehead or temple wound is too large for a linear closure or a local flap, partial closure and second intention healing of the shrunken defect is another consideration to mitigate excessive incisional tension. This offers the surgeon and patient an opportunity for a staged excision. After 3 to 6 months from the initial closure, the second intention wound that re-epithelialized may be excised to produce a less perceptible scar (▶ Fig. 4.2).

4.5.2 Linear Closure

Linear closure with side-to-side approximation of wound edges remains the workhorse repair for forehead and temple defects. Skin laxity varies among patients and by location in these cosmetic units, so pushing the wound edges together will determine if fusiform closure is possible. On the forehead, linear closures may be oriented horizontally or vertically. Horizontal linear closures should aim to place scars within RSTLs or at subunit junctions. Caution must be taken to avoid elevation of the brow, especially with lower forehead defects. Brow elevation of up to 1 cm may return to normal position over time, but patients may not appreciate prolonged asymmetry (▶ Fig. 4.3). Horizontal linear closures extending through the frontalis muscle risk transecting several branches of the STN and SON. This is likely to result in bothersome band of numbness extending to the scalp that may take up to a year to resolve. Vertical linear closures do not conform toRSTLs but may be the preferred option to prevent brow elevation and preserve natural contour (▶ Fig. 4.4, ▶ Fig. 4.5). Vertical closures run parallel to the sensory nerves and also provide the added benefit of maximal sensation preservation. Vertical closures in the central and paramedian forehead allow undermining deep to the frontalis muscle with minimal threat to sensory nerves.

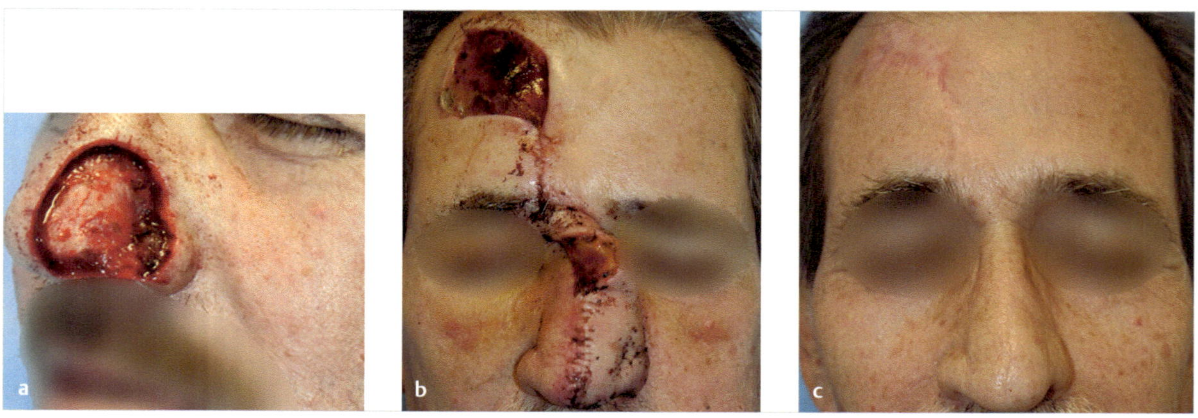

Fig. 4.1 Second intention healing. **(a)** Nasal tip/sidewall/ala defect. **(b)** Repair with a two-stage paramedian forehead flap elevated between dermis and frontalis muscle. Donor site defect allowed to heal by second intention above frontalis in order to reduce closure tension. **(c)** Four-month postoperative result. The forehead donor site has healed. If patients do not prefer the shinier textured skin, a staged excision of this smaller scar can be performed.

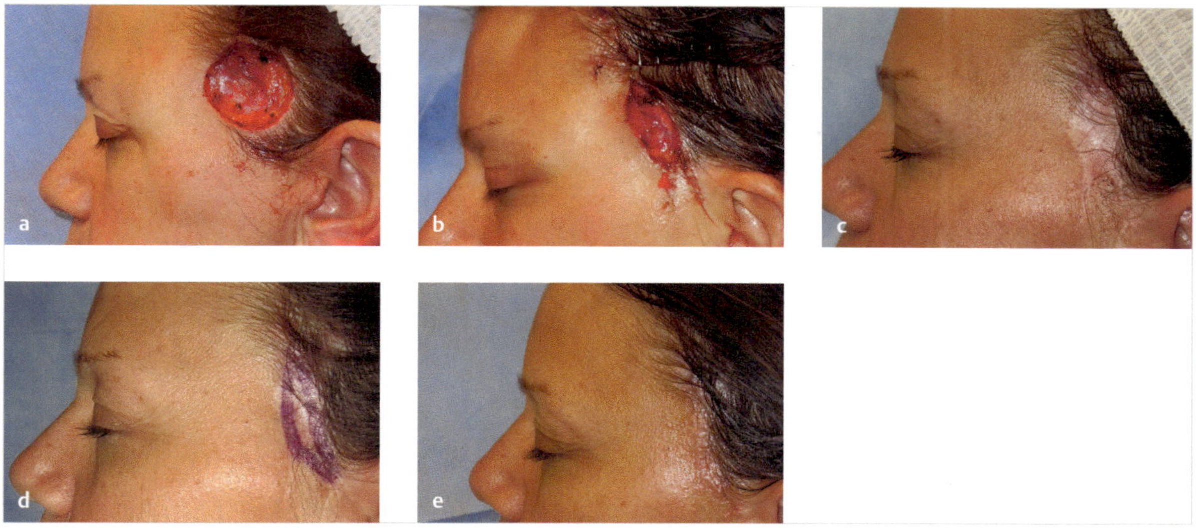

Fig. 4.2 Staged excision after second intention healing. **(a)** Original temple Mohs defect. **(b)** Partially closed defect with advancement flap. Given the large size of the defect, the center of the wound left to heal by secondary intent with plans for later scar revision. **(c)** Seven-week postoperative result with secondary intent healing of central defect. **(d)** Post staged excision of granulation scar tissue 6 months after initial MMS. **(e)** Final result 1 week after scar excision.

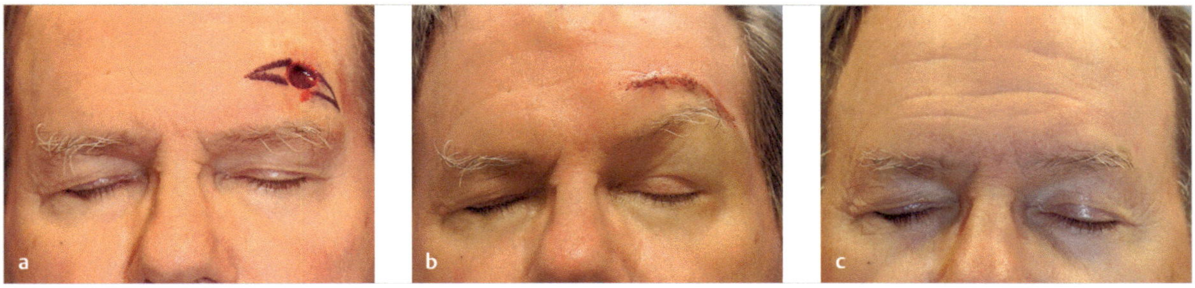

Fig. 4.3 Forehead horizontal primary closure with transient brow elevation. **(a)** Post-Mohs defect less than 1 cm in diameter with planned horizontal linear closure parallel to brow. **(b)** Site immediately post reconstruction demonstrating brow asymmetry. **(c)** Six-month postoperative result.

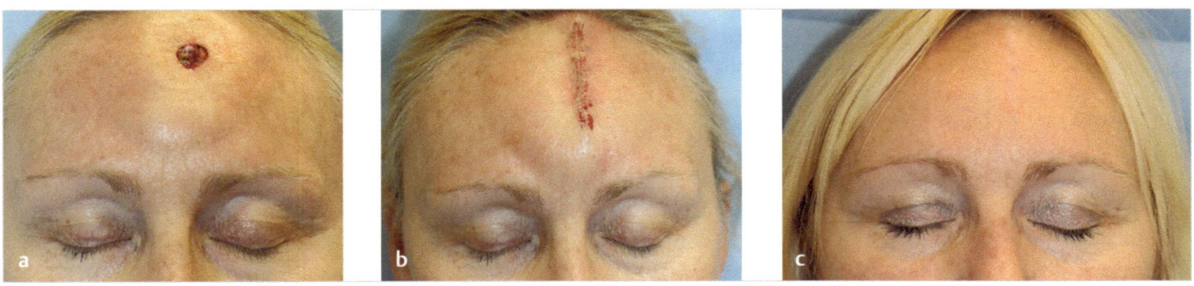

Fig. 4.4 Linear vertical forehead repair near frontal hairline. **(a)** Cephalad forehead Mohs defect near frontal scalp. There is minimal risk of brow position distortion in this location. **(b)** Defect repaired with vertical linear closure. **(c)** Three-month postoperative appearance.

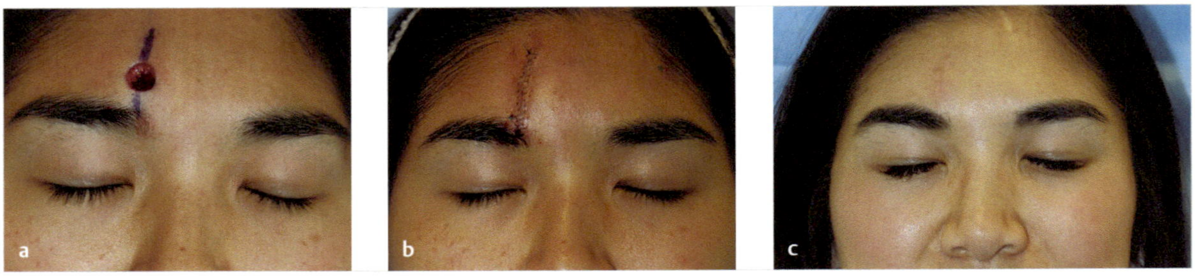

Fig. 4.5 Linear vertical forehead repair near brow. **(a)** Right paramedian forehead defect after MMS. **(b)** Vertically oriented repair to minimize displacement of eyebrow. **(c)** Two-month postoperative appearance.

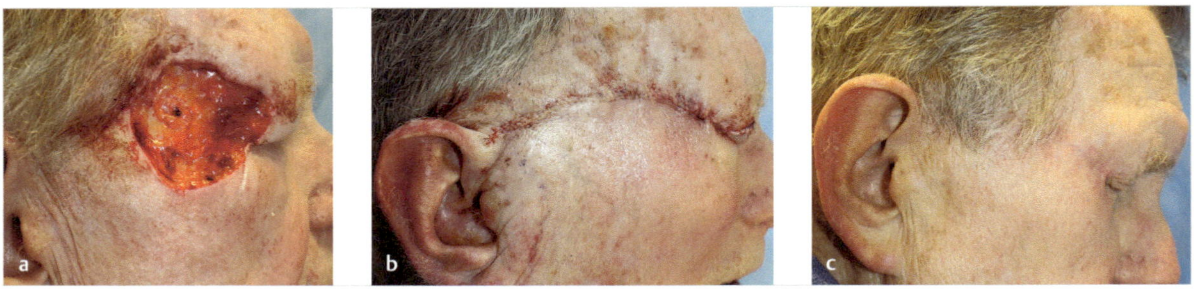

Fig. 4.6 Horizontal linear repair of the temple. **(a)** Moderately-sized right temple defect involving the lateral canthus and upper brow. **(b)** Due to the significant cheek laxity, a linear repair was possible. Orientation of the scar in this direction mitigates improper displacement of eyelid skin. **(c)** Four-month postoperative appearance.

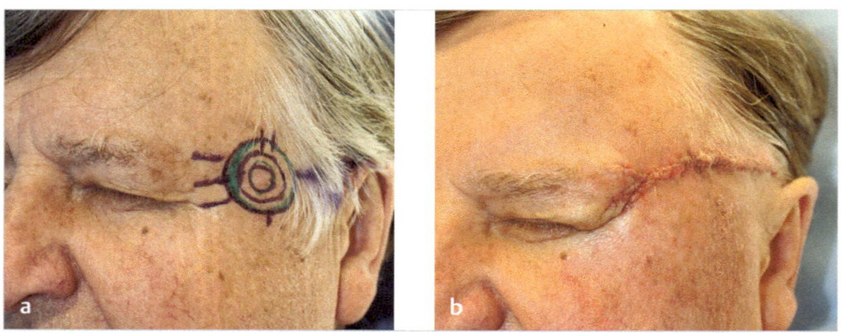

Fig. 4.7 Nested M-plasty repair for temple and lateral canthus. **(a)** Design of nested M-plasty prior to resection of skin cancer. **(b)** Immediate postoperative appearance of primary linear repair with M-plasty modification to minimize the encroachment of the scar on the lateral canthus.

On the temple, linear closures are usually oriented radial to the orbital rim as extensions of the crow's feet that can be elicited through forced closure of the eyelids and elevation of the zygomatic cheeks (▶ Fig. 4.6). M-plasty repair near the eyebrow or lateral canthus can minimize free margin displacement and reduce tissue redundancies (▶ Fig. 4.7). In contrast to the forehead subunit, verticallyoriented linear closures on the temple exhibit higher tension and may place inappropriate levels of tension on the lateral canthal skin.

4.5.3 Local Flaps

Forehead and temple defects are best repaired with a local flap in two common scenarios:

1. Defects greater than 3 cm in diameter.
2. Defects adjacent to a free margin where alternative repairs would cause its displacement.

Local flaps play a versatile role in temple and forehead reconstruction and deliver matching skin color and texture to the recipient area, providing excellent cosmetic outcomes. Local flaps may be simplified into two varieties: those that slide across a defect and those that lift over skin to close a defect. Advancement, rotation, and V-Y island pedicle flaps are categorized as sliding flaps, whereas rhombic and bilobed transposition flaps are the common lifting flaps utilized in these regions. Because of the limited adjacent skin reservoirs, position of cosmetic junction borders, and orientation of RSTLs, most flaps performed on the temple and brow are sliding flaps. The focus of the next section highlights key principles of flap design and execution.

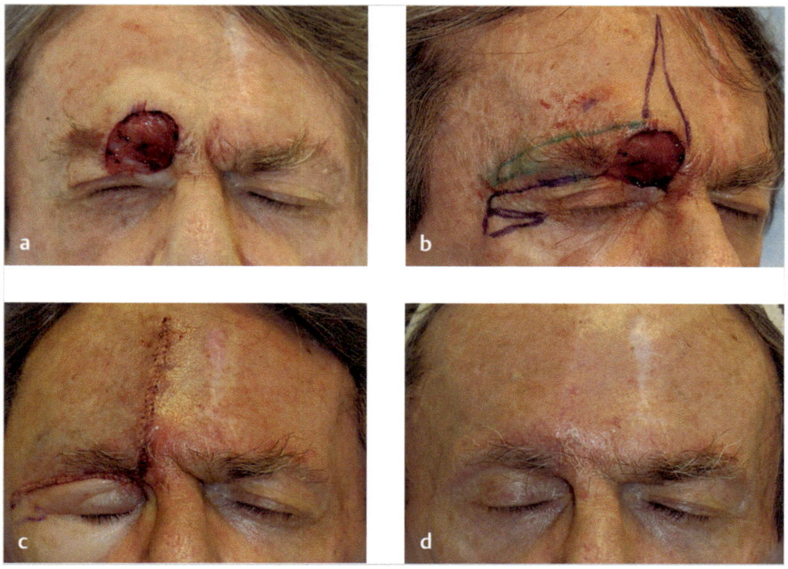

Fig. 4.8 Single-arm, laterally based advancement flap. **(a)** Mohs defect involving left brow and lower paramedian forehead. **(b)** Preoperative flap design. The incision under the eyebrow camouflages the scar in a cosmetic border. Movement of the flap from lateral to medial delivers a sufficient amount of skin to close the defect. **(c)** Immediate postoperative appearance. **(d)** Two-month postoperative appearance with preservation of brow position.

4.5.4 Sliding Flaps

Sliding flaps repair wounds by draping adjacent skin into the surgical defect. This category includes advancement, rotation, and V-Y island pedicle flaps. Sliding flaps are an excellent option for defects that are adjacent to a free margin such as the brow or eyelid. All three flap variations share a common tension vector that occurs at the leading edge of the flap where it meets the recipient area. It is important to note that tension is not displaced away from the wound and requires flap design to be mindful of possible free margin displacement. On the forehead, tissue movement is usually lateral to medial; thus, the lateral forehead often provides a reservoir of skin for the paramedian and medial forehead. On the temple, tissue is typically recruited inferiorly from the cheek.

Flaps that create a single incision off the inferior leading edge can parallel an RSTL or cosmetic subunit border in order to displace a redundant cone away from the defect (▶ Fig. 4.8). Incisions that arise from the inferior and superior edge of the defect can also mobilize a greater amount of tissue with enhanced vascularity (▶ Fig. 4.9). Smaller defects may be closed by flap undermining in the subcutaneous plane, but larger, more midline defects may necessitate submuscular undermining for flap release and enhanced vascularity.

These sliding flaps create 90-degree incisions, slide tissue medially or superiorly depending on location, and are most commonly used for midline and paramedian forehead defects. If tissue from one side of the defect is insufficient to close the wound, then a flap with bilateral arms can be created. Unilateral flaps are more commonly utilized for defects on the lateral forehead or paramedian forehead where looser reservoir tissue can be found. Bilateral flaps may be designed to repair larger defects in the midline forehead where decreased tissue laxity is compensated for by recruiting donor tissue from two ends.

Rotation flaps are sliding flaps designed with a sweeping curvilinear arc that pivots skin from lateral to medial. The skin should easily rotate flap tissue into the primary defect with the primary tension vector located at the leading edge of the flap. A larger flap arc may displace some tension away from the defect, but the key stitch under tension closes the leading edge of the flap and the recipient area of the defect. A redundant cone is typically removed from the pivot point but can be excised anywhere along the flap's longer side. Similar to advancement flaps, the flap's leading edge is typically hidden within parallel cosmetic borders such as the hairline. Rotation flaps may be designed unilaterally (▶ Fig. 4.10) or bilaterally (▶ Fig. 4.11). The surgeon should take care to avoid or minimize hair displacement from the temporal or frontal scalp onto non–hair bearing skin.

The V-Y island pedicle flap (IPF) is a modification of the traditional advancement flap. It involves the creation of a triangular flap adjacent to the primary defect that is completely separated from surrounding tissue while retaining an uninterrupted vascular supply on its undersurface. This central pedicle allows the flap to deliver thicker tissue to the surgical defect. Curvilinear incisions that follow natural lines of the face to improve final scar appearance are made through the dermis of both limbs of the flap, separating the flap from surrounding tissue and creating an island that is advanced with a key suture toward the primary defect. Circumferential undermining is performed to the point where 30 to 50% of the flap is tethered to the underlying tissue. The resultant secondary defect at the apex of the flap is closed primarily under minimal tension. This flap repair is an excellent option

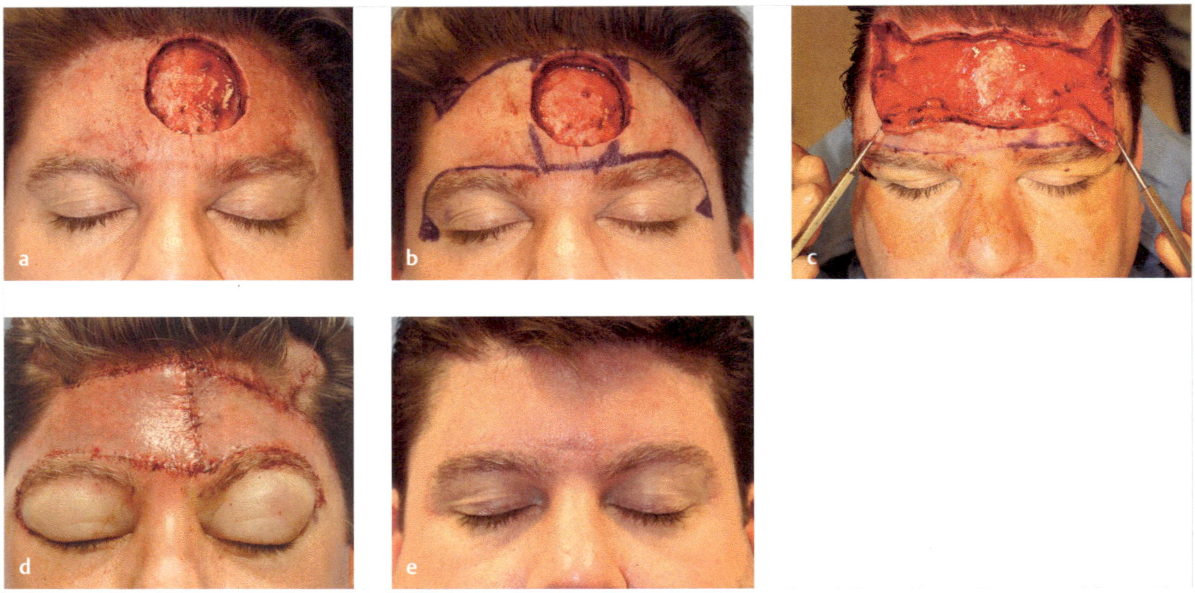

Fig. 4.9 Bilateral, double-arm advancement flap. **(a)** A 3.5-cm central forehead defect. **(b)** Flap designed with arms to hide along cosmetic junction borders of frontal hairline and eyebrows. **(c)** The flap retracted caudally demonstrating subfrontalis undermining. The inferior limbs of the flap were incised and undermined above the frontalis in order to preserve the neurovascular bundles. **(d)** Immediate postoperative appearance. **(e)** Four-month postoperative appearance.

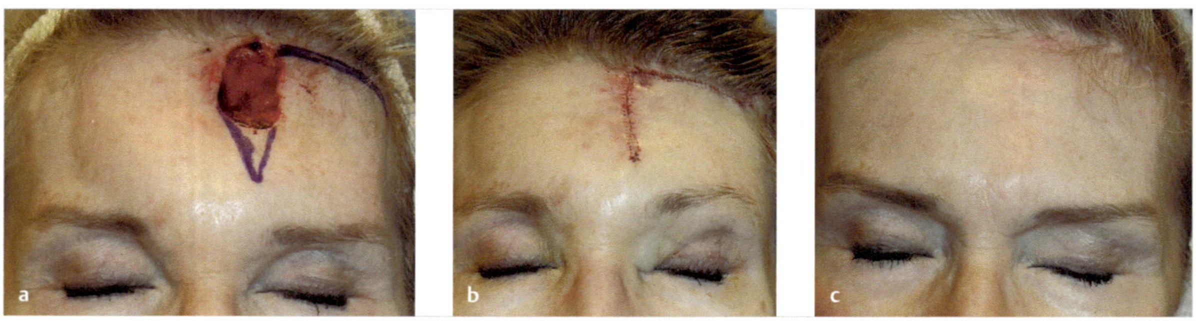

Fig. 4.10 Unilateral rotation flap. **(a)** Upper forehead defect with height greater than width is favorably shaped for a rotation flap repair. **(b)** Immediate postoperative appearance with one arm of flap camouflaged along frontal hairline. **(c)** Two-month postoperative appearance.

for small and medium-sized defects in the forehead and brow (▶ Fig. 4.12). It can also be used effectively for large upper forehead defects when based off of the supratrochlear artery (▶ Fig. 4.13). Trapdoor deformities may be minimized with appropriate undermining of the peripheral skin and sizing the flap to the size of the defect.

4.5.5 Transposition Flaps

Transposition flaps, unlike sliding flaps, lift and deliver tissue over an area of intervening skin and are best utilized in situations where excessive primary wound tension precludes the use of linear closure or a sliding flap. The benefit of transposition flap design is its displacement of the primary tension vector away from the defect to the tissue reservoir. It also permits delivery of more tissue to the defect for closure than sliding flaps.[15] Transposition flaps tend to be less frequently used on the temple or forehead because of unfavorable geometric scars and limited mobile skin nearby. When selected, transposition flaps are most commonly designed as rhombic flaps or bilobed flaps for larger defects on the temple when a single transposition flap would exert excessive tension on the wound closure.

Rhombic flaps are classically designed with a flap limb that extends off the midpoint of the defect and equals the diameter of the defect (▶ Fig. 4.14). The flap is made with a 60-degree angle that points toward the reservoir of skin to

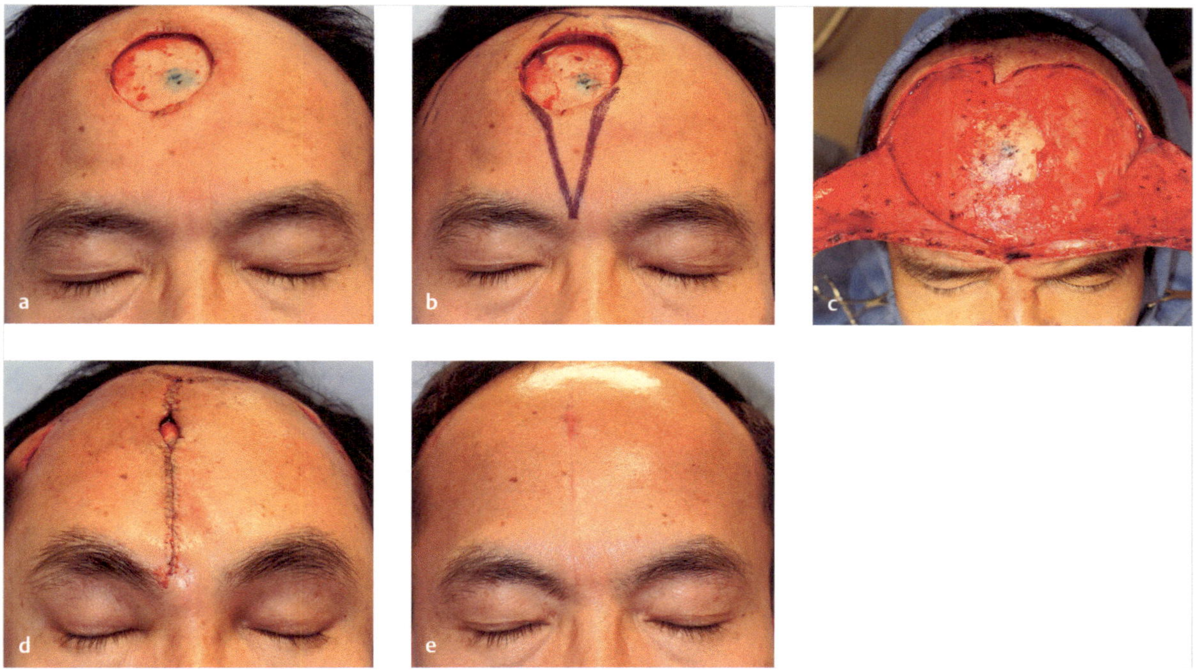

Fig. 4.11 Bilateral rotation flap. **(a)** Right paramedian forehead and frontal scalp defect. The exposed bone necessitates vascularized tissue coverage. **(b)** Planned bilateral rotation flap with limbs hidden along frontal hairline. **(c)** Bilateral flaps retracted laterally and caudally to show undermining plane prior to rotation toward one another. **(d)** Immediate postoperative appearance. A small area was allowed to heal by second intention in order to avoid excess tension on the leading edges of the flaps. **(e)** Three-month postoperative appearance.

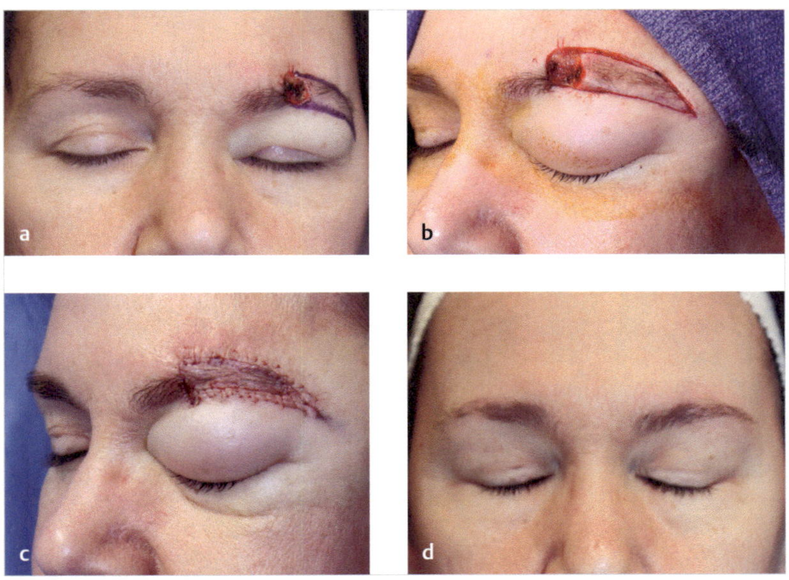

Fig. 4.12 V-Y advancement flap. **(a)** Mid-left brow defect. Planned V-Y pedicle flap with lateral to medial advancement. **(b)** Intraoperative photograph illustrating circumferential incision to release periphery of the flap with preservation of a central island pedicle. **(c)** Immediate postoperative appearance with flap incisions attempting to align with borders of the eyebrow. **(d)** Four-month postoperative appearance.

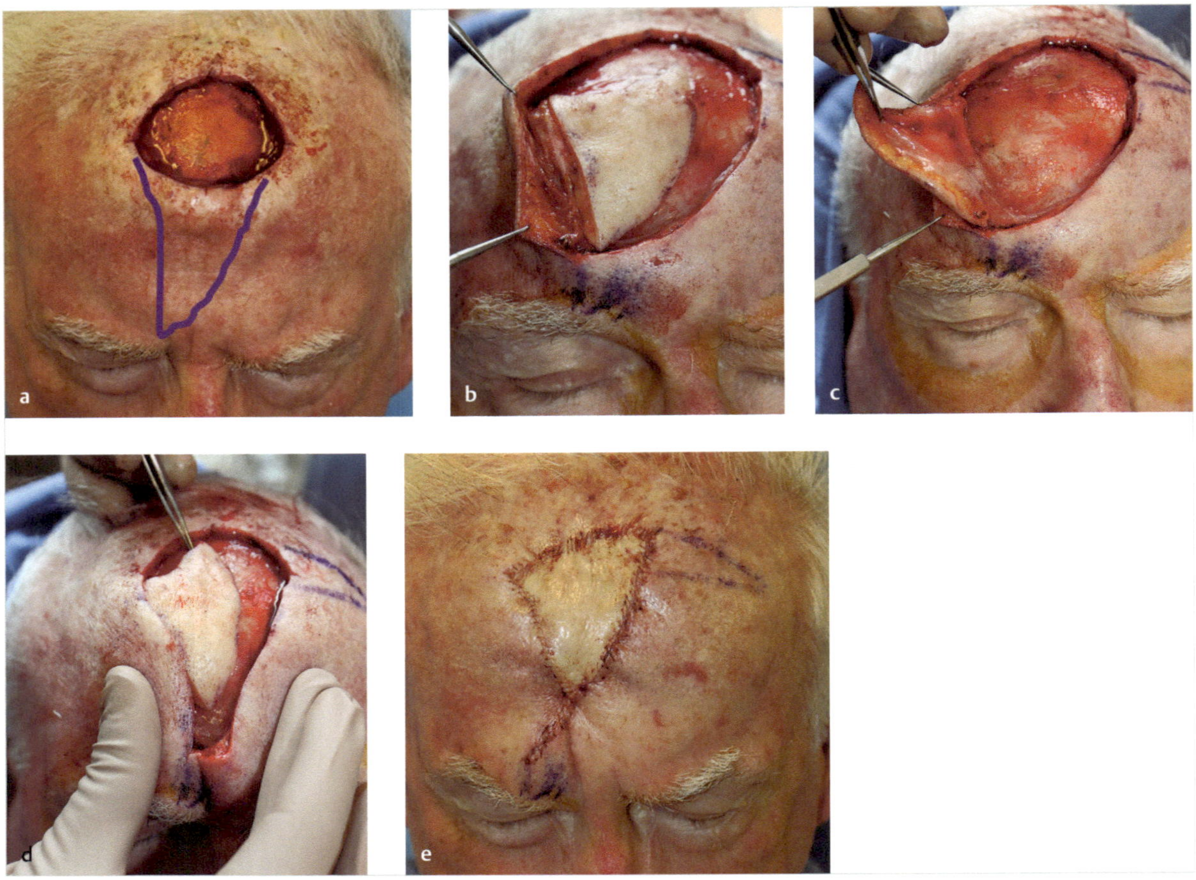

Fig. 4.13 Sling V-Y advancement flap. **(a)** Upper forehead defect to periosteum. V-Y flap designed inferiorly in order to recruit skin with a properly vascularized pedicle. **(b)** Skin retracted demonstrating incision of one limb of flap to the muscle. **(c)** Flap retracted demonstrating undermining of flap beneath the frontalis muscle. This bilevel undermining creates a sling flap based off the muscle and its perforating vessels. **(d)** Flap movement is an advancement to the recipient portion of the defect with horizontal tension vectors that do not result in displacement of the eyebrows. **(e)** Immediate postoperative appearance.

be lifted. Closure of the secondary defect occurs first, but this can often be challenging. The more commonly performed Webster's modification utilizes an elongated flap arm with a 30-degree angle pointing toward the flap reservoir. This modification permits easier closure of the secondary defect but can create an undersized flap requiring secondary motion from the recipient area for closure.

Bilobed transposition flaps recruit tissue more distally than rhombic flaps and distribute tension across a larger area away from the primary defect. A downside of this repair is that these flaps create broken line scars that can become perceptible over time, especially when crossing over RSTLs (▶ Fig. 4.15). It is this reason, along with the potential for flap "pincushioning," that makes them less commonly performed on the forehead and temple.

Defects greater than 3 cm that extend to bone on the forehead present unique challenges. Skin grafts may not survive due to an absent vascular bed, while traditional local flaps may not provide sufficient coverage. In these instances, axial transposition flaps can provide an effective solution (▶ Fig. 4.16). The tunneled transposed axial flap design and execution is similar to the paramedian forehead flap. A benefit of this flap is that the tunneled transfer precludes the need for future flap division.[16] The surgeon first designs the flap by mapping the path of an STA and places a template of the defect size on the forehead where movement of the flap allows the tissue to appropriately cover the defect. The template may be slightly undersized if secondary motion can be tolerated at the defect site. The pedicle of the flap should be approximately 1 cm in diameter at the flap's pivot point near the medial brow. The resulting flap is then elevated at a level immediately deep to the frontalis muscle, taking care that loose areolar tissue and periosteum remain at the secondary defect. Subsequently, a tunnel is created in the loose areolar tissue plane between the base of the flap pedicle and the primary defect. The flap is then carefully tunneled under and should move into the primary defect without tension. The flap tissue that is below the overlying bridge of skin is de-epithelialized at the

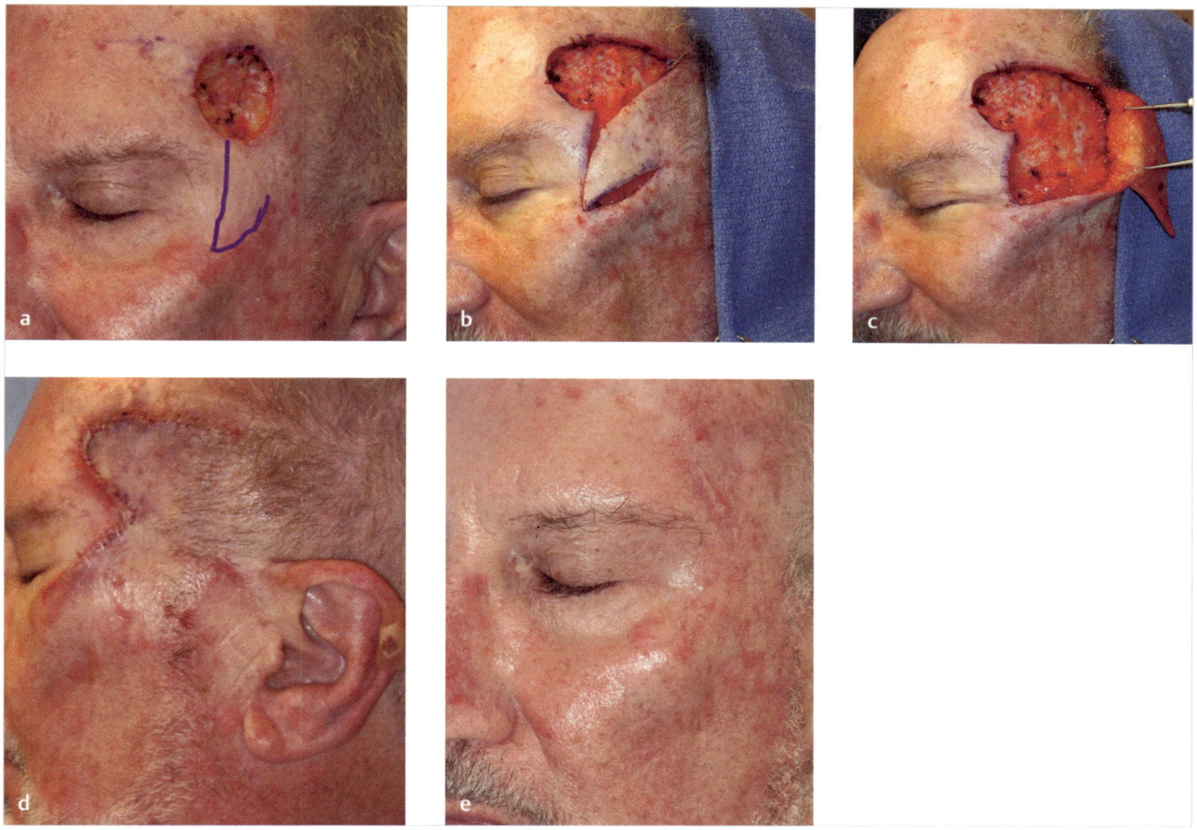

Fig. 4.14 Rhombic transposition flap. (a) Temple defect above the superficial temporal fascia. A superiorly based rhombic flap was designed in order to take advantage of the reservoir of skin inferior to the defect. (b) Rhombic flap incised with redundant tissue cone already removed into temporal hairline. (c) Flap undermined above superficial fascia and retracted back. (d) Immediate postoperative appearance. (e) Two-month postoperative appearance.

level of the adipose tissue. The flap is then sutured over the exposed bone in layers. The secondary defect is closed, if possible. If tension precludes closure of the forehead, then it may be allowed to heal by secondary intention.

4.5.6 Skin Grafts

Skin grafts can be considered for larger defects that are not amenable to linear repair or flap reconstruction. This is most common in areas of poor tissue elasticity such as the frontotemporal region and glabella (▸ Fig. 4.17). Grafting may also be considered after resection of high-risk tumors where ongoing surveillance is desired. Anticipated disadvantages to grafting the forehead and temple include poor color and texture matching with surrounding skin (▸ Fig. 4.18). The color and thickness mismatch is even more likely when thin grafts such as split-thickness skin grafts are used. Retroauricular, preauricular, forehead, and supraclavicular donor sites provide the closest tissue match for the temple and forehead. Burow's grafts from adjacent tissue and flap or linear repairs can be used to fill portions of defects still exposed. Delayed grafting after 1 to 2 weeks of granulation can improve survival, decrease wound contraction, and improve aesthetic outcomes. Alternatively, dermal skin substitutes can be secured into forehead and defects with delayed grafting, which may improve contour (▸ Fig. 4.19).

Full-thickness skin grafts harvested from hair-bearing sites such as the postauricular or temporal scalp may be mobilized to reconstruct eyebrow defects resulting in significant hair loss. The grafts should be lifted in the subcutaneous plane below the hair bulbs with care taken to incise parallel to the follicular units and avoid transection. The grafts should be sutured in such a way that the donor hairs align with the native eyebrow hairs. If hairs do not regrow, tattooing or stenciling should be sufficient to recreate symmetry. Hair transplantation to the brow is another option to restore hair to a graft that is alopecic.

4.6 Complications

Hematomas, infections, ischemia, and nerve injury are complications that may occur with forehead and temple

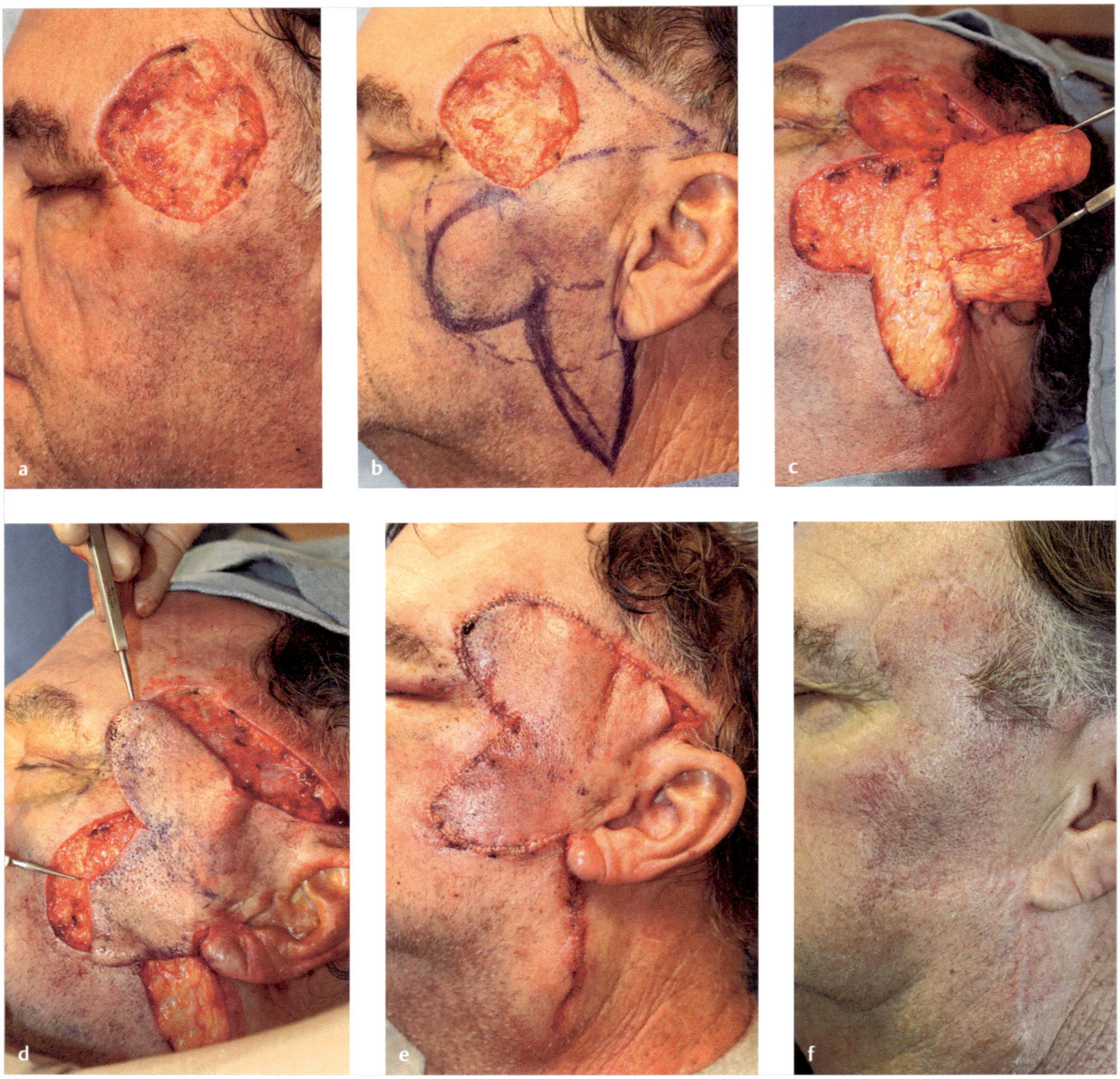

Fig. 4.15 Bilobed transposition flap. **(a)** Broad defect located on the left temple. **(b)** Bilobed flap design attempting to recruit tissue from the cheek. **(c)** Elevation of the flap in the supra-superficial musculoaponeurotic system plane. **(d)** Transposing the flap into the primary and secondary defects. **(e)** Closure of the flap displaces the primary vector toward the tertiary defect below the ear on the neck. A portion of the flap was left open to reduce tension in the hair-bearing skin. **(f)** Three-month postoperative appearance.

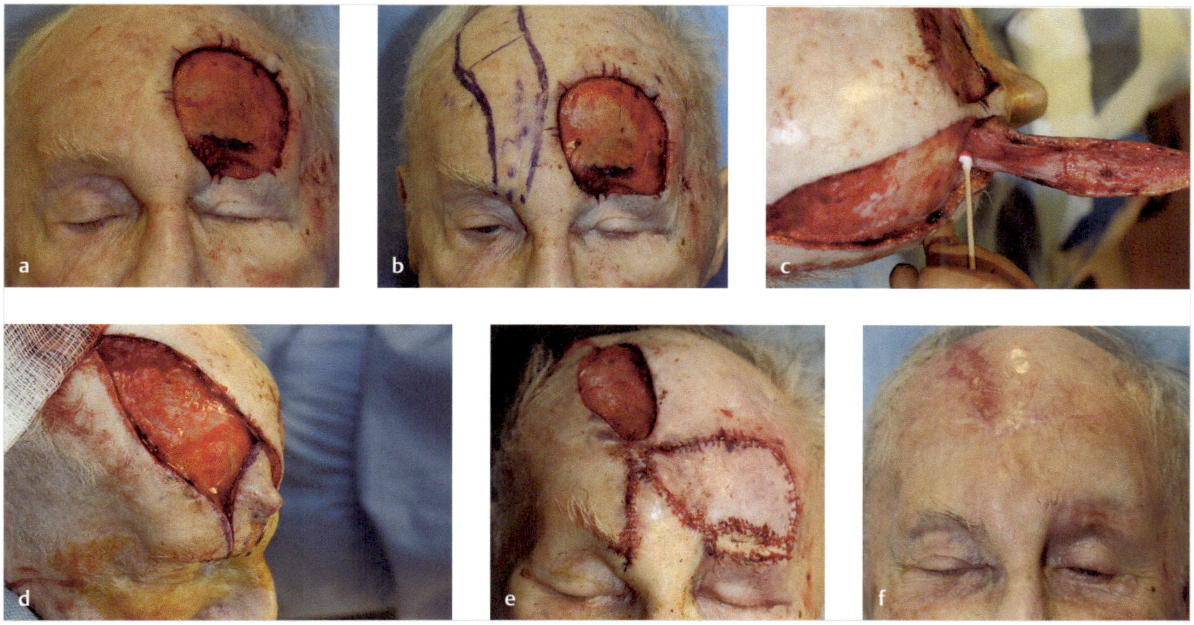

Fig. 4.16 Axial-based flap for large forehead defect with exposed bone. **(a)** Hemiforehead defect with areas devoid of periosteum. This wound requires repair with vascularized tissue. **(b)** Because a random-pattern flap is unlikely to cover the broad wound, an axial flap based off the contralateral supratrochlear artery is designed. **(c)** Elevation of the flap under the frontalis muscle. The cotton-tip applicator is pushing the corrugator muscle away from bone in an attempt to preserve the vessel. **(d)** Flap tunneled under the bridge of skin. The flap that remains beneath the bridge is subsequently de-epithelialized. **(e)** Immediate postoperative appearance. Much of the donor site was left to heal by second intention. **(f)** Four-month postoperative appearance.

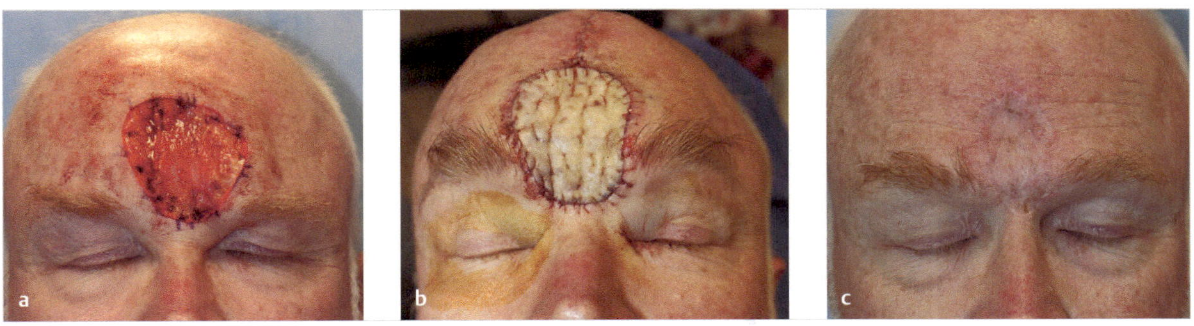

Fig. 4.17 Full-thickness skin graft. **(a)** Glabellar and mid-forehead defect with muscle preserved. **(b)** Thin clavicular graft sutured into place with numerous quilting sutures. **(c)** Three-month postoperative appearance.

reconstruction. A detailed understanding of the anatomy and tissue biodynamics can prevent some of these complications. Postoperative healing after a complication is usually poor and surgical revision of a reconstruction may be necessary.

Hematomas of the forehead or temple will present shortly after surgery as a tender, soft to firm palpable mass. They are relatively uncommon when a firm postoperative pressure dressing is applied because of buttressing to the underlying frontal or temporal bone. Meticulous hemostasis with electrocoagulation, careful surgical technique, and adequate pressure dressings will help mitigate most postoperative bleeding. Expanding hematomas require evacuation and hemostasis of active bleeding. Postoperative ecchymosis, on the other hand, is quite common when operating on the forehead and temples. Patients should be counseled that periorbital bruising after the first few days of surgery is not concerning. The edema and bruising fade while tracking caudally over the course of a week. Patients may be instructed to sleep in a reclined position and periodically ice the area to minimize bruising.

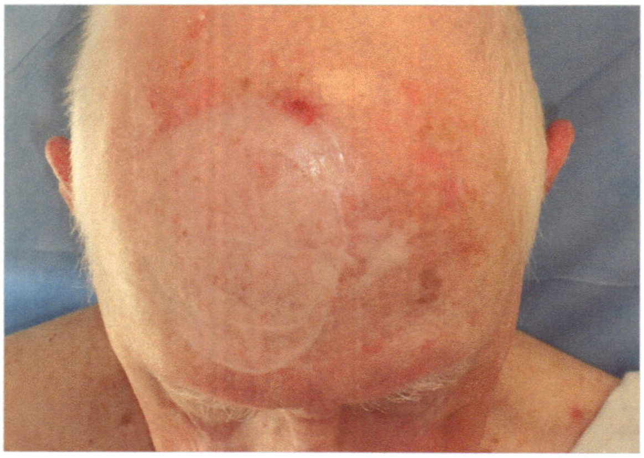

Fig. 4.18 Patient treated many years prior received a skin graft for a large forehead and scalp defect. The graft has healed with an expected color and contour mismatch.

Wound infections are uncommon with forehead and temple reconstruction. A surgical site infection typically presents within 1 week of surgery with tenderness, erythema, and sometimes drainage from the incision. Secondary wound dehiscence may be observed. Antibiotic prophylaxis is not indicated for most forehead and temple surgeries because of the lowrisk of infection.[17] Careful sterile technique and close follow-up serve to minimize infection risk.

Flap and graft ischemia and necrosis are minimized with appropriate patient selection and correct flap design and execution. Normally, the anastomotic blood supply in this region is rich and allows for successful local flap reconstruction. Excessive tension will strangulate the necessary blood supply to flaps, especially at the distal flap tips where distance from the vascular pedicle is greatest (▶ Fig. 4.20).

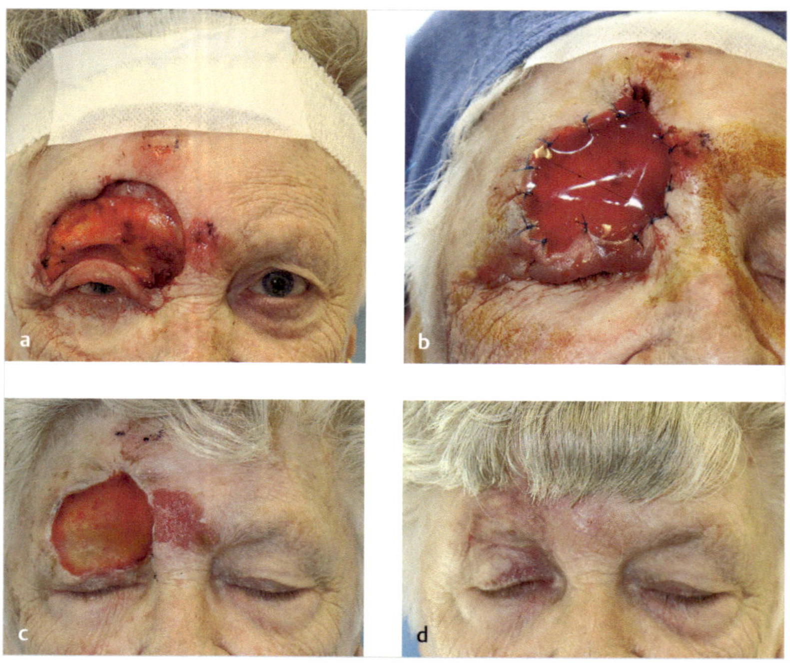

Fig. 4.19 Use of dermal skin substitute prior to grafting. **(a)** Broad upper eyelid/brow defect with some muscle removed. **(b)** Dermal bilayer collagen-silicone wound matrix sutured into wound provides a hospitable wound bed for grafting 3 weeks later. **(c)** Three-week postoperative appearance with silicone layer removed. A full-thickness skin graft was placed atop the new dermal bed. **(d)** Appearance 3 months after skin grafting.

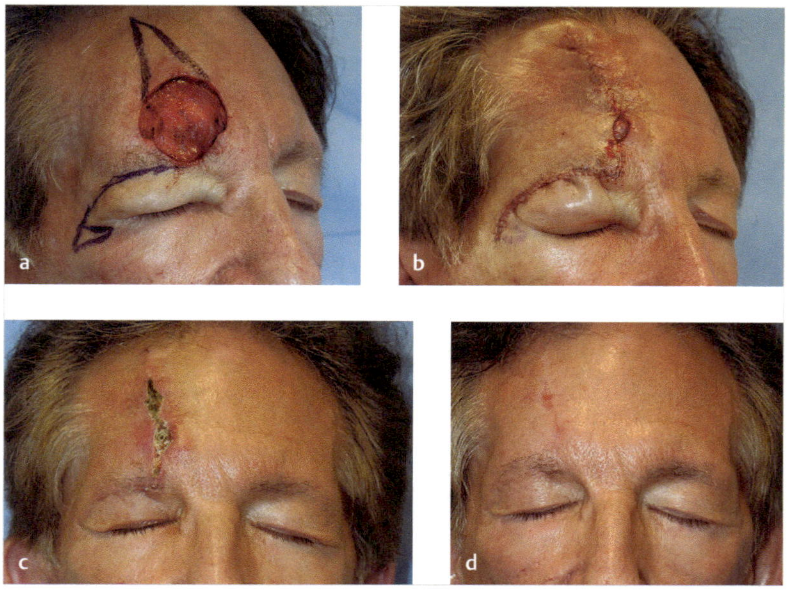

Fig. 4.20 Advancement flap under tension heals with ischemia. **(a)** Defect of the medial brow and forehead with planned laterally based advancement flap. **(b)** Appearance immediately after closure. Significant tension is seen at the flap's leading edge. A small area is allowed to heal by second intention in order to minimize flap tension. **(c)** Two-week postoperative appearance with incisional crusting due to ischemia and necrosis. **(d)** Three-month postoperative appearance. The partial-thickness necrosis resulted in a mildly hypertrophied erythematous scar. The patient declined revision.

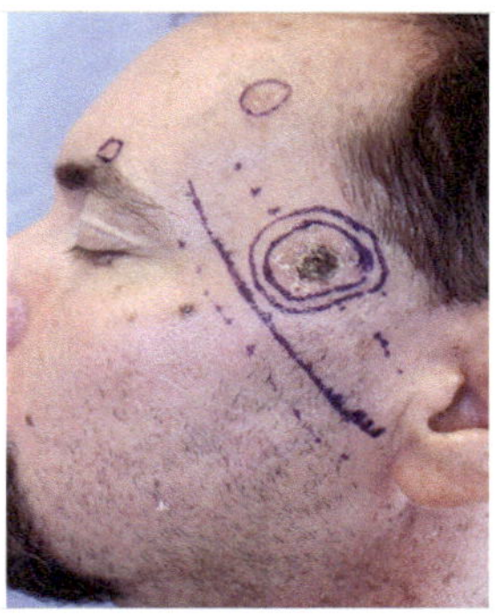

Fig. 4.21 Cancer outlined prior to Mohs resection. The anticipated path of the temporal branch of the facial nerve is marked along Pitanguy'sline (0.5 cm below tragus to a line 1.5 cm above lateral brow).

Another important consideration in this region is preservation of the temporal branch of the facial nerve. Nerve injury can be avoided with preoperative mapping of the temporal branch (▶ Fig. 4.21). An informed discussion regarding the implications of possible facial nerve transection should occur with the patient prior to tumor resection if nerve injury is anticipated. A comprehensive understanding of facial nerve trajectory across different tissue planes allows the surgeon to undermine skin with confidence in the temple and lateral forehead. If the temporal branch of the facial nerve is damaged, then an ipsilateral brow lift may be considered to restore brow symmetry (▶ Fig. 4.22). Damage to the STN and SON will lead to loss of sensation that usually returns within a year.

A final complication of forehead and temple reconstruction to note involves scarring at incision sites. Scar spreading can be revised on follow-up with future scar excisions or resurfacing laser therapy. These modalities are typically considered many months after the surgery and can help improve the final cosmetic outcome. Neuromodulator injected into the frontalis and corrugators at the time of repair or shortly after surgery may minimize wound tension and prophylactically minimize scar visibility.[18]

4.7 Conclusion

Forehead and temples perhaps are not as critical to facial appearance and function as the nose, eyelids, and lips, but they do play an important role in appearance. Reconstruction of defects in these locations should adhere to the fundamental principles of reconstruction. Sensory and motor nerves may be preserved and complications minimized with detailed knowledge of forehead and temple neurovascular anatomy.

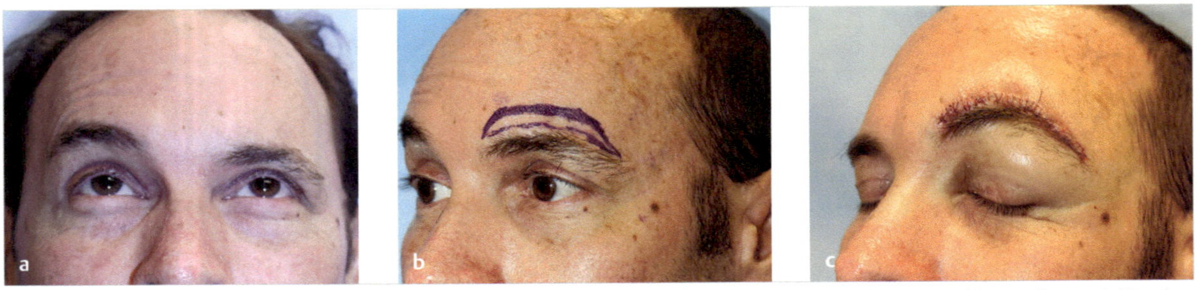

Fig. 4.22 Browlift after temporal branch injury. **(a)** Patient with left-sided facial nerve injury accentuated with raising of contralateral eyebrow. **(b)** Planned eyebrow lift via removal of crescentic island of skin. **(c)** Immediate postoperative appearance. The higher left brow likely settles with gravity over time in order to restore closer symmetry between eyebrows.

References

[1] Seline PC, Siegle RJ. Forehead reconstruction. Dermatol Clin. 2005; 23 (1):1–11, v

[2] Kleintjes WG. Forehead anatomy: arterial variations and venous link of the midline forehead flap. J Plast Reconstr Aesthet Surg. 2007; 60 (6):593–606

[3] Edizer M, Beden U, Icten N. Morphological parameters of the periorbital arterial arcades and potential clinical significance based on anatomical identification. J Craniofac Surg. 2009; 20(1):209–214

[4] Erdogmus S, Govsa F. Arterial features of inner canthus region: confirming the safety for the flap design. J Craniofac Surg. 2006; 17 (5):864–868

[5] Yu D, Weng R, Wang H, Mu X, Li Q. Anatomical study of forehead flap with its pedicle based on cutaneous branch of supratrochlear artery and its application in nasal reconstruction. Ann Plast Surg. 2010; 65 (2):183–187

[6] Reece EM, Schaverien M, Rohrich RJ. The paramedian forehead flap: a dynamic anatomical vascular study verifying safety and clinical implications. Plast Reconstr Surg. 2008; 121(6):1956–1963

[7] Vural E, Batay F, Key JM. Glabellar frown lines as a reliable landmark for the supratrochlear artery. Otolaryngol Head Neck Surg. 2000; 123 (5):543–546

[8] Erdogmus S, Govsa F. Anatomy of the supraorbital region and the evaluation of it for the reconstruction of facial defects. J Craniofac Surg. 2007; 18(1):104–112

[9] Christensen KN, Lachman N, Pawlina W, Baum CL. Cutaneous depth of the supraorbital nerve: a cadaveric anatomic study with clinical applications to dermatology. Dermatol Surg. 2014; 40(12):1342–1348

[10] Janis JE, Hatef DA, Hagan R, et al. Anatomy of the supratrochlear nerve: implications for the surgical treatment of migraine headaches. Plast Reconstr Surg. 2013; 131(4):743–750

[11] Jeong SM, Park KJ, Kang SH, et al. Anatomical consideration of the anterior and lateral cutaneous nerves in the scalp. J Korean Med Sci. 2010; 25(4):517–522

[12] Iwanaga J, Watanabe K, Saga T, Fisahn C, Oskouian RJ, Tubbs RS. Anatomical study of the superficial temporal branches of the auriculotemporal nerve: application to surgery and other invasive treatments to the temporal region. J Plast Reconstr Aesthet Surg. 2017; 70 (3):370–374

[13] Kochhar A, Larian B, Azizzadeh B. Facial nerve and parotid gland anatomy. Otolaryngol Clin North Am. 2016; 49(2):273–284

[14] Condie D, Tolkachjov SN. Facial nerve injury and repair: a practical review for cutaneous surgery. Dermatol Surg. 2019; 45(3):340–357

[15] Miller CJ. Design principles for transposition flaps: the rhombic (single-lobed), bilobed, and trilobed flaps. Dermatol Surg. 2014; 40 Suppl 9:S43–S52

[16] Sobanko JF, Portilla N, Etzkorn J, Shin T, Miller CJ. Repair of a hemiforehead defect with exposed bone. Dermatol Surg. 2018; 44 (12):1587–1590

[17] Wright TI, Baddour LM, Berbari EF, et al. Antibiotic prophylaxis in dermatologic surgery: advisory statement 2008. J Am Acad Dermatol. 2008; 59(3):464–473

[18] Zhang DZ, Liu XY, Xiao WL, Xu YX. Botulinum toxin type A and the prevention of hypertrophic scars on the maxillofacial area and neck: a meta-analysis of randomized controlled trials. PLoS One. 2016; 11 (3):e0151627

5 Scalp

David Zloty, Irèn Kossintseva, and Victoria Godinez-Puig

Abstract

Scalp reconstruction is commonly required after Mohs surgery. Creative use of a broad range of reconstruction options rewards both physician and patient with excellent cosmetic and functional outcomes. Excellence requires complete understanding of the anatomy of the scalp, including the location of multiple neurovascular bundles, and an appreciation of how the convex surface and relatively thick, poorly mobile skin make reconstruction challenging. Defect size, location, and presence or absence of hair or periosteum are important decision points when choosing a reconstructive option. Answers to these questions, when combined with patient factors (medical history, cosmetic desires, ability to care for the surgical site), allow the surgeon to develop a reconstruction ladder and algorithm. Second intention healing is useful for defects, even those without periosteum, in a range of defect sizes, in appropriately selected patients. Skin grafts, both full thickness and split thickness, are reserved for moderate to large defects in alopecic scalps when intact periosteum is present. In patients who are not able to care for a graft donor site, allogenic materials can serve as graft substitutes. The usefulness of primary closure can be extended to large defects by combining with pulley or purse-string sutures. Local flaps, either single or multiple, are a mainstay reconstruction option as they provide similar tissue and a secondary defect, which can be easily closed. Extensive defects not suitable for second intention healing or grafting require referral for placement of an internal tissue expander or consideration of free autologous tissue transfer.

Keywords: scalp, reconstruction, anatomy, second intention healing, skin grafts, autologous skin substitutes, local flaps, pulley sutures, purse-string sutures, free tissue transfer

Capsule Summary and Pearls

- The majority of undermining is at the subgaleal plane to minimize damage to overlying blood vessels, lymphatics, and nerves.
- Scalps have both tight and loose portions. Tight areas over the scalp vertex occur where the galea is thickest. Loose areas over the scalp periphery, especially occipital and parietal scalps, occur where the galea is less developed and blends with fascia of the scalp muscles.
- Second intention is a viable reconstructive option for scalp defects, especially if the scalp has had prior surgeries or a high-risk cancer requires close surveillance for recurrence.
- Second intention healing over bone is possible but requires prolonged and meticulous wound care in a moist environment.
- Mid-dermal placement of local anesthetic is most efficient and effective but requires high injection pressures.
- Anesthetic can be injected into the planned incision lines and standing cones while leaving the rest of the area to be bluntly undermined in the painless subgaleal plane.Galeal releasing incisions reduce tension only minimally and are performed parallel to the wound margin. Galeal releasing incisions are generally placed 1 to 2 cm apart.
- Deep suture placement must include the galea in the suture path for maximal tissue-holding properties.
- Proposed scalp incisions are based on the ability to encompass the greatest vascular supply and maintain hairline position, with less consideration given to the direction of relaxed skin tension lines.
- Primary closure in hair-bearing areas should only be used if low tensions are generated. Higher tensions can cause telogen effluvium or, less commonly, permanent hair loss.
- Primary closure for large defects in non-hair-bearing areas can be used with favorable cosmetic outcomes.
- Primary closure of large defects in non-hair-bearing areas can be aided by the use of pulley sutures. In hair-bearing areas, the use of pulley sutures can cause telogen effluvium or, less commonly, permanent hair loss.
- Purse-string suture closures are best employed in non-hair-bearing scalps. Purse-string and pulley sutures can be combined with second intention healing.
- Skin grafts require a placement on a base of periosteum and loose alveolar tissue to survive.
- Skin grafts will leave a larger contour deformity when compared to second intention healing.
- For large rotation flaps, incise incrementally, and then complete hemostasis before incising further. This increases control and visibility.
- Rotation flap arclengths must be designed at least four times longer than defect diameter to prevent necrosis at the flap edge and possible hair loss.
- Reduced elasticity and mobility of scalp skin limits the use of transposition and advancement flaps.
- Larger scalp defects may require combinations of second intention, rotation flap(s), and skin grafts.
- Small to moderate standing cones can be sutured out using rule of halves or allowed to settle spontaneously.

5.1 Relevant Anatomy

Scalp anatomy has many unique features. The convex curvature of the scalp necessitates larger sized flaps for comparable defects on other sites. Free margins, including hairline, eyebrows, and ears, must be maintained. Scalp movability and elasticity, a primary determinate in choosing a reconstructive option, is in turn influenced by location, age, degree of actinic damage, and, most importantly, individual genetic factors. The presence of large numbers of terminal hairs impacts reconstructive options, but it can also serve as a camouflaging benefit. The relative fragility of scalp dermis requires deep sutures to encompass additional tissue planes to ensure adequate holding tensions.

The cutaneous topography of the scalp relates to the underlying musculoskeletal framework (see ▶ Fig. 5.1). This framework determines scalp thickness and laxity and thus impacts strongly on reconstructive choices. Each topographic subunit of the scalp will have prominent neurovascular bundles originating peripherally, and coursing toward the scalp vertex. Anatomic knowledge of the position and plane of these bundles (as outlined later) helps direct flap design to maximize flap vascularity and minimize sensory changes. Reducing damage to terminal hairs requires careful consideration of incision angles to match hair follicle angles. In addition, undermining planes should be below hair bulbs, cautery has to be precise, and flap-closing tensions minimized to prevent permanent traction or scarring alopecia. Understanding all these variables inherent in scalp anatomy is required to optimize surgical outcomes.

The scalp comprises five tissue layers, with exceptions at the lateral and posterior peripheries, where three layers can be defined (▶ Fig. 5.2). The five layers, from superficial to deep, are: (1) skin, (2) subcutis, (3) galea aponeurotica, (4) loose connective fibroareolar tissue (subgaleal tissue/space), and (5) periosteum (pericranium). The presence of the subgaleal space, and the genetically determined degree of loose connective tissue within this space, allows the scalp to be a relatively glideable/mobile organ. However, at the posterior and lateral limits of the scalp, the absence of the subgaleal space restricts mobility. In these scalp areas, only skin, subcutis, and deep fascia are present.[1] The limits of galea extension are the occipitalis muscle posteriorly, the temporalis fascia laterally, and the frontalis and orbicularis oculi muscle anteriorly. The anterior extension of the galea allows both the frontal scalp and forehead to move as a unit and can account for periorbital ecchymosis sometimes seen after frontal scalp surgery. The five scalp layers are discussed in greater detail in the following sections.

5.1.1 Skin

The scalp skin, comprising epidermis and dermis, is a bit of a paradox from a surgical perspective. While the skin is thicker than anywhere else on the head and neck,[2] ranging from 3 mm on the vertex to 8 mm at the occiput, the structural integrity of the dermis is fairly friable, and consequently, does not hold deep sutures well. This necessitates that, if possible, placement of the deep sutures should include the more structurally robust galeal layer in the suture path. Dermal thickness varies according to patient age, ethnicity, and degree of actinic damage. Younger, sun-protected, Asian- or African-descent patients generally will have a thicker dermis. Langer's lines relate to collagen bundles arranged in the dermis, aligning with creases, and coinciding with lines of minimum tension.[3] On the scalp, they are mostly vertically longitudinal, until the occiput, where they become horizontal and circumferential (▶ Fig. 5.2). Although orientating incisions along Langer's lines can reduce closing tensions and scar width, location of scalp laxity and vascular bundles are generally more important variables to consider in flap design. Terminal hair follicles exit scalp skin at various angles according to location: almost horizontal over the central frontal scalp, sharply angled inferiorly at the scalp periphery, and more vertical as the vertex is approached. Hair bulbs are located at the dermal–subcutis junction averaging 4 to 6 mm below the skin surface. Minimizing hair follicle damage requires trichophytic incisions (the incision parallels the directional angle of the hair) and choosing an undermining plane below hair bulbs (deep subcutis or subgaleal). Careful attention to these variables avoids hair follicle transection and facilitates the narrowest possible scar with less chance of any ingrown hairs or cysts.

5.1.2 Subcutis

The subcutaneous fat is the second layer in the scalp. This layer is thick and houses a rich network of anastomosing arteries, veins, lymphatics, and coursing sensory nerves (▶ Fig. 5.3). The neurovascular and lymphatic supply to the scalp is centripetal (i.e., larger trunks run from the periphery medially and toward the center, becoming smaller and anastomosing), subcutaneous, and similar in distribution. Their distal ends are attached to the deep layers of the dermis at the subcutis junction. The rich vascular network at this level is responsible for what can be significant scalp hemorrhage after only superficial wounds.[1] The vascular supply is the anastomosed network between branches of external and internal carotid arteries. Where the scalp has five layers, there are no musculocutaneous perforators, and thus, a flap design that transects a significant portion of the peripheral vasculature can reduce flap tip perfusion and increase necrosis risk. Of note, the vascularity and relative perfusion of central scalp is decreased in male-patternbaldness,[4] presumably related to the association between relative tissue hypoxia and hair loss. This may partially explain why surgery on bald scalp is usually less bloody

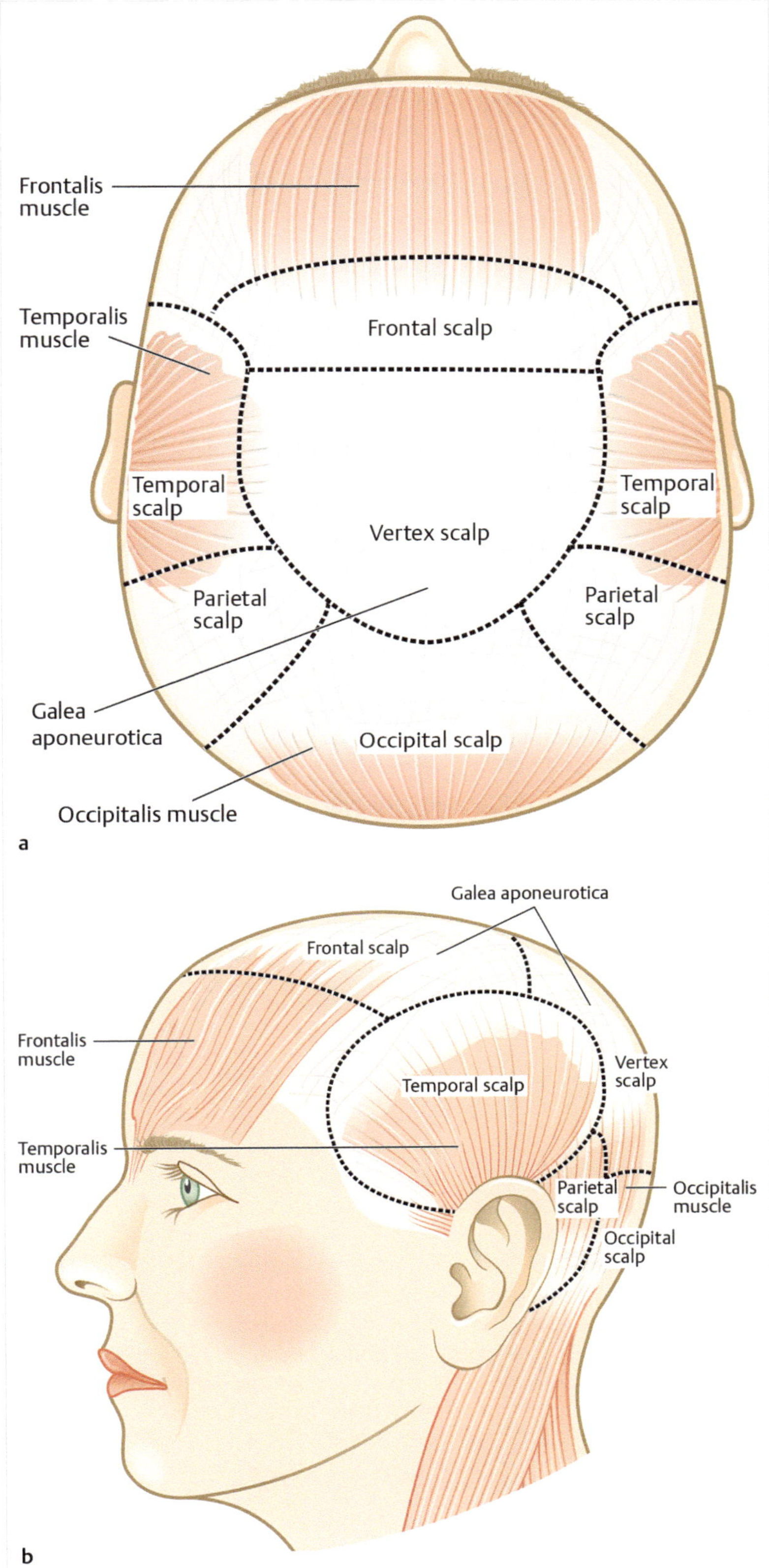

Fig. 5.1 (a, b) Musculoskeletal scalp anatomy and cosmetic subunits.

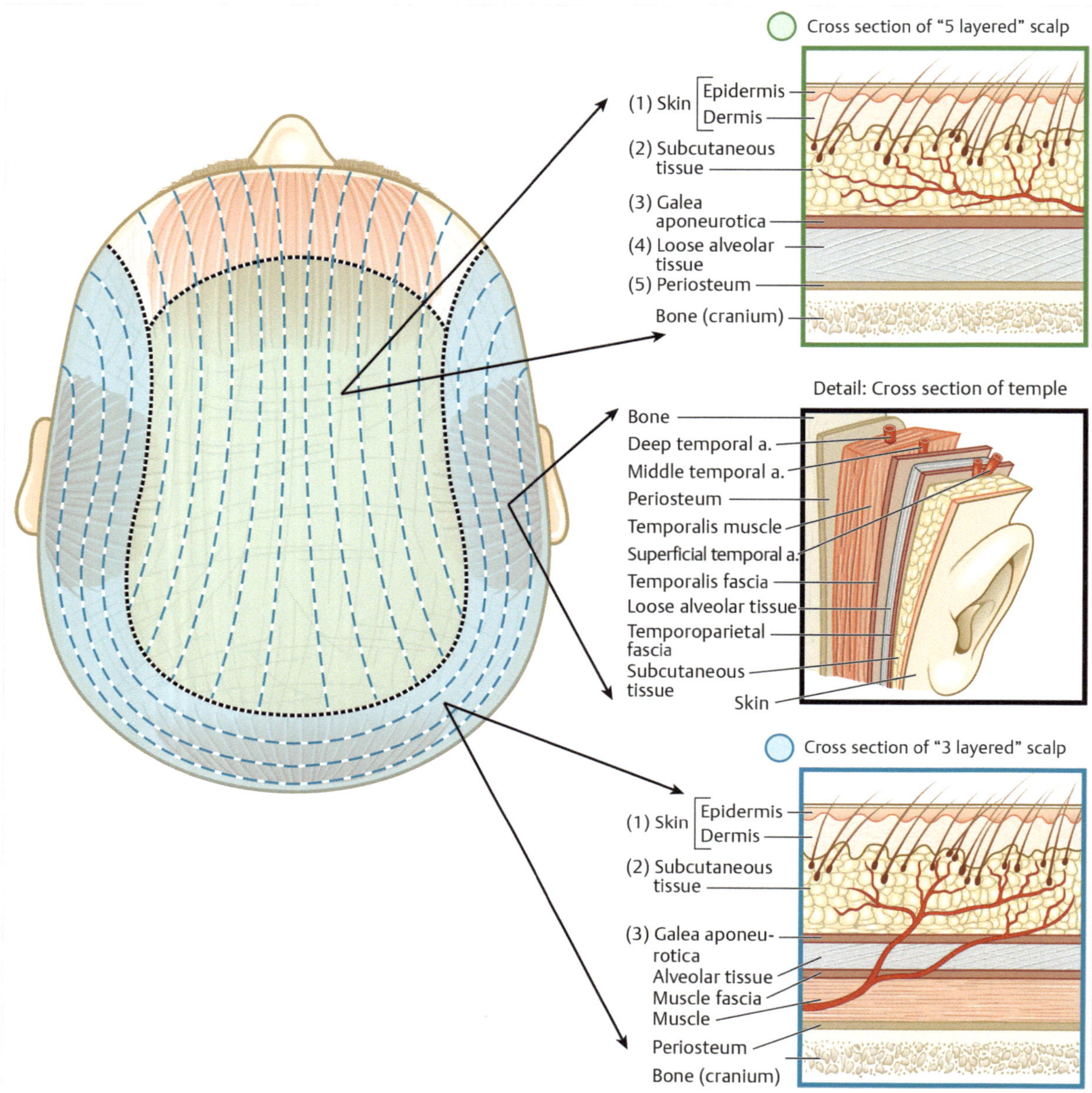

Fig. 5.2 Layers of the scalp, planes of dissection and incision lines.

than in patients who have no hair loss. Surgeons must be mindful that arterioles can be closely apposed to hair-bulbs. Consequently, hemostasis has to be judicious and precise to reduce collateral damage to hair follicles and lessen the potential for permanent scarring alopecia. Sensory nerves in the subcutis have a similar course to that of the vascular system and peripheral incisions for flap design can transect larger nerve trunks resulting in sensory changes that can take an extended time to resolve. Rarely, sensory changes can be permanent. Lymphatics bear the same "snakelike" distribution, lying deep in the subcutaneous tissue. The dense network of lymph-collecting vessels arises from precollectors within 2 cm of the midline and runs obliquely down and backward to reach the first-tier lymph nodes. On average, four frontal-collecting, six parietal-collecting, and six occipital-collecting lymph vessels are found in the scalp.[5]

5.1.3 Galea Aponeurotica

Galea, the third layer in the scalp, is a 1- to 2-mm-thick, very dense, inelastic fibrous sheet. It is stretched under tension between the frontalis muscle anteriorly, moving over the vertex and extending to the occipital muscle

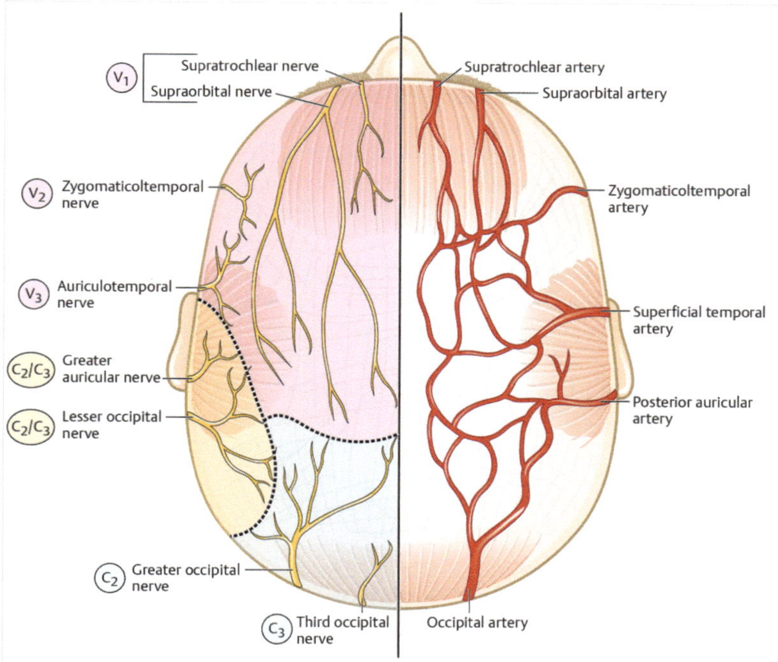

Fig. 5.3 Neurovascular scalp anatomy.

posteriorly. The frontal and occipital muscle bellies are inserted directly into the galea. It fades out laterally by blending with the temporal fascia (▶ Fig. 5.2).[1] The frontalis muscle arises from the front of the aponeurosis and is inserted into the superior part of the orbicularis oculi. This allows the subaponeurotic/subgaleal space to extend anteriorly beneath the orbicularis oculi into the eyelids, yielding an effective dissection plane. As outlined earlier, this plane allows anterior and inferior movement of surgical blood, leading to periorbital ecchymosis and swelling. The fibrous nature of the galea imparts three important qualities. First, the high-tensile strength allows the galea to support buried or pulley sutures under very high tension. If galea is not captured in a suture path, closure of moderate- to high-tension reconstructions becomes difficult. Second, because the galea is stretched under tension between the frontal and occipital poles, an incision made in the galea can lead to retraction away from the wound edge. Surgeons must be mindful of this concept and ensure their suture path is angled to include the galea should retraction be evident. Third, as galea is significantly resistant to stretching, a practice of galeotomy, or linear galeal transection (serial relaxing incisions), is still used to reduce scalp tension and facilitate greater stretch.[6] The effectiveness of galeotomies in reducing closure tension remains debated. In addition, galeotomies can increase the risk of vascular damage. In the author's practice, galeotomies have given only minimal additional tissue length and are used only rarely in an attempt to gain maximal tissue length when reconstructions are under very high tension.

5.1.4 Subgaleal Loose Connective Tissue

The loose fibroareolar tissue makes up the fourth layer and presents as a potential space underneath the densely packed scalp layers above. This layer allows for the overlying scalp to glide over the periosteum and accounts for scalp movability. In scalps where this layer is well developed and relatively "thick," the gliding phenomenon can be generous, while scalps that have a relatively poorly developed fibroareolar layer are found to be "tight." The subgaleal space is avascular and easily separated by blunt dissection. As such, it presents the primary plane for scalp undermining. The extent of subgaleal loose connective tissue is the most important factor that determines scalp laxity and the ease with which scalp tissues can be moved during reconstructions.[1] To a lesser degree, scalp laxity is accounted for by the ability of scalp to elasticize, which relates to its pliability along the Langer's lines.

5.1.5 Periosteum

Periosteum (pericranium) is the fifth layer of the scalp and covers all the skull bones. It is a dense fibrous sheet, readily separable from the overlying loose subgaleal space, but relatively adherent to the underlying skull. However, periosteal stripping is possible, bloodless, and can be accomplished with blunt dissection. The periosteum is untethered from the bone in a rolling fashion using a periosteal elevator or equivalent. The minimal blood supply to periosteum comes from tiny bone perforators derived from meningeal vessels. During dissection, any bleeding is controlled with careful and precise cautery. Periosteal "toughness" allows consideration to suspend heavy or high-tension flaps from this dense layer in order to avoid widened scars. Although placement of periosteal supporting sutures is possible, the authors rarely practice this technique. Of note, the top layer of the skull, the outer table, just deep to the periosteum is often removed when a tumor is not able to be cleared within the periosteum or margins are not contiguous enough to be confident in tumor clearance.

5.2 Reconstructive Options

5.2.1 Algorithm for Scalp Reconstruction

Presenting a comprehensive algorithm for scalp reconstruction is challenging as patient preferences substantially impact on the chosen reconstruction option. A primary patient factor is their level of cosmetic concern. For those patients willing to tolerate loss of hair-bearing scalp, the reconstructive algorithm expands dramatically. Similarly, patients with multiple medical comorbidities may mandate or request a less involved reconstruction. Local tissue factors, including previous surgeries, past radiotherapy, and loss of periosteum, can all lead to reconstructive choices outside the defined algorithm. Surgeon experience influences the decision process, and any algorithm will exhibit a personal and institutional bias.

Many author groups have published effective algorithms for scalp reconstruction.[7,10] The presented algorithm represents the author's primary decision pathway when deciding on a reconstructive choice in an outpatient setting using local anesthesia. Four components populate the author's algorithmic approach. This includes defect size, which in the author's experience can be divided into small (< 2 cm in longest dimension assuming a circular defect; ▸ Fig. 5.4), moderate (3–5 cm in longest dimension; ▸ Fig. 5.5), and large or extensive (> 6 or 9 cm in longest dimension, respectively; ▸ Fig. 5.6). Scalp tension/scalp mobility, which can be both site and patientdependent, has been separated into high, moderate, or low. The potential for a reconstruction to distort hairline position and the location of the defect in hair-bearing or alopecic scalp comprise the final two decision pathways. As previously outlined, patient and surgeon preferences can lead to a chosen reconstruction, which was not within the algorithmic outline.

5.2.2 Second Intention Healing

Second intention healing (SIH) is a valuable scalp reconstructive option in a diffuse range of defect scenarios. The prevalence of SIH in scalp reconstruction is unknown. A British study estimated overall SIH prevalence at 41/1,000 population,[11] while a U.S. private Mohs micrographic surgery center repaired 37.9% of wounds (at variable sites) using SIH.[12] In the senior author's (DMZ) practice, 15% of scalp defects are repaired with SIH. An

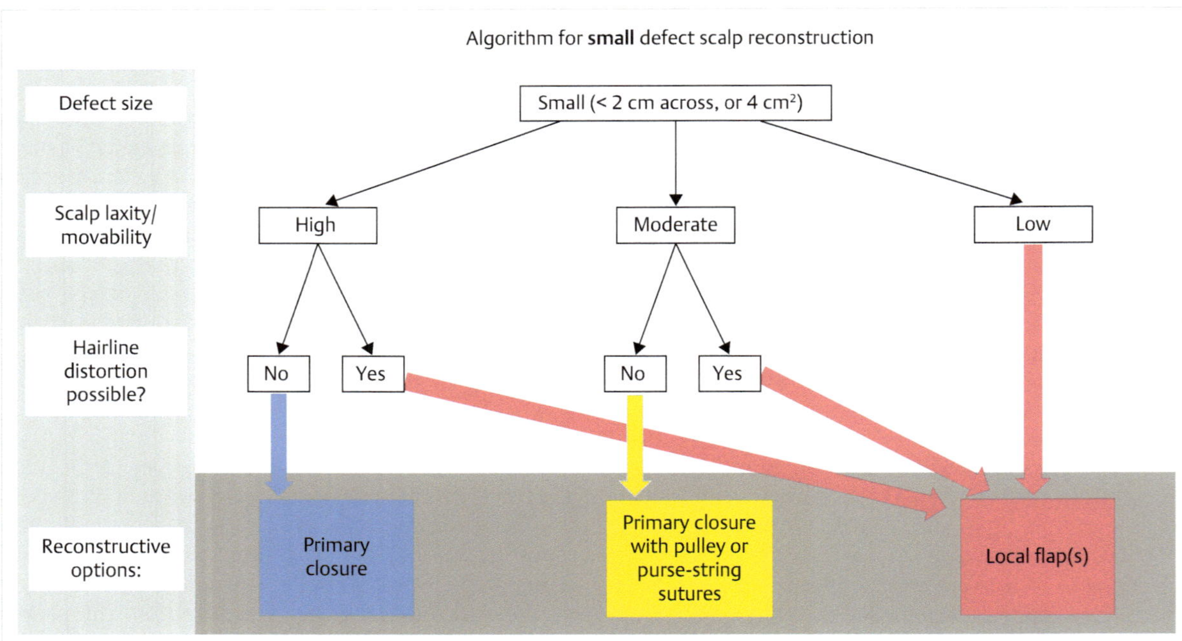

Fig. 5.4 Algorithm for reconstruction of small flap defects. The algorithm must be implemented in accordance with individual patient factors. Further information is found in the chapter text.

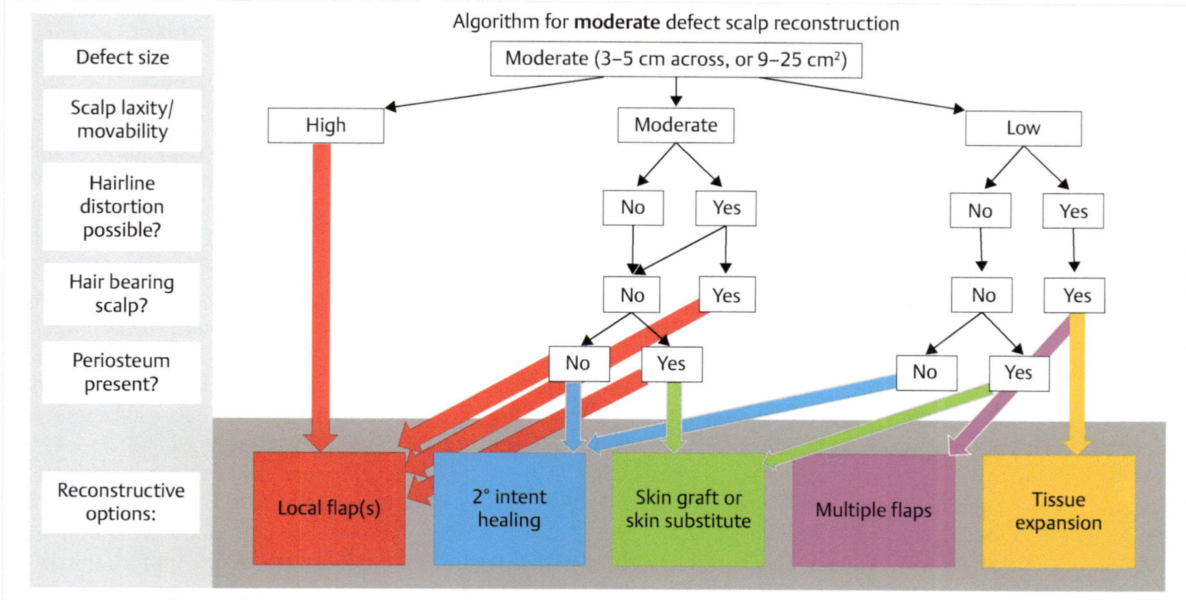

Fig. 5.5 Algorithm for reconstruction of moderate flap defects. The algorithm must be implemented in accordance with individual patient factors. Further information is found in the chapter text.

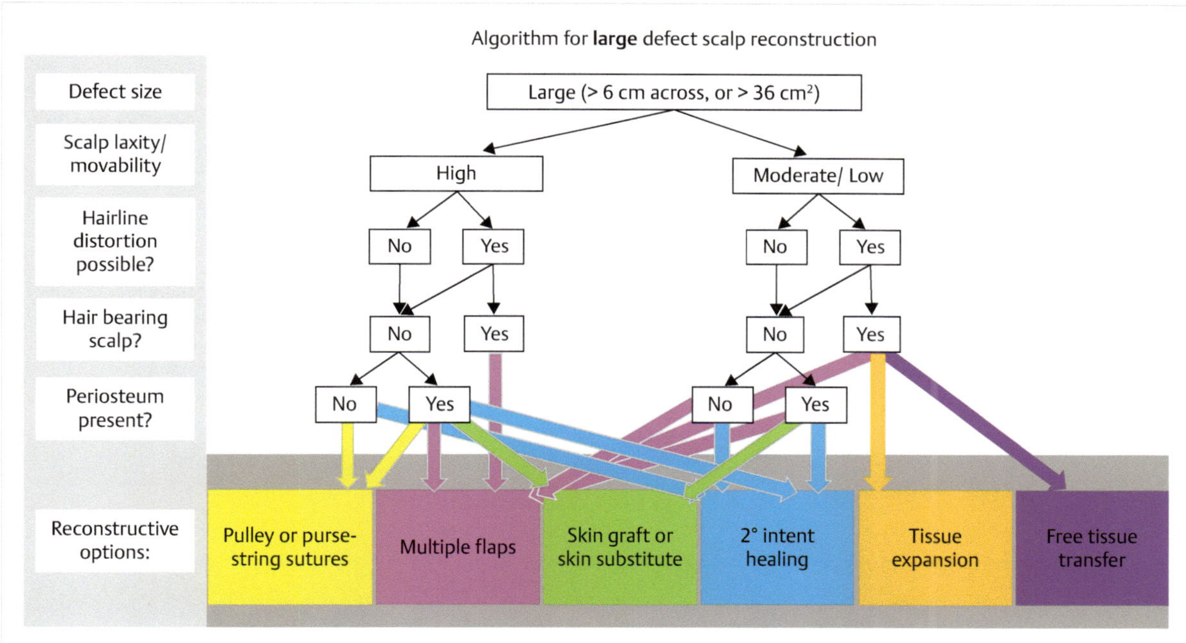

Fig. 5.6 Algorithm for reconstruction of large flap defects. The algorithm must be implemented in accordance with individual patient factors. Further information is found in the chapter text.

interesting survey study found that the most experienced surgeons were significantly more likely to heal deep and larger wounds secondarily.[13] The use of SIH as a reconstructive option remains very physician and institution dependent as evidenced by a systematic review[7] where SIH was part of a reconstructive ladder, but not listed as surgical option in a 105-patient, single-institution study.[14] The editors find SIH to be ideal for partial-thickness defects or shallow full-thickness defects in non-hair-bearing locations.

SIH should be considered in large defects where local flap(s) would not be sufficient and the patient does not wish a skin graft secondary donor defect, or the morbidity of freetissue transfer. SIH allows easy surveillance for possible recurrence in high-risk skin cancers. In cases where patients wish to avoid any additional surgery after cancer resection because of medical or social concerns, SIH is the only viable option. In an environment of minimizing medical costs, SIH allows good functional and cosmetic results in carefully selected patients. Although care of an SIH wound can be time-consuming and prolonged, there is no restriction on exercise, bathing/showering, or other activities of daily living.

The ideal scalp sites for SIH are areas of alopecia, away from hairlines, with an intact periosteum, although any area of the scalp can be considered.[15] Hair-bearing areas can be repaired with SIH, if the patient is less cosmetically concerned, or is willing to change their hairstyle to allow camouflage of the hairless scar. SIH over areas of absent periosteum or compromised vascular supply has been well documented.[16,17] The authors have successfully used SIH in over 30 cases where periosteum was absent, including 1 case in a previous radiotherapy field. No infections occurred within the surrounding soft tissue or bone, and the postoperative course was well tolerated by patients. One additional case did not heal after 15 months, leading to sequestration of the outer table, requiring removal, and placement of a split-thickness skin graft (STSG).

The primary criterion that must be met before choosing SIH is the need for the patient and/or family member to care for an open, potentially draining wound, for a prolonged period of time. A study of 38 patients with a mean area of exposed soft tissue of 15.75 cm^2 and mean area of exposed bone of 10.74 cm^2 showed a mean time to epithelialize of 7 and 13 weeks, respectively.[16] These parameters do not mirror the authors' experience. In our patient population, time to complete healing with periosteum present averaged 14 weeks, and with periosteum absent 24 weeks (▶ Fig. 5.7, ▶ Fig. 5.8). The authors' mean size of scalp defect with periosteum present was 40.8 cm^2, while mean size of defect with periosteum absent was 54.5 cm^2. These larger defects partially explain the authors' longer healing times. However, SIH is not linear, and larger wounds can heal quicker than expected given logarithmic wound contraction.[18] Differences in wound care protocols, or patient factors, may also have played a role. Longer healing times for SIH compared to other reconstructive options can delay postoperative adjuvant therapy should this be required.

Care of an SIH scalp wound requires meticulous attention to keeping a moist wound bed, especially if periosteum is absent. After excision, an occlusive ointment is placed on the wound bed, followed by application of an absorbent pressure dressing. The authors leave the dressing in place for 48 hours, at which time the patient removes the dressing, showers the site with warm water and a mild shampoo, and then the site is redressed with liberal application of an occlusive ointment and a light nonadherent membrane. This process is repeated from twice a day to every 2 to 3 days depending on the quantity of drainage. The authors have not used more advanced wound dressings. The use of oral antibiotics has not been required, and minimal postoperative discomfort is easily controlled with acetaminophen or equivalent.

Various adjuvant treatments have been used to speed healing or promote granulation tissue over exposed bone.

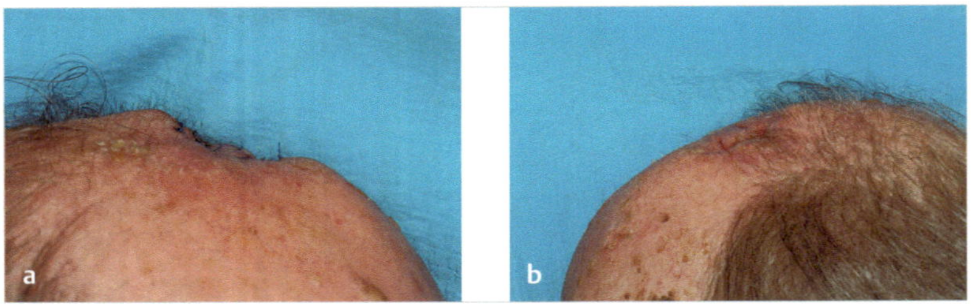

Fig. 5.7 Resolution of moderate standing cone in an 80-year-old man with a 3.2 × 2.7 cm defect over the central parietal scalp closed with pulley sutures. **(a)** immediately postsurgery. **(b)** Two weeks postsurgery.

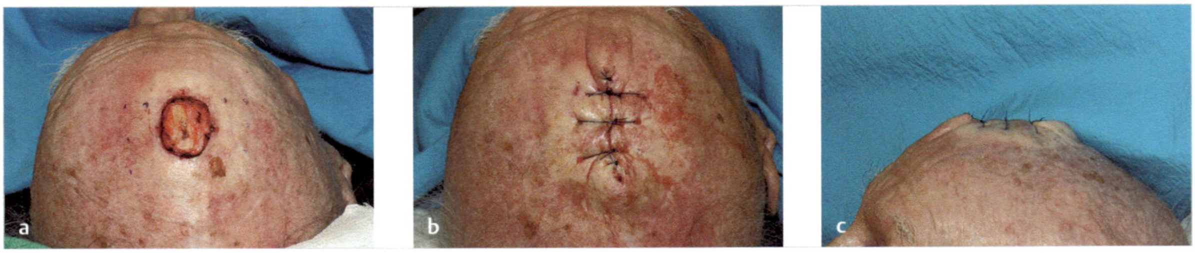

Fig. 5.8 Closure of a 4.2 × 3 cm defect over central parietal scalp in an 81-year-old man with two previous cerebrovascular accidents. **(a)** immediately prior to closure. **(b)** immediately after placement of three pulley sutures. **(c)** lateral view. Cutaneous redundancies will be allowed to settle spontaneously.

The creation of fenestrations in the outer table can stimulate new granulation tissue.[19] The authors have had some anecdotal success with minocycline 100 mg once or twice a day for up to 3 months. The sharp removal of fibrin from the wound edge or base can stimulate granulation tissue formation and hasten epithelialization. Epithelial migration arrest is successfully treated with a mid-potency topical steroid twice a day for 1 week. Many other modalities have been promoted in the literature including silicone gels,[20] negative pressure wound therapy,[21] 0.5% timolol solution,[22] and various allogenic dressings. The authors have no direct experience with these therapies.

In the editors' experience, wounds extending to the cranium with absent periosteum are at high risk for epithelial migration arrest. This can be mitigated by the use of iodoform-impregnated gauze changed every 2 to 3 days. Dermabrasion of the outer table with a diamond fraise can also increase blood supply and granulation tissue from the perforations. The application of a wound-vac or negative-pressure dressing changed every 2 to 3 days can also promote granulation tissue and vascularity to support delayed application of a skin graft.

A scalp wound, which will be repaired using SIH, can be reduced in size by the use of purse-string[23] or pulley sutures.[24] Although the effectiveness of these modalities is debated in the literature, the authors have found they reduce the size of a defect by approximately 20%, but there appears to be only minimal impact on overall healing time (▶ Fig. 5.9, ▶ Fig. 5.10). Combining partial closures with Burow's triangle grafting can provide a shorter healing time and improve contour in some cases.

The usual cosmetic result is fully evident by 12 to 18 months after complete SIH. Over this time period, scar thickness and erythema settle into a pale, shiny, hairless area. The contour match to the surrounding skin is good and can be better than what can be achieved with skin graft healing.

5.2.3 Skin Grafts

Split- or full-thickness skin grafting is commonly used to reconstruct medium to extensive scalp defects where periosteum is present and patient cosmetic concerns are minimal. Skin grafting is advantageous in patients who have marked concurrent medical morbidities where more complex reconstructions are not practical. Skin grafts are also a valuable option after high-risk cancer excisions as the ease of surveillance for possible recurrence is increased. Studies have shown that skin grafts comprise upward of 20 to 52% of scalp reconstructions.[14, 24] STSG are favored over full-thickness skin grafts (FTSG) given the former's reduced nutritional demands and larger potential size. The authors, however, do favor FTSG, if practical, as the donor site can be closed primarily, reducing donor site care. Furthermore, an FTSG can be harvested and thinned as needed to be the same thickness as STSG. FTSG also have the potential for an improved final cosmetic result (▶ Fig. 5.11, ▶ Fig. 5.12).

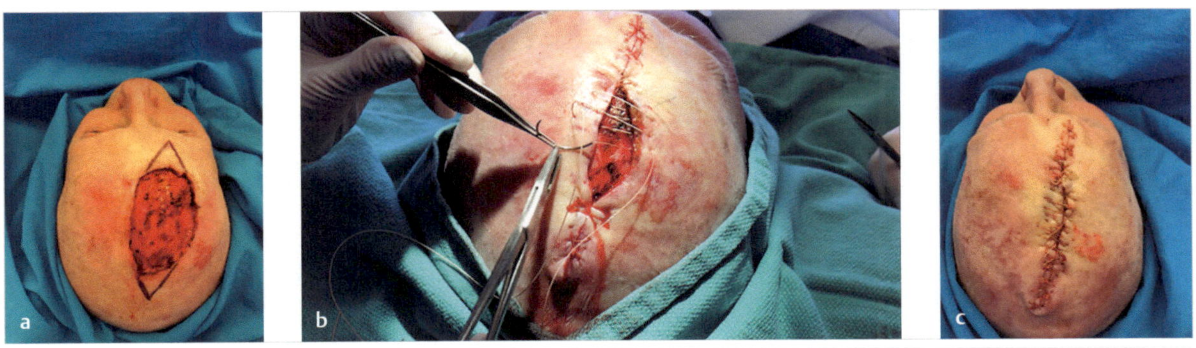

Fig. 5.9 Large primary closure using running pulley sutures in an 86-year-old man with a 9.7 × 6.0 cm defect in a tight parietal scalp. **(a)** immediately prior to closure. **(b)** intraoperative placement of the running pulley suture. **(c)** immediately after complete closure.

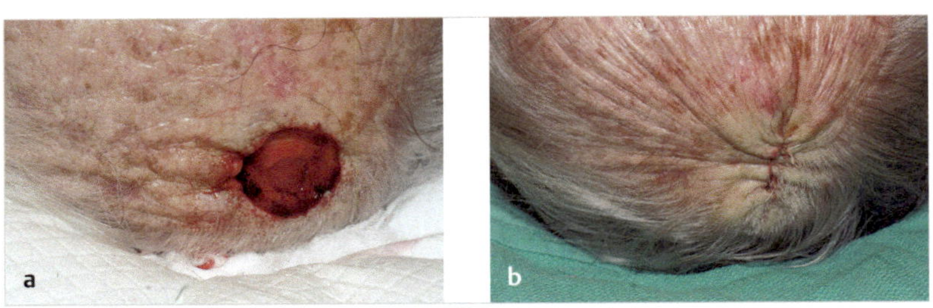

Fig. 5.10 Purse-string suture placement in a 93-year-old old man with a 4.1 × 2.9 cm defect on the posterior scalp vertex. **(a)** immediately prior to closure. **(b)** immediately postplacement. Folded cutaneous redundancies will resolved spontaneously.

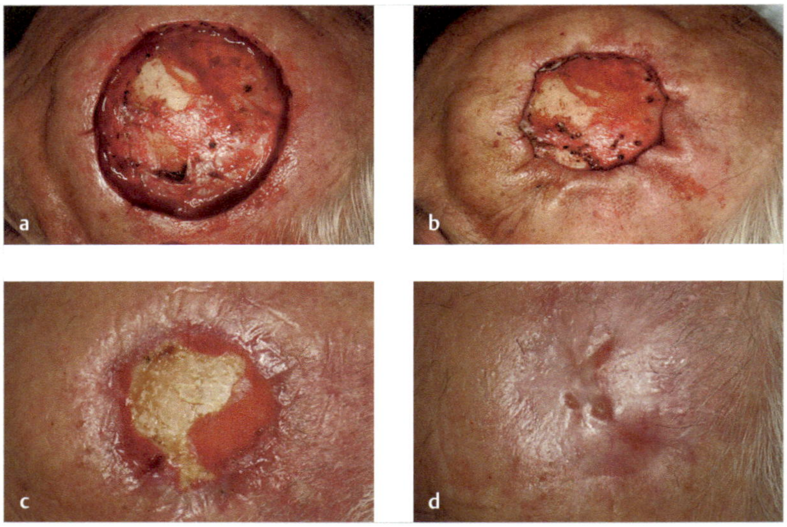

Fig. 5.11 Purse-string placement and second intention healing in a 78-year-old man with a 7 × 7 cm defect. **(a)** immediately prior to closure. **(b)** immediately post-placement of purse-string suture defect size reduced to 5 × 5 cm. **(c)** Six weeks postoperative. **(d)** Eight months postoperative.

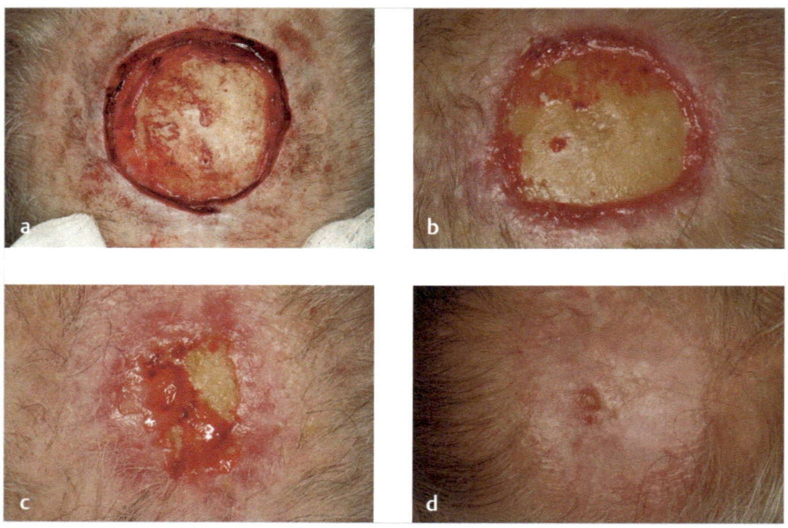

Fig. 5.12 Second intention over bone in a 69-year-oldman with a 7 × 7 cm defect over the central frontal scalp. **(a)** immediately postoperative. **(b)** One month postoperative. **(c)** 4.5 months postoperative. **(d)** Ten months postoperative.

Fixation of skin grafts can be completed with sutures or staples, and in the authors' experience, have led to equivalent results.

In an outpatient setting, STSG are commonly harvested using a Weck blade with a thickness of 12 to 20 µm. Preferred donor sites are the anterior thighs, lower abdomen, and upper medial arm. Successful harvesting of an intact, uniform graft requires operator skill in directing forward and downward pressures with the Weck blade, liberal use of a skin lubricant, as well as an assistant who is able to stabilize and flatten the donor area. Given these technical concerns, a potentially painful donor site, and the need for prolonged donor site care, the authors prefer using FTSG. The FTSG can be thinned aggressively and, as for an STSG, can be fenestrated to increase size.

An intact periosteum is required for skin graft survival. Rarely, direct placement of an STSG over exposed bone will survive if scalp emissary veins are patent and present in adequate numbers. If periosteum is absent, options to provide a vascularized bed include a technique known as backgrafting in which an adjacent flap of adequate size to cover the primary defect is elevated (either in the subcutaneous plane or in the subgaleal plane) and rotated or transposed into the primary defect. The donor site of the flap has periosteum and/or galea and subcutaneous tissue at the base and can be grafted. Another option is to raise an adjacent flap at the subperiosteal plane, separate the periosteum and loose alveolar tissue from the galea, rotate these tissues into the bony defect, immediately apply a graft over these tissues, and then reset the skin, subcutaneous tissues, and galea of the flap to their original location (▸ Fig. 5.13). Delayed grafting after successful stimulation of granulation tissue through SIH protocols can be considered. Finally, the bare bone can be

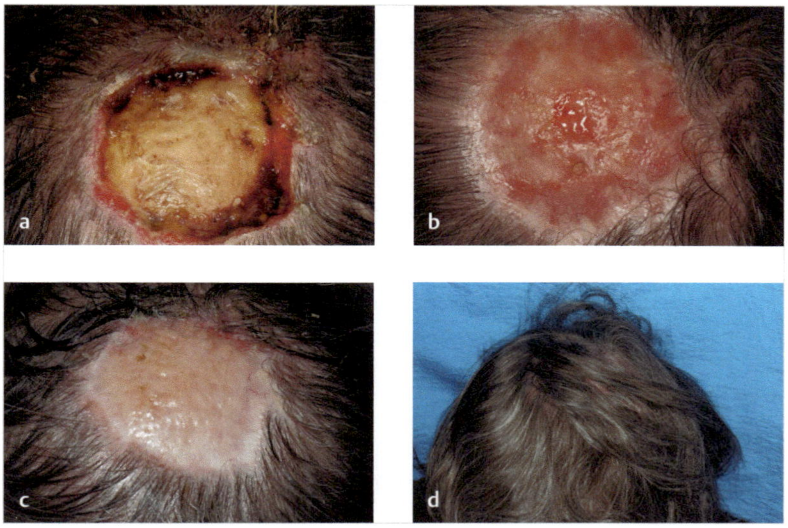

Fig. 5.13 Second intention over bone in an 85-year-old woman with a 7.6 × 7.5 cm defect over the hair-bearing scalp vertex. She did not wish for a more complex repair. **(a)** One week postoperative. **(b)** Five months postoperative. **(c)** Ten months postoperative. **(d)** Ten months postoperative with hairstyle modified to camouflage scar.

fenestrated or removed completely to expose the vascular diploic space, with a graft then immediately placed over the diploe. Full removal of the outer cortex is not performed in an outpatient setting.

Assuming an adequate vascular bed, skin grafting on scalp sites has success rates for complete healing in greater than 90% of the author's cases. If the defect is deep, grafts must be designed 10 to 20% larger to prevent tenting and loss of direct contact with the recipient bed. Given the large size of most scalp defects repaired with skin grafts, the authors aggressively thin FTSG to the mid-reticular dermis to reduce metabolic requirements and increase survival. Although the value of bolster dressings for skin graft fixation has been debated,[25] the author's preference is to apply a fixation dressing given the large size and depth of many scalp defects. Wound care includes only liberal application of an occlusive ointment at the periphery of the bolster, and avoidance of prolonged exposure to water over the treatment area for 2 to 4 weeks postoperative. Analgesics include acetaminophen or a nonsteroidal anti-inflammatory drug, individually or combined. Narcotic analgesics are rarely used. Sutures are removed at 1 week, and the occlusive ointment continues until complete healing is evident, generally in 2 to 4 weeks.

Complications in scalp skin grafts are uncommon, less than 5% of the author's cases. This has included small areas of graft necrosis, treated using a second intention wound healing protocol. Superficial crusting does not mean the entire graft is not taken—usually the base of the graft is viable and only the surface requires mild debridement, followed by local wound care to prevent scab or crust from re-forming. Small seromas or hematomas have occurred and are easily treated with a 19-gauge needle aspiration or expression through a no. 15 blade stab incision. Infection has occurred in less than 1% of patients, cultures have shown *Staphylococcus aureus*, or *Streptococcus pyogenes*, which have responded quickly to an oral first-generation cephalosporin.

The expected cosmetic result is an alopecic, hypopigmented, shiny, atrophic scar, with moderate contour deficit if used in thick-skinned temporal or occipital areas. However, for patients with moderate to severe hair loss and atrophic skin, the cosmetic results can be good, and in some cases, better than what could be achieved by a large flap(s).

In a limited number of cases, the use of skin substitutes can prove helpful to further decrease operative time and wound care commitments in debilitated patients or those patients who simply wish to avoid reconstruction with large flaps or freetissue transfer. Examples include acellular dermis graft (Alloderm,LifeCell Corporation)[26] or dermal regenerative template (Integra, Integra Life Sciences).[27,28] Both require a vascularized bed, so periosteum must be present, or if absent, the outer table will have to be fenestrated or removed. The material is sutured lightly into the defect and both stimulate a healthy granulating bed, which can then be allowed to continue to complete healing, or secondarily grafted with an STSG. Care required is daily application and changing of an occlusive ointment and nonadherent dressing.

5.2.4 Local Flaps

Operative wounds on the scalp can be classified based on their size (assuming a circular defect and measuring diameter) as small (< 2 cm), medium (3–5 cm), large (6–8 cm), and very large (> 9 cm). When planning for scalp reconstruction, one has to account for the differences between regions of loose and tight attachment of the scalp to the cranium. Small operative wounds on the occipital, temporal, and the most anterior regions of the frontal scalp are easily closed with advancement and transposition flaps, as the galea is thin and blends into the temporoparietal or occipitofrontal muscle fascia in these regions. In contrast, the parietal and posterior regions of the frontal scalp have a dense galeal layer, no underlying muscle, and poor distensibility, making such repairs less effective.[29]

Scalp flaps should ideally be dissected below the galea, as larger blood vessels, lymphatics, and nerves run superficial to this plane. This allows for their preservation and prevents resultant flap ischemia. The absence of large vessels in the subgaleal plane offers the advantage of a relatively bloodless plane of dissection and minimal requirements for hemostasis. Although the risk for hair follicle injury and subsequent hair loss is also decreased when dissecting within the subgaleal plane, such flaps can be quite inelastic and nondistensible. Therefore, a large surface area relative to the size of the defect must be accounted for when designing scalp flaps.

Whenever possible, the simplest reconstruction technique should be used to provide the most functional and aesthetic results with the least complexity. Local flaps are ideal to achieve these goals as they replace the defect with similar tissue and produce a donor area that is easily closed. When reconstructing the scalp with flaps, a primary functional consideration should be to ensure adequate coverage of the calvarium in order to prevent desiccation and infection.[7] Cosmetic considerations include preservation of free margins such as the anterior hairline and ears. Flap size should be sufficient to minimize tension on wound edges and limit postoperative iatrogenic alopecia. In order to further minimize hair follicle injury, incisions should be made parallel to the direction of hair growth (trichophytic incision), and cautery used judiciously on wound margins.

Linear/Primary Reconstruction

Small Primary Closures

Primary linear closures can be employed to repair small defects in the looser regions of the scalp. Although the convex shape of the scalp limits mobility gain, generous undermining (carried out up to 5 cm based on the author's experience) is required to achieve a tension-free closure. Additional mobility can be obtained with galeal releasing incisions, which are placed parallel to the incision line on the galeal surface of the advancing repair surface and spaced 15 to 20 mm apart. When performing such incisions, caution should be taken to avoid injury to the vasculature, which increases the risk for subsequent hematoma and flap ischemia.

A bilayered technique should be followed, with closure tension directed mainly to the galea to minimize tension on the skin and limit resultant alopecia. In order to achieve this, deep interrupted sutures at the level of the galea utilizing suture material of proper strength and thickness should allow for complete approximation of the wound edges. For this purpose, the authors favor the use of 2–0 or 3–0 polyglactin 910 (Vicryl). Well-placed deep sutures should allow the overlying skin to be approximated with minimal tension. Skin sutures can be used in an interrupted or continuous fashion with sutures such as 3–0 or 4–0 nylon (Ethilon), or staples, according to physician preference. Any resulting small to medium standing cutaneous deformities can be tolerated on the scalp, as they will significantly flatten over time (▶ Fig. 5.14). The editors often use the same suture types for deep and skin sutures in scalp primary closures including 3–0 polyglactin 910 on an RB-1 needle for an additional curve, making wrist action for eversion and deeper galeal bites easier. In addition, the 3–0 polyglactin 910 RB-1 typically has a longer thread, which is helpful in larger scalp reconstructions.

Moderate Primary Closures

Although medium and large defects are usually less amenable to primary repair, linear closure of larger defects has been reported and can be achieved in selected cases where wounds are located on the looser areas of the scalp where there is underlying musculature.[30] Extensive undermining, up to 15 cm, has been described to successfully distribute the wound closure tension over a wide area.[31] As in small primary closures, galeal releasing incisions can be considered to further increase wound edge mobility.

Alternatively, pulley sutures, which are effective in areas of high tension and poor local tissue mobility, can be used for medium defects, even when these are located on tight regions of the scalp. Pulley sutures allow for reduction in tension along the suture length, and provide efficient hemostasis, as well as overall reduction in time and cost to perform the closure with similar cosmetic and functional outcomes[32] (▶ Fig. 5.15, ▶ Fig. 5.16). One technique first

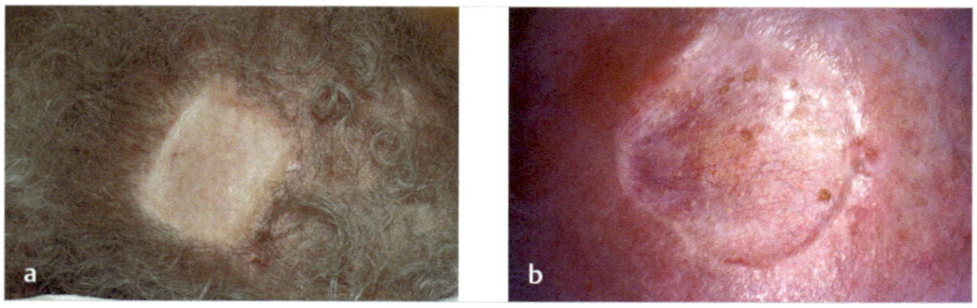

Fig. 5.14 Split-thickness skin graft's long-term cosmetic results. **(a)** Atrophic depressed alopecic shiny result 10 years postoperative (graft was not placed by authors). **(b)** Atrophic depressed result 4 years postoperative in a 75-year-old man with a 6.1 × 5.7 cm defect.

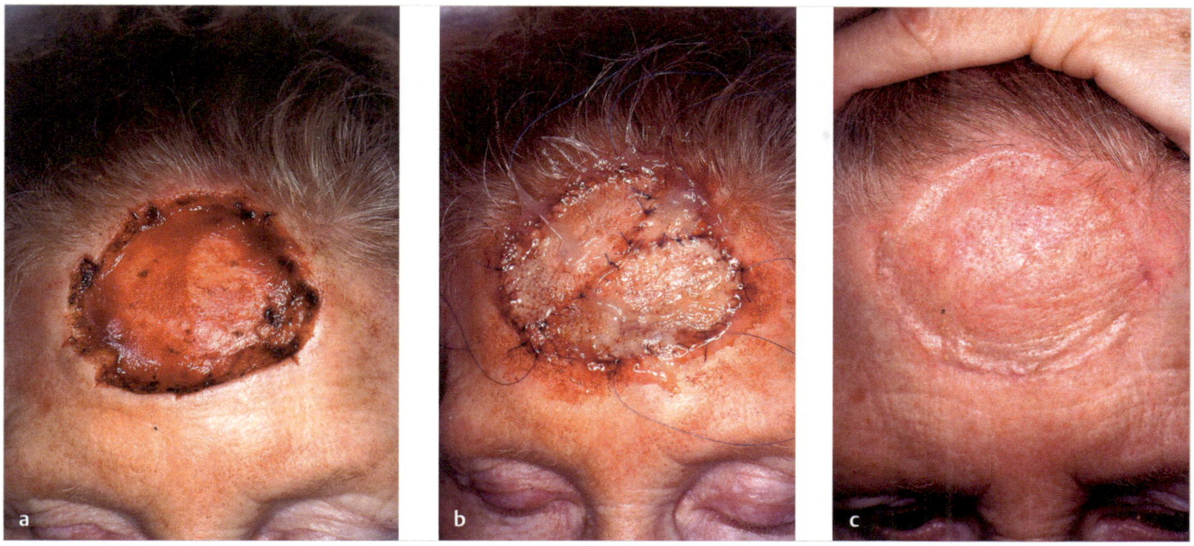

Fig. 5.15 Full-thickness skin graft in a 67-year-old woman with a 5.5 × 4.7 cm defect. She did not wish more involved reconstruction. **(a)** Immediately prior to graft placement. **(b)** immediately after graft placement. Donor sites were left and right clavicular areas. **(c)** 2.5 months postoperative.

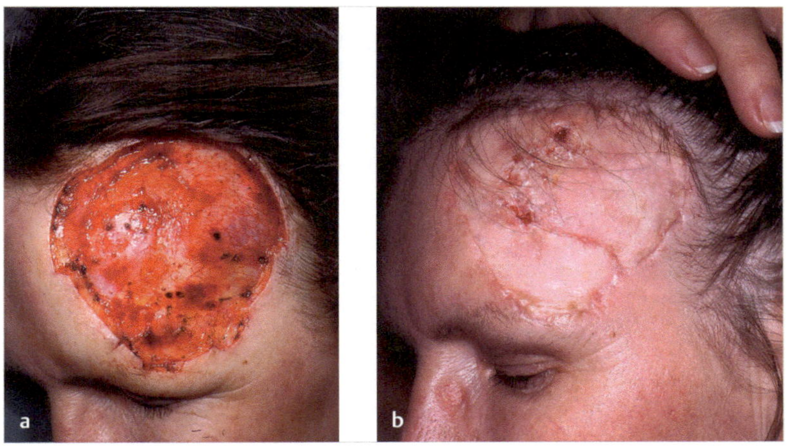

Fig. 5.16 Full-thickness skin graft on the left temporal/parietal scalp in a 51-year-old woman with a 7.5 × 7.1 cm defect after Mohs excision of a basal cell carcinoma.The patient did not wish more advanced reconstruction. **(a)** Immediately prior to graft placement. **(b)** Six weeks postoperative.

requires undermining of wound edges. One or more pulley sutures are then placed in a "far-near-near-far" technique including galea at the base, in which the needle enters "far" from one wound edge and exits "near" the opposite wound edge, after which it re-enters "near" the initial wound edge and exits "far" from the opposite wound edge, so that two loops are completed. Once all sutures are placed, an assistant exerts tension while the surgeon ties one or more sutures serially.[24] In addition, pulley sutures can serve as external tissue expanders by providing progressive tissue expansion (intraoperative tissue creep). With this technique, suture tails are left long after initial pulley placement. Pulley sutures are left in place for 1 week, after which wound edges are sharply debrided and a hemostat is attached to the loop connecting the "far" bites of the pulley suture, with the suture being cut between the hemostat and the knot. Once this is performed, the suture is advanced and retied, allowing for additional would edge advancement. This is repeated on a weekly basis until the wound is effectively closed.[24]

Purse-String Closures

Purse-string closures allow for partial closure of round or oval-shaped small to medium defects, regardless of their location on the scalp. By reducing scar area, healing time is expedited, and hemostasis is enhanced. With this technique, little to no undermining is performed. A running subcuticular suture parallel to the plane of the skin and going around the entire perimeter of the wound is placed, after which tension is directed to the ends of the suture, so that they effectively decrease scar area, and the knot is

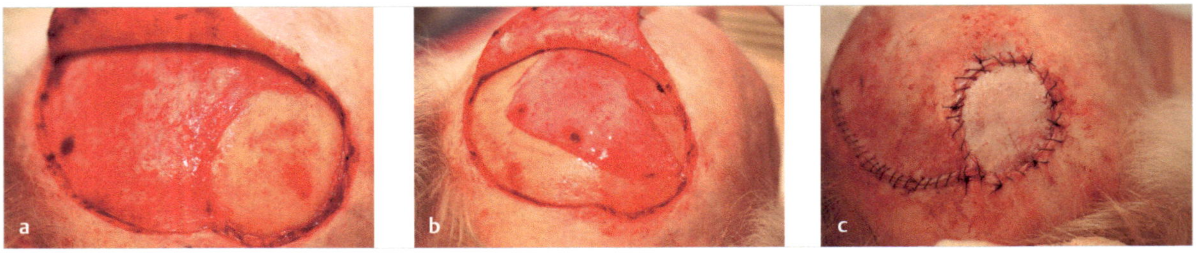

Fig. 5.17 Use of a periosteal flap to allow placement of a skin graft over a 4.1 × 3.7 cm defect with exposed bone in an 82-year-old man. The tumor removed was a high risk and graft coverage allows easier assessment for possible recurrence compared to flap closure. **(a)** Rotation flap raised in the subgaleal plane with loose alveolar tissue and periosteum exposed. **(b)** Periosteal flap incised, rotated, and partially sutured into the primary defect. **(c)** Rotation flap returned to the original position and graft applied.

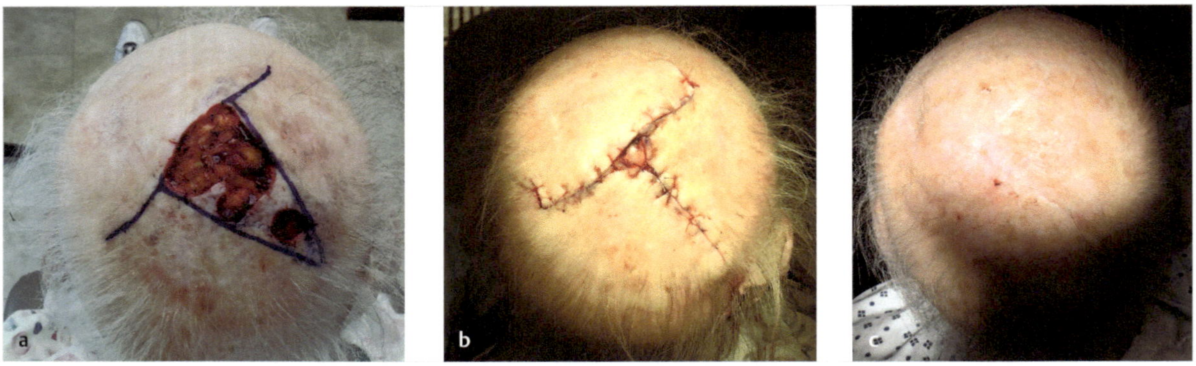

Fig. 5.18 (a–c) Multiple full-thickness defects of the scalp closed with one A-T advancement flap. **(a)** Multiple defects placed in an elongated A-T advancement flap. **(b)** Bilateral advancement flap closed with a small area left to heal by second intention. **(c)** One-year follow-up. (These images are provided courtesy of Stanislav N. Tolkachjov, MD.)

tied externally to the wound[33] (▶ Fig. 5.17). In some cases of partial closure, the area of the wound that is left open is allowed to heal by second intention.

Other Advancement Flaps

Other types of advancement flaps (e.g., H-plasty flaps or O-T flaps) have a limited role in scalp reconstruction due to the inelastic nature of the scalp. Similar to primary linear closures, modified advancement flaps are mainly used for small defects located on the loose regions of the scalp. Less commonly, bilateral advancement flaps (such as O-T flaps) can be used for moderate sized defects if scalp mobility is adequate (▶ Fig. 5.18).

Rotation Flaps

Rotation flaps have a major role in scalp reconstruction as the natural convexity of the scalp is well suited for curvilinear incisions. Simple rotation flaps can be used for small (9 cm^2) scalp defects (▶ Fig. 5.19). Generally, incisions should be roughly four to six times the length of the original surgical defect to account for the intrinsic inelasticity of the scalp. A standing tissue cone is designed adjacent to the operative wound to create a triangulated defect, after which a curvilinear incision is designed along an arc adjacent to the defect and directed toward a tissue reservoir. The arc of rotation can be vertically oversized superiorly, so the distance from the pivot point to the flap tip equals the distance from the pivot point to the most distal aspect of the defect. This allows for compensation of pivotal restraint, minimizes tension on the flap, and eliminates the need for secondary motion around the operative defect.[34] The flap should be widely undermined, particularly around the point of pivotal restraint. As the flap is elevated, it is rotated to fill the surgical defect. Once this occurs, a secondary defect is created along the entire arc of the flap, which is closed in a fashion allowing for tension to be evenly distributed along its span. Discrepancies in length between each side of the arc may be created and require the removal of standing cutaneous deformities[35] or can be sewn out using the rule of halves principle. In the editor's experience, large single-arm rotation flaps can effectively cover a large defect (▶ Fig. 5.20).

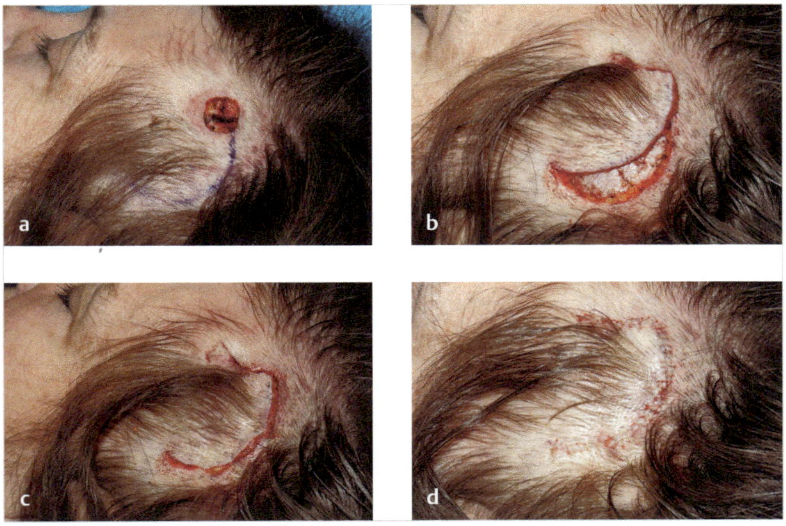

Fig. 5.19 Small rotation flap in a 70-year-old woman with a 2.0 × 1.6 cm defect over the left parietal scalp. **(a)** Flap designed to encompass greatest vasculature and maintain hairline position. The length of the flap is four times the defect diameter. **(b)** Flap rotated into position to ensure both primary and secondary defects can be closed under low tension. **(c)** Primary and secondary defects closed with deep sutures. **(d)** Final flap trimming and epidermal sutures placed.

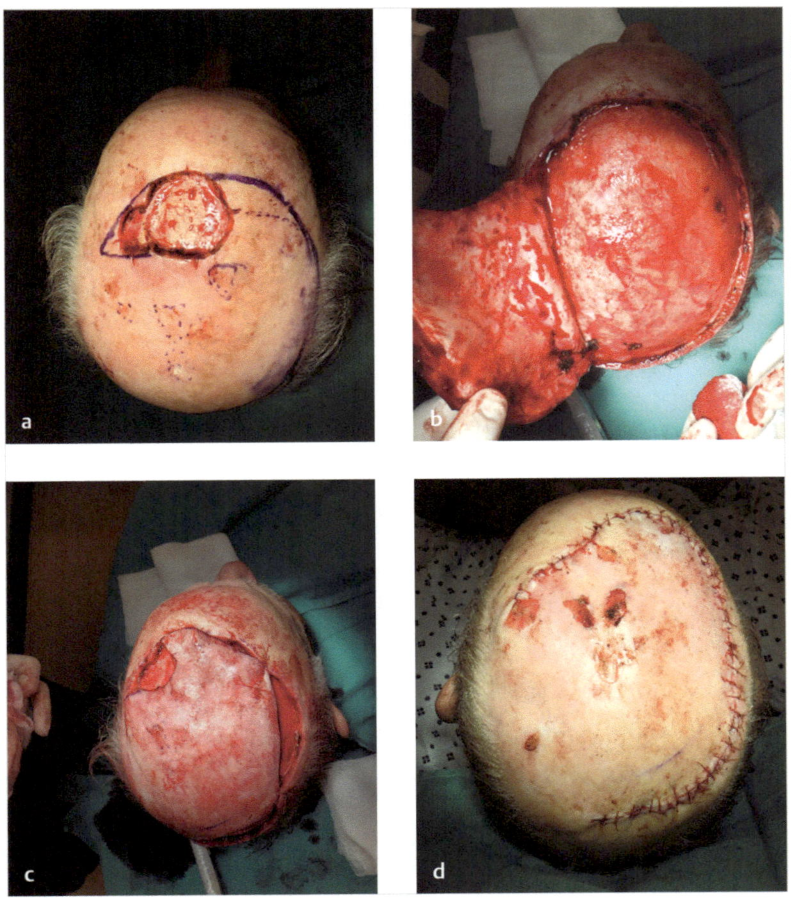

Fig. 5.20 **(a–d)** Single-arm scalp rotation flap. **(a)** Flap design showing a wide and long arc of at least 4 times the area as the defect width. This allows for a wide base for flap perfusion and a long arc of rotation to minimize tension along the arc path. **(b)** Flap undermined at the subgaleal plane. The flap can be undermined quickly in this plane without having to use cautery during the undermining process. However, some surgeons prefer to cauterize as the flap is being incised. **(c)** Key sutures align the anterior end of the flap as well as a midpoint pulley suture to allow the flap to be anchored at the high tension points. **(d)** A few more deep 3-0 polyglactin 910 sutures on an RB-1 needle are placed to minimize tension and ensure approximation of the galea and dermis/subcutis. Epidermal sutures are then used. Running or interrupted sutures are effective. (These images are provided courtesy of Stanislav N. Tolkachjov, MD.)

Double Rotation Flaps

O-to-Z Rotation Flaps

O-to-Z rotation flaps are particularly wellsuited for small to large vertex defects when insufficient laxity exists for closure with a single-sided rotation flap. Rather than pure rotational movement, these flaps can incorporate varying amounts of advancement into the design. Two distinct arcs are created, each originating 180 degrees opposite one another, with both extending in the same direction.

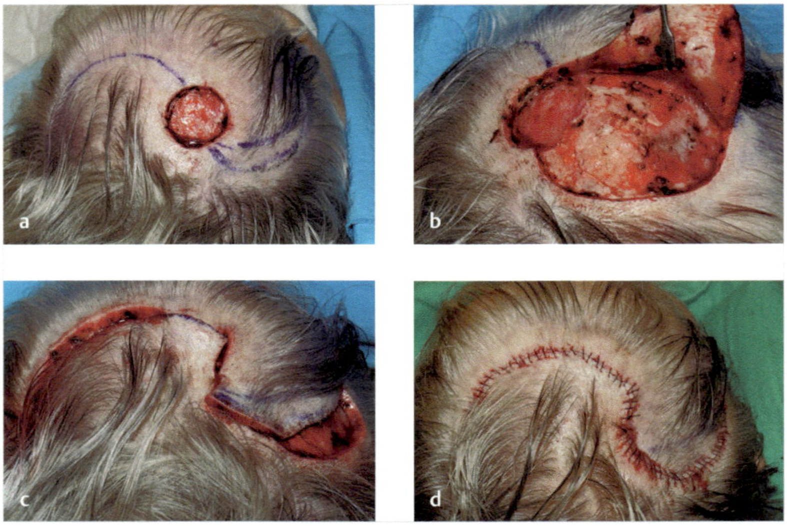

Fig. 5.21 O-Z rotation flaps in a 70 year old female with a 3.9 × 3.6 cm defect over the central parietal scalp. **(a)** Flap incision lines in place with each arc four times the length of the defect diameter. **(b)** One flap has been raised in the subgaleal plane. **(c)** Primary defect is closed first. **(d)** Primary and secondary defects closed and epidermal sutures placed.

Each flap follows the same principles as the single rotation flaps. Once elevated, each flap is rotated in the same direction (either clockwise or counterclockwise), converting the circular "O"-shaped defect into a "Z"-shaped suture line.[35] The key suture approximates the leading edge to each rotation flap, and then the redundancy along the corresponding area is sewn out by the "rule of halves" technique (▶ Fig. 5.21).

Double Hatchet Flaps

Double hatchet flaps are a variant of O-to-Z rotation flaps incorporating further advancement into the design. Two triangular flaps that would otherwise be utilized as standing cones for a primary linear closure are created with the shape of a hatchet, with each flap originating 180 degrees opposite one another, and extending in the same direction. Once incised and raised, each flap is rotated so that the leading edge of each hatchet is approximated into the other, thus closing the primary defect. Secondary defects are then closed in a V-Y fashion.[36,37]

Multiple Rotation Flaps

Generally, large to very large defects or medium defects in very inelastic scalps are reserved for this indication as their implementation is time-consuming and will lead to extensive scalp scarring.

Pinwheel Flaps

Pinwheel flaps are composed of four rotation flaps, each separated 90 degrees from one another (see ▶ Fig. 5.22). These flaps converge centrally after being raised and rotated, thereby allowing closure of the operative defect.[38] In the editors' experience, if four rotation flaps are required to close the defect rather than only two, then

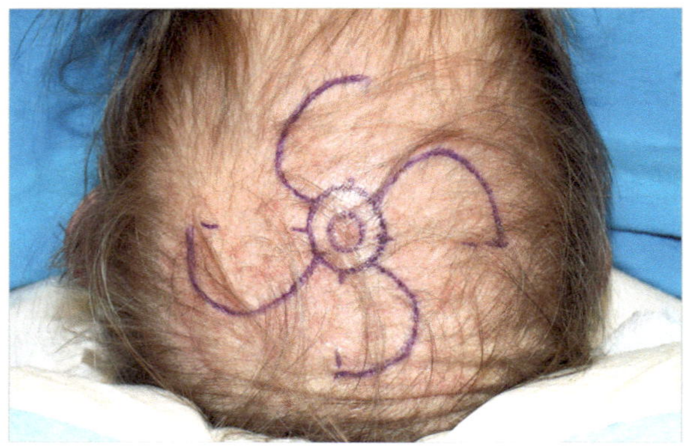

Fig. 5.22 Pinwheel flap. Design of the pinwheel flap drawn. This flap is used in tight scalps when a single arc or O-Z rotation flaps are not enough to close the defect.

a better option is four rhomboid or Limberg's flaps (as discussed in the next section) or a large single-arm rotation flap.

Orticochea Flaps

Orticochea flaps are composed of three or four rotation and/or advancement flaps and are used for medium (10–50 cm^2) or large (> 50 cm^2) vertex scalp defects. The scalp is divided into vascular territories that should be included in each flap: temporal, occipital, and supraorbital/supratrochlear territories. Three to four flaps are appropriately designed around the operative wound following the same principles of single rotation or advancement flaps. Extensive undermining is undertaken to mobilize the entire scalp, and galeal releasing incisions are utilized to further expand mobility of each flap.[16,39]

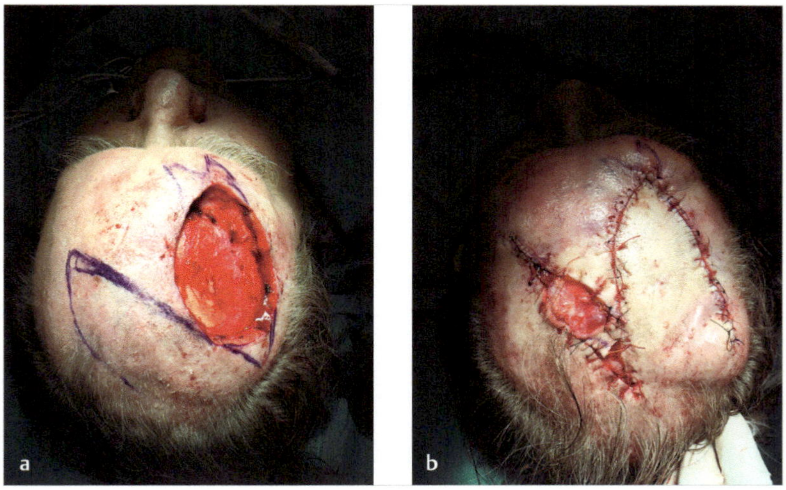

Fig. 5.23 Scalp banner transposition flap. **(a)** Large vertically-oriented defect with some bone exposed. **(b)** Banner flap transposed to cover the defect. Note that the galea of the flap was left intact over the secondary defect allowing FTSG placement and pulley sutures to partially close the secondary defect and improve granulation. (These images are provided courtesy of Stanislav N. Tolkachjov, MD.)

Transposition Flaps

In the author's experience, transposition flaps are of limited usefulness for closing operative wounds on the scalp. In selected cases where rotation flaps are not suitable, bilobed, trilobed, rhomboid, and Banner flaps can be considered. Transposition flaps can be used to cover large defects with exposed calvarium lacking periosteum while leaving an intact periosteum and some galea in the secondary defect for a backgraft, which can often be taken from the excised standing tissue cone of the transposition flap itself (▶ Fig. 5.23).

Rhomboid Flaps

Multiple Limberg's flaps can be used in selected cases where the operative wounds are located on loose regions of the scalp, such as the frontal scalp of bald male patients. With this technique, the wound is projected into a hexagon fitting three distinct rhombi, so that three consecutive rhombic flaps allow for repair of the wound. Of note, such flaps have the disadvantage of leaving a multiplicity of scars that may be aesthetically undesirable.[40]

Microvascular Free Flaps

Although beyond the scope of dermatologic surgery, microvascular free flaps, also known as free autologous tissue transfers, are usually performed by plastic surgeons for the reconstruction of large to extensive defects that cannot be repaired otherwise. For scalp reconstruction purposes, free flaps may be composed of muscle only or may contain skin, subcutaneous tissue, and muscle. These flaps are completely separated from their original vascular supply at the donor site. The flap can now be moved to a distant recipient site, where the vascular pedicle is anastomosed with appropriate recipient arteries and veins through microsurgical techniques. These flaps offer the advantages of bringing a bulk of vascularized tissue allowing for appropriate contouring of the calvarium, and in the case of flaps containing muscle only, providing a healthy recipient site for subsequent skin grafts. The superficial temporal artery and vein are common recipient vascular pedicles, though facial vessels and the external jugular vein can be used as well. Donor tissues may include the radial forearm, anterolateral thigh, gracilis, lateral arm, parascapular, rectus abdominis, and latissimus dorsi. These flaps have been shown to have a very high success rate in the literature and have been shown to be safe in the elderly population.[7]

5.3 Complications

Complications after scalp reconstruction are uncommon. Two primary complications in any skin surgery are necrosis and infection. The robust blood supply of the scalp reduces the incidence of both, even after large reconstructions. In the author's practice, scalp reconstructions have a 0.6% incidence for infection and 2% for necrosis. This is in comparison to 0.8% and 5%, respectively, when all reconstructive sites are combined. Infections, when culture was possible, most commonly grew *S. aureus*. The patients generally respond to a 2-week course of a first-generation cephalosporin. Necrosis is treated with careful serial debridement of any fully declared full-thickness loss, followed by the use of protocols as outlined under Chapter 5.2.2.

Surprisingly, given the high scalp vascularity, hematomas after scalp surgery in the author's practice are also uncommon, but the incidence is not tracked. The low occurrence of hematomas may relate to the higher closure tension of scalp reconstructions, which could serve as a form of vessel tamponade. Hematomas, should they arise, are treated as per standard well-defined and published protocols.

Multiple larger blood vessels supplying the scalp can increase the risk for significant intraoperative bleeding. A thorough understanding of vessel anatomy, including location and plane, is mandatory. This knowledge can alert the physician and allow visualization and ligation of the vessel, before it is inadvertently transected. The author's preference in larger scalp reconstructions is to incise the outline of each flap in small sections, complete hemostasis, and then continue. This allows excellent visualization for undermining and accurate incision angles to preserve hair follicles.

When reconstructions are performed in hair-bearing scalps, the possibility of telogen effluvium and permanent traction alopecia exists. As previously outlined, incision angles matching the angle of hair follicles, and low-tension closures, minimize the chance of hair loss. In many cases postsurgery, differentiating temporary from permanent hair loss can only occur with the passage of time. Up to 2 years can be required for scalp hair to return to a clinically meaningful number around the surgery site. This is especially true in patients of advanced age. Hair loss can also occur in areas of previous necrosis or dehiscence. Initial treatments include changing the patient's hairstyle, use of scalp dyes, or hair-thickening agents, all to camouflage or give the illusion of greater hair density. Permanent improvement requires serial excisions of the alopecic scalp, or the use of internal tissue expanders with subsequent removal of the alopecic scalp and then movement of the expanded skin into the defect. Hair transplantation using modern techniques can be a very effective method to improve scarring hair loss secondary to surgery. There is a large body of evidence outlining high survival rates for follicular unit grafts in scars.

Larger incisions in the scalp to allow full flap movement and accurate undermining commonly lead to transection of cutaneous sensory nerves. This can lead to numbness, paresthesias, or dysesthesias. Patients with damage to scalp nerves generally report numbness first, primarily with hair grooming. In the majority of cases, this is not of great concern to the patient. However, as nerve repair begins, secondary paresthesias and dysesthesias can occur, with patients finding this bothersome. In the author's experience, 85% of patients have resolution of symptoms by 1 year, without the need for active treatment. By 2 years, almost all patients have had complete resolution of symptoms, again without the need for active treatment such as oral neuroleptics.

Given the large size and higher closure tensions of many scalp reconstructions, hypertrophic and, more prominently, widened scars occur in 5 to 10% of the author's patients. Hypertrophic scars, if still problematic 6 months postsurgery, can be treated with intralesional triamcinolone acetonide (or equivalent) at concentrations of 20 to 40 mg/mL with on average 0.05 mL deposited every 1 cm of the scar length. Widened scars, if of cosmetic concern, can be serially excised or undergo hair transplantation as outlined earlier.

Milia, keratin cysts, and ingrown hairs are easily extracted with a 19-gauge needle (or equivalent), if requested by the patient for cosmetic reasons. Folliculitis of limited degree, if bothersome to the patient, can be treated with a 19-gauge needle evacuation or more aggressive scalp massage during shampooing. Larger areas will require good scalp hygiene, and less commonly a 1-month course of an oral antibiotic in the cephalosporin or tetracycline families.

In patients undergoing SIH, very uncommonly, bony sequestration can occur. This requires removal of the involved bone and application of a skin graft (or equivalent) over the diploic space. This is not commonly performed in an outpatient surgical setting. Referral to the appropriate specialist is required. Rarely arteriovenous malformations (AVMs) can occur along an incision margin. They present as subtly pulsatile red-blue nodules or plaques. If located away from prominent bony suture lines, they can be safely excised in an outpatient setting under local anesthesia. Larger AVMs or AVMs located directly over a bony suture line should be assessed radiologically or referred to an appropriate specialist to ensure there is no continuity with the dural space through the epiploic veins. Very rarely, a venous air embolus could occur in a seated patient when a large scalp resection requires removal of periosteum and air enters the CNS through epiploic veins.[41] The presentation is sudden onset of neurological symptoms. Treatment requires awareness of the possibility, recognizing symptoms, supportive emergency care if required, and immediate transfer to hospital.

References

[1] Seery GE. Surgical anatomy of the scalp. DermatolSurg. 2002; 28 (7):581–587

[2] MatloubH, MolnarJ, et al. Anatomy of the scalp. In: Stough D, Haber R, eds. Hair replacement. St Louis, MO: Mosby;1996:20

[3] GibsonT. Physical properties of the skin. In: Converse JM, ed. Reconstructive plastic surgery. 2nd ed. Philadelphia, PA: WB Saunders;1977:70

[4] Klemp P, Peters K, Hansted B. Subcutaneous blood flow in early male pattern baldness. J Invest Dermatol. 1989; 92(5):725–726

[5] Pan WR, Le Roux CM, Briggs CA. Variations in the lymphatic drainage pattern of the head and neck: further anatomic studies and clinical implications. PlastReconstrSurg. 2011; 127(2):611–620

[6] Raposio E, Santi PL, Nordström RE. Serial scalp reductions: a biomechanical approach. DermatolSurg. 1999; 25(3):210–214

[7] Desai SC, Sand JP, Sharon JD, Branham G, Nussenbaum B. Scalp reconstruction: an algorithmic approach and systematic review. JAMA Facial PlastSurg. 2015; 17(1):56–66

[8] Leedy JE, Janis JE, Rohrich RJ. Reconstruction of acquired scalp defects: an algorithmic approach. PlastReconstrSurg. 2005; 116 (4):54e–72e

[9] Shestak KC, Jones NF, Wu W, Johnson JT, Myers EN. Effect of advanced age and medical disease on the outcome of microvascular reconstruction for head and neck defects. Head Neck. 1992; 14(1):14–18

[10] Lipa JE, Butler CE. Enhancing the outcome of free latissimusdorsi muscle flap reconstruction of scalp defects. Head Neck. 2004; 26 (1):46–53

[11] Chetter IC, Oswald AV, Fletcher M, Dumville JC, Cullum NA. A survey of patients with surgical wounds healing by secondary intention; an

assessment of prevalence, aetiology, duration and management. J Tissue Viability. 2017; 26(2):103–107
[12] Ravitskiy L, Brodland DG, Zitelli JA. Cost analysis: Mohs micrographic surgery. DermatolSurg. 2012; 38(4):585–594
[13] Vedvyas C, Cummings PL, Geronemus RG, Brauer JA. Broader practice indications for Mohssurgical defect healing by secondary intention: a survey study. DermatolSurg. 2017; 43(3):415–423
[14] Rysz M, Grzelecki D, Mazurek M, Starościak S, Krajewski R. Surgical techniques for closure of a scalp defect after resection of skin malignancy. DermatolSurg. 2017; 43(5):715–723
[15] Olson MD, Hamilton GS , III. Scalp and forehead defects in the post-Mohssurgery patient. Facial PlastSurgClin North Am. 2017; 25 (3):365–375
[16] Becker GD, Adams LA, Levin BC. Secondary intention healing of exposed scalp and forehead bone after Mohs surgery. Otolaryngol Head Neck Surg. 1999; 121(6):751–754
[17] Snow SN, Stiff MA, Bullen R, Mohs FE, Chao WH. Second-intention healing of exposed facial-scalp bone after Mohs surgery for skin cancer: review of ninety-one cases. J Am AcadDermatol. 1994; 31(3, Pt 1):450–454
[18] Lam TK, Lowe C, Johnson R, Marquart JD. Secondary intention healing and purse-string closures. DermatolSurg. 2015; 41 Suppl 10:S178–S186
[19] Enei ML, Machado Filho Cd. Closure of chronic ulcer localized on the scalp previously irradiated using a fenestration technique. DermatolSurg. 2015; 41(10):1196–1198
[20] Monk EC, Benedetto EA, Benedetto AV. Successful treatment of nonhealing scalp wounds using a silicone gel. DermatolSurg. 2014; 40 (1):76–79
[21] Chang YY, Tay AC. A case series on management of complex scalp wounds. Wound Practice and Research.. 2015; 23(4):174–177
[22] Beroukhim K, Rotunda AM. Topical 0.5% timolol heals a recalcitrant irradiated surgical scalp wound. DermatolSurg. 2014; 40(8):924–926
[23] Joo J, Custis T, Armstrong AW, et al. Purse-string suture vs second intention healing: results of a randomized, blind clinical trial. JAMA Dermatol. 2015; 151(3):265–270
[24] Malone CH, McLaughlin JM, Ross LS, Phillips LG, Wagner RF , Jr. Progressive tightening of pulley sutures for primary repair of large scalp wounds. PlastReconstrSurg Glob Open. 2017; 5(12):e1592
[25] Steiner D, Hubertus A, Arkudas A, et al. Scalp reconstruction: a 10-year retrospective study. J CraniomaxillofacSurg. 2017; 45(2):319–324
[26] Shimizu I, MacFarlane DF. Full-thickness skin grafts may not need tie-over bolster dressings. DermatolSurg. 2013; 39(5):726–728
[27] Leclère FM. The use of Integra® dermal regeneration template versus flaps for reconstruction of full-thickness scalp defects involving the calvaria: a cost-benefit analysis. Aesthetic PlastSurg. 2017; 41 (2):472–473
[28] Sand JP, Diaz JA, Nussenbaum B, Rich JT. Full-thickness scalp defects reconstructed with outer table calvarial decortication and surface grafting. JAMA Facial PlastSurg. 2017; 19(1):74–76
[29] HoffmanJF. Reconstruction of the scalp. In: Baker S, ed. Local flaps in facial reconstruction. 3rd ed. Philadelphia, PA: WB Saunders;2014:641
[30] Ibhler N, Ziegler MC, Penna V, Eisenhardt SU, Stark GB, Bannasch H. An algorithm for oncologic scalp reconstruction. PlastReconstrSurg. 2010; 126(2):450–459
[31] Raposio E, Nordström RE, Santi PL. Undermining of the scalp: quantitative effects. PlastReconstrSurg. 1998; 101(5):1218–1222
[32] Kannan S, Mehta D, Ozog D. Scalp closures with pulley sutures reduce time and cost compared to traditional layered technique:a prospective, randomized, observer-blinded study. DermatolSurg. 2016; 42 (11):1248–1255
[33] Weisberg NK, Greenbaum SS. Revisiting the purse-string closure: some new methods and modifications. DermatolSurg. 2003; 29 (6):672–676
[34] Dzubow LM. The dynamics of flap movement: effect of pivotal restraint on flap rotation and transposition. J DermatolSurgOncol. 1987; 13(12):1348–1353
[35] LoPiccolo MC. Rotation flaps: principles and locations. DermatolSurg. 2015; 41 Suppl 10:S247–S254
[36] Emmett AJ. The closure of defects by using adjacent triangular flaps with subcutaneous pedicles. PlastReconstrSurg. 1977; 59(1):45–52
[37] Sowerby LJ, Taylor SM, Moore CC. The double hatchet flap: a workhorse in head and neck local flap reconstruction. Arch Facial PlastSurg. 2010; 12(3):198–201
[38] Simsek T, Eroglu L. Versatility of the pinwheel flap to reconstruct circular defects in the temporal and scalp region. J PlastSurg Hand Surg. 2013; 47(2):97–101
[39] Badhey A, Kadakia S, Abraham MT, Rasamny JK, Moscatello A. Multiflap closure of scalp defects: revisiting the orticochea flap for scalp reconstruction. Am J Otolaryngol. 2016; 37(5):466–469
[40] JacksonIT. Forehead reconstruction. In: Jackson IT, ed. Local flaps in head and neck reconstruction. 1st ed. St Louis, MO: The C.V. Mosby Company;1985:63
[41] Spence NZ, Faloba K, Sonabend AM, Bruce JN, Anastasian ZH. Venous air embolus during scalp incision. J ClinNeurosci. 2016; 28:170–171

6 Cheek

Jonathan Cappel

Abstract

The cheek is a common site of Mohs surgery and subsequent reconstruction. It is a large subunit with complex topography that borders many other facial subunits. Thus, many factors must be considered while operating in this area. This chapter addresses relevant anatomy such as the facial nerve and parotid gland and duct that one must take into account prior to performing surgery on the cheek. Illustrations are shown of the vascular, neural, and glandular anatomy and in addition the relaxed skin tension lines. A unique subunit principle of the cheek, with illustration, is presented including the considerations for these different subunits. An algorithm for approaching reconstruction of a cheek defect is laid out based on location and size of the defect. Reconstructions are discussed and shown with complimentary photographs especially of the more challenging repairs. This chapter ends with a discussion of possible complications that may occur subsequent to a surgery in this area and things to consider in minimizing complication risk.

Keywords: cheek anatomy, Mohs, skin cancer, cheek defects, flap, repair, cheek reconstruction

Capsule Summary and Pearls

- The cheek is a large subunit bordering many other complex facial subunits that must be taken into account when performing surgery in this area.
- Beware of the well-known danger zones where damage of branches of the facial nerve is of higher likelihood (▶ Fig. 6.1).
- The relaxed skin tension lines (RSTLs) of the cheek as well as dynamic and static lines from the muscles of facial expression run parallel and often defects are sutured in this plane to minimize appearance of scarring (▶ Fig. 6.3).
- The cheek can be divided up into eight subunits based on location with each having different skin quality and considerations given proximity to different neighboring facial subunits (▶ Fig. 6.4).
- A reconstructive algorithm can be used as a guide when faced with a cheek defect (▶ Fig. 6.5).
- There are minimal naturally occurring lines on the cheek; if equivocal repair options, consider the repair with the least number of lines (i.e., linear repair has one).
- Curvilinear repairs on the cheek are of great value given convexity and allowing one to minimize tissue redundancy and tension on the eyelid.
- Advancement flaps, including the V-Y advancement flap, are very useful on the cheek given large reservoir of mobile skin on lateral cheek and superior neck.
- Suspension sutures to the medial canthal tendon or periosteum of the nasion or orbital rim are of great value to minimize risk of ectropion.
- The bilobed transposition flap, as utilized on the nose, can be used for very large defects on the cheek with success when reconstructive options are limited.
- Eversion, while still utilized on the cheek, may take a longer time to resolve than other facial sites.
- Standing tissue cones at the inferior pole of a curvilinear repair may persist, while those falling superiorly in the eyelid will often relax.

6.1 Introduction

The cheek is a common area of treatment in Mohs micrographic surgery (MMS) and subsequent reconstruction. It is also one of the larger subunits and borders many other complex structures and subunits (ocular, auricular, oral, nasal, temporal, neck) and defects often may have significant overlap with other facial subunits. The first thing to consider in evaluating and treating a tumor with MMS, and then ultimately the reconstruction of the resulting defect, is the relevant anatomy of a particular area. The relevant anatomy of the cheek is discussed in the following section.

6.2 Relevant Anatomy

In discussing the anatomy of the cheek, we will start by addressing the anatomical structures deep to the surface of the skin. Then we will go on to discuss the superficial peripheral borders and boundaries of the cheek along with the aesthetic subunits of the area.

The superficial fascia, also known as the superficial muscular aponeurotic system (SMAS), of the cheek contains many important anatomic structures. These include the parotid gland and duct, muscles of facial expression as well as branches of the facial and trigeminal nerve, and

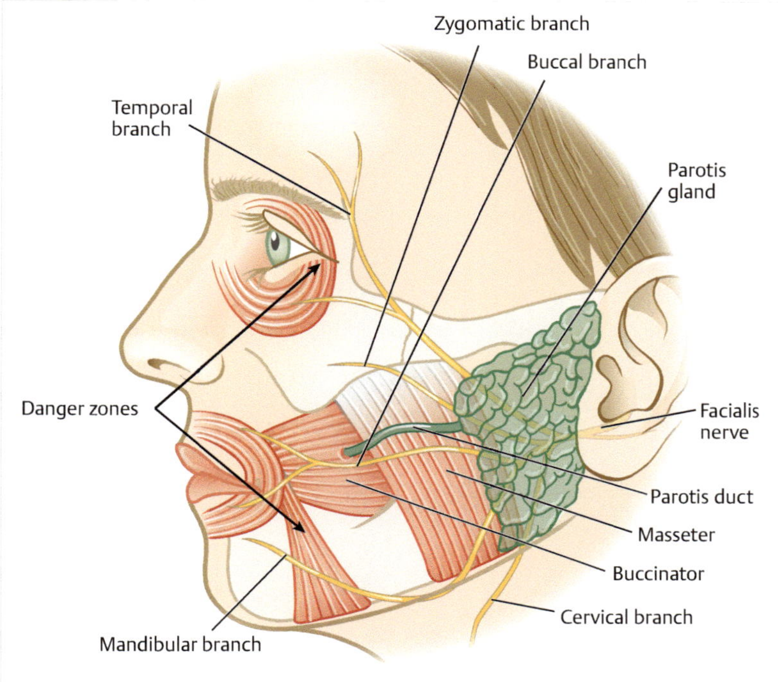

Fig. 6.1 Please note the above anatomy of the cheek including the parotid duct and facial nerve. Specifically pay attention to the danger zones where the temporal and mandibular branches of the facial nerve lie more superficially and are at higher risk of damage in these areas. The mandibular branch of the facial nerve is found in the cheek and its course parallels the inferior margin of the mandible.

the facial artery and vein. The parotid gland lies in the inferolateral portion of the cheek in the superficial fascia. The branches of the facial nerve and of course the parotid duct arise from the anterior border of the parotid gland. The parotid duct courses anteriorly from there lying atop the masseter muscle and can be found about 2 cm inferior to the zygomatic arch. The transverse facial artery and buccal branch of the facial nerve can often be found in close proximity to the parotid duct as well. As the parotid duct continues more anteriorly/medially, it eventually pierces the buccinator muscle of the cheek and drains into the oral cavity. The branches of the facial nerve (temporal, zygomatic, buccal, mandibular, and cervical) arise from within the parotid, and a diagram of these branches, the well-known danger zones,[1] and parotid gland and duct anatomy is seen in ▶ Fig. 6.1.

The facial artery crosses the mandible at the anterior border of the masseter muscle lying deep to the platysma in this location. As it progresses proximally at the angle of the mouth, it gives off the inferior labial and superior labial branches and once it reaches the lateral nose it becomes the angular artery. The infraorbital artery enters the cheek through the infraorbital foramen of the maxilla and anastomoses with branches of the facial artery listed earlier.[2] The vascular anatomy of the cheek is shown in ▶ Fig. 6.2.

The relaxed skin tension lines (RSTLs) begin at the nasolabial fold (NLF) and run parallel to the NLF and eventually parallel to the inferior lateral canthal lines upon progressing more laterally. At the lateral cheek, they begin to no longer run parallel to aforementioned lines and run vertically parallel to the preauricular crease. The RSTLs are important to consider in reconstruction given reconstruction in these planes has the least amount of tension.[3] Additionally, in particular for cheek reconstruction, the RSTL plane is also the same plane that all naturally occurring dynamic and static lines (rhytids) are formed over time from movements of the muscles of facial expression. Thus, reconstructions can be performed and can be best hidden if placed within already formed lines or lines that will form in the future. These RSTLs are shown in ▶ Fig. 6.3.

6.3 Aesthetic Subunits and Defects

The cheek's peripheral borders are the infraorbital rim and zygomatic arch superiorly and the border of the mandible inferiorly. The medial border is the nasofacial junction, NLF, and labiomandibular crease medially and the preauricular crease laterally.[4] For the purposes of this text, we will divide the cheek up into eight subunits all approximately 3 to 4 cm^2 in size. These are the superomedial cheek, medial cheek, inferomedial cheek, superior central cheek, central cheek, inferior central cheek, superior lateral cheek, and inferior lateral cheek. These different subunits have different quality of skin with medial subunits being thicker and more sebaceous and superior and lateral subunits being more thin and nonsebaceous when approaching eyelid and preauricular skin. Different repairs are considered in each of these areas primarily based on size and location but also certainly considering differing skin qualities, proximity to other facial subunits

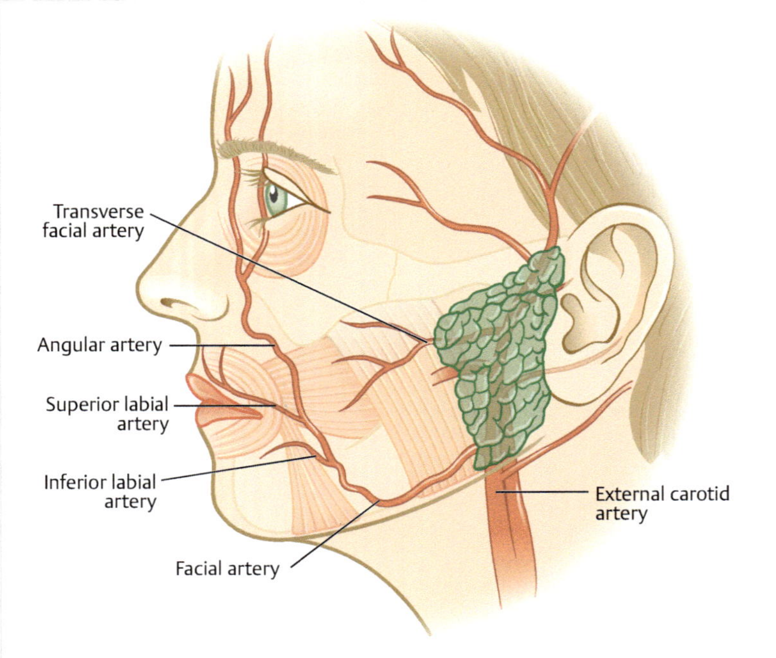

Fig. 6.2 The figure above illustrates the vascular anatomy of the cheek. Relevant branches of the external carotid artery are shown including the transverse facial artery and facial artery and its branches. Please note the infraorbital artery is not shown in this illustration.

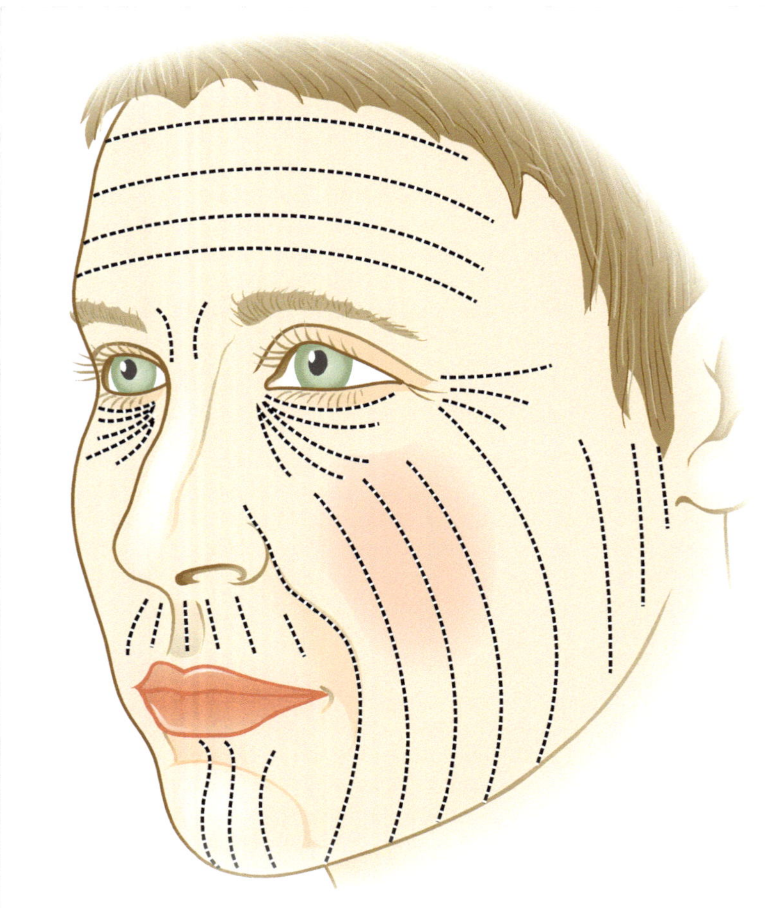

Fig. 6.3 The relaxed skin tension lines (RSTLs) are shown above. Specially pay attention to the parallel nature of these lines to the nasolabial fold as they progress laterally and how they change as they approach the auricular and ocular areas.

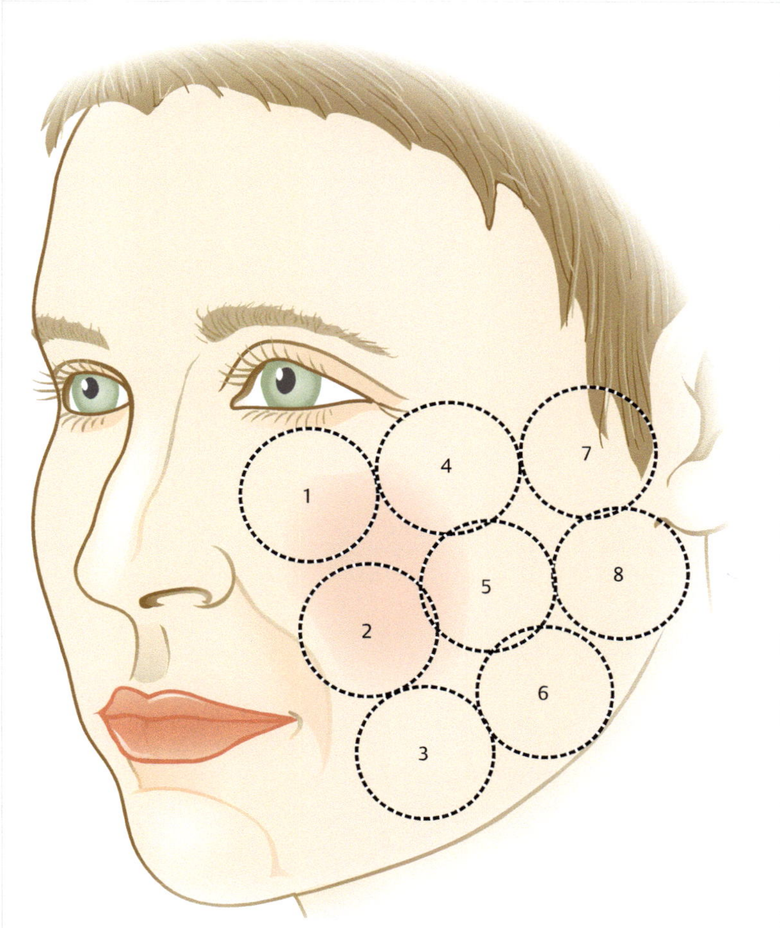

Fig. 6.4 This figure divides the cheek into the eight different proposed subunits shown. These subunits each have unique skin quality and different considerations to take into account while operating in these areas.

and topography of each specific area. These different subunits are displayed in ▶ Fig. 6.4.

This figure nicely diagrams these different cheek subunits and the overlap and borders they have with other subunits of the face (ocular, auricular, oral, nasal, temporal, neck). This clearly is a very important consideration in reconstruction of the cheek given defects often are not contained to just one of the facial subunits. Each of the other (noncheek) facial subunits have their own considerations, which are addressed elsewhere in this text, that one must take into account when faced with a cheek defect that overlaps into, approximates, or closely approximates another facial subunit.

6.4 Reconstructive Options

The reconstruction options on the cheek are vast given the diverse areas of the cheek that border many unique structures such as the nose, mouth, eye, and ear. Additionally, the cheek has a large surface area among the facial subunits, thus allowing for larger tumors solely involving the cheek and sometimes necessitating very large repairs. The algorithm shown in ▶ Fig. 6.5 has been constructed as a basic guide when approaching a cheek defect. The variables addressed are size and location of the defects, which then guide one to some possible repairs to consider given those variables. Further discussion of different repairs and other considerations are included in the text in the sections to follow.

6.4.1 Primary Closures

The most common repair for optimal outcome on the cheek is the curvilinear repair.[5] The cheek has convexity with minimal other topographical changes compared to other facial subunits while having few naturally occurring lines. Since additional lines are difficult to hide, the curvilinear repair, in most circumstances, allows for the best result given the minimal cosmetic footprint of a single line. These repairs are best suited to run in the RSTLs, given most naturally occurring lines on the cheek are parallel to those lines. ▶ Fig. 6.6 and ▶ Fig. 6.7 are an example of a curvilinear closure repaired parallel to the RSTLs and dynamic facial lines.

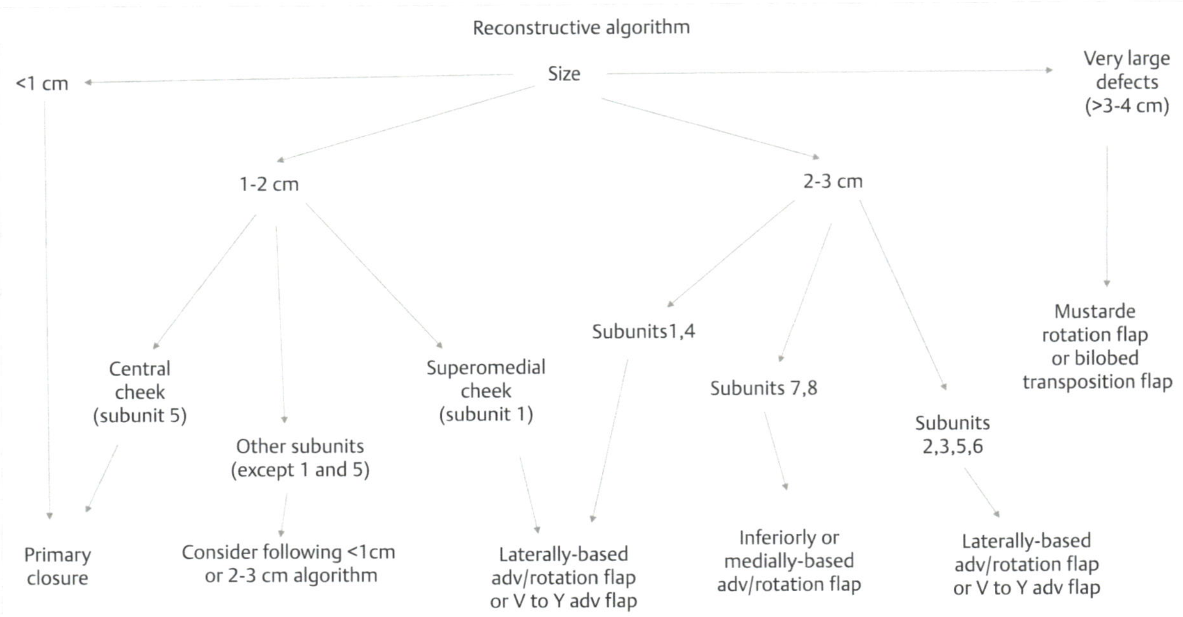

Fig. 6.5 A basic preliminary algorithm to consider while approaching a cheek defect. This algorithm is primarily based on size and location. Of course, each cheek defect is quite unique and this should only be used as a basic starting point of repairs to consider when faced with a defect.

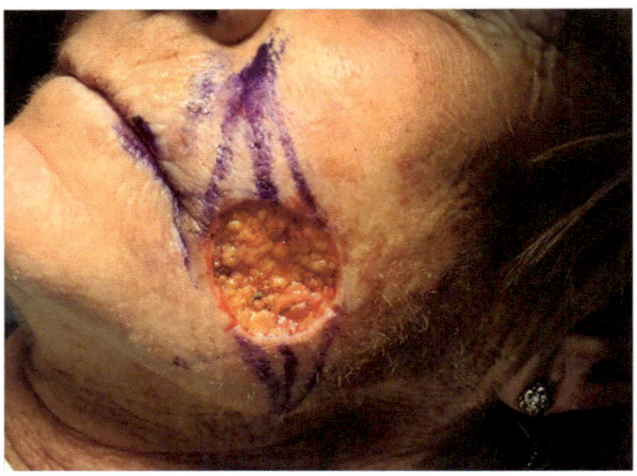

Fig. 6.6 Moderate-sized defect approximating subunit 2. Primary curvilinear repair was chosen. Please note parallel nature to dynamic lines of facial expression and relaxed skin tension lines (RSTLs). (This image is provided courtesy of Stanislav N. Tolkachjov, MD.)

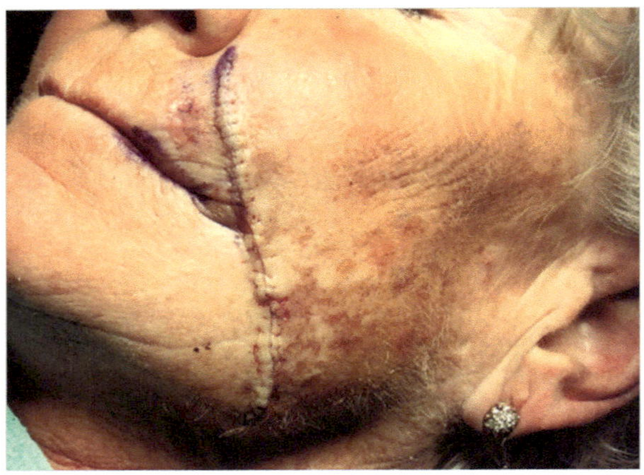

Fig. 6.7 Immediate postoperative photograph. (This image is provided courtesy of Stanislav N. Tolkachjov, MD.)

Additionally, curvilinear repairs are often used on the cheek to accomplish several goals, of which the most obvious is allowing one to repair parallel with RSTLs. Additionally, they are used on the convex surface of the cheek to allow for minimizing the length of the repair due to tissue redundancy. Finally, curvilinear repairs may be utilized to minimize tension placed in the vertical direction to avoid excessive tension on the eyelid and a resulting ectropion. ▶ Fig. 6.8 and ▶ Fig. 6.9 are other examples of curvilinear repairs.

Curvilinear repairs are most often done on the medial cheek with a stepwise approach of design and execution. The concavity of the superior and inferior Burow's triangles is directed medially and laterally, respectively, with the apex of the triangles directed vertically. After removal of the Burow's triangles and hemostasis, an assistant can place skin hooks in the tips of defect with tension in a vertical vector. Then the first suture is placed centrally in the defect perpendicular (with a horizontal tension

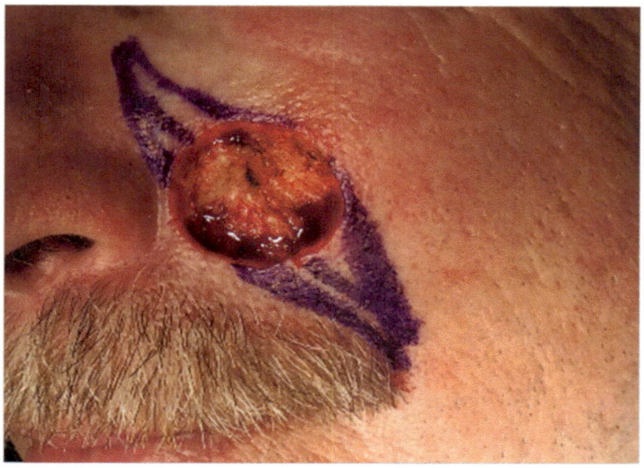

Fig. 6.8 Moderate defect approximating subunits 1 and 2. Primary curvilinear repair was chosen. Please note how repairs can be hidden in lines of facial expression as well as borders between subunits. (This image is provided courtesy of Stanislav N. Tolkachjov, MD.)

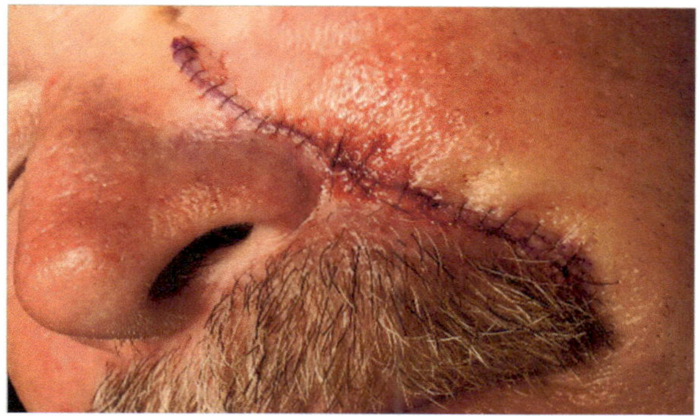

Fig. 6.9 Immediate postoperative photograph. (This image is provided courtesy of Stanislav N. Tolkachjov, MD.)

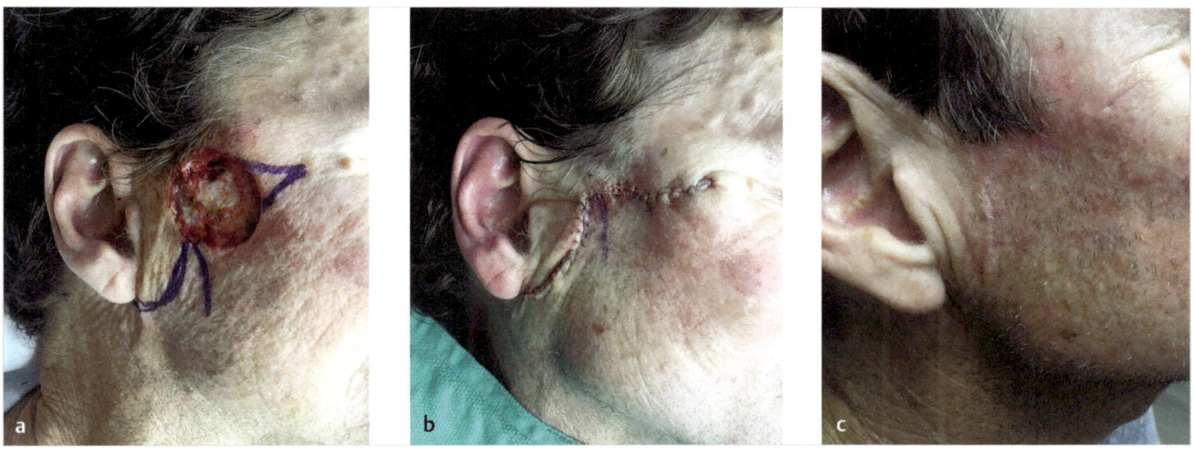

Fig. 6.10 (a) Moderate-sized defect approximating subunit 7 for which inferiorly based advancement/rotation flap is drawn with tissue redundancy removed from the post auricular area. (b) Immediate postoperative photograph. (c) Outcome 1 month postoperatively.

vector) to the now vertical orientation of the defect to prevent any tension on the lower eyelid. Skin hooks can be kept in place for placement of at least the next two sutures, and a suture can be placed at the midpoint of the remaining superior and inferior defects in the same fashion as above. This style of suturing can be continued until all dermal sutures are placed. This allows the redundancy of the unequal lengths of the medial and lateral portion of the removed Burow's triangles to be sutured out, thus minimizing the length of the repair.

6.4.2 Flaps

Advancement and/or Rotation Flaps

When linear or curvilinear repairs are not an option, the next best options, in the author's opinion, are repairs that produce only two lines. In this situation, ideally one and/or two suture lines run in an RSTL or natural border of the cheek to minimize appearance. The most common repair to produce such is an advancement and/or rotation flap. These two flaps are very similar, especially on the cheek. The major difference is that the advancement flap movement is in the same vector along the length (advancing edge) of the flap, while the movement in a rotation flap changes vectors ("rotates") along the course of the flap. Rotation flaps are of great utility especially when working in the periocular, perinasal, and periauricular regions. This allows for rotation around these structures, without involving them in the flap, while also sometimes allowing one to remove and hide areas of tissue redundancy in the natural cosmetic borders just lateral to the nose or in the preauricular fold. These flaps may be used for large reconstructions on the superior cheek (bordering eyelid) or lateral cheek (bordering ear). ▶ Fig. 6.10, ▶ Fig. 6.11, ▶ Fig. 6.12 are examples of the aforementioned flaps with ▶ Fig. 6.10 specifically illustrating removing and hiding areas of tissue redundancy in the periauricular skin

Advancement and rotation flaps are raised in the plane of the mid-subcutaneous tissue, and care is taken to avoid undermining deeper where the potential of damaging important anatomic structures is of higher likelihood. Undermining large areas should be performed while alternating between reflecting the flap and then retracting the flap over the scissors or scalpel to observe that the plane of undermining is running parallel to the surface of the skin rather than diving too deeply. After undermining to achieve flap mobility, the first few sutures are placed. It is essential that these sutures are meticulously placed especially in large flaps that are close to and/or involving the eyelid. An important point in performing flaps on the superior cheek (bordering the eyelid) is the utility of sutures to suspend the flap to the periosteum of the orbital rim, nasion, or medial canthal

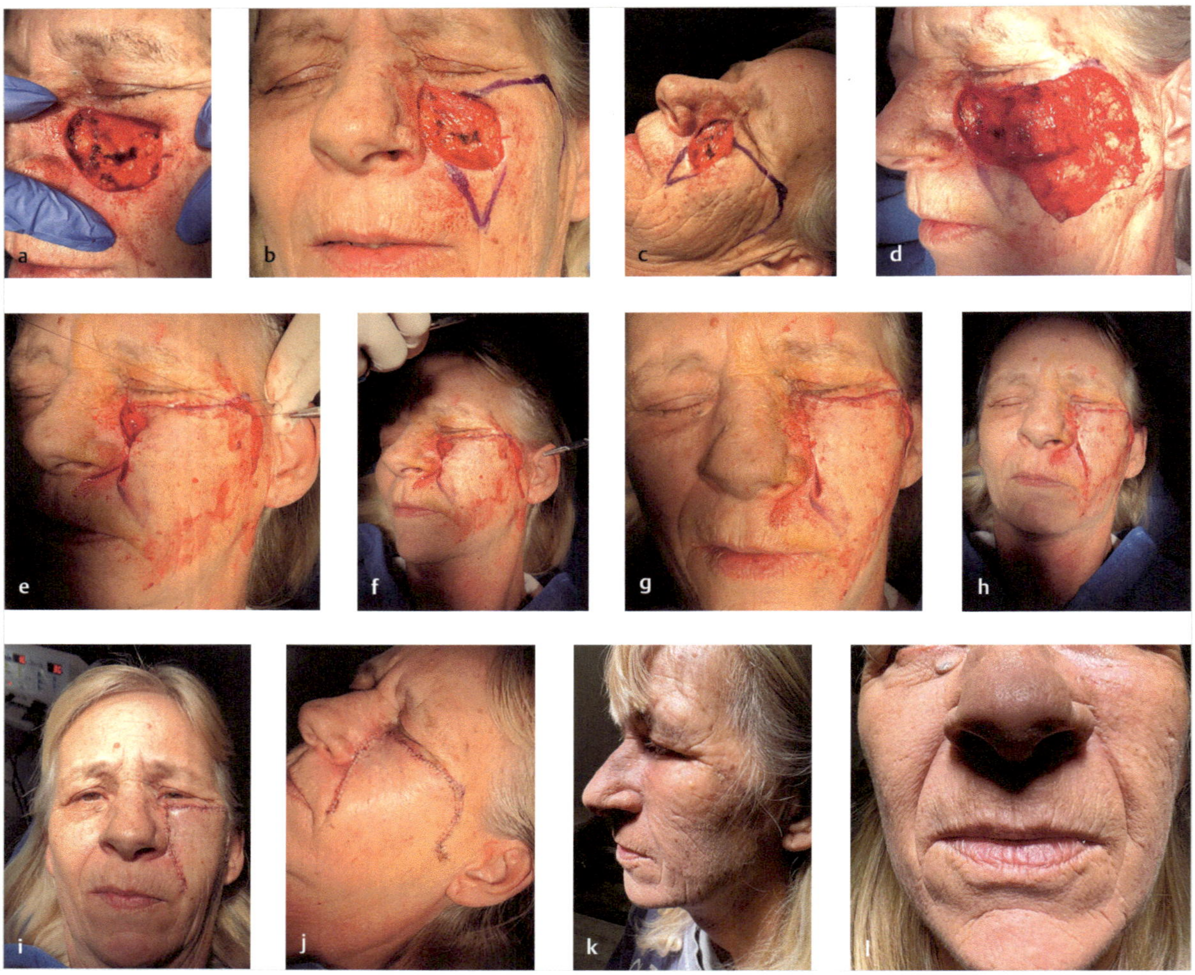

Fig. 6.11 (a–l) Superiorly-based cheek rotation flap. **(a)** Moderately-sized defect involving the medial malar infraorbital cheek. **(b)** Anterior view showing design with take-off point of the flap starting at the level of the highest point of the defect and flap drawn superolaterally toward the laterally-based tissue reservoir. Inferior standing tissue cone planned with the melolabial fold. **(c)** Lateral view of the design. **(d)** Flap undermined enough to allow tension-free movement. **(e)** Key stitches at the apical triangle horizontally and the temple superolaterally. This allows redistribution of tension medially and superolaterally, respectively, and avoids tension on the eye superiorly. The flap is suspended with these tension vectors. Some surgeons choose to place tacking sutures to the periosteum of the lateral orbital rim and the medial canthal ligament. **(f)** Sewing out the rest of the flap to redistribute tension. **(g)** Flap mostly sewn in place leaving an inferior standing tissue cone (STC). **(h)** Inferior STC excised with the melolabial fold. **(i)** Immediate postoperative result (anterior). Note the upward push of the flap to properly suspend the eye prior to relaxation. **(j)** Immediate postoperative result (lateral). **(k)** 2-month followup showing normal eye position with the patient's preoperative age-related eyelid ptosis (lateral view). **(l)** Anterior view. (These images are provided courtesy of Stanislav N. Tolkachjov, MD.)

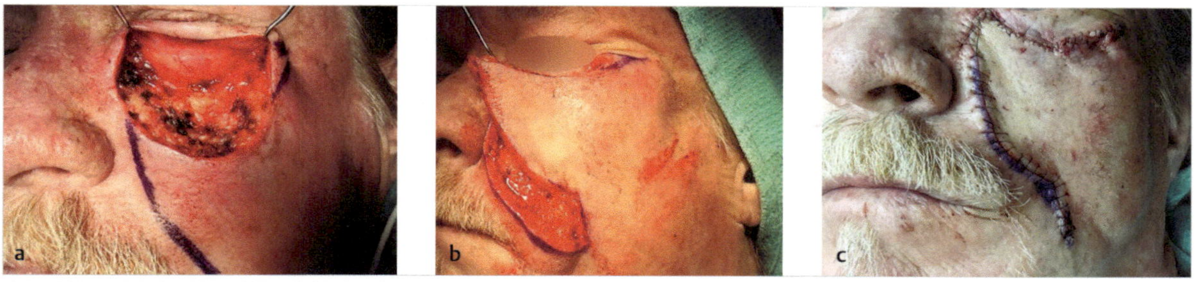

Fig. 6.12 **(a)** Large defect approximating subunit 1 for which inferiorly based advancement/rotation flap is drawn. **(b)** Flap raised and being pulled into place with skin hooks. **(c)** Immediate postoperative photograph. Once again, the load-bearing sutures were placed with a horizontal tension vector and also suspension sutures can prove helpful to prevent ectropion. (These images are provided courtesy of Stanislav N. Tolkachjov, MD.)

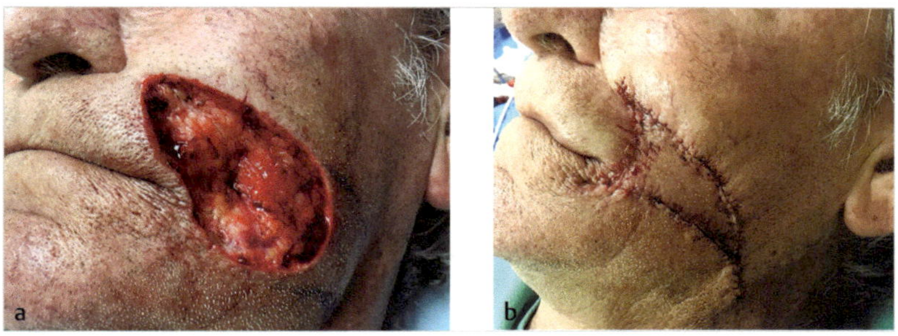

Fig. 6.13 **(a)** Large defect approximating subunits 2 and 3 for which V-Y advancement flap is drawn. **(b)** Immediate postoperative photograph. Please note initial sutures on the leading edge were at superior portion of the medial part of flap. Placing the initial load-bearing sutures at this location minimized tension on the lip medially and the eye superiorly.

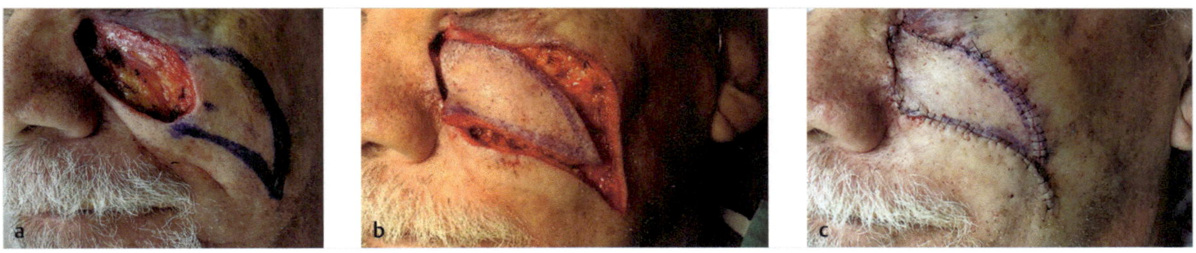

Fig. 6.14 **(a)** Large defect approximating subunit 1 for which V-Y advancement flap is drawn. **(b)** Intraoperative photograph after initial suspension suture placed. **(c)** Immediate postoperative photograph. (These images are provided courtesy of Stanislav N. Tolkachjov, MD.)

tendon depending on the location.[6] The size and weight of these flaps, coupled with the effect of gravity and scar contraction over time in proximity to the eyelid, can put excessive tension on the eyelid and cause ectropion over time. Thus, suspension sutures are often utilized to allow for tension to be on the periosteum and not on the eyelid itself. This was deemed necessary in several of the periocular flaps shown in this chapter.

After the periosteal sutures, if utilized, the goal of the next several key sutures is to move the flap entirely into place with the tension vectors of the sutures running parallel to the eyelid. For example, inferior to the eye the suturing tension vectors run mediolaterally, while lateral to the eye the tension is in the cephalocaudal direction. One or two sutures in both these locations do the majority of the work to place the flap in the correct location, while the remainder are placed for fine-tuning and perfect approximation.

The specific type of advancement flap known as the V-Y advancement flap has great utility on the cheek given highly mobile lateral cheek skin and robust subcutaneous blood supply for flaps in this location. This flap does have four lines associated with it, so it may have a substantial cosmetic footprint, but it can be very helpful for repair of large defects. This repair is of great benefit when the defect is bordering the nose and NLF. In this location, two of the four lines of this repair can be hidden in the naturally appearing creases of the NLF and the lateral alar groove.[7,8] ▶ Fig. 6.13, ▶ Fig. 6.14 are examples of the utility of the V-Y advancement flap for large defects or defects in challenging locations.

The V-Y advancement flap is incised to the deep subcutaneous tissue to take advantage of the mobility and

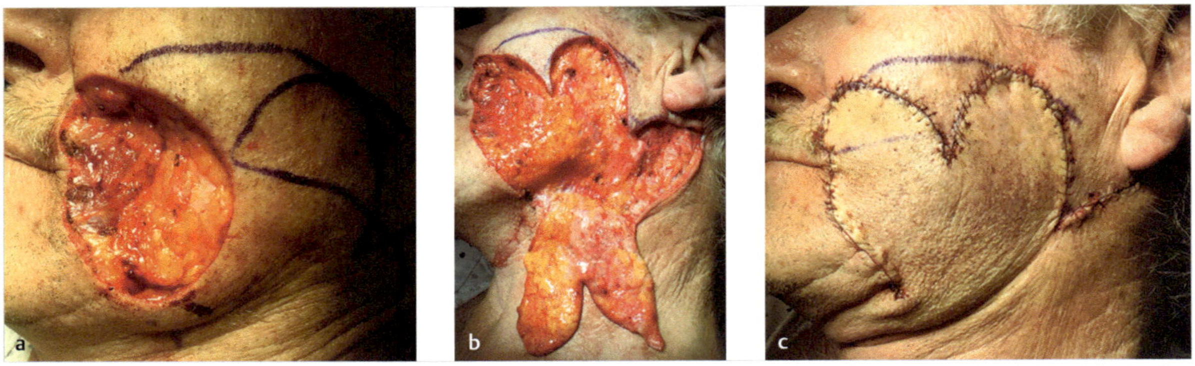

Fig. 6.15 (a) Large defect approximating subunits 2 and 3 for which bilobed transposition flap is drawn. **(b)** Flap raised showing proper plane prior to suturing into place. **(c)** Immediate postoperative photograph. Minimal tension on adjacent lip. Initial load-bearing sutures placed in horizontal direction to avoid tension on the eyelid.

vascularity of subcutaneous tissue in this location. Undermining is performed in all directions outwardly underneath the skin adjacent to the flap. Additionally, vertical releasing of the deep subcutaneous tissue at the leading and trailing edge of the flap can be performed if extra mobility in needed. Mobility is enhanced by dissecting down into the subcutaneous tissue of the buccal fat pad to lengthen the pedicle of the flap, allowing for greater movement. The flap can be pulled into place with a skin hook and a suture can be placed at the apex of the V where the skin adjacent to the flap can be sutured linearly. This may in effect support the flap to a degree and can minimize tension on the suture on the leading edge of the flap. Finally, the leading-edge sutures are directed with horizontal tension vectors and suspension sutures, such as those to the lateral nasal sidewall periosteum, can be used if there is concern about tension on a free margin such as the eyelid.

Transposition Flaps

Transposition flaps, in the author's hands, are used less frequently on the cheek given cosmetic footprint, but they can certainly be useful in the periocular area or for very large defects on the cheek without many other good options. The plane utilized for the flap is the same as that for advancement and/or rotation flaps. The advantage of transposition flaps is they virtually just fall into place with minimal tension other than from the weight of the flap. ▶ Fig. 6.15 is an example of a bilobed transposition flap on the cheek for a large defect. The design for the bilobed transposition flap on the cheek is the same basic design utilized for nasal defects[9,10] and recruits mobility from loose skin on the neck or jowls. The intent for this flap is to hide as many of the lines from the lobes in the naturally occurring borders between subunits, such as the jawline or postauricular skin. In some instances, the lobes are taken from the neck and moved superomedially to cover the medial cheek or superolaterally to cover the preauricular cheek. If the preferred reservoir for a large preauricular defect is postauricular skin, the first lobe of the bilobed flap can transpose over the ear, hiding the second lobe in the postauricular skin and the tertiary defect in the hairline or lateral neck. Care should be taken not to transpose postauricular hair-bearing scalp; instead, the design may originate inferolaterally or involve more than two lobes, which creates a longer arc of transposition while recruiting a more distant skin reservoir.

6.4.3 Second Intention Healing

Second intention healing is used minimally on the cheek given convexity of this subunit. It could be considered for small defects in locations that are concave such as the nasofacial junction or the preauricular crease. It should generally be avoided for defects close to the free margins of the eyelid or mouth given risk for contraction and distortion of those subunits.

6.4.4 Full-Thickness Skin Graft

The use of the full-thickness skin graft (FTSG) should be avoided on the cheek unless there are no other options for very large defects. Defects involving either an entire subunit of the cheek or highly immobile skin, especially in patients who have had several previous reconstructions on the cheek resulting in surrounding scar tissue, would be a reasonable situation in which an FTSG could be utilized. FTSGs on the cheek are often cosmetically unacceptable compared to a primary closure or flap repair. FTSGs may be used in combination with other repairs on the cheek for large defects such as in combination with primary closures or flaps that partially reduce the defect and leave a smaller area to receive a graft taken from a Burow's triangle or from the redundancy of a point of rotation (see Chapter 11). However, if an FTSG is utilized on the cheek with a suboptimal result, revision can be done with excision of that FTSG and subsequent primary or flap closure or serial excisions to remove the FTSG entirely.

6.5 Complications and Revisions

Complications on the cheek do occur, and one must be aware of them to prevent such complications. Complications can be categorized into infection, bleeding, nerve or other anatomical structure damage, and finally poor cosmetic result.

Infection prevention and infection complications will be minimally addressed given it is outside the scope of this text; however, please refer to Chapter 12 of this book for such information and also see the resources mentioned at the end of this chapter. Infection prevention and treatment are crucial to improve surgical outcomes and to minimize morbidity and even mortality.[11]

The importance of anatomical knowledge is crucial to effective surgery on the cheek to minimize risk of damaging vital anatomic structures. Please refer to earlier section on relevant anatomy of the cheek for further details. Appropriate consent should be obtained when working in a particular area (i.e., subunit 3 due to the superficial nature of the mandibular branch of the facial nerve). Certainly, at times, damage to relevant anatomical structures, such as the facial nerve or parotid gland/duct, cannot be avoided when operating on aggressive tumors. Extirpation of deep tumors in the mid cheek can involve removal of the superficial parotid gland and/or the parotid duct. Incision lines of flaps or primary closures of these defects can drain clear salivary fluid with gustation. Usually these temporary fistulas will close and resolve without further interception as healing continues and scar formation contracts. If it persists or sinus tract formation ensues, then referral to an otolaryngologist or other head and neck surgeon specializing in nerve damage repair would be warranted.[1]

Bleeding complications do occur; however, they can be minimized. Generally speaking, the smaller the defect and repair (i.e., less cut tissue), the lower the risk of having bleeding complications. In addition to repair size, sound hemostasis is probably the single most important factor to minimize bleeding complications. The cheek may have higher risk of bleeding complications than many other subunits, especially if patients are on an anticoagulant. This is likely due to the size of the subunit, potentially large tumors solely involving the cheek, and large flap repairs with broad dead spaces resulting in higher risk of bleeding or hematoma formation. Further discussion of bleeding and hematoma complications is outside of the scope of this text.[12,13]

The poor cosmetic outcome can result from and may be related to any of the prior complications listed earlier. Also, it can be related to any number of other factors including the patient's skin and postoperative care as well as surgical technique. The biggest modifiable risk for poor cosmetic outcome, outside of smoking, is surgical technique, including choosing the appropriate repair addressed elsewhere in this text. The author hopes that the algorithm in ▶ Fig. 6.5 and accompanying text will be of assistance in achieving good surgical outcomes with fewer surgical revisions.

References

[1] Condie D, Tolkachjov SN. Facial nerve injury and repair: apractical review for cutaneous surgery. Dermatol Surg. 2019; 45(3):340–357

[2] TankPW. Grant's Dissector. 13th ed. Baltimore, MD: Lippincott Williams and Wilkins; 2005

[3] Borges AF. Relaxed skin tension lines (RSTL) versus other skin lines. Plast Reconstr Surg. 1984; 73(1):144–150

[4] Dobratz EJ, Hilger PA. Cheek defects. Facial Plast Surg Clin North Am. 2009; 17(3):455–467

[5] Soliman S, Hatef DA, Hollier LH , Jr, Thornton JF. The rationale for direct linear closure of facial Mohs' defects. Plast Reconstr Surg. 2011; 127(1):142–149

[6] Robinson JK. Suspension sutures in facial reconstruction. Dermatol Surg. 2003; 29(4):386–393

[7] Zook EG, Van Beek AL, Russell RC, Moore JB. V-Y advancement flap for facial defects. Plast Reconstr Surg. 1980; 65(6):786–797

[8] Peled IJ, Wexler MR. The usefulness and versatility of V-Y advancement flaps. J Dermatol Surg Oncol. 1983; 9(12):1003–1006

[9] Zitelli JA. The bilobed flap for nasal reconstruction. Arch Dermatol. 1989; 125(7):957–959

[10] Giacomarra V, Renco M, Bianchi M, Tirelli G, Russolo M. Bilobed flap in the reconstruction of cheek defects. Acta Otorhinolaryngol Ital. 2001; 21(6):356–360 Italian

[11] Wood LD, Warner NM, Billingsley EM. Infectious complications of dermatologic procedures. Dermatol Ther (Heidelb). 2011; 24(6):558–570

[12] Bunick CG, Aasi SZ. Hemorrhagic complications in dermatologic surgery. Dermatol Ther (Heidelb). 2011; 24(6):537–550

[13] Delaney A, Diamantis S, Marks VJ. Complications of tissue ischemia in dermatologic surgery. Dermatol Ther (Heidelb). 2011; 24(6):551–557

7 Auricular Reconstruction

David G. Brodland and Molly Powers

Abstract

This chapter focuses on preservation of the symmetrical projection of the ear (which is the top aesthetic concern in auricular reconstruction, followed by maintaining the nautilus shape), and preservation of the helical rim and special considerations for the same. This chapter also discusses several reconstructive options, and cartilage flaps and grafts that may be needed to prevent auricular distortion. The authors also consider here that not all wounds necessitate reconstruction; many wounds on the anterior and posterior surfaces, not involving the helical rim, heal well by second intention.

Keywords: Auricular reconstruction, cartilage flap, cartilage graft, helical rim advancement, external auditory canal stenosis, retroauricular interpolation

Capsule Summary and Pearls

- Preserving the symmetrical projection of the ear is the top aesthetic concern in auricular reconstruction followed by maintaining the nautilus shape.
- Preservation of the helical rim is important and special considerations should be taken to preserve it.
- When there is significant structural loss, cartilage flaps and grafts may be needed to prevent auricular distortion.
- When there are significant defects involving the external auditory canal (EAC), caution must be taken for stenosis.
- Lastly, it is important to consider that not all wounds necessitate reconstruction. Many wounds on the anterior and posterior surfaces, not involving the helical rim, heal well by second intention.

7.1 Introduction

The structure and form of the ear itself has many complex intricacies, while its functions are simple and basic. The ear has many variations in the quality of the cartilage, skin, and soft tissue that make each auricle unique to reconstruct. The two primary goals of any reconstruction are to maintain the function, and secondarily, preserve the aesthetic form. When reconstructing the auricle, preserving auditory function and maintaining the normal projection of the ear will help attain these primary goals. The cartilage of the ear provides the foundation for its structure and identifiable shape. The anterior and lateral profiles comprise each ear's unique appearance such that their preservation is critical for a successful reconstruction. When contemplating a reconstruction of the ear, it is often simplest to approach each anatomical zone separately. ▸ Table 7.1 lists each of the anatomical zones of the ear. It is best to approach the aesthetics of reconstruction based on the hierarchy listed in ▸ Table 7.2. Each auricular defect is unique and calls for careful consideration for each reconstructive option.

The topographical anatomy of the ear is unique (see ▸ Fig. 7.1a). An interesting feature of the ear is the variation in its components. Cartilage ranges from soft and delicate to rigid. Skin ranges from elastic on the earlobe to rigid anteriorly. Therefore, it is important to assess and appreciate each ear's unique features.

7.2 Relevant Anatomy

The topographical anatomy of the ear is noteworthy and unlike any other anatomical site on the body. These

Table 7.1 Anatomical zones

Superior helix
Mid helix
Lobule
Antihelix
Concha
Tragus
Remainder of anterior ear
Remainder of posterior ear

Table 7.2 Hierarchy of aesthetic concerns

1. Symmetrical projection
2. Smooth, nautilus-like shape of the helix
3. Color/texture of skin
4. Anterior/posterior dimension
5. Vertical height
6. Presence and symmetry of tragus
7. Contour of antihelix and conchal bowl

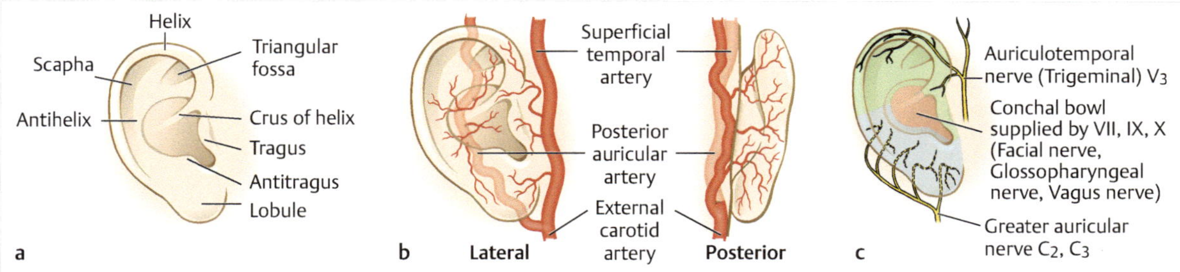

Fig. 7.1 **(a)** Anatomic subunits of the ear. **(b)** Vascular supply of the lateral and posterior ear. **(c)** Cutaneous innervation of the ear.

topographical landmarks are illustrated in ▶ Fig. 7.1a. Not only are there multiple anatomical subunits of the ear, but there are also many anatomical variations within each subunit, such as rigid and soft cartilage. The skin on the earlobe is relatively elastic while the skin on the anterior surface has no elasticity. With the multiple convexities and concavities involving the auricle, as well as varying characteristics of the skin and subcutaneous tissue, it is important to assess and appreciate each ear's unique structure.

Despite the ear's intricate architecture, its primary functions are quite basic: hearing, maintaining EAC patency for the conduction of sound, and holding eyeglasses.

While the ear is relatively inconspicuous in its lateral location with limited visibility from the frontal view, change of its projection from the head can lead to noticeable deformities. There is a well-established hierarchy of aesthetic concerns of the ear that are listed in ▶ Table 7.2. We recommend prioritizing each concern as listed to obtain the best cosmetic outcome.

The ear has many complexities while its framework is relatively simple. The cartilage serves as the foundation that is then draped by the perichondrium, subcutaneous tissue, then the skin. On the posterior ear, the skin and subcutaneous tissue remains relatively loose and nonadherent as compared with the anterior ear. As a result, the posterior ear has more mobility and, to some degree, can serve as a skin reservoir for flaps and grafts. When performing these procedures, the undermining plane on the ear remains superficial to the perichondrium. If undermining is necessary on the lobule, it is best to do so in the mid fat.

Relaxed skin tension lines are not important for ear reconstructive strategy. Due to the complex topography of the ear, the scars of reconstruction remain relatively camouflaged and inconspicuous and are more dependent on reconstruction design and suturing technique.

The arterial supply of the auricle is from the external carotid artery with two main branches: the superficial temporal artery and the posterior auricular artery (see ▶ Fig. 7.1b.) These two networks have extensive anastomoses providing a very rich blood supply. This makes random patterned flaps dependable and relatively low risk with appropriate execution.

Cutaneous innervation of the ear is supplied by both cranial and spinal nerves (see ▶ Fig. 7.1c). Cranial nerves VII, IX, and X innervate the conchal bowl. The greater auricular nerve, arising from C2 and C3, innervates the lower half of the ear. The superior ear anteriorly is innervated by the auriculotemporal nerve, a branch of CN V3. The remainder of the superior ear posteriorly is innervated by the lesser occipital nerve (C2, C3).

7.3 Reconstructive Options (▶ Fig. 7.2)

7.3.1 Superior Helix

As the most iconic component of the auricle, the helix is responsible for the normal shape and position of the ear. It is comprised of delicate cartilage that can be easily deformed during reconstructions. In addition, it is the most common location of skin cancers of the ear. For these reasons, the proper reconstruction of the helix is paramount to maintaining its normal contour.

We propose the algorithm in ▶ Fig. 7.3 to approach defects on the superior helix. First, it is necessary to determine if there is infrastructural compromise. If there is none, we recommend a simplified closure. If the defect remains small (< 1 cm), does not involve the helical groove, and adequate soft tissue remains, a simple primary closure may be performed with excellent results. After undermining above the perichondrium, an elongated linear or curvilinear closure oriented diagonally to the helical rim is a simple method to prevent standing vertical cones and flattening of the helical curvature. This elongated closure often has a larger length-to-width ratio than the typical 3:1 observed at other anatomic locations.

Additional options for the superior helix without structural deficits are second intention, full-thickness skin grafts (FTSGs), and flaps. Second intention is best reserved for wounds that are shallower and have intact perichondrium. They have a smaller risk of auricular distortion from wound contraction as compared with deeper and larger wounds. If the wound is larger and

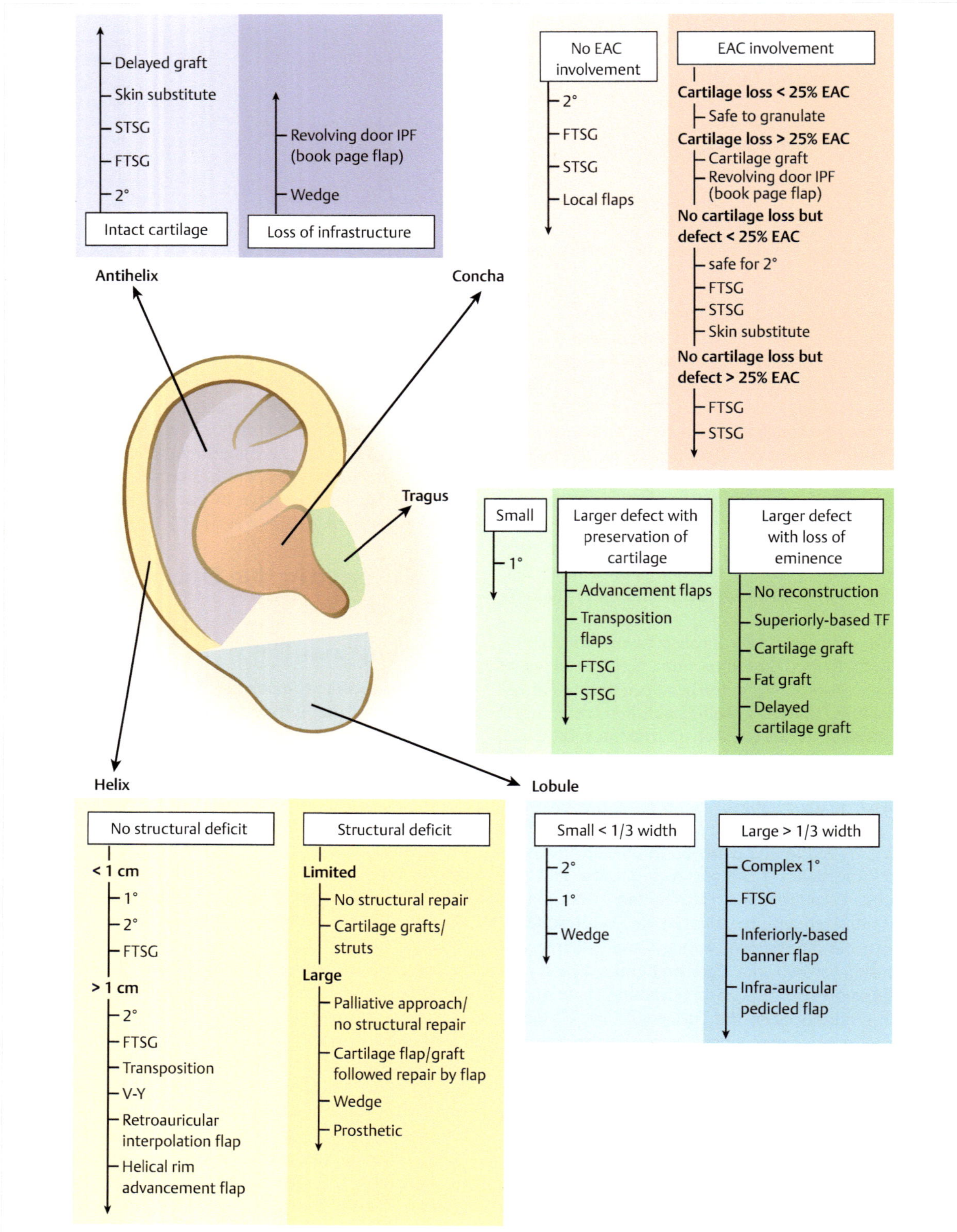

Fig. 7.2 Division of the ear and reconstructive options for anatomical subunit. (STSG, split thickness skin graft; FTSG, full thickness skin graft; 1°, primary; 2°, secondary; EAC, external auditory canal; TF, transposition flap; IPF, island pedicle flap.)

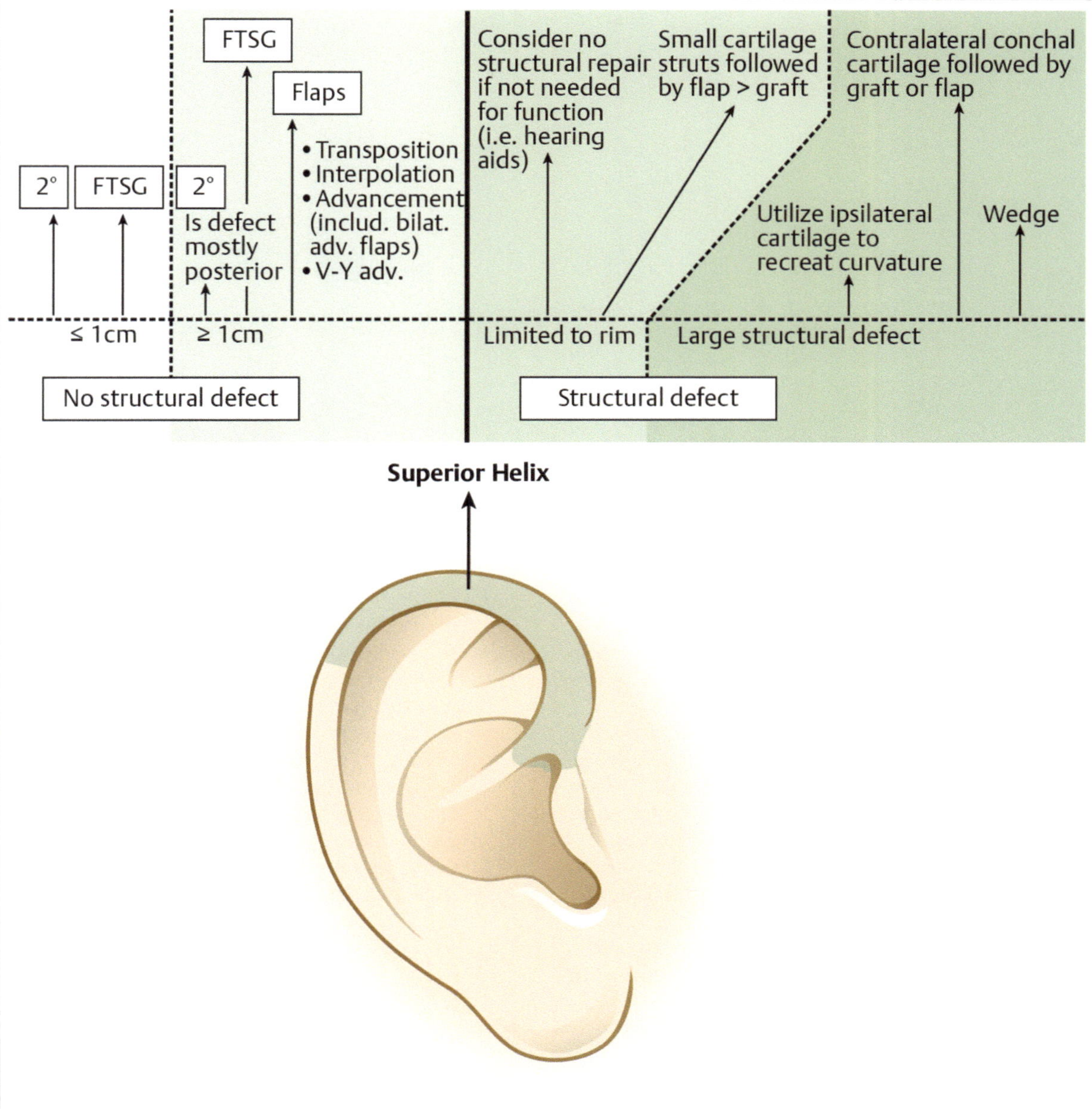

Fig. 7.3 Reconstruction algorithm of the superior helix. (2°, second intention; FTSG, full thickness skin graft.)

adjacent to the less rigid cartilage of the helical rim, distortion may be more likely. If the wound is more posterior where tissue is looser and supported by underlying rigid structural cartilage, distortion is less likely. FTSGs from the postauricular area, preauricular area, or the conchal bowl are excellent options for repair of superior helical defects without extensive infrastructural compromise. Assessing the wound bed's vascular base is also important. FTSGs are better utilized with intact perichondrium and structurally insignificant loss of cartilage. Flaps (as listed in the superior helix reconstructive algorithm) should be considered when defects are larger, the wound bed has a poor vascular base, or when larger cartilage grafts have been used for structural support.

Repairs of superior helical defects with loss of structural integrity require more careful planning and discussion with the patient. Patient discussion should detail the types of reconstructions and review the goals and expectations of each option. For example, if the patient depends on the integrity of the auricle for hearing aids, reading glasses, etc., then discussing the need to preserve this function may be necessary. In the case of a larger

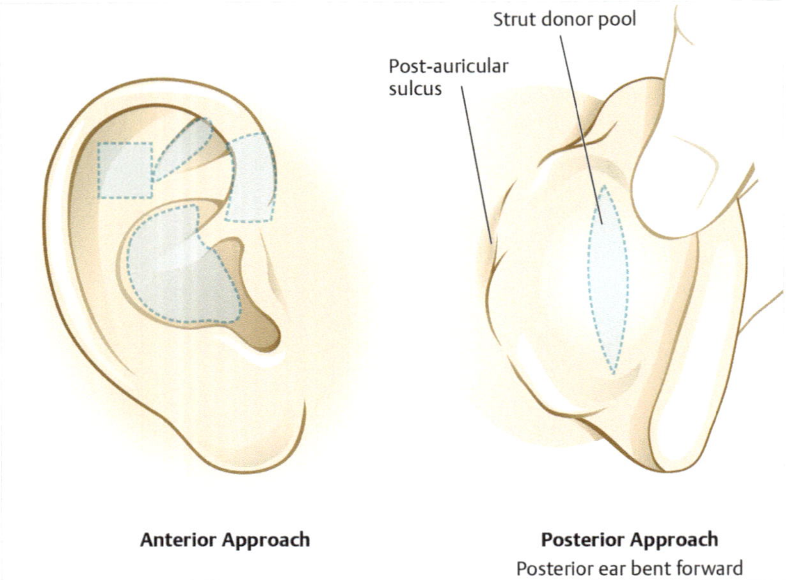

Fig. 7.4 Illustration of cartilage donor sites of the ear.

structural defect, cartilage grafts or struts may be used to optimize auricular restoration and cosmesis.

Donor sites for cartilage grafts are demonstrated in ▶ Fig. 7.4. For larger structural defects, there are several reconstructive options. If the nautilus shape of the auricle is compromised, harvesting the entire ipsilateral or contralateral conchal bowl cartilage can be used to recreate this shape nicely. In addition to cartilage grafts, cartilage flaps can be performed. It is possible to transpose or advance cartilage with the aid of a muscular or subcutaneous vascular base. In ▶ Fig. 7.5 and ▶ Fig. 7.6, a transposition of cartilage is utilized to provide structural support for the helical rim. For defects of the superior helical rim that are deep but remain less than 1.0 to 1.5 cm in width, a wedge closure is an alternate option for repair. If a defect is too large for an aesthetic wedge closure, reestablishing structural support with a cartilage graft and performing a multistaged flap, such as a retroauricular interpolation flap or a tube flap, may yield the most optimal cosmetic results.

Superior helix: most visible subunit/iconic feature

I. No structural deficit.
   1. ≤ 1 cm:
      a) Primary closure.
      b) Second intention.
      c) FTSG.
   2. > 1 cm:
      a) Second intention.
      b) FTSG.
      c) Flaps.
      - Transposition.
      - Interpolation.
      - V-Y advancement.
      - Helical rim advancement.

II. Structural deficit.
   1. Limited to the cartilaginous rim.
      a) No structural repair.
      b) Small cartilage grafts/struts.
   2. Large structural deficit.
      a) Palliative approach to expedite wound healing without structural repair.
      b) Cartilage graft.
      c) Cartilage flap with muscular/subcutaneous base.
      d) Wedge closure (defect deep and width < 1.5 cm).
      e) Cartilage graft/flap with multistage repair (defect > 2.5 cm).

Reconstructive Steps for Repairs Suitable for the Superior Helix

Cartilage Grafts

- Select donor site.
  - Ipsilateral vs. contralateral.
    - Prefer ipsilateral to simplify wound care and minimize number of wounds when practical.
    - If cartilage adjacent to wound is accessible (due to exposure) and its use as a cartilage graft would not compromise auricular structure, consider as a potential donor site.
    - Contralateral if the donor pool is absent from tumor removal or if ipsilateral harvest would cause structural or aesthetic compromise.
  - Conchal bowl.
    - Anterior approach.
    - Posterior approach.
  - Anterior helix.
  - Scaphae.
  - Crus of antihelix.

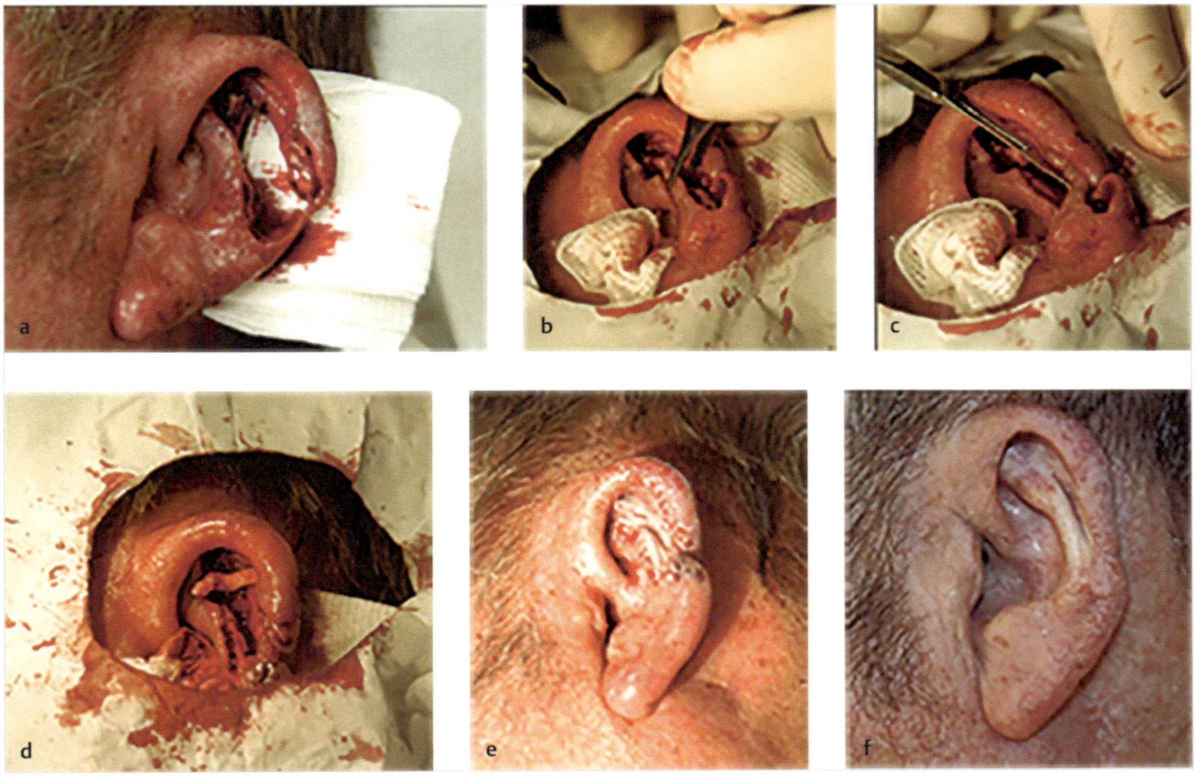

Fig. 7.5 **(a)** Through-and-through defect necessitating structural support to maintain the nautilus shape of the helix. **(b,c)** Transposition of cartilage utilized to provide structural support for the helical rim. **(d)** Cartilage strut supporting the superior helix. **(e)** Immediate postoperative photo with skin graft on the anterior ear. **(f)** Three-month postoperative photo.

Step-by-step:

- Cleanse entire ear including posterior ear and the most external portion of the EAC (not chlorhexidine due to possible ototoxicity).
- Select donor site.
- Create single incision.
  - Linear for long, narrow strut-like grafts.
  - U-shaped for larger, broader grafts.
- Dissect skin off the underlying cartilage in the perichondrial plane.
- Incise precisely measured cartilage needed.
- Using forceps, carefully stabilize cartilage and dissect cartilage off the undersurface of the skin from the other side of the ear within the perichondrial plane.
  - Remember the cartilage is extremely fragile and can fracture easily. This dissection must be performed with caution.
- After cartilage is harvested, place in saline, obtain hemostasis of the donor site.
- We recommend closing the skin on the ear with simple interrupted sutures.
  - Interrupted 5–0 chromic or 5–0 fast-absorbing gut suture may be used; may also use nonabsorbable suture (5–0 polypropylene).

Spoke and Wheel Cartilage Struts (▶ Fig. 7.5a–f)

Goals:

- **The wheel:** Reestablish structure of outer ear margin (helical rim).
- **The spoke:** Provide structure radiating from the EAC/conchal bowl (the hub).

Step-by-step:

- Evaluate the defect and determine where the strut would provide the most benefit for infrastructural support.
- Factors to consider:
  - Size of the defect.
  - Likely direction of maximal wound contraction.
  - Size of cartilage strut available.
- Harvest cartilage as previously outlined.
- Harvest strip of cartilage with appropriate curvature to simulate the helix and straight cartilaginous struts to serve as radial structure (the spokes).
- Helical cartilage will need to be enveloped within residual helical skin or well-vascularized flap.
- The radial spokes are typically 3 to 4 mm in width and need to be securely seated in soft tissue pockets on the

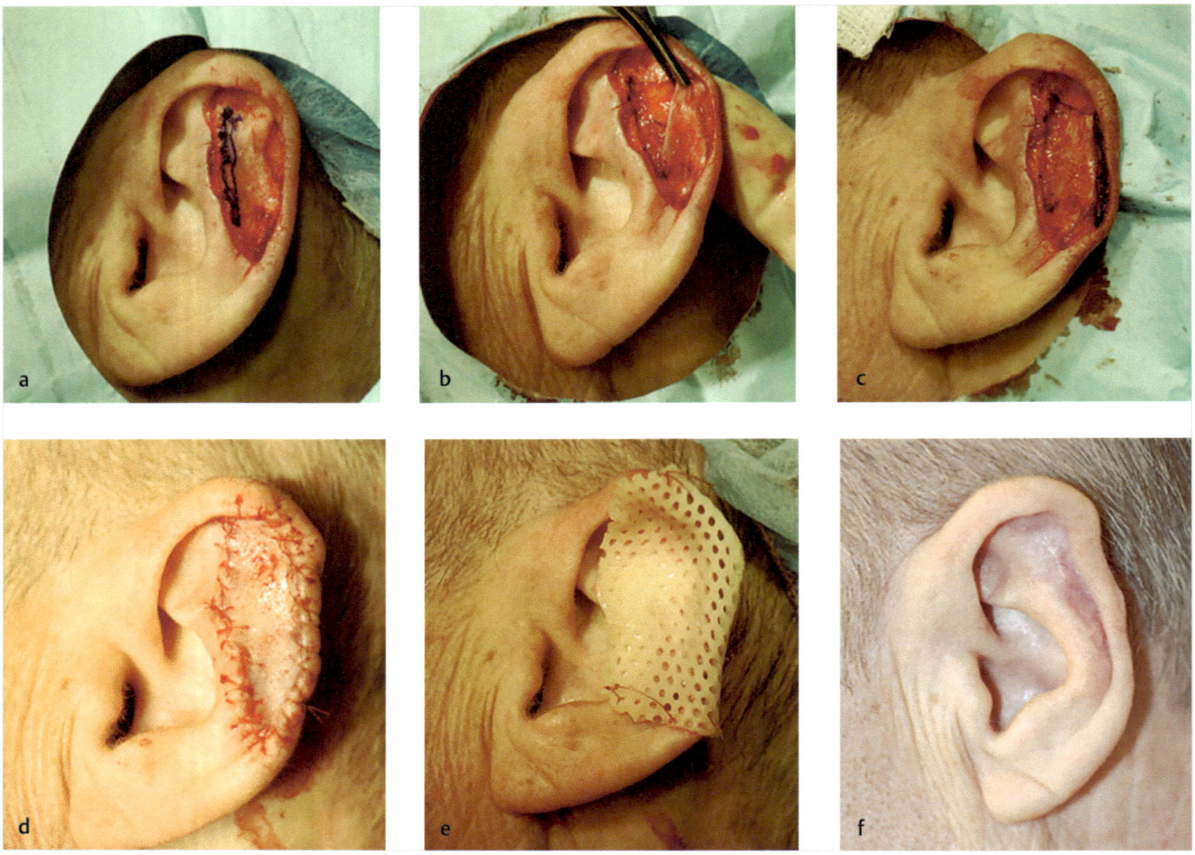

Fig. 7.6 **(a)** Donor pool for flap anterior to helix. Cartilage flap for helix outlined anterior to plane of incision for cartilage transposition flap. **(b)** Cartilage flap being transposed posteriorly to support antihelical skin. **(c)** Cartilage flap and graft sutured into recipient beds of antihelical and helix, respectively. **(d)** Full-thickness skin graft (FTSG) sutured over cartilage flap and graft. Cartilage graft is thoroughly enveloped by residual skin of the helix. Sutures tuck the cartilage graft and surround it on three sides for vascular supply. **(e)** Molded thermoplastic dressing sutured over the entire reconstruction site for 1 week. **(f)** Four-month postoperative result.

central end created by sharp and/or blunt dissection. The peripheral end and, if possible, the midportion of the strut must be fixated to the underlying tissue. This end should also be affixed to the helical cartilage by lashing-type suturing or if possible, direct suturing to the cartilage.

- With a vascularized base of either remnant ear tissue or flap tissue, the exposed side of the spoke and wheel structure may be covered with a split-thickness skin graft (STSG). An STSG is preferred because its lower metabolic requirement is preferred as graft coverage.
- A tightly compressed bolster dressing is key to the secure immobilization of the new structure to avoid dislodgement and to assure survival of the graft. Extreme care for ideally one month postoperatively is critical to avoid dislocation of the cartilage components and should be emphasized to the patients.

Cartilage Flap (► Fig. 7.6a–f)

Step-by-step:

- Determine where the infrastructural support is needed as described in the spoke and wheel instructions.
- Identify donor source.
  - Ideally cartilage can be transposed or slightly rotated on a perichondrial or subcutaneous base.
- Ideal to recreate the natural architecture of the helix.
  - Important to be mindful of the contractile forces of healing and provide structural support to maintain the natural shape of the ear.
- Once donor site is identified, incise the cartilage, again leaving the subcutaneous base intact.
  - There are effectively two methods to executing a cartilage flap depending on the flexibility/rigidity of the cartilage.

    - If cartilage is more flexible, may perform a rotation or transposition of the cartilage without completely separating the flap from the adjacent cartilage.
    - If cartilage is more rigid, it may require complete separation from the auricle, remaining embedded within the skin flap with the posterior surface as a vascular base (serving as an island pedicle flap).
- Very gently move cartilage to desired location.
  - Important to acknowledge the fragility of the cartilage and ease with which this may fracture.
- Suture into place with 5–0 or 4–0 absorbable suture or clear nylon.
- May place graft or flap over the cartilage flap.
  - Important for cartilage to have a vascular base to optimize survival.
- We recommend the use of a bolster or even a moldable thermoplastic splint to further immobilize and shape the flap + /− graft for 1 week.
  - After removal of the bolster, may preserve the thermoplastic splint and continue to use as a formal brace for one or more additional weeks thereafter.
  - Recommend bandaging the area for protection from accidental distortional injury for up to one month postoperatively.

*In this case, adequate movement of flap could be obtained without completely incising and separating the cartilage flap from the inferior antihelix (▶ Fig. 7.6b, c).

Full-Thickness Skin Grafts (FTSGs)

Donor sites:

- < 1.5 cm:
  - Consider postauricular sulcus (relatively easy to close primarily).
  - Conchal bowl (donor site heals by second intention).
- > 1.5 cm:
  - Postauricular.
  - Preauricular.
  - Conchal bowl.
  - Supraclavicular.
  - Upper inner arm.
  - Burow's triangle from closure of another defect.

Step-by-step:

- Create template of defect.
- Place template at the donor site over taut skin.
- Trace template/score skin with scalpel.
- Pearl: keep template on sterile tray to use in "right sizing" nonstick gauze to be placed over the graft at the conclusion of the procedure.
- Raise the graft in the subdermal plane with scissors or scalpel.
- Defat the graft to visualize glistening, white dermis; thin as needed, tailored to the wound depth.
- Place graft in saline.
- Obtain hemostasis and suture donor site.
  - 4–0 or 5–0 dermal + /− epidermal sutures.
- Suture graft in place.
  - Recommend 6–0 or 5–0 fast-absorbing gut with interrupted sutures placed in key locations (4 corners on a < 2-cm graft) to secure the orientation of the graft in the defect.
  - Running 6–0 or 5–0 fast-absorbing gut around the perimeter of the graft focusing on perfect edge approximation and contact of the graft with the wound bed.
    - May need basting suture(s) to maximize wound bed contact and/or recreate natural topography of the ear (i.e., helical groove, etc.).
- Apply a thin layer of Vaseline to the graft.
- Create bolster dressing utilizing the template for sizing the nonadherent gauze (Telfa) on the graft and folded gauze overtop. Vaseline gauze is also an effective bolster material.
- Tie bolster with remainder of dermal suture or other nonabsorbable suture.
- Consider thermoplastic splint in lieu of gauze bolster dressing.

Split-Thickness Skin Graft (STSGs) (▶ Fig. 7.7a–d)

Donor sites:

- < 3.5 cm: Consider over the mastoid process.
- > 3.5 cm:
  - Consider the upper, outer thigh.

Step-by-step:

- Create template of defect utilizing suture pack material or non-stick gauze.
- Place template at the donor site with skin taut.
- Trace template/score skin with scalpel.
- Keep template on sterile tray to help create accurate dressing for nonadherent gauze dressing.
- Harvest the graft with scalpel, Weck blade, or other STSG harvesting tool (Dermatome).
  - Lubricate donor site with ointment to aid in harvest.
- Place graft in saline after wiping ointment and removing hair if necessary.
  - Temporarily cover/dress donor site.
  - Allow to heal by second intention.
- Prepare the wound bed.
  - If cartilage is void of perichondrium, perforate cartilage every 1.0 cm^2 with 3- to 4-mm punch through full thickness of cartilage exposing vascularized tissue from other side of cartilage through perforations.
- Suture graft in place.
  - Recommend placing a 6–0 fast-absorbing gut with interrupted sutures at the key locations to keep the graft in the optimal orientation.
  - Running 6–0 or 5–0 fast-absorbing gut around the perimeter of the graft focusing on perfect edge

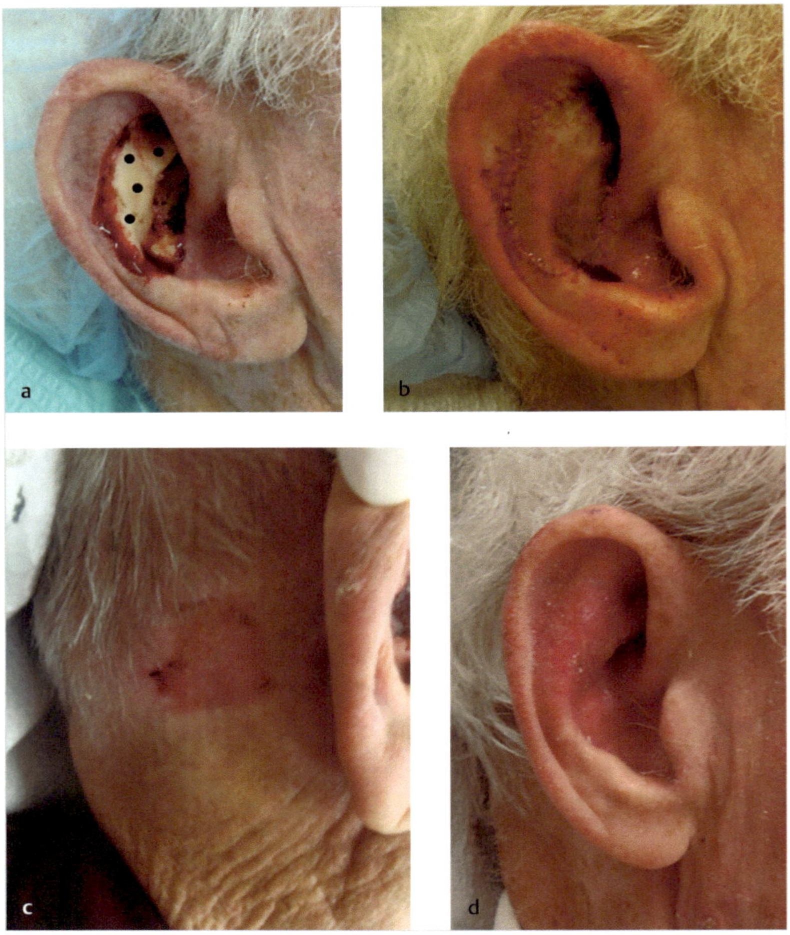

Fig. 7.7 **(a)** Post-Mohs wound with significant absence of the perichondrium. To create vascular source to graft, perforate cartilage with 3- to 4-mm punch to (but not through) the soft tissue of the posterior ear. Perforations shown as *black circles*. **(b)** Split-thickness skin graft (STSG) sutured into place. **(c)** One-week postop picture of donor site. **(d)** Four-month postop result.

approximation and contact of the graft with the wound bed. Watch for and avoid "rolling" of STSG edges.
- Pearl: Create nonadhering dressing with the template using nonadherent gauze.
- Thin layer of petrolatum to the graft.
- Tie bolster with nonabsorbable suture or remaining absorbable dermal suture.
- Considered thermoplastic splint for shaping of the ear in lieu of bolster dressing.

Transposition Flaps (One-Stage Pre- or Postauricular to the Superior Helix) (▶ Fig. 7.8a–f)

Step-by-step:
- Select donor site from pre- or postauricular skin.
- Carefully measure the length of the flap needed to cover the defect.
- Incise the flap.
  - May need to remove skin on the more proximal superior portion of the ear as a rotation Burow's triangle to allow for one-stage transposition.
- Lift the flap in the subcutaneous plane and trim after assuring adequate length.
- Utilizing 5–0 or 6–0 absorbable suture, close secondary defect, then place suture at the tip of the flap to set the flap into its ideal position.
- Layered suturing of the remainder of the flap.

7.3.2 Mid Helix

Similar to the superior helix, reconstruction of the mid helix is essential to maintaining the normal curvature of the helical rim. In contrast to the superior helix, the cartilage of the mid helix may be more rigid and provides more structural support though this is variable. In addition to the structural difference, the mid helix has a more limited cutaneous donor pool for reconstruction. The superior helix, inferior helix, posterior ear, and postauricular area serve as the mid helical donor pools.

Reconstruction of the mid helix requires assessment of several key factors. First, it is important to note whether there is a structural deficit that needs repair. Second, involvement of the helical groove may necessitate special consideration for the repair of the defect. The algorithm to repair the mid helix (▶ Fig. 7.9) is similar to the superior helix. However, the primary donor pools for the mid

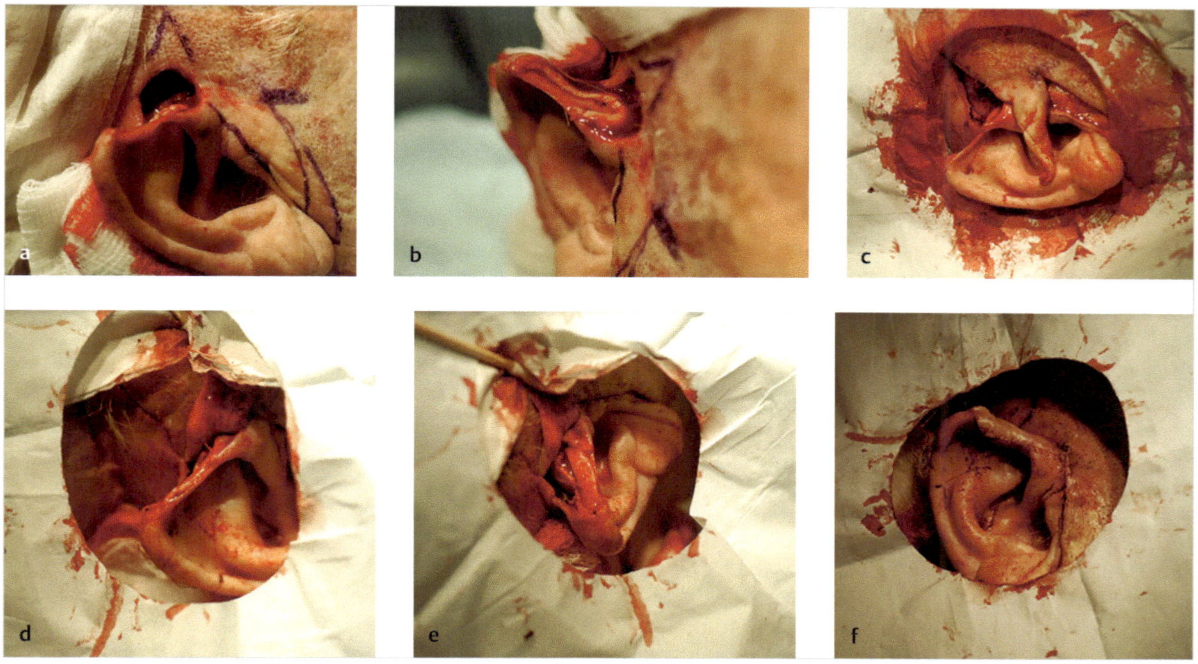

Fig. 7.8 **(a)** Postoperative defect. **(b)** Substantial cartilage loss of the superior helix. **(c)** Preauricular flap raised for transposition. **(d)** Cartilage graft from contralateral conchal bowl tacked into place. **(e)** Superior view of cartilage graft. **(f)** Flap transposed and tacked into place.

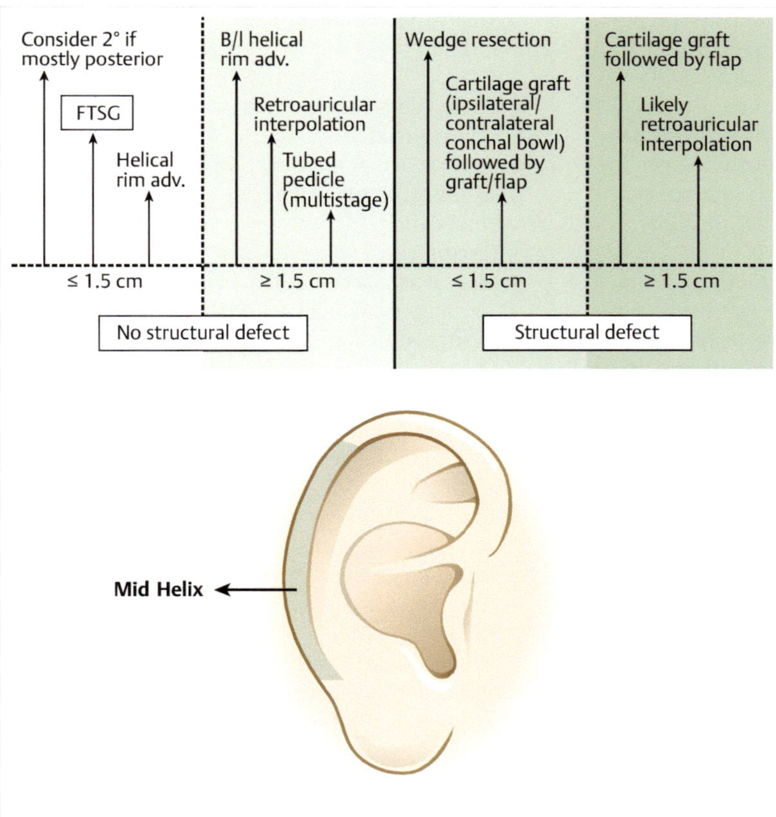

Fig. 7.9 Reconstruction algorithm of the mid helix. (2°, second intention; adv., advancement; FTSG, full thickness skin graft; b/l, bilateral.)

helix are inferior lobular, postauricular, and retroauricular skin. As a result, helical rim advancement and retroauricular interpolation flaps are more commonly performed in this location.

After assessing the wound and discovering no structural deficit, the size of the wound must be taken into account. Wounds that are smaller than 1.5 cm and limited to the rim may be considered for a primary closure as described in the superior helix section. Second intention is another option for defects that are mostly posterior to minimize the likelihood of helical rim deformation as the wound heals and contracts. In addition, if the wound involves the helical groove, second intention may not be advisable as this may cause fusion and therefore noticeable distortion of the helical rim. An FTSG and a helical rim advancement flap are also excellent options and probably the most commonly used options for reconstruction. In addition, these may be better suited than second intention if there is more involvement of the helical rim. Both a graft and the helical rim advancement flap may help to reestablish this very important cosmetic unit of the ear if executed carefully. If the wound is larger than roughly 1.0 cm in width, primary closure may be difficult to perform, and second intention is more likely to lead to auricular deformity. We prefer FTSGs, helical advancement flaps, retroauricular interpolation flaps, or multistaged tubed pedicle flaps. Each patient has unique anatomy and tailoring the repair for each defect is crucial. For example, a helical rim advancement flap may not be the best option for even a smaller wound if the lobule is too small or nonexistent to recruit skin for the closure. Helical rim advancement flaps are an excellent option for small- to medium-sized wounds, especially when they do not cross the helical groove. A retroauricular interpolation flap is preferred when the wound is larger or if the wound crosses the helical groove. This interpolation flap provides excellent vascular supply, and therefore is very reliable.

Repair of the mid helix with a structural deficit, again, is similar in principle to the repairs of superior helix necessitating structural support. Given the iconic curvature of the helix from the most superior aspect to the lobule, irregularities of this curved contour can be quite noticeable. For optimal cosmesis, it is advised to repair structural deficits to minimize these irregularities in the curvature of the helix. For smaller defects, a helical advancement flap (unilateral or bilateral) that is inclusive of cartilage (chondrocutaneous) may help to restore the appearance of the ear. Excision of a crescentic Burow's triangle including cartilage from the superior scapha can be utilized when advancing the superior rim inferiorly to improve reach and avoid a cupping deformity. It is important to note that this may shorten the height of the ear. As with the superior helix, a cartilage graft followed by FTSG or STSG or retroauricular interpolation flap is considered the workhorse repair for structural mid helical defects. Lastly, a wedge resection may be considered, although this will lead to size discrepancy between the patient's ears and can cause "cupping" if not performed with extreme care.

When there is involvement of the helical groove, special considerations must be taken. If the wound is small (< 0.5 cm) and involves minimal cartilaginous loss, reconstruction without structural support is an option. A flap or graft may be used; however, the helical groove should be maintained with the aid of external supports such as a bolster, thermoplastic cast, spiral suture, etc. When performing the spiral suture, we recommend the needle entering from the anterior helical groove through to the posterior aspect of the ear, then looping from the posterior aspect of the helix around the helical rim and reentering on the anterior helical groove. This spiral suture will help guide and form the appropriate shape of the healing repair. Other external stabilizing tools may be utilized to help maintain or recreate the helical groove. Defects greater than 0.5 cm that involve cartilaginous loss will likely require support with cartilage graft followed by soft tissue repair and, again, strategies to maintain the helical groove.

I. No structural deficit.
   a) ≤ 1.5 cm:
      1. Primary closure.
      2. Second intention.
      3. FTSG.
      4. Helical advancement flap.
   b) > 1.5 cm:
      1. FTSG.
      2. Helical advancement flap (may consider bilateral advancement).
      3. Retroauricular interpolation.
      4. Multistaged tubed pedicle.
II. Structural deficit.
   a) ≤ 1.5 cm:
      1. Helical advancement flap inclusive of cartilage.
      2. Cartilage graft followed by flap or graft.
      3. Wedge resection.
   b) > 1.5 cm:
      1. Cartilage graft followed by flap. May consider graft if there is adequate vascular supply.
III. Involvement of the helical groove.
   a) ≤ 0.5 cm:
      1. May be able to reconstruct the groove without structural support.
      2. Maintain groove with spiral suture, bolsters, thermoplast, etc.
   b) > 0.5 cm:
      1. Will likely need cartilaginous support with graft or flap (with supporting soft tissue bridge).
      2. Advancement of composite cartilage/skin.
      3. Maintain groove with spiral suture, bolsters, thermoplastic splint, etc.

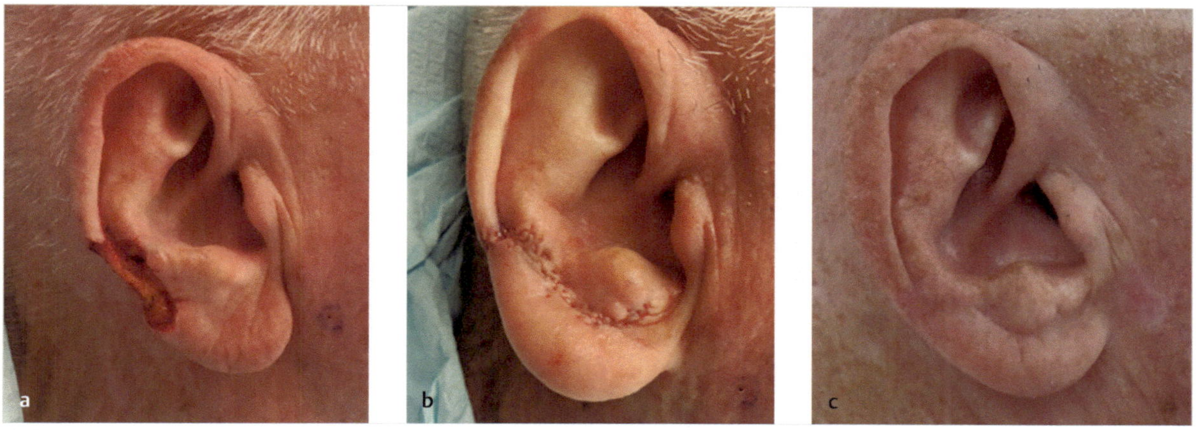

Fig. 7.10 **(a)** Post-Mohs defect on the mid- to lower helix. **(b)** Anterior view of the immediate postop helical rim advancement flap. **(c)** Three-month postop picture.

Reconstructive Steps for Repairs Suitable for the Mid Helix

Helical Advancement Flap[1] (Antia-Buch) (▶ Fig. 7.10a–c; ▶ Video 7.1)

Step-by-step:

- Mark key anatomy on patient ear (helical groove).
- Incise inferiorly along the helical groove.
- Incise the Burow's triangle on the posterior aspect of the ear.
  - Extends from the wound margin to a point just before the postauricular sulcus.
- Undermine posteriorly in the perichondrial plane until more inferiorly where the cartilage ends. Then remain in the mid subcutaneous tissue.
  - Be sure to keep scissors firmly toward the cartilage posteriorly in order to maintain maximum flap vascularity.
- Minimally undermine all the wound edges of the defect between 1 and 3 mm.
- Move the flap from inferior to superior and remove the anterior Burow's triangle from the lobule as needed.
- Close the anterior Burow's triangle defect with 5–0 or 6–0 absorbable suture.
- Place the key suture(s) that advance(s) the flap to cover the defect.
  - Important to remember that wound eversion on the helix of the ear is key to preventing an inversion of the scar.
- Suture the remaining flap into place.
- Top sutures: running 6–0 or 5-0 fast-absorbing gut.

Retroauricular Interpolation Flap[2–4] (▶ Fig. 7.11)

Step-by-step:

- Make template of the defect.
- Identify donor site.
  - May consider raising the flap immediately posterior to the defect, utilizing the posterior skin of the ear to become the leading edge of the flap.
  - For smaller defects, start the leading edge of the flap in the sulcus or even the postauricular skin depending on how much reach is needed.
- When designing, imagine tucking the denuded auricle under the flap of skin.
  - Base of flap is often just peripheral to what would be the shadow of the helix.
- Incise the flap.
- Lift the flap at the depth needed to fill the defect and gradually deepen the level of undermining to assure a robust vascular base.
- Suture the flap into place (5–0 or 6–0 absorbable dermal sutures) with the goal to minimize tension along the leading edge of the flap then with 6–0 fast-absorbing gut on top.
- May need to recreate the helical groove depending on the defect.
  - Running suture originating from the anterior aspect of the helical groove, through the helix then from the posterior helix to reenter the helical groove anteriorly creating a spiral along the helix.
  - May use bolsters with cardstock from the suture packs to recreate the groove.
  - May use thermoplastic splints to help reshape the groove.
- After 3 weeks or longer if needed, the pedicle is severed and the posterior aspect of the flap is sutured into place.
- Donor site can be left to heal by second intention or repaired via skin graft.

7.3.3 Lobule

The lobule is the only anatomical subunit of the ear that is devoid of rigid infrastructure. For this reason, defects on the earlobe tend to be simpler to repair than defects

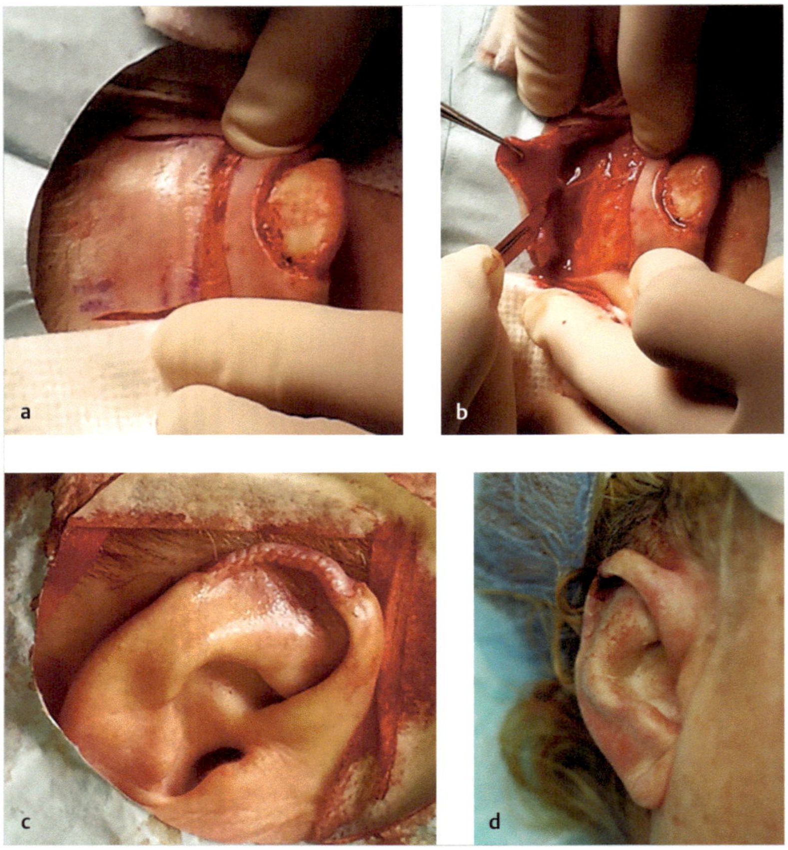

Fig. 7.11 **(a)** Posterior view of the post-Mohs defect with retroauricular flap incised and leading edge of the flap on the posterior ear. **(b)** Flap being lifted on the posterior ear. **(c)** Immediate postop picture. **(d)** Anterior view demonstrates preservation of the helical rim contour.

on the superior and midhelix. Due to the pliability of the skin on the lobule, the tissue redundancy, and laxity of the pre-and postauricular skin, the most common reconstructions of the earlobe are relatively simple. However, when defects of the lobule are larger, they may necessitate structural support. The most important aspect of the lobule's reconstruction is to maintain the semicircular configuration of the earlobe. If this is maintained, the repair is often unnoticeable to the casual observer even if the lobule size differs somewhat from the contralateral lobe (see ▶ Fig. 7.12).

When defects of the lobule are small (less than one-third the horizontal width of the lobule), their repairs can remain simple. It is reasonable to let smaller, superficial defects heal by second intention; however, caution is advised when the defect is located on the anterior aspect of the lobule as they may demonstrate more noticeable scar contraction or hypertrophy. One of the most common methods to repair the lobule is with a primary or wedge closure. Approximating the remaining unaffected skin is often possible and yields excellent results. Some important concepts to remember when suturing the lobule is to maintain the natural semicircular curvature of the lobule and to create maximum wound eversion to avoid depressed scar lines.

Larger defects (greater than one-third the horizontal width of the lobule) often require more innovative and creative reconstructions. Often, a complex primary closure, such as folding the lobule upon itself to recreate the natural curvature, is sufficient (see ▶ Fig. 7.13). At times, cartilage grafts should be considered if there is a risk of significant tissue contraction and distortion of the lobule. An FTSG is a reasonable option; however, they do run the risk of contraction and may lead to shriveling or pincushioning of the lobule. Avoidance of undersizing the graft may help to mitigate this risk. Utilizing the pre-, post-, and infra-auricular skin to repair the lobule should not be overlooked. It is sometimes simple and effective to use a single-staged transposition from these donor pools to repair the lobule (see ▶ Fig. 7.14). Also, the use of a two-stage interpolation repair from the infra-auricular skin may provide excellent results and lessen the risk of contraction (see ▶ Fig. 7.15).

Lobule

1. Small (≤ 1/3 horizontal width of lobule).
   a) Second Intention.
   b) Primary closure.
   c) Wedge.
   d) Single-arm or O-Z rotation flaps.

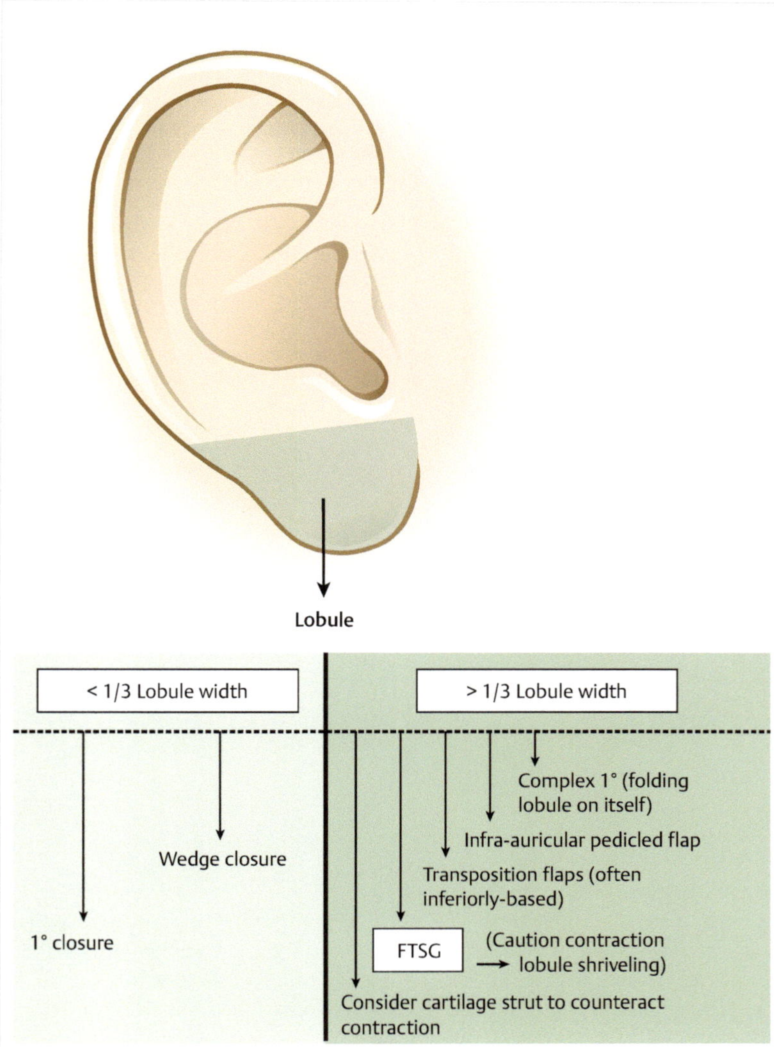

Fig. 7.12 Reconstruction algorithm of the lobule.

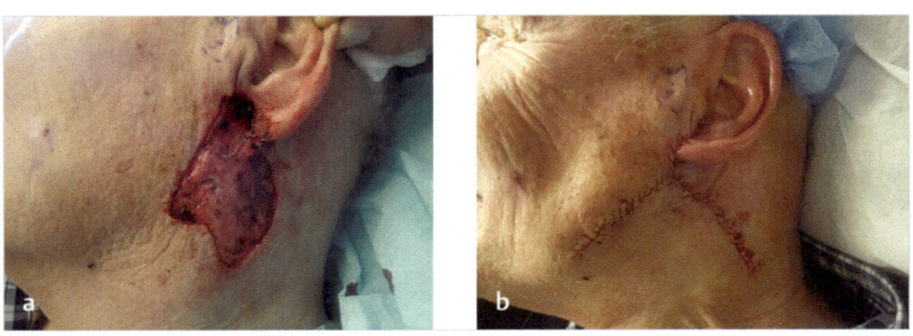

Fig. 7.13 **(a)** Large post-Mohs site of a basal cell carcinoma involving the ear lobule, preauricular area, infra-auricular area, extending on to the neck. **(b)** Inferior skin on the neck was advanced superiorly. Ear lobule was advanced and reattached to the preauricular skin. Caution was taken to maintain the natural curvature of the lobule inferiorly.

2. Larger (> 1/3 horizontal width of the lobule); consider cartilage grafts.
   a) Complex primary.
   b) FTSG.
   c) Superiorly based transposition flaps. See ▶ Fig. 7.14.
   d) Inferiorly based transposition flaps.
   e) Infra-auricular interpolation flap. See ▶ Fig. 7.15.

Reconstructive Steps for Repairs Suitable for the Lobule

Complex Primary: Folding the Lobe on Itself and Closing Remaining Defect (▶ Fig. 7.13)

Step-by-step:

- Assess the anatomy of the unaffected ear.

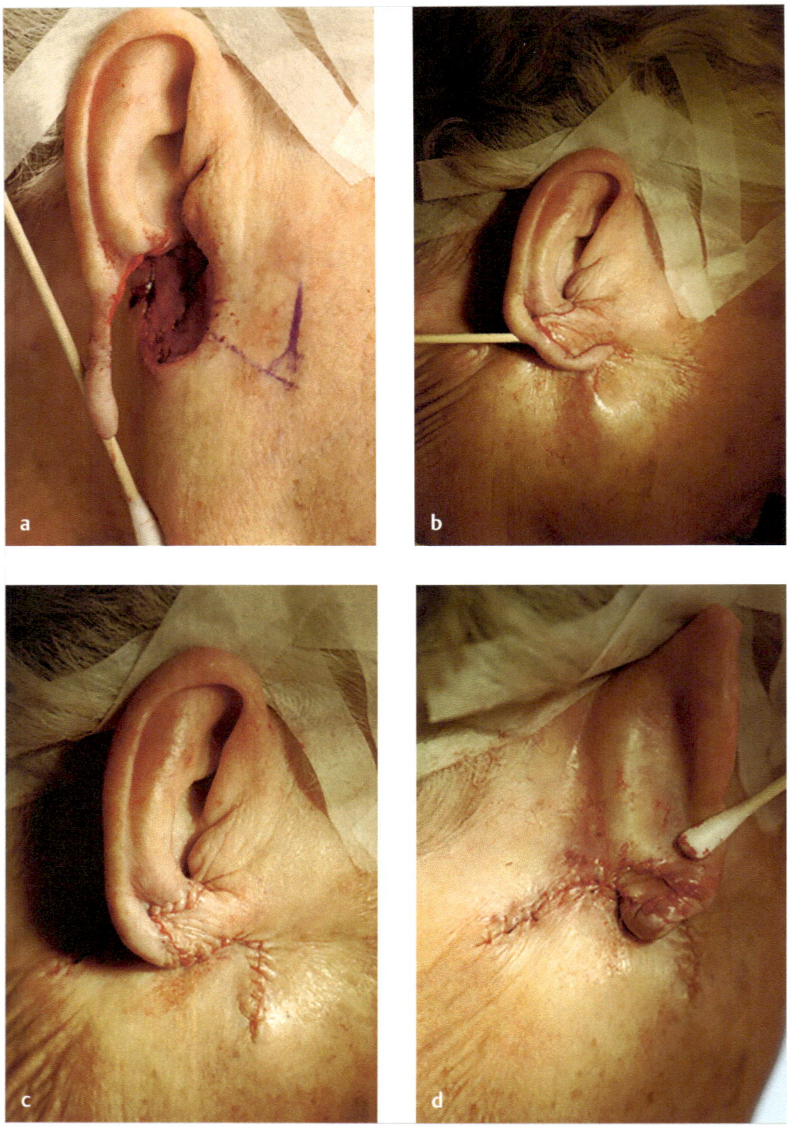

Fig. 7.14 **(a)** Post-Mohs defect demonstrating complete through-and-through loss of the central lobule with preservation of the inferior border. Defect also extends in the infra-auricular region. Transposition flap design from the preauricular area drawn. **(b)** Preauricular skin transposed to form the lobule, with remaining rim of lobule extending along the inferior border, recreating the natural curvature of the lobule. **(c)** Anterior view immediately postop. **(d)** Posterior view immediately postop. Can appreciate the Burow's graft from repair of the infra-auricular defect was utilized to repair the posterior aspect of the lobule.

- Free vs. attached lobule.
- Recommend using hooks to move tissue to discover best tissue configuration.
- Place key sutures with 5–0 absorbable to maintain tissue configuration.
- Wound eversion is necessary to prevent inversion of the scar on the lobule.
- Running top sutures with 5–0 or 6–0 fast-absorbing gut.
  - May need occasional vertical mattress to create maximal wound eversion.

Transposition Flaps

Step-by-step:
- Assess anatomy of unaffected ear for symmetry.
- Assess defect on the lobule and size of flap needed.
  - May be able to utilize native ear lobule skin if possible.
- Identify donor site of flap.
  - Commonly preauricular, infra-auricular, and postauricular skin.
- If lobular defect is full-thickness, may need FTSG to repair the underside of the transposed flap (▶ Fig. 7.14d).
  - Consider using Burow's triangles, preauricular, or postauricular skin.

Inferiorly Based Interpolation (▶ Fig. 7.15)

Step-by-step:
- Create template of the defect.
- Select donor site and incise within the shadow of the earlobe or from the postauricular skin.
- Raise an inferiorly based pedicle.

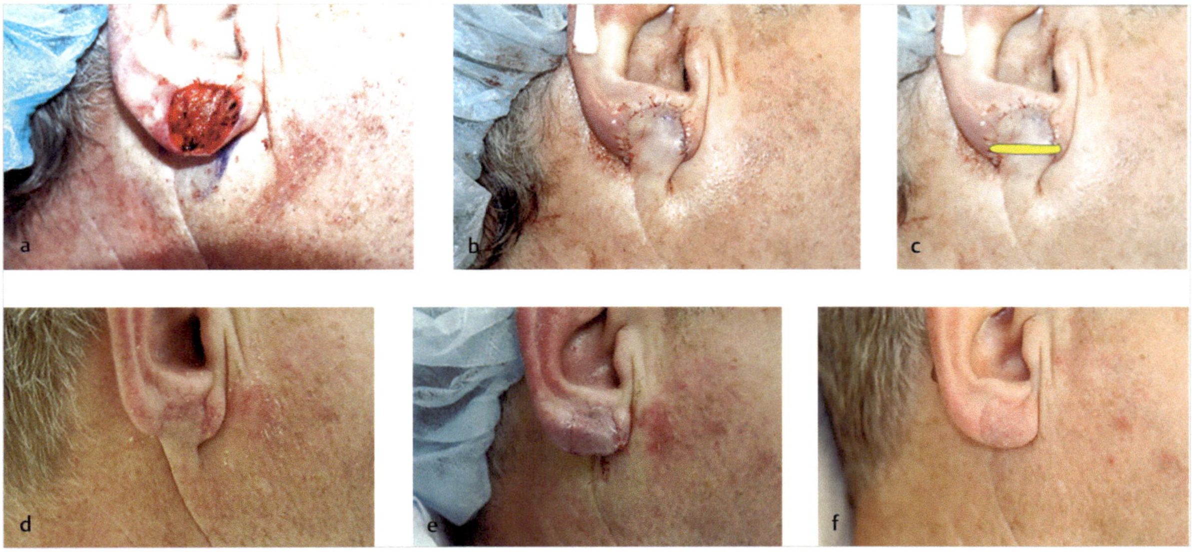

Fig. 7.15 (a) Post-Mohs partial-thickness defect limited to the lobule without loss of adipose tissue. (b) Immediate postop picture of the interpolation flap from the inferior postauricular skin over horizontally oriented strut of cartilage harvested from the postauricular ear. (c) Illustration of the cartilage strut placed horizontally across the defect at the point of possible maximum contraction and therefore wound distortion. The strut is 2 to 4 mm wider than the exposed width of the defect and 2 to 4 mm in diameter. It is inserted into pockets created by a scalpel. The strut is fixed with one or two looping absorbable sutures near the inferior margin of the lobule. (d) Three-week postop from first stage of interpolation flap. (e) Immediate postop from interpolation flap take-down. (f) Three-month follow-up picture.

  - Pedicle should be at least 50% width of the flap.
- Suture flap onto ear with 5–0 or 6–0 absorbable sutures then epidermal sutures.

7.3.4 Antihelix

Due to the complex topography, defects of the antihelix can seem difficult and intimidating to repair. However, even with large defects in this region, healing by second intention often produces acceptable results. Assessing the necessity of structural repair of the antihelix and discussing reconstruction goals with the patient will help guide selection of repair options.

As with the helix, we recommend concentrating on two distinct categories of antihelical reconstruction: intact infrastructure and loss of infrastructure. Defects of the antihelix without infrastructural loss are simple. The majority of the defects heal well by second intention. If perichondrium has been lost, one may consider 3- to 4-mm punch fenestrations per 1.5 cm^2 to expose vascularized tissue from the opposite side of the ear and therefore increase the vascular supply to the base of the wound. An STSG is an excellent option for thin defects. In our hands, STSGs are preferred in this area owing to their decreased metabolic requirement, their ability to survive exposed cartilage more readily than an FTSG, and their excellent skin match to the antihelix. However, an FTSG can also be considered if the vasculature of the wound base is adequate. Punch fenestrations may be considered prior to placement of STSGs and FTSGs to increase the vascular supply. They can also be used to augment second intention healing. Skin substitute products are another option to help stimulate granulation tissue in the absence of a well-vascularized wound bed. The placement of a skin substitute may be followed up by placement of an STSG or an FTSG after adequate granulation tissue formation.

When there is loss of infrastructure of the antihelix, repairs need to be individualized to each patient's defect, ear architecture, healing preferences, and cosmetic goals. Often, loss of cartilage on the antihelix with preservation of the helical rim does not necessitate specific repair. If healing by second intention will lead to distortion of the nautilus-like shape of the ear, then reconstruction with cartilage replacement may be necessary. Wounds with loss of cartilage that are relatively smaller (< 1.5 cm) may be closed with a simple wedge excision. A stellate wedge excision may help mitigate the risk of ear cupping. Larger infrastructural defects of the antihelix may require cartilage grafts, including spoke-and-wheel, followed by a flap or graft. Flaps provide a vascular supply and are better suited for larger defects necessitating cartilage replacement. Flap options in this area include retroauricular interpolation flaps, revolving door island pedicle flaps, book flaps, etc.

Antihelix (including scaphoid and triangular fossae) (▶ **Fig. 7.16**)

1. Intact cartilage.
   a) Second intention.

Intact cartilage	Loss of infrastructure
• **Second Intention** – perforation of cartilage in absence of perichondrium • **STSG** – thin defects – exposed cartilage +/- punch fenestration • **FTSG** – vascular base needed • **Skin substitute products** – in absence of perichondrium to induce granulation • **Delayed FTSG** – after granulation +/- skin substitute	• **Wedge Excision** – stellate → to prevent cupping – traditional • **Revolving Door Island Pedicle Flap/ Book Page Flap**

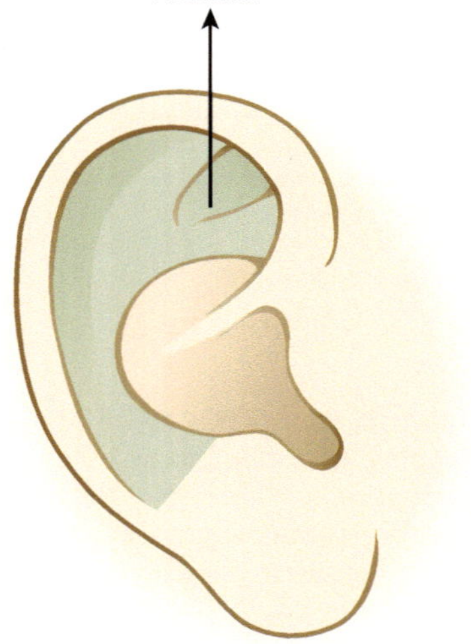

Fig. 7.16 Reconstruction algorithm of the antihelix.

b) FTSG.
c) STSG.
d) Xenograft.
e) Delayed FTSG.

2. Loss of infrastructure.
   a) Wedge excision (stellate, traditional).
   b) Revolving door island pedicle flap, book page flap.
   c) Retroauricular interpolation.

Reconstructive Steps for Repairs Suitable for the Antihelix (▶ Fig. 7.16)

Wedge Excision

Step-by-step:

- Mark a simple V-shape extending from the defect into the concha.
  - This may be modified to a stellate configuration with two elongated triangles of cartilage excised superiorly and inferiorly parallel to the helix.
- Remove this portion of the ear entirely (including cartilage).
  - It is important to remove a portion of the concha to minimize tension and the risk of cupping or deformation.
- Obtain meticulous hemostasis.
- Approximate cartilage with 4–0 or 5–0 absorbable suture.
  - This step is imperative to prevent deformation of the ear.
- Place dermal sutures with 5–0 or 6–0 absorbable suture then top sutures with 6–0 fast-absorbing gut.
- May need thermoplastic splint, bolsters, sutures, or other shaping to recreate the helical groove.
  - In ▶ Fig. 7.17b, the use of a nylon suture helps to recreate the helical groove.

Book Flap (▶ Video 7.2)

Step-by-step:

- Identify donor skin on the posterior ear.

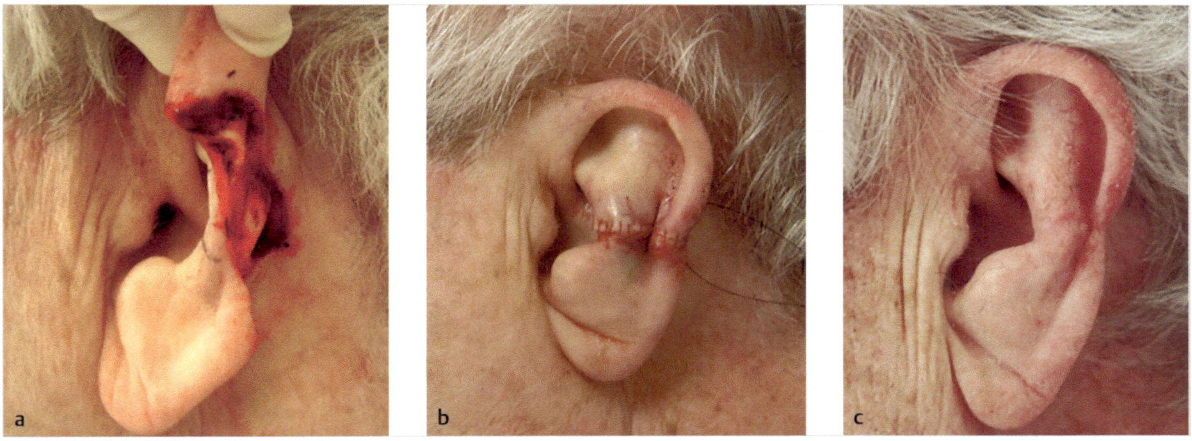

Fig. 7.17 Ear wedge resection. **(a)** Defect after tumor extirpation with Mohs surgery. **(b)** Immediate postoperative picture of wedge closure of the mid helix. Note the nylon suture placement to maintain the helical groove. **(c)** Long-term postoperative picture with preservation of the helical groove and slight auricular rim contraction.

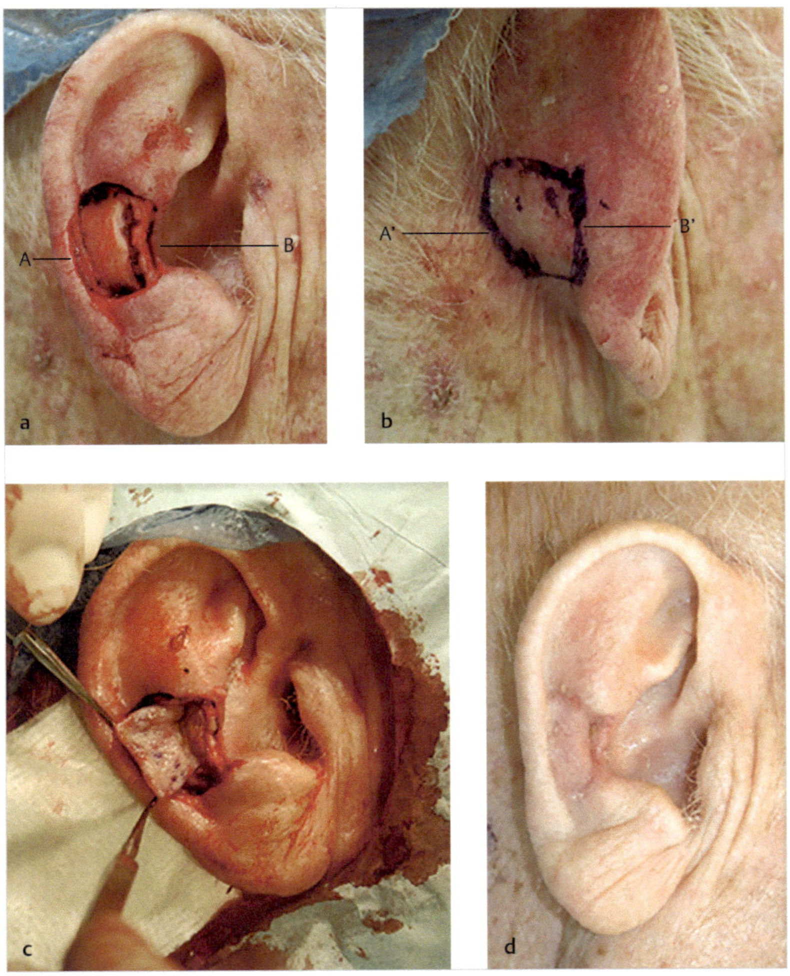

Fig. 7.18 Book flap. **(a)** Posttumor extirpation from Mohs surgery. **(b)** Postauricular donor site. **(c)** Intraoperative movement of the flap prior to suturing. **(d)** Three-month postoperative photo. The wound edge **A** will be sutured to the edge of the flap **A'**; while **B** will be sutured to **B'**.

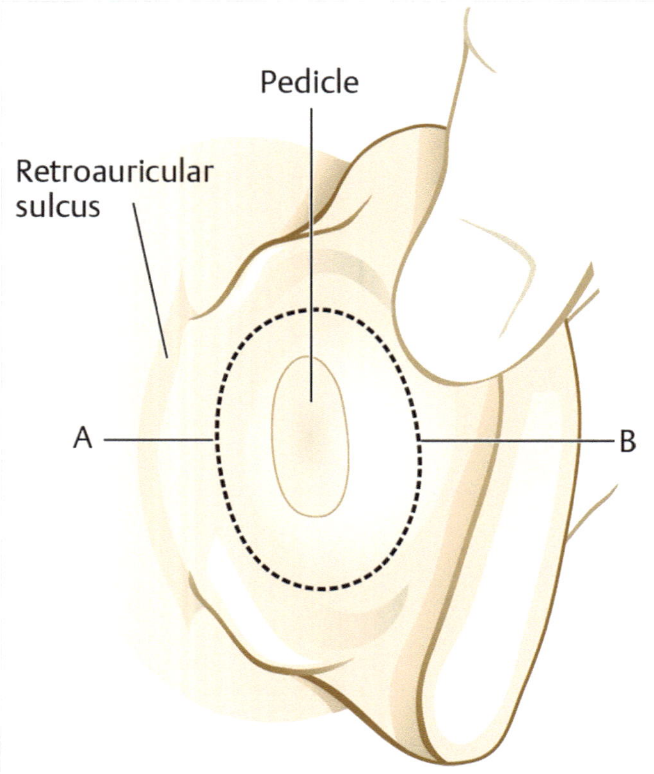

Fig. 7.19 Illustration of the posterior ear revolving door IPF or book page flap design. On the posterior ear illustrated here, the area closest to the sulcus, A, will be turned like the page of a book to be the most lateral edge (or closest to the helical rim) on the anterior ear. The opposite side of the flap, B, will abut the wound edge adjacent to the rim of the conchal bowl.

- Make incision through the posterior ear through which the flap will pass to the anterior surface of the ear.
- Create template with sterile suture pack and place on the donor skin site.
- Incise template on the donor skin on the posterior ear. On the posterior ear, the area closest to the helical rim will be flipped to become the medial (conchal bowl) edge on the anterior surface of the ear, while the flap edge originating from near the postauricular sulcus will be positioned nearest the helical rim anteriorly. See ▸ Fig. 7.18 and ▸ Fig. 7.19; ▸ Video 7.2.
- Develop vascular pedicle from region of the postauricular sulcus.
- First, pass the conchal bowl edge of the flap (lateral aspect on the posterior ear) through the full-thickness incision.
- The helical rim edge of the flap (created from the area closer to the sulcus on the posterior ear) follows. This is then turned like a book page into the anterior wound.
- Suture into place with dermal 5–0 or 6–0 absorbable suture and epidermal 6–0 fast-absorbing gut.
- May allow donor site to heal by second intention or apply graft as needed.

7.3.5 Concha

Repairs of the concha are relatively simple to plan and execute with the majority of defects healing well by second intention (▸ Fig. 7.20). It is best to simplify conchal bowl repairs into two distinct categories: involving the EAC or not. When defects do not involve the EAC and the perichondrium is intact, there is no risk of the EAC stenosis. These defects of the concha can heal well with second intention regardless of their size. One may consider STSGs or FTSGs to speed healing. Other options include placement of skin substitutes or tissue importation flaps. To augment healing, 3- to 4-mm punch fenestrations of the cartilage can be utilized. When the perichondrium is not intact, healing can be delayed. In this circumstance, an STSG and punch fenestrations through large areas of perichondrial loss, placement of skin substitutes, and/or a book page flap can be employed for speedier wound healing.

When the defect involves the EAC, there is risk of EAC stenosis, and caution must be taken to avoid this complication. For cartilaginous defects involving the EAC, it is safe to granulate when defects are < 25% of the EAC circumference. Larger cartilaginous defects involving > 25% of the EAC circumference will require a repair with an FTSG or flap +/− cartilage graft to prevent stenosis. For lesions that are limited to the skin, it is safe to granulate wounds involving up to 50% of the circumference of the EAC without the risk of stenosis. Defects larger than 50% would be best reconstructed by skin grafting and possibly cartilage grafting to prevent stenosis.

Patient discussion regarding the healing options of second intention or placement of a graft is critical. Grafting

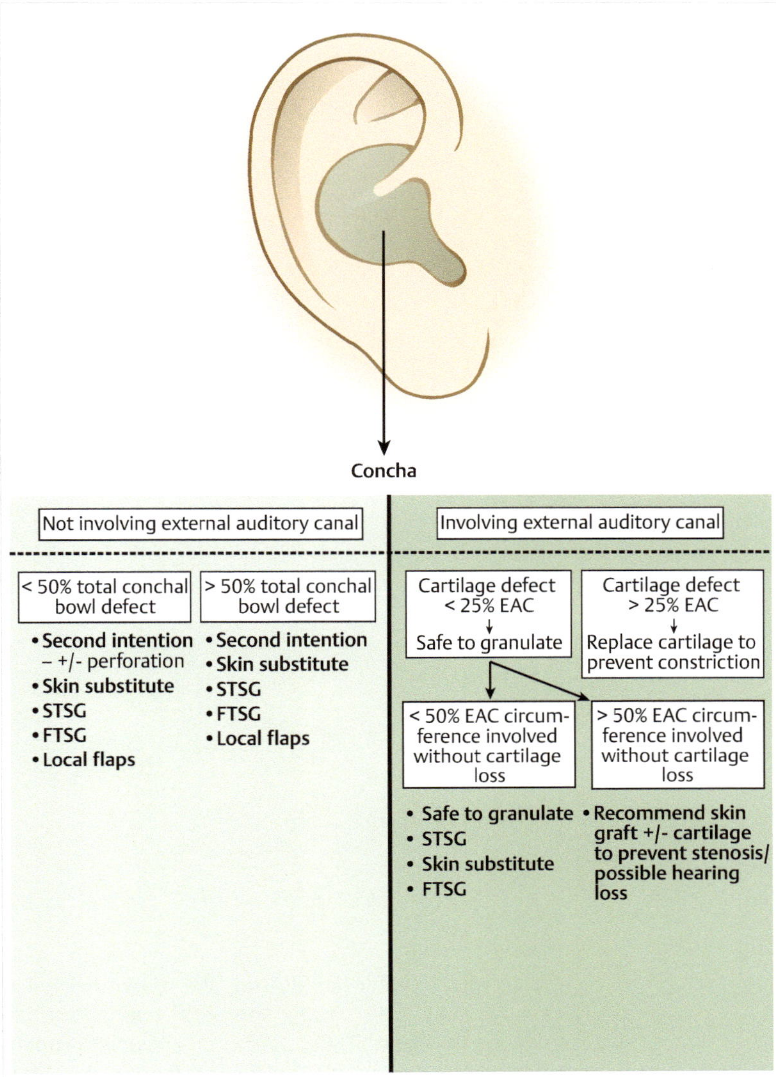

Fig. 7.20 Reconstruction algorithm of the concha.

in the conchal bowl has several considerations. First, grafts are considered for expediting healing and inhibiting scar contraction. Assessing the size of the defect and the vascularity of the bed is important for choosing the most appropriate graft. We use STSGs on the anterior ear, given an excellent cosmetic match and tenuous vascularity of these defects. STSGs are preferred if there is exposed cartilage. FTSGs are also a good option in this area assuming there is an adequate vascular base. Punch fenestrations through the cartilage may be utilized to provide vascular base from the opposing perichondrium. In addition, thinning the FTSG may be beneficial, especially near the EAC. If there is a wound base with a large proportion of exposed cartilage, one may consider placement of a skin substitute to expedite healing or to build more of a vascular base for a delayed graft.

Concha

I. Involving EAC.
   1. Cartilage defect.
      a) < 25% of EAC circumference → safe to granulate.
      b) > 25% of the EAC.
         - STSG.
         - FTSG.
         - Tissue importation flaps.
   2. No cartilaginous defect.
      a) < 50% EAC circumference involved without cartilaginous defect.
         - Safe to granulate without worry of stenosis.
         - STSG.
         - FTSG.
         - Skin substitutes.
      b) > 50% EAC circumference involved—recommend skin grafting to prevent stenosis and possibly conductive hearing loss.

II. Not involving EAC.
   1. ≤ 50% of total conchal bowl defect.

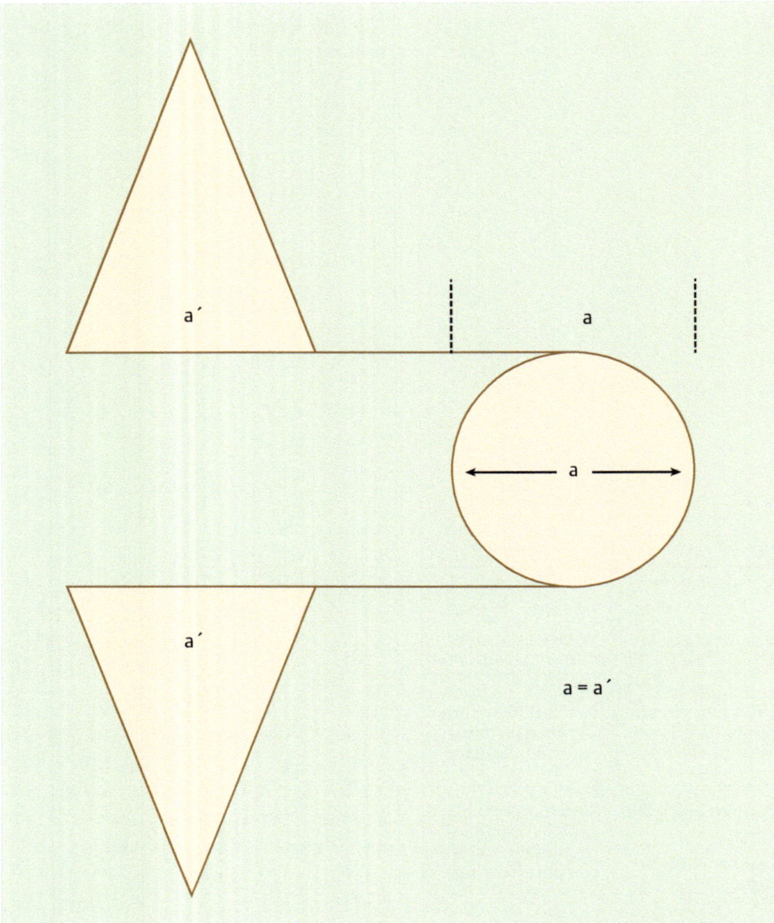

Fig. 7.21 Illustration of the tragal advancement flap. A similar flap can be used on the posterior ear recruiting tissue from the postauricular crease.

a) Second intention.
b) STSG.
c) FTSG.
d) Local flaps.
- Transposition from preauricular/tragal area.

2. > 50% of total conchal bowl defects.
a) Second intention.
b) STSG.
c) FTSG.
d) Tissue importation flaps such as postauricular island pedicle flap or book page island pedicle flap as discussed in the antihelix section.

7.3.6 Tragus

While the tragus is a relatively minor component of the ear, its absence can be quite noticeable. The primary goal of reconstruction of the tragus is to maintain projection that is symmetrical from the anterior perspective. Tragal reconstruction depends on whether or not there is compromise to the tragal cartilage. If the defect is relatively small with preservation of the cartilage, a simple primary closure can be utilized. Larger defects can be repaired with an advancement flap utilizing the preauricular skin (see ▶ Fig. 7.21, ▶ Fig. 7.22). Additional options include transposition flaps, FTSGs, STSGs, or a partial primary closure of the preauricular sulcus using a Burow's FTSG for the tragus.

When there is substantial cartilaginous loss of the tragal eminence and optimal aesthetic closure is desired, recreating this prominence is the key for a successful reconstruction. Transposition flaps are one way of repairing this defect without the use of a cartilage graft. Superiorly based transposition flaps can recreate the prominence by intentionally designing tissue redundancy and anticipating dependent edema due to the "trapdoor defect" phenomenon. This flap can be intentionally developed with excess soft tissue located within the flap covering the tragal site. A cartilage graft may be used at the time of repair or can be delayed. Lastly, a soft tissue or adipose graft can be utilized to recreate this tragal eminence.

1. Small defects with preservation of cartilage → consider primary closure.
2. Larger defects with preservation of cartilage.
a) Advancements flap (▶ Fig. 7.21, ▶ Fig. 7.22).
b) Transposition flap.

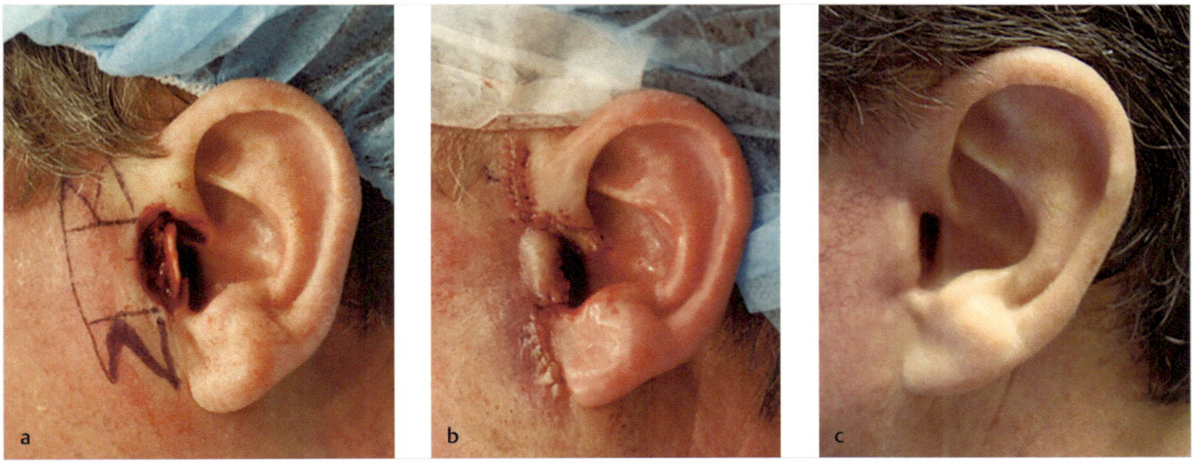

Fig. 7.22 Tragal advancement flap. **(a)** Tragal defect with flap outline. **(b)** Immediate postop picture of flap with the crus of the helix repaired via Burow's graft from the preauricular area. **(c)** Three-month postop picture.

   c) FTSG.
   d) STSG.
3. Loss of tragal eminence (determine if aesthetically important to the patient).
   a) Consider closure without specific reconstruction of the eminence.
   b) Superiorly based transposition flap.
   c) Intentionally thicker flap.
   d) Cartilage graft.
   e) Delayed cartilage graft.

Reconstructive Steps for Repairs of the Tragus

Tragal Advancement Flap (▶ Fig. 7.22)

Step-by-step:

- Identify length of skin needed to wrap around posterior to the anterior tragus.
- Mark this length as the width of the flap in the preauricular area.
  - May also design the base of the Burow's triangle to be equal to the horizontal width of the defect. See ▶ Fig. 7.21.
- Mark the inferior and superior Burow's triangles. Save the skin for possible graft if needed.
- Incise the flap and undermine in the superficial fat.
- Close secondary defects first with 5–0 absorbable suture.
- Thin the flap as needed.
- Then suture the flap into place (5–0 absorbable suture), adequately enveloping the tragal cartilage followed by 6–0 or 5–0 fast-absorbing gut.

7.3.7 Remainder of the Posterior Ear

The majority of the defects on the posterior helix can be managed by second intention healing. Defects impinging on the helical rim or those bridging across the sulcus will require other considerations to avoid distortion of the helical rim or pinning back of the ear, respectively. Grafting may be the best repair option, when necessary. Fortunately, the posterior ear has more laxity than other subunits, and for this reason smaller defects may be closed primarily. Partial closures or purse-string closures are other considerations to help reduce the size of defect and expedite the healing process. Assuming there is an adequate vascular base, an FTSG is another option. If there is exposed cartilage on the posterior surface, often an STSG would be a superior option. A flap may also be considered when there is a poor vascular bed for grafting. Often a transposition or a rotation flap may be well utilized in this location. Superior defects are best repaired with the postauricular donor pool, and inferior defects can often utilize the laxity of skin on the posterior ear itself or the retroauricular sulcus. Cartilage grafts are rarely needed in this location, but should be considered if there is compromise to the helical rim.

Remainder of posterior ear (including through-and-through defects)

1. Second intention.
2. FTSG.
3. STSG.
4. Skin substitutes.
5. Replace cartilage if structurally necessary.
6. May consider transposition flaps.

7.4 Complications and Revisions

Complications of the ear are not uncommon and can be classified as during (intraoperative), immediate (first 2 wk postop), midterm (2 wk–2 mo postop), and long-term (greater than 2 mo postop). Immediate postoperative complications are mostly related to bleeding or infection. Uncontrollable bleeding is rarely a problem, given the ability to directly apply pressure and cauterize vessels. After the epinephrine from the local anesthesia wears off, patients may experience some minor bleeding from the surgical site that can be controlled with pressure in the majority of cases. Antia-Buch helical rim advancement flaps and retroauricular interpolation flaps are at the highest risk of bleeding, especially in patients on anticoagulants. Uncontrolled bleeding may lead to wound dehiscence, infection, and eventual failure of the closure (primary, graft, or flap). In addition to intraoperative meticulous hemostasis, we recommend limited activity for the first 48 hours and a pressure dressing for the first 24 to 48 hours.

Infections are another immediate complication most commonly noted about one week postoperatively. Given the unique flora on the ear, especially near the EAC, it is important to culture wound infections and have a high suspicion for gram-negative infections. Appropriate antibiotics should be prescribed depending on the culture. Some surgeons use dilute white vinegar soaks and topical gentamicin ointment as part of wound care for the ear.

As with any reconstruction within the first 2 weeks of surgery, it is also possible to see infections, skin necrosis, failed grafts/flaps, and rarely maggot infestation of wounds healing by second intention. However, there are several complications that are unique to the ear. For example, retainment of foreign bodies in the EAC can not only lead to significant pain and discomfort, but may also cause pressure on the tympanic membrane and possible temporary conductive hearing loss. Prior to bandaging, assess the EAC for retained gauze, bleeding that may lead to thrombotic impactions, and other foreign objects. Sterile chondritis is another unique complication of auricular reconstruction. It is most likely to occur in the setting of second intention healing with exposed cartilage. We recommend petrolatum jelly or other occlusive ointments to the wound and coverage with a nonstick gauze to prevent desiccation of the cartilage. Nonsteroidal anti-inflammatory drugs may be taken on schedule to alleviate pain and reduce the inflammation of the cartilage. A wound culture should generally be obtained in the setting of chondritis. It is imperative to rule out infectious chondritis as the two can be clinically indistinguishable. For patients that are strictly one-sided sleepers, sleeping on the affected side can compromise the reconstruction or be painful. We encourage alternate sleeping positions or a donut pillow to avoid direct pressure to the site.

Midterm and long-term complications of the ear occur between 2 to 8 weeks and 2 months after surgery, respectively. There is often overlap with the timing of these potential complications. One example of a mid- to long-term complication is the formation of a keloid. This can begin to occur as soon as 6 weeks postoperatively. It is important to obtain a history of keloids from the patient and treat early and aggressively if there is any sign of keloid formation. Other long-term complications should be considered when choosing the appropriate repair. Long-term complications include contractures and distortion of the helical rim, cupping of the ear, and EAC stenosis. With the chronic use of protective equipment masks that tightly fit around the ears having become commonplace, the Editor (SNT) recommends patients to avoid wearing masks that tie around the ear. Instead, he recommends the use of masks that tie over the head and neck, removing tension that would chronically pull down on ears after reconstructive surgery. In patients who have had superior helical rim or helical crus reconstruction, especially with limited structural support, this tension can lead to contracture and even helical rim collapse. These complications can be revised; however, an effort to avoid them proactively is the best strategy whenever possible through careful planning of the reconstruction and follow up in the early postoperative period.

References

[1] Zilinsky I, Cotofana S, Hammer N, et al. The arterial blood supply of the helical rim and the earlobe-based advancement flap (ELBAF): a new strategy for reconstructions of helical rim defects. J Plast Reconstr Aesthet Surg. 2015; 68(1):56–62

[2] Ellabban MG, Maamoun MI, Elsharkawi M. The bi-pedicle post-auricular tube flap for reconstruction of partial ear defects. Br J Plast Surg. 2003; 56(6):593–598

[3] Fernández-Palacios J, de Armas Díaz F, Alvarado Benítez R, Rodríguez Aguirre M. [Helix reconstruction by tubular flap]. Acta Otorrinolaringol Esp. 1997; 48(1):81–84

[4] Dujon DG, Bowditch M. The thin tube pedicle: a valuable technique in auricular reconstruction after trauma. Br J Plast Surg. 1995; 48 (1):35–38

8 Lip (Perioral) Reconstruction

Nicola A. Quatrano and Thomas E. Rohrer

Abstract

This chapter presents an algorithmic approach to reconstructive options for repairing perioral defects after Mohs micrographic surgery with a focus on cosmetic subunits. These algorithms represent common reconstructive techniques and their variations utilized within each subunit in the perioral region serving as general principles. Perioral anatomy, key principles, practical pearls, and common pitfalls are reviewed to offer a solid foundation for successful perioral reconstruction.

Capsule Summary and Pearls

- Know the perioral anatomy including cosmetic subunits, neurovascular supply, musculature, and tissue reservoirs.
- Restoration of the oral sphincter is prioritized, followed by preservation of motor and sensory innervation and optimizing cosmesis.
- Mark cosmetic subunits, vermilion border, and favorable lines of closure with ink prior to local anesthesia.
- Respect the various cosmetic subunits when designing closures.
- Maintain the position and alignment of the vermilion-cutaneous junction (VCJ) and the philtrum at the midline.
- Place closures along relaxed skin tension lines and at the junction of cosmetic subunits.
- Do not distort the free margin.
- The vermilion is not an inviolable structure.
- Recruit tissue from lateral reservoirs on the lip or adjacent cheek.
- Consider extending surgical defects to subunit boundaries or removing an entire subunit in order to better conceal the incision lines of the repair.
- Repair defects within a single subunit when possible.
- Divide defects that bridge the VCJ into vermilion and cutaneous defects and repair each individually.
- Avoid pincushioning by appropriately sizing and adequate thinning of flaps and undermining the surrounding tissue.
- Achieve thorough hemostasis of the lip prior to closure.
- Recreate the alar crease at the isthmus and the melolabial fold with a periosteal stitch.
- Close vermilion–vermilion and vermilion–cutaneous wound edges with braided interrupted sutures.
- Close full-thickness defects in four layers, starting with reapproximation of the orbicularis oris sphincter.
- Always consider individual factors in selecting the best method of repair.
- Limit mobility of the perioral region postoperatively to avoid complications and maximize cosmetic results.

8.1 Introduction

The upper and lower lips are the predominant feature of the lower face and carry considerable aesthetic significance. Beyond this, the lips have important motor and sensory functions including facial expression, oral competence and articulation of speech, as well as the protective perception of touch, pain, and temperature. The variations in texture, color, and contour between its numerous cosmetic subunits add to the complexity of the perioral region. Given these significant functional and aesthetic considerations, perioral surgical defects present reconstructive challenges from which innovation has led to a multitude of repair options. The goal in all lip reconstructions is to preserve or restore the function and aesthetics of this unique structure. Key principles for successful perioral reconstruction are detailed in Capsule Summary and Pearls at the beginning of this chapter.

8.2 Cosmetic Subunits and Relevant Anatomy

The perioral region is comprised of five distinct cosmetic subunits: two cutaneous lateral upper lip subunits, the philtrum, the cutaneous lower lip and chin, and the vermilion lip (▶ Fig. 8.1). Together, the philtrum and two lateral subunits form the cutaneous upper lip. The nasal base, defined by alar creases, the alar sill, and the columella border the upper lip superiorly. The melolabial fold and the labiomandibular crease (marionette lines) serve as the lateral boundaries of the upper and lower lips, respectively. Although considered a single subunit, the lower lip and chin can be divided at the labiomental crease, which serves as the inferior limit to the lower cutaneous lip. A small triangle of skin, the isthmus or the hairless triangle, exists in the superolateral corners of both cutaneous lateral upper lip subunits adjacent to the

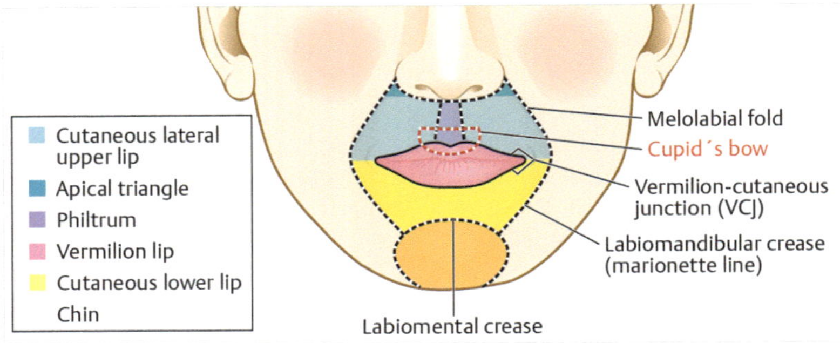

Fig. 8.1 Perioral cosmetic subunits and junctions.

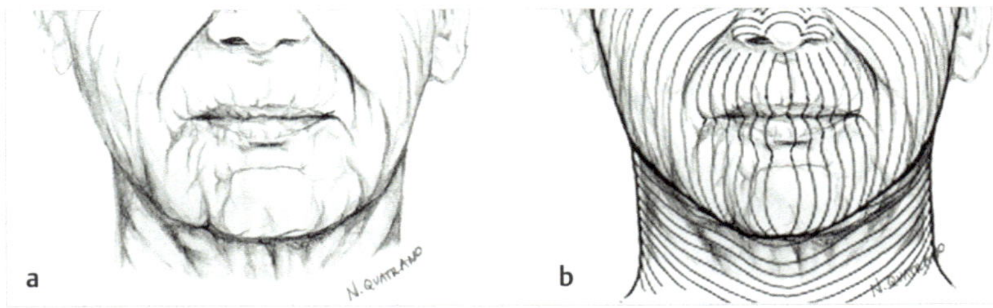

Fig. 8.2 Perioral relaxed skin tension lines **(a)** and overlying Langer's lines **(b)**.

nasal ala. These apical triangles warrant special consideration during reconstruction, as their preservation is essential to optimize cosmetic outcomes. Of similar aesthetic importance, the philtrum is a concave subunit bounded by parallel convex philtral columns in the medial upper lip and is defined inferiorly by the Cupid's bow of the vermilion lip.

The transition from cutaneous upper and lower lips to vermilion takes place at the vermilion-cutaneous junction (VCJ). A well-defined line, referred to as the mucocutaneous or anterior vermilion line, and its rolled border represent an important landmark in lip reconstruction. The combination of thin, nonkeratinizing epithelium and abundant underlying vasculature gives the vermilion a characteristic pink hue. The modified mucosa of the vermilion covers the free margin of the lip and is adapted for external exposure, with relatively few salivary glands compared to the multitude found deep to the labial and buccal mucosa.[1] Its surface is divided into internal (wet) and external (dry) components and the innermost point of contact between the upper and lower lips is defined as the posterior vermilion line.

From superficial to deep, lip tissue is comprised of skin, muscle, and mucosa. The body of the lip is predominantly formed by the orbicularis oris muscle, which is concentrically oriented and inserts directly into the skin's undersurface. The relaxed skin tension lines (RSTLs) of the upper and lower lips are oriented in a radial fashion about the oral stoma coursing perpendicularly to the underlying orbicularis muscle. These radial lines are accentuated with pursing and are ultimately paralleled by the wrinkle lines of older patients and enhanced by chronic sun damage and smoking (▶ Fig. 8.2). The radial RSTLs, the melolabial fold, and the labiomental crease are favorable sites to conceal incisions in lip reconstruction.

In bilaterally paired sets, the muscles of facial expression attach radially along the outer margin of the orbicularis oris, marked by the melolabial fold and labiomental creases. Motor innervation to these lip elevators and depressors originates primarily from the buccal and marginal mandibular branches of the facial nerve, respectively. Although rarely damaged due to their location beneath the musculature, injury to the marginal mandibular nerve anterior to the angle of the jaw during undermining as the nerve becomes more superficial over the bony prominence can lead to significant functional and cosmetic deformity due to the inability to laterally depress the lower lip.[2] This inability is most notable when smiling due to the resulting asymmetry but can also effect speech.

Many of these muscle fibers converge at the modiolus just lateral to the commissure and, as a group, provide the orbicularis oris with an indirect connection to the facial skeleton. This lack of direct connection allows for the advantage of lip tissue to be significantly stretched during reconstructive surgery.[1] Even with larger defects slightly more than half of either lip, reconstruction can be accomplished in most cases without causing excessive microstomia. When the orbicularis oris muscle is compromised, priority is placed on restoration of the muscle sphincter. The orbicularis oris muscle sphincter of the lower lip is crucial given its greater role in the retention of intraoral contents.[3]

Sensory innervation of the upper lip originates from branches of the infraorbital nerve, while branches of the mental nerve provide that of the lower lip. Both infraorbital and mental nerves arise from foramens along the midpupillary lines in the maxilla and mandible, respectively, and can be reached percutaneously or via an intraoral route for regional blocks if needed (▶ Fig. 8.3).

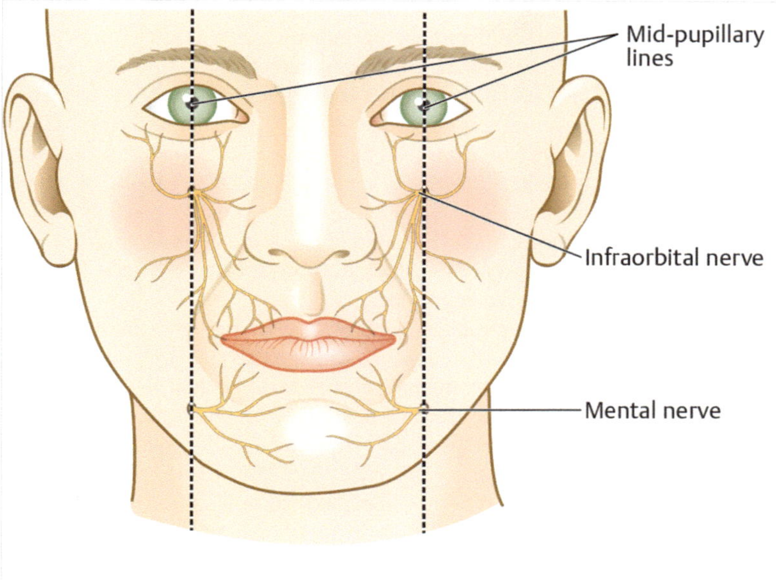

Fig. 8.3 Sensory innervation to the upper and lower lips.

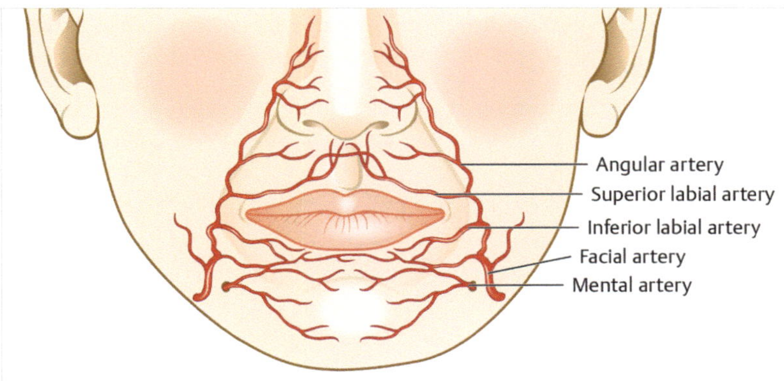

Fig. 8.4 Arterial anatomy of the upper and lower lips.

Superior and inferior labial arteries provide the principal vascular supply to the lips. Both arteries originate from the facial artery along its course beneath the orbicularis oris muscle about 10 to 12 mm from the oral commissure.[4] Often with a tortuous course, the labial arteries run horizontally in the submucosal plane, just beneath the orbicularis and at approximately the level of the anterior vermilion line. While the superior labial artery gives off septal and alar branches medially, the lower labial artery anastomoses with the mental artery through a variable pattern of labiomental branches often vertically oriented across the lower lip and chin (▶ Fig. 8.4).[5,6,7]

8.3 Reconstructive Algorithm

When planning reconstruction of the perioral region, great effort should be made to maximize cosmesis; however, priority should always be placed on the preservation of function. Careful marking of the vermilion border, aesthetic subunits, and favorable lines of closure, such as the RSTL and subunit junctions, is essential prior to executing any perioral reconstruction and preferably done prior to local anesthetic infiltration. One of the most important considerations in lip reconstruction is preservation of lip position. Pushing or pulling the upper or lower lip out of place, pulling the Cupid's bow off center, or creating any misalignment of the vermilion border can be aesthetically devastating and all efforts must be made to plan reconstructive options that minimize these outcomes. Over time, the high mobility of the perioral region tends to organize tissue in this region back toward baseline positioning and, therefore, even large repairs can result in excellent final outcomes. In addition, it is better to confine reconstructive design to within a single subunit using tissue from within the respective aesthetic region of the lip. With larger defects or those that span multiple subunits, repairs are more likely to involve tissue from the adjacent regions of the cheek or chin.

Certain repairs are more commonly utilized within specific subunits as their closure lines are favorably hidden in the lines of that subunit. The location, size, shape, and depth of the defect will influence the choice of closure within a given subunit. Individual patient characteristics such as skin texture, thickness, and laxity (often influenced heavily by age and sun damage) should also be taken into consideration when choosing the optimal closure. However, an algorithmic approach based on region can be helpful as common patterns of repair within certain aesthetic subunits can serve as a guideline for reconstructive design.[8]

8.3.1 Vermilion

The vermilion lower lip is most commonly plagued with squamous cell carcinomas (SCC), often in the setting of actinic damage and tobacco exposure. While SCC of the vermilion upper lip tend to involve the cutaneous lip, those of the lower vermilion often have little to no cutaneous involvement, unless they are allowed to progress before treatment. For this reason, defects limited to the vermilion lower lip are considered separately (▶ Fig. 8.5), while defects involving the vermilion upper lip are included in the algorithms described below for the cutaneous upper lip.

After tumor extirpation, second intention healing can be considered for partial-thickness defects restricted to the vermilion. Superficial defects limited to the mucosal lip are often best left to heal with granulation alone and even some larger defects with partial resection of the orbicularis can heal by second intention with satisfactory results.[9,10] With an abundant vascular supply, defects of the mucosal lip re-epithelialize rapidly. A visible stellate scar may result from and represent a disadvantage of second intention healing but can be easily revised with minimal recovery (▶ Fig. 8.6).

The remaining vermilion after tumor extirpation often consists of actinically damaged tissue. For defects in this setting, a complete vermilionectomy, followed by repair of the entire vermilion subunit is preferred. The favored method of vermilion restoration is the mucosal advancement flap (▶ Fig. 8.7). With any vermilion repair, the design, wet–dry line, and vermilion border should be marked prior to local anesthesia. When performing the vermilionectomy, the anterior incision lines extend laterally from the defect along the VCJ, while the posterior incision lines extend laterally from the most posterior aspect of the defect to meet the anterior incision lines at the commissures with removal of mucosal Burow's triangles as

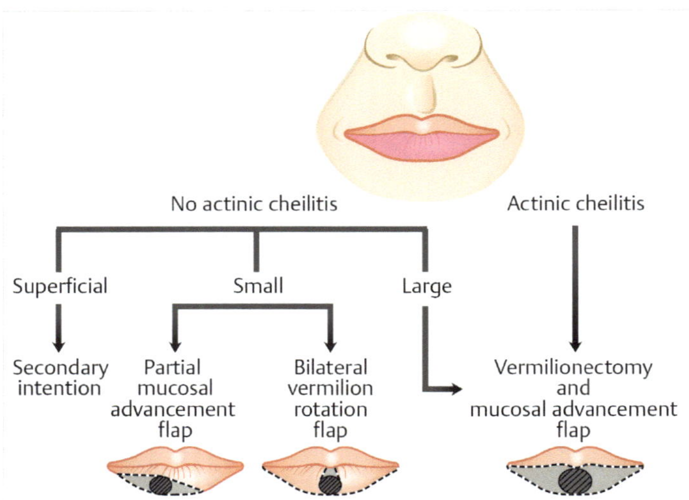

Fig. 8.5 Vermilion lower lip reconstruction algorithm.

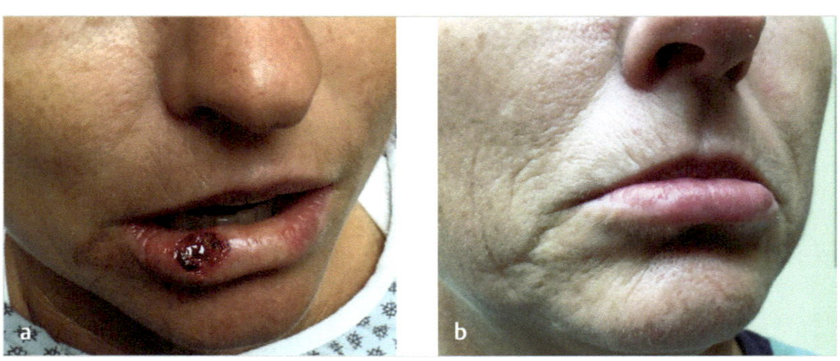

Fig. 8.6 Second intention healing. **(a)** Defect limited to vermilion lower lip. **(b)** Final result with subtle stellate scar. (These images are provided courtesy of Stanislav N. Tolkachjov, MD.)

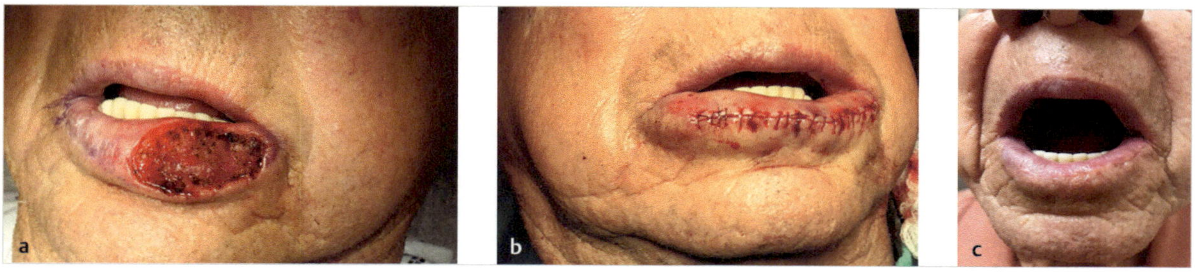

Fig. 8.7 Mucosal advancement flap (complex layered closure). **(a)** Vermilion lower lip defect. Vermilionectomy design marked. **(b)** Mucosal flap advanced and sutured. **(c)** Final result (1-year follow-up). (These images are provided courtesy of Stanislav N. Tolkachjov, MD.)

necessary. The vermilion is then removed with care to minimize trauma to the underlying orbicularis muscle. The mucosal advancement flap utilizes the mucosa lining the inner surface of the lip and is elevated by undermining within the submucosal plane deep to the minor salivary glands and immediately superficial to the orbicularis muscle. To allow sufficient anterior advancement under minimal tension, dissection may need to be extended along the vertical length of the lip to the apex of the gingivolabial sulcus, but this is often not required. The flap is then advanced anteriorly over the free margin of the lip to the anterior vermilion line where a key suture is placed in the middle of the advancing edge. Soft braided absorbable suture, such as polyglactin 910, is used to place interrupted sutures along the remainder of the flap's leading edge and reestablish the VCJ. The editors often use nonabsorbable epidermal sutures only if sufficient undermining has been done to relieve tension. Accurate positioning of the VCJ is of upmost importance for optimal aesthetic outcome and can be challenging especially in the setting of an adjacent cutaneous lip defect. Inherent contraction of the mucosal flap with wound maturation may distort the anterior vermilion line despite best efforts to properly align and require subsequent revision surgery. If needed, additional excision of the normal tissue of adjacent cutaneous lip may allow for proper alignment.

In addition to accurate positioning of the anterior vermilion line, the mucosal advancement flap can present other challenges. Although the vermilion is a modified mucosal surface, the labial mucosa often results in a slightly deeper red vermilion substitute that may be disfavored, especially by male patients. Some degree of touch, pain, and temperature sensation is expected to return to the vermilion over several months following mucosal advancement flap repair; however, in some patients the restoration of sensation is inadequate. Care can be taken to preserve small neurovascular structures encountered during dissection by gentle blunt spreading rather than sharply undermining when possible. This limited undermining of the mucosal lip provides two advantages: limiting sensory disruption and minimizing subsequent flap contraction.

For small defects restricted to the vermilion where there is minimal adjacent actinic cheilitis, a partial mucosal advancement flap and a bilateral vermilion rotation flap are excellent reconstructive options. Both techniques allow preservation of the healthy vermilion and favorable placement of closure lines along the VCJ. A partial mucosal advancement flap may be favored for defects with a long axis aligned with the anterior vermilion border. An ellipse is designed that places the anterior incision along the vermilion border without extending the incisions from commissure to commissure. After removal of the vermilion cones, a partial mucosal advancement flap is elevated and brought anteriorly to meet the VCJ as described earlier.

A bilateral vermilion rotation flap is designed with bilateral incisions off of the anterior aspect of the defect along the VCJ (▶ Fig. 8.8). The flaps are elevated superficial to the orbicularis and a mucosal Burow's triangle is taken posterior to the defect. Incisions along the VCJ may be extended to the commissures to allow adequate rotation under minimal tension but may not be required. Soft, braided absorbable interrupted sutures allow precise VCJ and flap alignment. The main advantage of a bilateral vermilion rotation flap is the tension is largely displaced laterally and therefore does not pull the lower cutaneous lip up superiorly, making the lower lip appear smaller (as can occur with mucosal advancement flaps).

8.3.2 Cutaneous Lateral Upper Lip

The cutaneous lateral upper lip can be further divided into apical and mid-lower regions, which are helpful to consider when debating reconstructive options. Second intention healing on the cutaneous lateral upper lip is limited to superficial defects located in concavities such as that of the isthmus or apical triangle.[11] Granulation of deeper defects often creates a hypertrophic scar. Full-thickness skin grafts (FTSG) are rarely used in this area as they are often complicated by pincushioning, offer a poor color and texture match, and are an unacceptable alternative for the hair-bearing upper lip of men. Primary linear closures are useful for small defects in the mid-lower

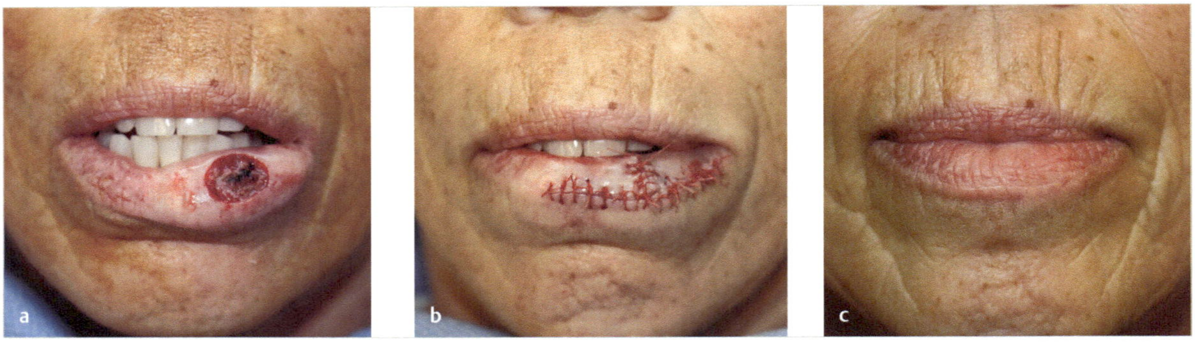

Fig. 8.8 Bilateral vermilion rotation flap. **(a)** Vermilion lower lip defect. **(b)** Bilateral rotation flaps sutured in place. **(c)** Final result.

lateral subunit. For apical or larger defects, a variety of local flaps can be utilized to tap into regional or distant laxity and displace tension, thereby avoiding displacement of the free margin. Local skin redundancy offers excellent texture, thickness, appendage, and color match. Most local flaps in the perioral region are advancement or rotation flaps that slide tissue, almost always, from a laterally based reservoir along natural motion vectors and stay within the cosmetic unit. Depending on the location of the defect, specific flaps are used in particular regions of the cutaneous lateral upper lip to best hide suture lines (▶ Fig. 8.9). Ultimately, individual variation in tissue laxity and size of the cosmetic subunits will heavily influence the reconstructive method chosen.

Small defects, less than 1 cm in diameter, on the lateral subunit can be closed primarily with a linear closure without the concern of free margin distortion.[8,12] A fusiform defect is first created by removing Burow's triangles with the optimum angle of 30 degrees at the apices above and below the primary defect. Closure lines should deliberately be placed along the radial RSTLs or at the junction of cosmetic subunits to both minimize tension on the wound and improve cosmetic results. With a linear closure, the distance between the two ends of the defect will lengthen to match that of the fusiform's arc. The superior portion of the closure should not cross the melolabial fold, and if approaching this boundary, the scar line should be redirected along the alar crease for better camouflage. If the inferior portion of the closure ends near or on the vermilion border, extension of the incision through the upper vermilion to the mucosal portion of the lip is often required to avoid standing cones (▶ Fig. 8.10). This is favored over the use of an M-plasty, which extends outside of the RSTLs and is therefore less well camouflaged and, with all of the very small and acute angles, is more prone for tissue mismatch and minor step-off deformities. Minimal tension on the closure is achieved through undermining laterally above the orbicularis oris. During layered suturing, emphasis is placed on maintaining alignment of the VCJ as even small offsets yield poor aesthetic results. Once again, careful marking of this important landmark prior to local anesthetic infiltration is essential to aid in precise repositioning. Suturing technique to optimize wound eversion is critical on the upper lip, especially on the hair-bearing lip of men where decreased collagen density between hair follicles reduces suture grip and increases the risk of scar inversion.[13]

Apical Triangle

Apical defects are best reconstructed with flaps that hide suture lines within the perialar groove or melolabial fold. Crescentic advancement flaps are ideal for small defects in the apical region that borders the inferior alar crease or lateral nostril sill. With this repair, the inferior Burow's triangle is placed along the RSTLs of the upper lip, identical to that in primary closure; however, the superior Burow's triangle is displaced along the alar crease in a crescentic fashion to facilitate medial advancement of tissue (▶ Fig. 8.11). After excision of both triangles, the flap is undermined laterally in the subcutaneous tissue and advanced medially to bring together the inferior aspect of the crescent and the superior aspect of the defect with a key suture. For larger defects that have more tension on the closure, deep tacking sutures from the flap to periosteum below the ala help advance the flap medially without pulling the ala laterally. The crescent may be excised after advancement and closure of the lip in order to minimize the excised tissue.[14] Strategic placement of incision lines within the RSTLs and the alar groove consistently results in well-concealed scars and excellent cosmetic outcomes.

Rotation flaps offer an excellent reconstructive option for similarly sized defects of the apical region that border the melolabial fold (▶ Fig. 8.12). Once again, the inferior Burow's triangle is designed along the RSTLs of the upper lip. The arc of the rotation flap is designed from the superior aspect of the defect and extends inferolaterally along the melolabial fold. The incision should be designed outside of the fold and then follow its curvature in order to maintain both lip height and proper position of the melolabial fold upon medial rotation and closure. Undermining

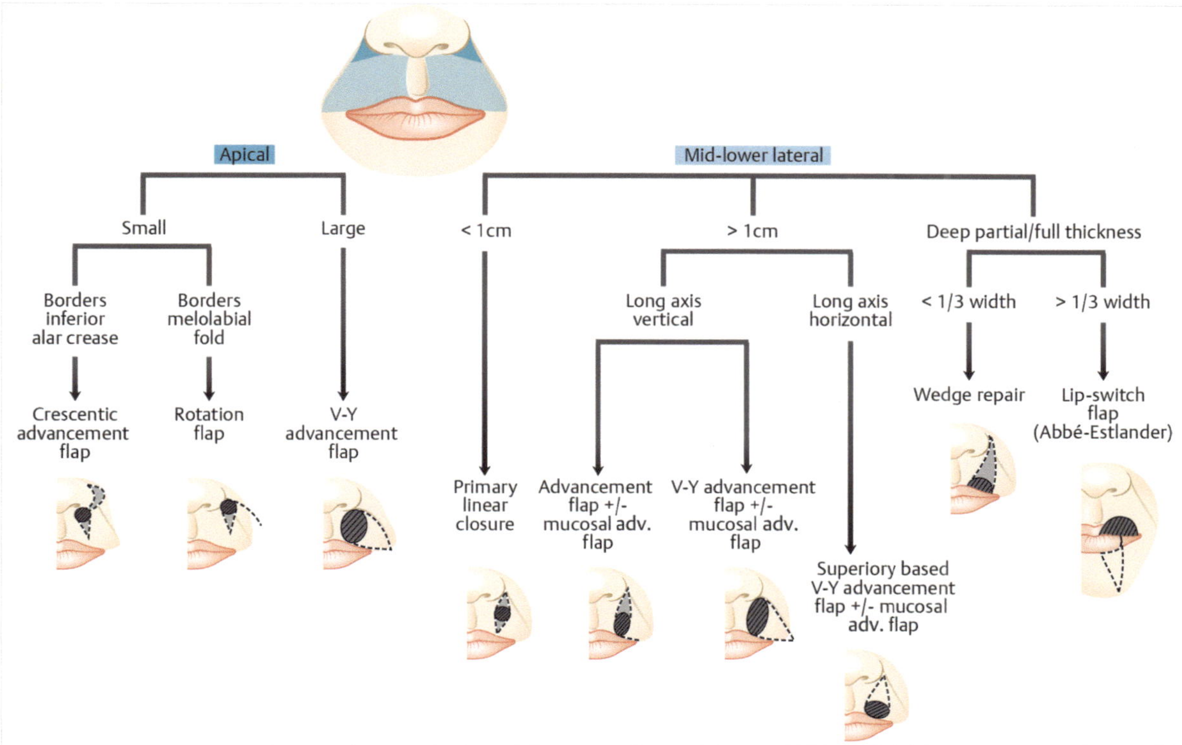

Fig. 8.9 Cutaneous lateral upper lip reconstruction algorithm. adv., advancement.

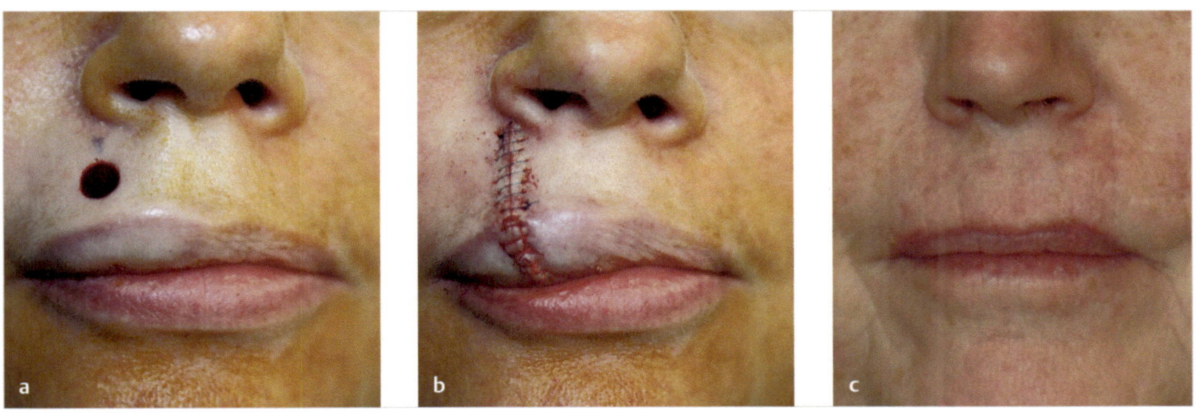

Fig. 8.10 Primary linear closure. **(a)** Cutaneous upper lip defect. **(b)** Linear repair with suture line extended into the apical triangle and mucosal vermilion. **(c)** Final result.

takes place laterally in the subcutaneous–orbicularis oris junction of the lip and the flap is both rotated and advanced medially to close the defect. The repair is confined within the cutaneous lateral upper lip subunit and suture lines are well camouflaged within the melolabial fold offering excellent cosmetic outcomes. A variation on this repair displaces the inferior Burow's triangle along the lateral alar crease extending to the alar sill, offering superior camouflaging of incision lines along subunit junctions.

Both the crescentic advancement and rotation flaps can be utilized for larger defects of the apical region by extending the inferior Burow's triangle through the VCJ and onto the vermilion as described for primary linear closure earlier. However, for larger defects of the apical region, specifically those that abut the nasal ala and the melolabial fold, V-Y advancement flaps, traditionally referred to as island pedicle flaps (IPF), may be better a reconstructive option.[15] Unlike other advancement flaps

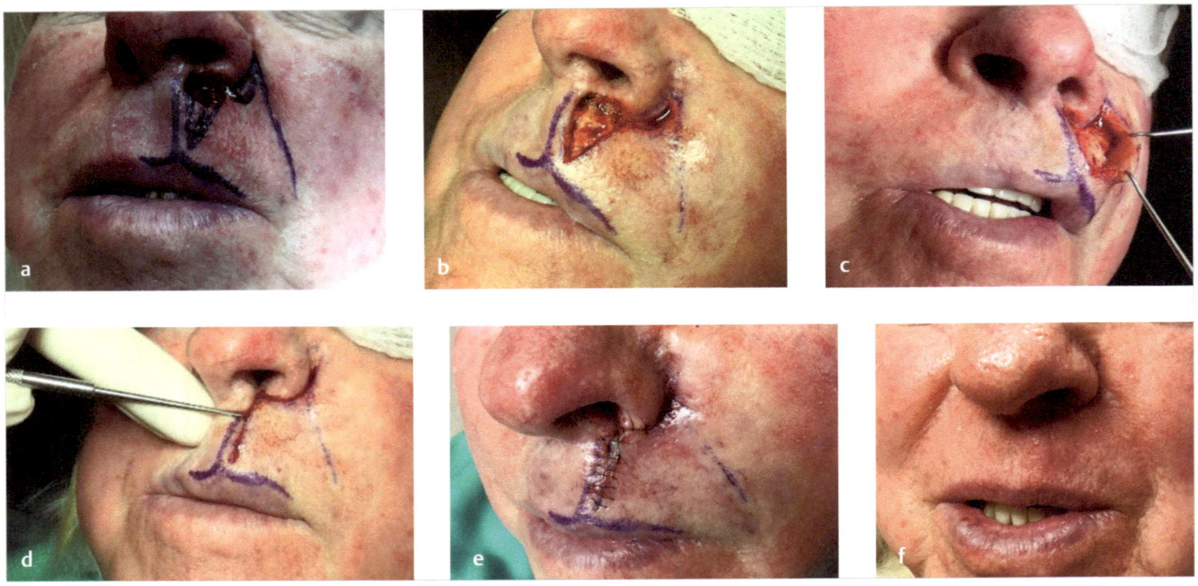

Fig. 8.11 Crescentic advancement flap. (a) Apical region defect bordering the lateral nostril sill. Subunit boundaries and flap design marked. (b) Crescentic and inferior Burow's triangles removed. (c) Flap undermined in the subcutaneous tissue. (d) Flap advanced medially. (e) Flap sutured. (f) Final result (4-week follow-up). (These images are provided courtesy of Stanislav N. Tolkachjov, MD.)

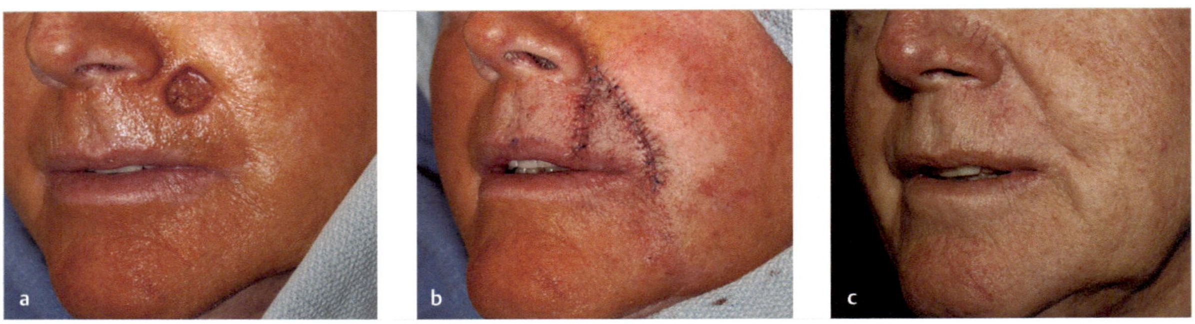

Fig. 8.12 Rotation flap. (a) Apical region defect bordering the melolabial fold. (b) Flap sutured. (c) Final result.

that are pulled into place, the V-Y flap is mobilized as a subcutaneous island that is pushed toward the primary defect through closure of the secondary defect. The V-Y flap is designed with its leading edge along the inferolateral aspect of the defect and its axis parallel to the melolabial fold. The two limbs of the triangular incision should be placed along boundary lines whenever possible. The superior lateral limb of the V-Y flap is placed along the melolabial fold to preserve this boundary and for optimal camouflage. The incision should be carried outside of the fold and then mimic its curvature in order to both maintain lip height and properly position the melolabial fold upon closure. Depending on the proximity of the defect's inferior margin to the vermilion, the inferior limb can be well camouflaged along the VCJ (▶ Fig. 8.13). Expanding the defect superiorly to the alar base or inferiorly to the vermilion through removal of intervening skin may be necessary to facilitate this placement and avoid transection of the RSTLs by the inferior scar line. The width of the flap should match the widest diameter of the defect and its length should be at least twice that diameter along the axis of the flap.[16] Gradual tapering of the limbs to meet at an angle no more than 30 degrees minimizes any upward or lateral tension on the oral commissure upon closure.

Perforators from the facial artery as it follows along the melolabial fold prior to becoming the angular artery offer an abundant vascular supply to the V-Y flap in this region. The flap is incised and undermining of the surrounding skin just above the orbicularis muscle allows for optimal wound eversion and limits potential for a trapdoor effect.[8] Because of the robust vascularity of the perioral tissue, the superior and inferior edges of the pedicle can be thinned to both match the depth of the defect and

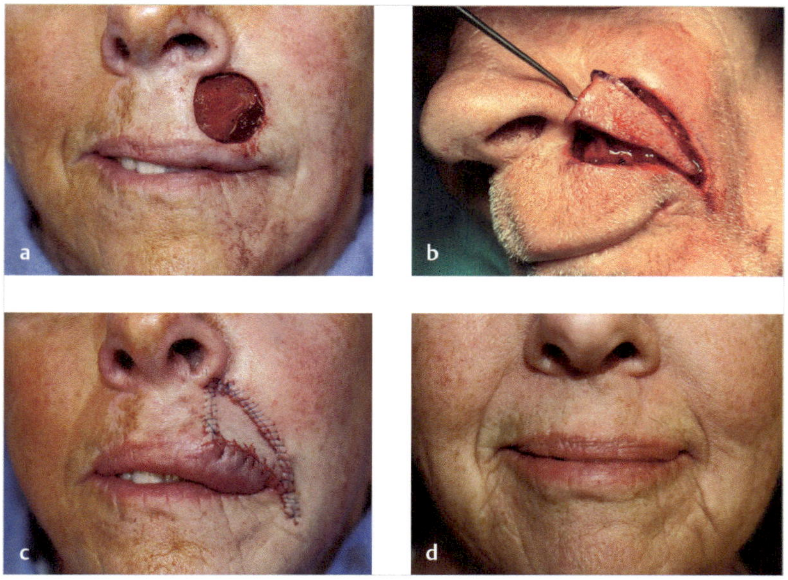

Fig. 8.13 V-Y advancement flap. **(a)** Cutaneous upper lip defect bordering both nasal ala and vermilion border. Intervening skin between the defect and vermilion-cutaneous junction (VCJ) may be excised if necessary to allow flap design with incisions along cosmetic subunit borders. **(b)** Incised and undermined pedicle flap demonstrating movement parallel to the melolabial fold for a similar type defect. (This image is provided courtesy of Stanislav N. Tolkachjov, MD.) **(c)** Flap sutured in place. **(d)** Final result with incision lines wellhidden along the melolabial fold and VCJ.

maximize mobility, without compromising the flap. The centrally located blood supply makes the V-Y flap more resistant to ischemia compared to other random-pattern flaps. A skin hook is used to carefully elevate the flap to assess mobility and ensure a tension-free reach. The advancing edge of the flap and/or the defect is rounded or squared off to create the best fit and minimize pincushioning. After meticulous hemostasis, the flap's leading edge is first sutured to the superomedial margin of the defect with a single 6–0 polypropylene suture to ensure flap position. The dermal edges of the primary and secondary defects are then approximated with 5–0 polyglactin 910 suture. This dermal suturing pushes the flap tissue into the defect, equally distributing the tension along both limbs of the flap, supporting the weight of the flap, and minimizing upward or lateral tension on the oral commissure. The epidermis is closed with 6–0 polypropylene suture to perfect epidermal approximation. Absorbable, braided sutures such as polyglactin 910 are used to place epidermal sutures at the VCJ if applicable.

The excellent tissue match, inconspicuous placement of incisional scars, and abundant vascular supply make the V-Y advancement flap a reliable repair in both viability and aesthetic results. When not placed along the VCJ, the visibility of the scar from the inferior limb represents a potential disadvantage of the V-Y flap, as does the potential for a trapdoor effect. However, this can be minimizing with adequate undermining and debulking of the flap. Mild pincushioning can be treated postoperatively with intralesional steroid and 5-fluorouracil injections.

Mid-Lower Lateral Subunit

Defects adjacent to the vermilion border and larger defects greater than 1 cm of the mid to lower lateral subunit are best reconstructed with flaps that hide suture lines within the RSTLs, vermilion border, and the melolabial fold. A variety of advancement flaps can be utilized to tap into tissue laxity of the lateral lip, melolabial fold, and cheek. Depending on the defect size and proximity to the vermilion border or alar crease, the defect may be expanded to these boundaries to improve flap movement and scar camouflage.

Similar to primary closure, advancement flaps involve tissue movement horizontally but almost exclusively use lateral laxity as to minimize distortion of the philtral columns (▶ Fig. 8.14). After careful marking of the vermilion border prior to anesthetic, the advancement flap is designed with an inferior horizontal incision extending laterally from the defect's inferior edge along the vermilion border with approximately a 3:1 length-to-width ratio. The flap is then undermined just above the orbicularis on the cutaneous lip and within the subcutaneous plane on the cheek to provide adequate flap mobility and allow closure under minimal tension as to avoid distortion of the philtrum. The superior Burow's triangle is placed parallel to the radial RSTLs of the upper lip and can be taken prior to or after flap advancement to better exact the amount of redundant tissue. The variations of advancement flap include those with excision of both superior and inferior Burow's triangles, which can be excised in a variety of positions and those which avoid excision of the inferior, or secondary, triangle through suturing out the tissue redundancy.[17] Placement of the secondary Burow's triangle can strategically be placed along the lower lip's VCJ, marionette line, or taken in crescentic fashion along the horizontal incision (▶ Fig. 8.15).

The flap is advanced medially and a key suture is place at the inferior aspect of the defect and leading edge of the flap just above the vermilion, taking care to properly align

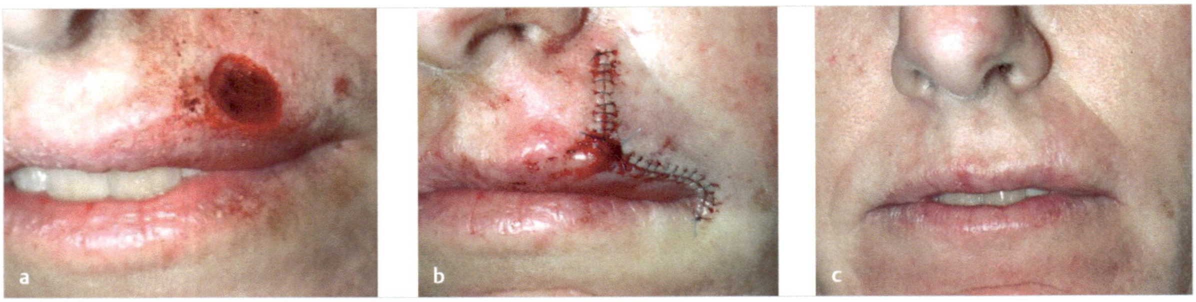

Fig. 8.14 Advancement flap. **(a)** Cutaneous upper lip defect bordering the vermilion-cutaneous junction (VCJ). **(b)** Advancement flap sutured in place with superior Burow's triangle incision along the radial relaxed skin tension lines (RSTLs) and inferior Burow's triangle incision along the lower lip VCJ. **(c)** Final result with incision lines well hidden in the RSTLs and cosmetic subunit borders.

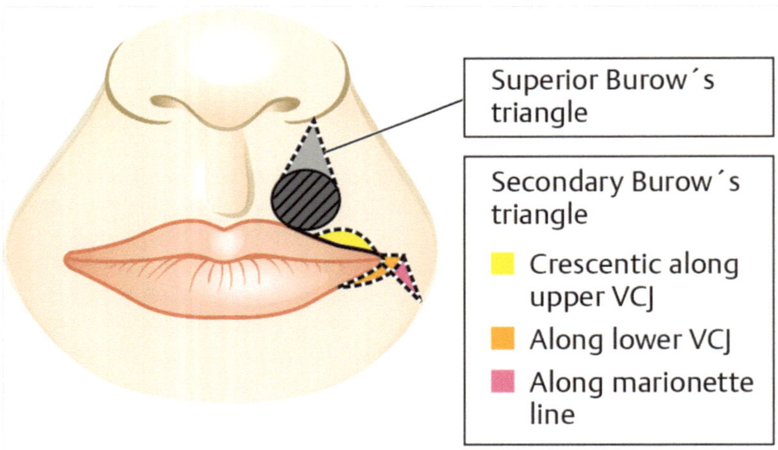

Fig. 8.15 Traditional advancement flap on the cutaneous upper lip with variable placement of the inferior, or secondary, Burow's triangle.

the VCJ. Dermal sutures are placed with 5–0 polyglactin 910 to bring together the subcutaneous tissues of the vertical wound edges followed by an epidermal running suture with 6–0 polypropylene. At the VCJ, 5–0 polyglactin 910 is used to place interrupted epidermal sutures using the rule of halves to evenly distribute any redundancy.

Larger defects that require significant medial advancement may require extension of the horizontal incision laterally beyond the vermilion and inferior to the commissure following the melolabial fold for adequate movement while the superior Burow's triangle can be carried into the perialar crease in a crescentic fashion. This allows even greater flap mobility and camouflaging of scars (▶ Fig. 8.16; ▶ Video 8.1).

Because laterally based flaps are slightly wedgeshaped, there is a tendency for the vermilion border to be pushed down with medial advancement along the vermilion border. This becomes most important with larger advancement flaps and may require trimming of their inferior edge to avoid distortion of the vermilion border. Blunting of the melolabial fold may occur when cheek skin is advanced into the upper lip. This can be limited by placement of a periosteal suture that tacks the undersurface of the flap to the underlying periosteum of the pyriform aperture of the maxilla to reestablish the melolabial fold at its original position.[18,19] In the editors' experience, the melolabial fold does have an inherent tendency to reestablish over time; however, this is not universal.

Defects of the cutaneous lateral upper lip can often involve the adjacent vermilion and provide a reconstructive challenge. In these cases, adjunct flaps are best used to repair each cosmetic subunit and properly reposition the VCJ. An advancement flap or a V-Y advancement flap in combination with a partial mucosal advancement flap is an ideal reconstructive option to repair both cutaneous and vermilion defects, respectively. This method of closure ensures optimal tissue match for the respective subunits as well as precise recreation of the VCJ in its proper location. The advancement flap is designed in typical fashion as described earlier. After the cutaneous defect is repaired, acute Burow's triangles are taken laterally off the vermilion defect and the mucosa is undermined just above the orbicularis oris to allow advancement of the mucosa to meet the cutaneous flap edge at the newly established VCJ. In the cases where the defect's long axis is horizontally oriented, a superiorly based V-Y flap can be used in combination with mucosal advancement with excellent results.[20] Incision lines are well hidden along

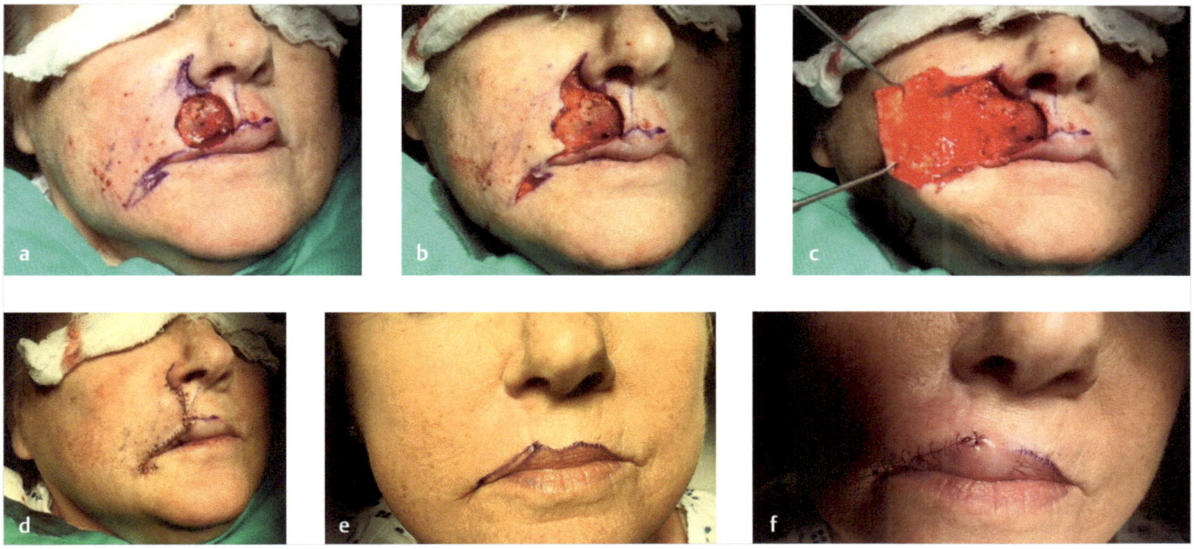

Fig. 8.16 Crescentic advancement flap. (a) Cutaneous upper lip defect and flap design. (b) Vermilion border incised and superior crescentic and inferior Burow's triangles removed. (c) Flap undermined and elevated. (d) Flap sutured in place. (e) Slight hooding of the upper lip due to large flap transfer, as seen at follow up. (f) Repair of hooding. (These images are provided courtesy of Stanislav N. Tolkachjov, MD.)

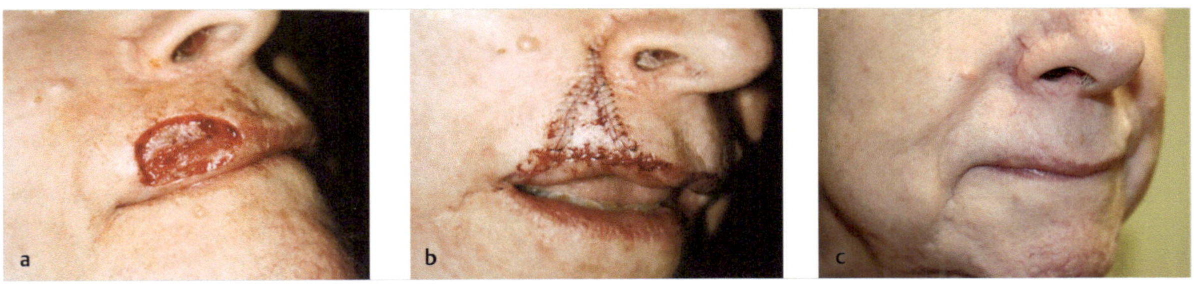

Fig. 8.17 V-Y advancement with partial mucosal advancement flap. (a) Cutaneous upper lip defect with vermilion involvement. (b) Superiorly based V-Y advancement flap and partial mucosal advancement flap sutured into place with precise recreation of the vermilion-cutaneous junction. (c) Final result.

the VCJ inferiorly and in the RSTLs of the upper lip and melolabial fold superiorly (▶ Fig. 8.17). A mucosal graft can be used as an alternative to a mucosal advancement flap and is typically harvested from the wet mucosa of the lower lip. However, disadvantages of the graft include creation of an additional wound to close and heal at the harvest site and the enforcement of strict limitations in lip movements for up to 2 weeks to minimize disruption of the graft–bed contact.

A wedge repair of the lip is a modification of a primary linear closure where intervening muscle and subcutaneous tissue are excised to prevent bulging at the closure line. This technique is particularly useful for larger defects (1–2 cm) on the lower half of the upper lip that are full-thickness or deep partialthickness, especially when the vermilion is involved or closure of only the cutaneous defect will push down the VCJ. Partial-thickness wedge resection can be used for defects where the muscular defect is smaller than the cutaneous defect. A wedge of muscular tissue is removed to create straight wound edges of muscle prior to approximation with an absorbable plication suture. An advancement flap can then be used to repair the cutaneous defect.[21]

Full-thickness wedge repair entails a multilayer primary V-shaped closure (▶ Fig. 8.18). This method can be safely utilized for defects up to one-fourth to one-third the width of the upper lip, depending on an individual's skin laxity, with minimal risk of microstomia or distortion.[13,22] A composite, full-thickness wedge of mucosa-muscle-skin is resected to a varying height depending on the defect size. Larger defects may require resection extending to the gingival sulcus. Inherent elasticity of the lip tissue obviates the need for undermining during lip wedge repair. The three layers of tissue are best approximated with four layers of suture: mucosa with fast-absorbing suture, muscle with long-acting absorbable

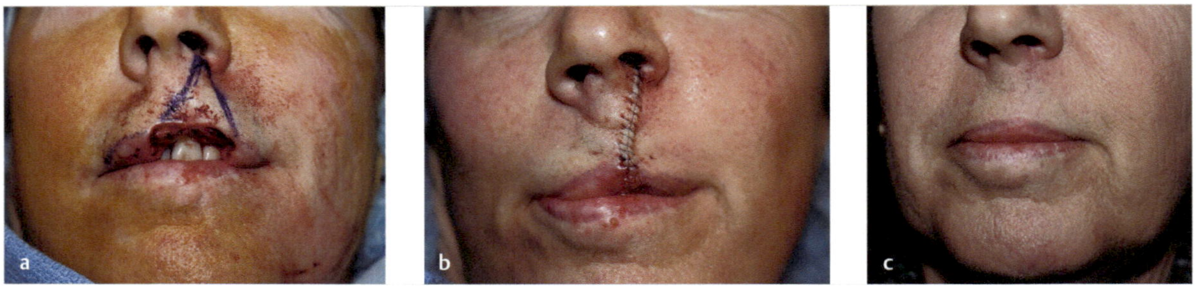

Fig. 8.18 Wedge repair. **(a)** Vermilion-cutaneous, full-thickness upper lip defect involving both philtral and lateral subunits. Wedge resection marked. **(b)** Wedge repair sutured in place with four-layer technique. **(c)** Final result with blunting of Cupid's bow and mild philtral distortion.

suture, dermis and subcutaneous tissue with long-acting absorbable sutures, and the dermis and epidermis with nonabsorbable sutures.[23] Typically the muscle is repaired first to facilitate approximation of the wound edges and minimize tension during closure of the remaining layers. When reapproximating the muscle, it is important to incorporate the most superficial portion that lies just beneath the vermilion in order to avoid notching. Next, the subcutaneous tissue is closed with dermal sutures, followed by placement of the mucosal and epidermal sutures. As with primary linear closure, precise placement of dermal sutures to realign the VCJ is essential for an acceptable cosmetic outcome. While braided absorbable sutures are used epidermally to approximate the vermilion, nonabsorbable polypropylene sutures are used for the cutaneous closure. Disadvantages of the lip wedge repair include bleeding due to transection of the labial arteries, a time-consuming four-layer repair, and the potential for lateral distortion of the philtrum due to excess tension at closure.

Full-thickness defects that involve more than one-third the width of the upper lip represent a reconstructive challenge. Repair by wedge resection or local cutaneous flaps for these large defects risks microstomia, free margin distortion, ischemia, and dehiscence due to excessive tension. In these cases, the lip-switch flap is a better repair option, as it offers a full-thickness tissue substitution with appropriate thickness, restoration of the orbicularis oris sphincter, and its own vermilion and mucosa to match that of the recipient site (▶ Fig. 8.19). The design, originally described by Sabattini, has undergone several modifications and is commonly referred to as the Abbe–Estlander flap.[24,25,27]

For upper lip defects, the Abbe interpolation flap is designed as a triangular full-thickness segment of tissue from the lower lip with a width slightly smaller than half of the defect and a height that matches that of the defect. By designing a flap half the width of the defect, the length of the upper and lower lip remain proportional. The labial artery is left intact on one side to provide a pedicle, either medially or laterally based to best facilitate flap transfer. For very laterally located defects involving the commissure, the pedicle should be based medially and then transposed around the oral commissure so that the reconstruction can be achieved in a single stage, as described by Estlander.[27] It is important to remember the labial artery courses between the mucosa and orbicularis oris just beneath the posterior vermilion line as to not transect the vascular supply during flap incision. The pedicle includes a cuff of tissue around the artery to ensure venous drainage. The flap is rotated almost 180 degrees about its pedicle to insert into the upper lip defect. Both the donor site and the flap are sutured in the standard four-layer fashion, described earlier, to carefully approximate the tissue layers, especially the muscle, and realign the VCJ. As with other staged interpolation flaps, the pedicle is divided and the flap inset at 3 weeks. Food intake is limited to liquids and soft foods to avoid chewing while the pedicle is attached.

Although the return of quality muscle movement to the flap is variable, motor reinnervation begins after a few months and becomes increasingly normal during the first year.[28,29] By 1 year after transfer, sensory function returns to near normal with the exception of temperature detection, which can remain impaired.[28] The prolonged phase of denervation and distortion of the oral commissure, often requiring commissure plasty, are major disadvantages to the lip-switch repair. Although lip-switch flaps can also be utilized for full-thickness defects of the lower lip, they are not an ideal reconstructive method in these cases due to philtral distortion if the upper lip donor site is used.

8.3.3 Philtrum

As the focus point of the upper lip, the philtrum carries significant aesthetic importance. This delicately shaped subunit is formed by the decussation of the orbicularis oris muscle and consists of a central concavity bounded by parallel convex philtral columns representing the insertion points of the contralateral muscles.[30,31] Defects involving the philtrum pose a significant challenge for the reconstructive surgeon. The philtrum is relatively void of crease lines found elsewhere on the upper lip and

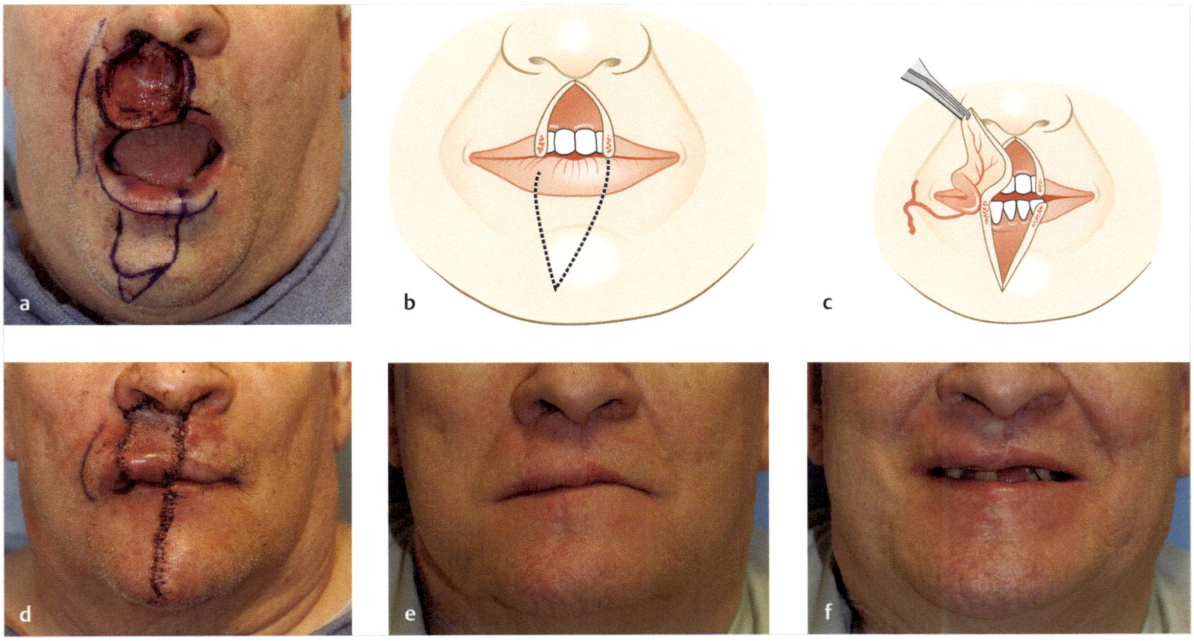

Fig. 8.19 Lip-switch flap (Abbe–Estlander flap). **(a)** Near full-thickness defect involving more than one-third the length of the upper lip. Abbe flap design marked along with the melolabial fold and vermilion subunit boundaries. **(b)** Full-thickness defect completed and flap incised. **(c)** Flap pivoted nearly 180 degrees on a lateral pedicle containing the labial artery. **(d)** Flap and donor site sutured. **(e,f)** Final result (after pedicle divided and flap inset at 3 weeks). Patient declined revision of upper vermilion-cutaneous junction step-off. (These images are provided courtesy of Christopher J. Miller, MD.)

has a limited reservoir of available skin for reconstruction and a dynamic topography, all of which add to the complexity of its repair. The approach to defects of the philtral subunit (▶ Fig. 8.20) and the most common reconstructive options are reviewed in the following.

Secondary intention can be an option for small defects within the philtral concavity; however, this option is rarely chosen, given the risk of excessive contraction leading to hypertrophic scarring, philtral distortion, and/or eclabium, especially near the vermilion border.

Primary linear closure can be utilized for small defects less than 50% the philtral width. The addition of an M-plasty at the inferior pole of the closure can be used to keep the incision lines within the philtral subunit, avoiding the extension onto the vermilion and preserving the Cupid's bow (▶ Fig. 8.21). Linear closure can be considered for larger defects; however, their use can result in blunting or flattening of the Cupid's bow. Additionally, given the lengthening between the two ends of the defect with linear closures, larger defects closed in this fashion risk distortion of the free margin by depressing the underlying lip. This is referred to as a fish-mouth deformity if the inferior pole of the primary closure obliterates the Cupid's bow and draws the VCJ to a point. Therefore, if a linear closure necessitates extension past the VCJ, thereby defacing the Cupid's bow, an alternative repair option should be chosen.

Similar-sized defects that are located over the philtral columns can be repaired with traditional or crescentic advancement flaps when they border the vermilion or nasal sill, respectively (▶ Fig. 8.22, ▶ Fig. 8.23). These are performed in the same fashion described earlier for the lateral subunits with special care to accurately reposition the VCJ. Despite extension into adjacent subunits, the flap is designed so that incision lines are placed along the subunit junctions yielding excellent cosmetic results.

The Cupid's bow of the vermilion lip defines the inferior region of the philtrum, and its intricate contour is marked by a concavity in the lower philtrum and a distinctive curvilinear vermilion border. It is a central structure at the junction of multiple subunits (vermilion, cutaneous lateral upper lip, and philtrum), and so, defects in this area often involve more than one subunit. Importantly, when repairing defects of the central cutaneous lip that reside in or involve the lower portion of the philtrum, this distinctive landmark must be recreated. An ideal repair will restore the original contour, shape, and position of the Cupid's bow, which vary between individuals based on age, race, actinic damage, smoking, and previous alternations including intradermal fillers and/or surgery.

A modification of the mucosal advancement flap, referred to as the "Seagull flap," is a reconstructive option for defects involving the Cupid's bow that are less than

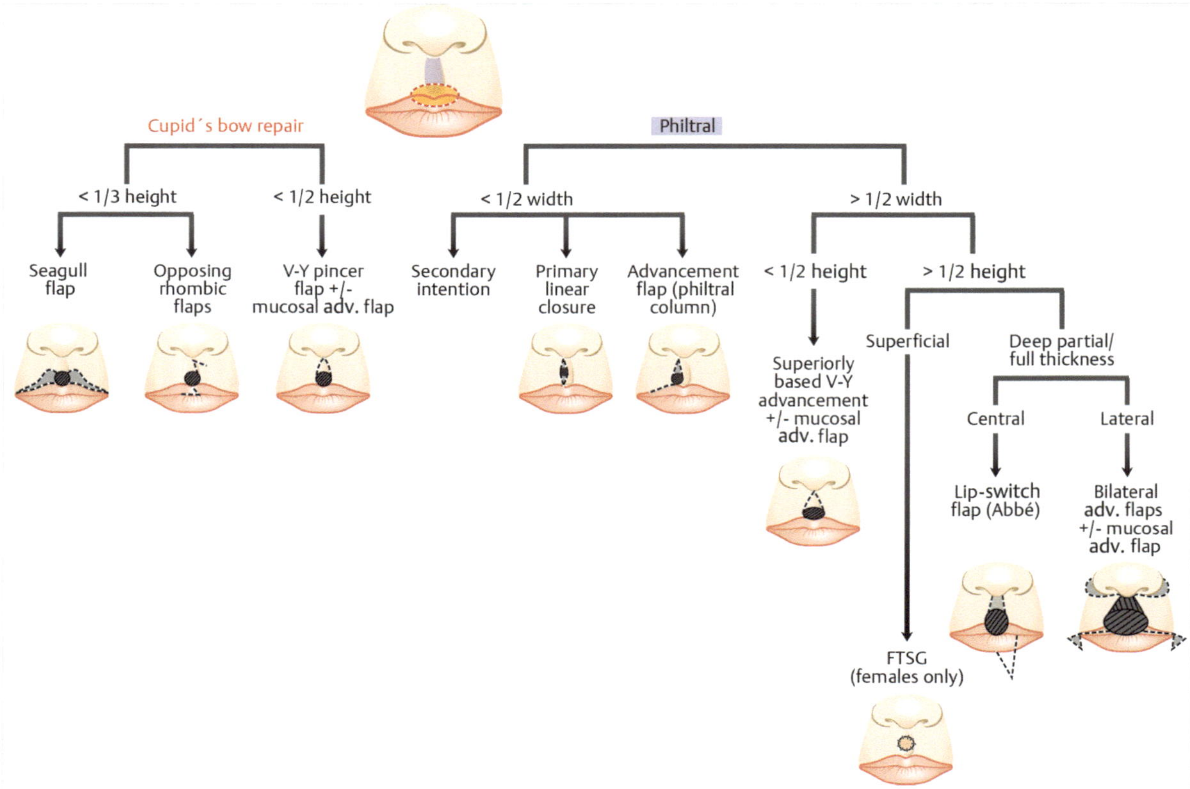

Fig. 8.20 Philtrum reconstruction algorithm. adv., advancement.

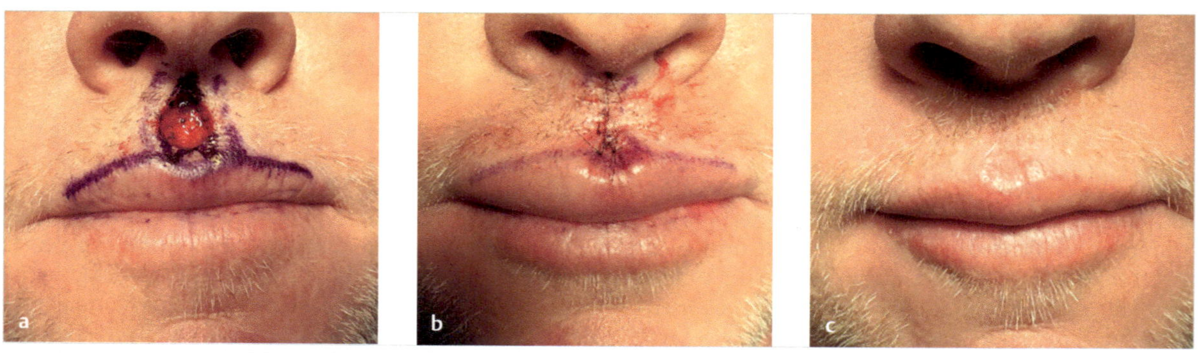

Fig. 8.21 Primary linear closure with M-plasty. **(a)** Small philtral defect approximating the philtral column. **(b)** Linear repair with M-plasty preserving Cupid's bow. **(c)** Final result. (These images are provided courtesy of Stanislav N. Tolkachjov, MD.)

one-third the philtral height (▶ Fig. 8.24).[32] Design of the flap begins with careful marking of the VCJ and philtral columns for orientation, followed by a redrawing of the Cupid's bow emanating from or incorporating the superior aspect of the defect. Bilateral apices align with the philtral columns, while the concavity is maintained at midline. Lateral incisions are extended and brought together at 30 degrees to avoid standing cones. After excision of two lateral Burow's triangles, superficial undermining is performed predominantly above the orbicularis on the superior cutaneous flap and to less extent submucosally on the vermilion as to avoid excessive elevation of the vermilion lip. The key suture is placed midline and reestablishes the position of the notch of the Cupid's bow. The advancement flaps are then brought together with a single layer of interrupted soft braided absorbable sutures (5–0 polyglactin 910) along the remainder of the flap's leading edge to recreate the VCJ.

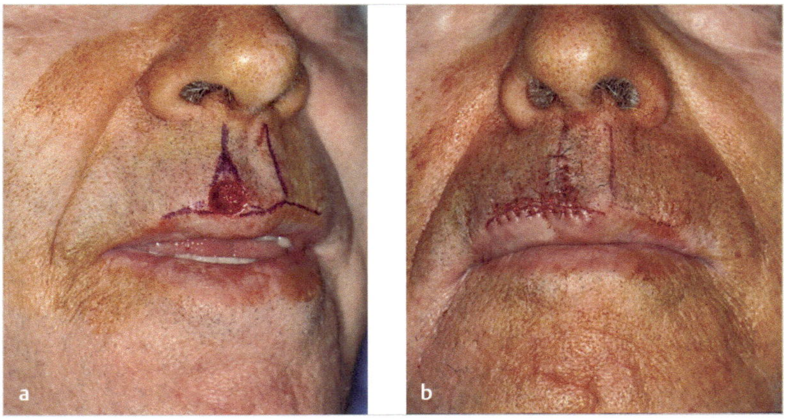

Fig. 8.22 Advancement flap. **(a)** Philtral column defect bordering the vermilion. Superior Burow's triangle and vermilion-cutaneous junction marked. **(b)** Advancement flap sutured with incision lines along cosmetic subunit borders.

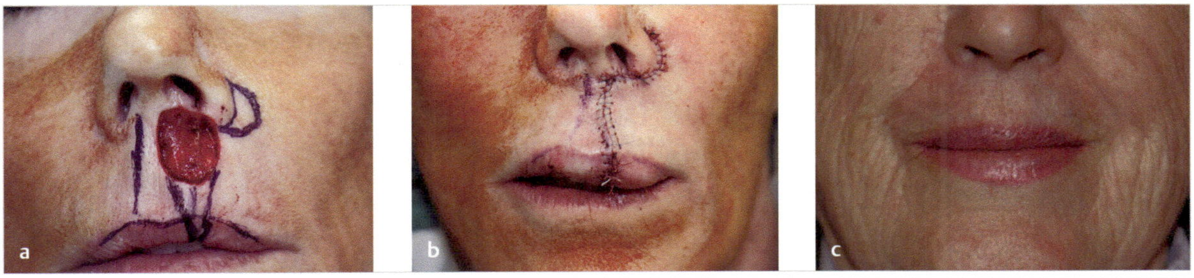

Fig. 8.23 Crescentic advancement flap. **(a)** Philtral column defect bordering the nasal sill. Inferior Burow's triangle extending to mucosal vermilion and perialar crescent marked. **(b)** Advancement flap sutured in place. **(c)** Final result.

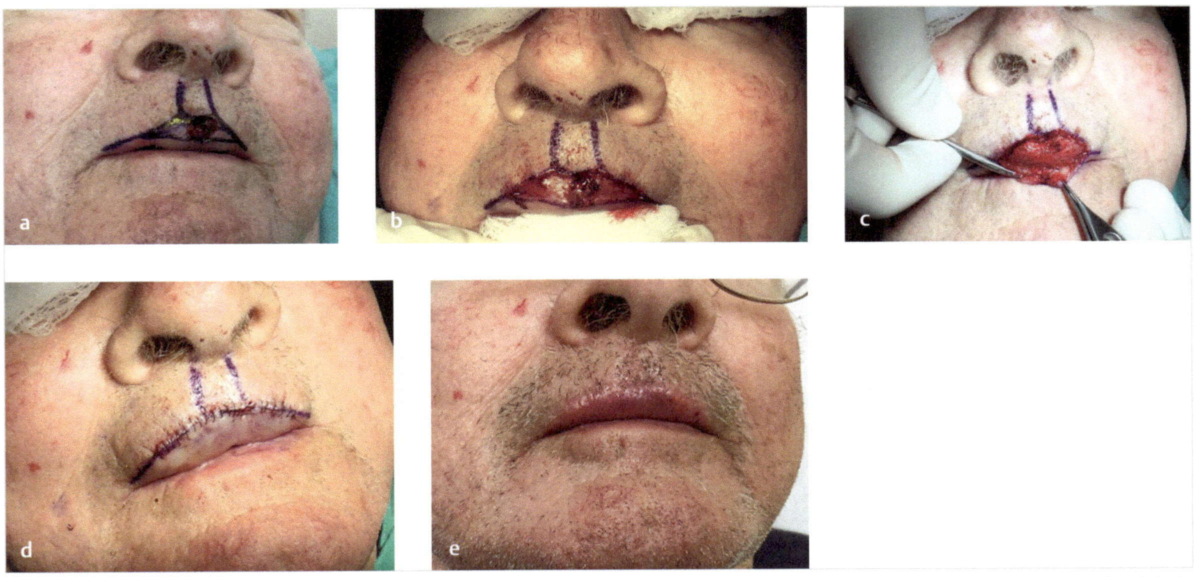

Fig. 8.24 Seagull flap. **(a)** Cupid's bow defect. Cupid's bow redrawn with subunit borders and lateral Burow's triangles marked. **(b)** Lateral Burow's triangles excised. **(c)** Superficial undermining above the muscle. **(d)** Flap sutured. **(e)** Short-term result (1-week follow-up). (These images are provided courtesy of Stanislav N. Tolkachjov, MD.)

Accurate positioning of the VCJ is of upmost importance for optimal aesthetic outcome, as described earlier. Increased gum showing when smiling is a potential downside to this repair.

Repair of the Cupid's bow using two opposing rhombic flaps has also been described.[33] Each flap is designed with a vertical incision extending outward from the center of the superior or inferior edge of the defect and a lateral incision. The superior rhombic flap is elevated from the cutaneous lip and transposed to replace the cutaneous portion of the defect, while the inferior rhombic flap is elevated and transposed, from either the ipsi- or the contralateral side, to replace the vermilion portion of the defect. Placement of a half-buried horizontal mattress stitch (5–0 polypropylene) at the point of maximum tension is used to close the secondary defect of each flap before trimming of their abutting edges to recreate the curvilinear vermilion border. While subcutaneous sutures are placed with 5–0 polyglactin 910, epidermal sutures are placed using polypropylene for the superior flap and 5–0 silk or polyglactin 910 for the inferior flap. This repair offers an alternative approach for effectively recreating the philtral curvature and curvilinear border of the Cupid's bow.

V-Y advancement flaps are an excellent reconstructive option for defects of the philtrum that are too wide for primary linear closure (up to 1.5 times the philtral width) but are still less than 50% the philtral height (▶ Fig. 8.25).[34] The flap is designed as a triangle extending superiorly off the defect with its apex at or even slightly onto the columella if necessary. The triangle is incised, and undermining takes place in the superficial subcutaneous plane laterally. The editors often undermine deeply with a combination of blunt and sharp undermining to achieve appropriate flap movement. The inferior and superior edges of the flap can be freed from the underlying muscular attachments to a small extent to allow movement without compromising the vascular supply. If there is still inadequate mobility, it may be necessary to eliminate the muscular attachments entirely and convert the triangular flap into a Burow's graft rather than risk distortion of the vermilion under excessive tension. The V-Y flap is advanced inferiorly and a key suture is placed between the leading edge of the flap and the inferior aspect of the defect. If a defect lies above the VCJ, it may be necessary to first remove the cutaneous tissue between the defect and the vermilion as to optimally camouflage the suture line along the VCJ. Subcutaneous sutures are occasionally needed; otherwise, the secondary defect and lateral edges of the flap are closed primarily with nonabsorbable running or interrupted epidermal sutures (6–0 polypropylene), and the VCJ is reestablished with absorbable interrupted epidermal sutures (5–0 polyglactin 910). If the defect also involves the vermilion lip, a mucosal advancement flap should be performed in addition to the V-Y advancement, as described earlier. This ensures proper positioning of the VCJ, well-camouflaged suture lines, and optimal aesthetic results. Alternatively, a mucosal V-Y flap can be designed inferiorly to repair the vermilion defect, meeting the cutaneous flap to recreate the VCJ.[35,36] The mucosal V-Y is designed inferior to the defect onto the vermilion, and its execution is identical to the superior V-Y, except undermining is within the submucosal plane, and interrupted epidermal absorbable braided sutures (5–0 polyglactin 910) are used to close the secondary defect and secure the flap in a single layer.

As with V-Y advancement flaps in other locations, there is risk of pincushioning, which can be minimized with adequate undermining, proper sizing, and insetting, and treated with intralesional corticosteroid or 5-fluorouracil injections. Particular to philtral repair, excessive upward tension can displace the vermilion and/or cause eclabium. Limiting selection of this repair for defects less than 50% the philtral height will decrease this risk, as will adequate undermining and conversion to Burow's graft if needed. The incision lines within the relatively smooth surface of

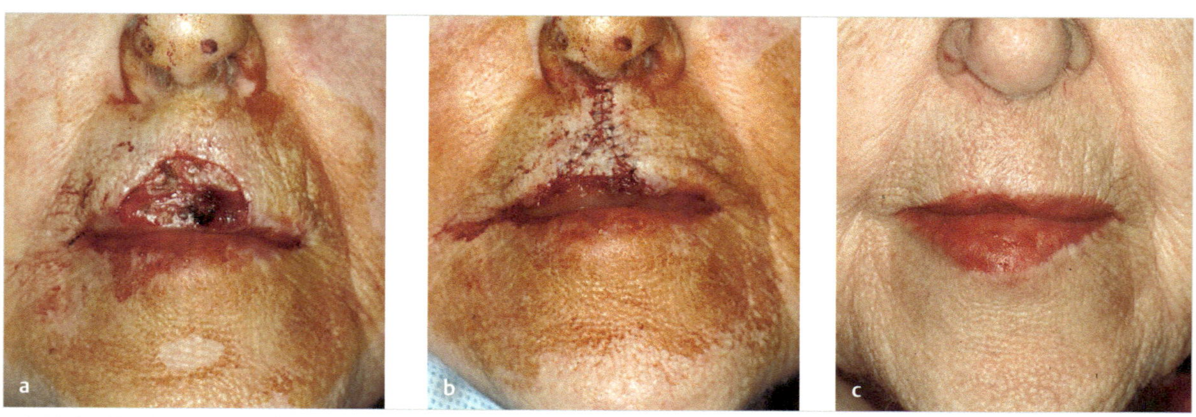

Fig. 8.25 V-Y advancement with partial mucosal advancement flap. **(a)** Philtral defect with vermilion involvement. **(b)** Superiorly based V-Y advancement flap and partial mucosal advancement flap sutured into place with precise recreation of the vermilion-cutaneous junction and Cupid's bow. **(c)** Final result.

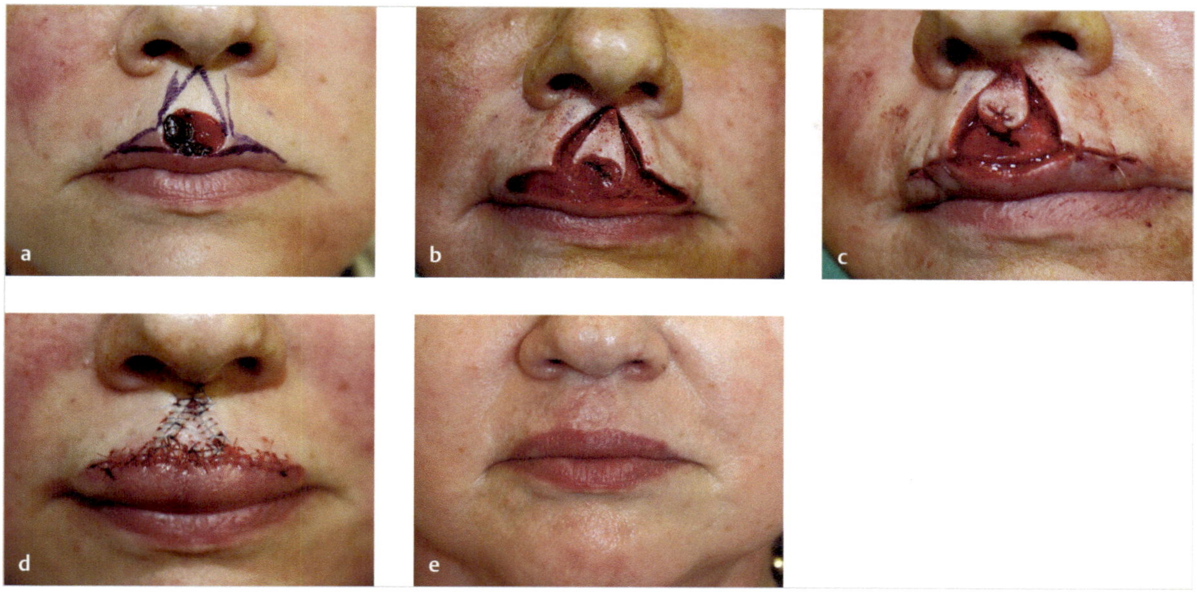

Fig. 8.26 Pincer flap with partial mucosal advancement flap. **(a)** Cupid's bow defect with superiorly based V-Y advancement flap and lateral vermilion Burow's triangles marked. **(b)** Flap incised and lateral Burow's triangles removed. **(c)** Two corners of the advancing edge are rotated medially and sutured together creating a concavity. Partial mucosal advancement with key sutures placed. **(d)** Flaps sutured in place. **(e)** Final result.

the sulcus can sometimes be cosmetically displeasing and improved with laser resurfacing or manual dermabrasion.

A variation of the V-Y advancement flap referred to as the "pincer flap," originally described by Dr. David Brodland, can be used to reconstruct the Cupid's bow when defects of the lower sulcus are too large for repair by the seagull flap but still less than 50% of the philtral height (▶ Fig. 8.26).[37] The repair is designed and executed identically to that of the superiorly based V-Y flap, but the two corners of the advancing edge are rotated medially and sutured together. This both increases the size of the flap and tethers the flap down to better reconstruct the concavity of the Cupid's bow.

Larger defects of the philtrum, greater than 50% the philtral height, are at increased risk for eclabium development.[22] When unable to be repaired with local skin flaps, FTSGs can be utilized for these defects; however, it is important to recognize several considerable limitations. Color and texture match of tissue in this cosmetically sensitive area is difficult, unless the defect is small enough to utilize a Burow's graft, which offers an excellent match.[8] In order to obtain adequate tissue, grafts are typically harvested from the pre- or postauricular skin. These sites offer a less-than-ideal match in many cases and yield an unacceptable cosmetic result for the hair-bearing upper lip in men. Although less common in the concavity of the philtrum, FTSGs are at risk for pincushioning and contraction that threatens eclabium, particularly with deeper defects.[34] For this reason, the use of FTSGs is limited by the depth of the defect.

When appropriate, the defect can first be expanded to enhance symmetry or to remove the entire subunit to best conceal scar lines along cosmetic borders. FTSGs can also be used in combination with repairs of the lateral subunit to limit the recipient bed within the confines of the philtral subunit (▶ Fig. 8.27). Once harvested, subcutaneous fat is trimmed from the undersurface of the flap and it is shaped to match the defect. Meticulous suturing with 6–0 polypropylene both secures the grafts and approximates the dermis of the graft with that of the wound edge, maximizing viability and cosmesis.[38]

Large, full-thickness defects of the philtrum that are restricted to the central portion of the upper lip can be repaired with a lip-switch flap of similar size transferred from the lower lip to provide restoration of the complete aesthetic unit and restore the subunit's cosmetic borders, as described earlier.[39] Large philtral defects that extend onto the adjacent lateral lip or are too deep for FTSG can be repaired with bilateral advancement flaps. The details of their execution are also described earlier. It is important to remember that the flap is undermined above the orbicularis on the cutaneous lip and extensively within the subcutaneous plane on the medial cheek as needed for adequate mobility. With large advancement flaps, incisions may be extended inferiorly beyond the vermilion below the commissure and superiorly into the perialar crease in crescentic fashion to both avoid distortion and camouflage scar lines. If there is vermilion involvement, a mucosal advancement flap is used to repair the vermilion subunit independently. When necessary, a

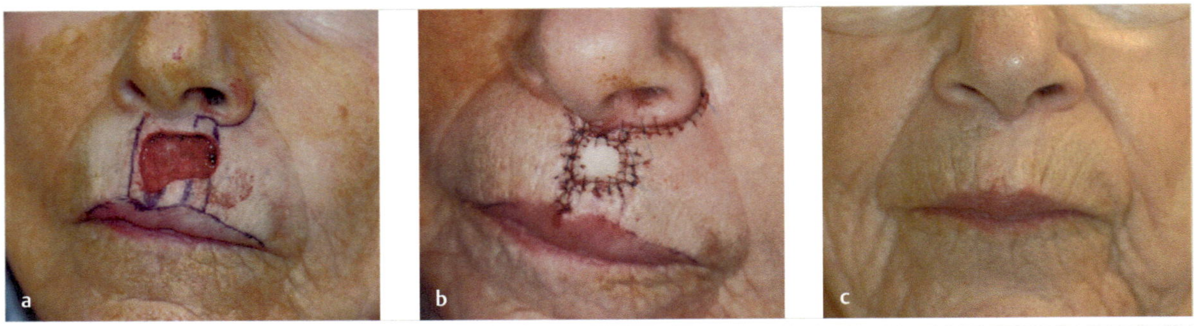

Fig. 8.27 Perialar advancement flap with full-thickness skin graft (FTSG). (a) Philtral defect extending beyond subunit borders. Philtral columns and perialar advancement flap marked. (b) Advancement flap performed to align wound edge with philtral column. FTSG sutured in place. Note FTSG limited to philtral subunit. (c) Final result.

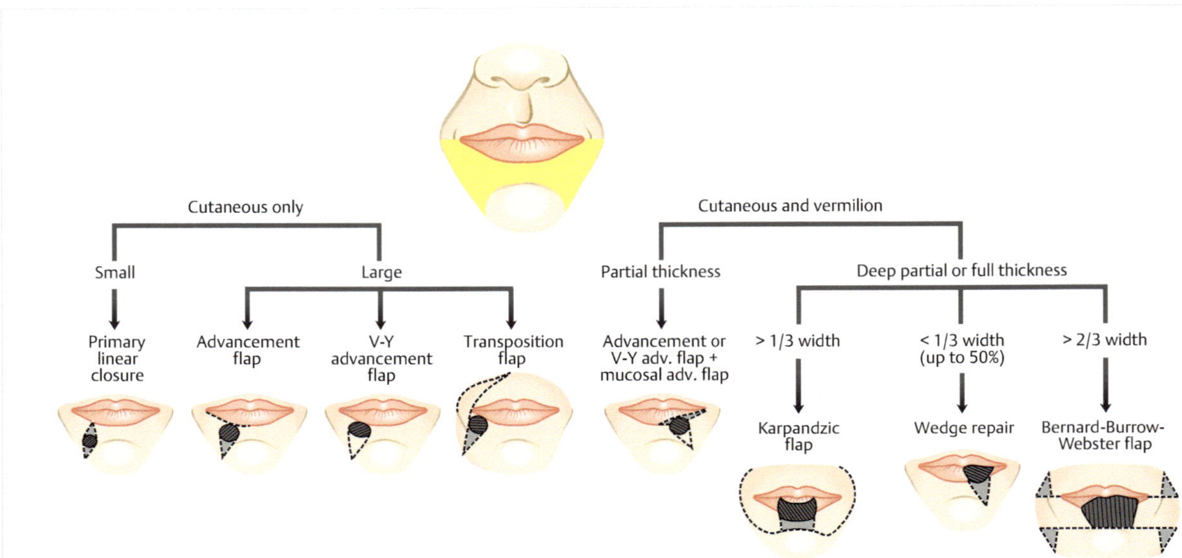

Fig. 8.28 Cutaneous lower lip reconstruction algorithm.

periosteal stitch can be used to reestablish the melolabial fold and prevent its blunting with cheek advancement.

8.3.4 Cutaneous Lower Lip

The approach to cutaneous lower lip reconstruction is relatively simplified when compared to that of the cutaneous upper lip and can be divided into defects with and without vermilion involvement and further by defect depth (▸ Fig. 8.28). Many of the repair techniques described for the upper lip are also excellent options in this subunit.

Similar to primary linear closures of the cutaneous lateral upper lip, those of the cutaneous lower lip should be positioned along the RSTL, however, subtle they may be. The length of the incision can be shortened with the use of an M-plasty, particularly when avoiding extension past the VCJ or labiomental crease. Chin repair options are discussed in Chapter 9 of this book.

When primary linear closures cannot be contained within the subunit, advancement flaps are an ideal option. Although the tissue reservoirs on the cutaneous lower lip differ slightly from that of the upper lip, traditional and V-Y advancement flaps similarly tap into inferolateral laxity of the cheek or chin and are designed to hide incision lines along the radial RSTL, vermilion border, and melolabial fold or marionette line (▸ Fig. 8.29). If there is vermilion involvement of the defect, a mucosal advancement flap is used to repair the vermilion defect in conjunction with the cutaneous flap (▸ Fig. 8.30). The execution of these flaps is identical to that described for the cutaneous upper lip. Although often unnecessary, a bilateral A-T advancement flap can also be utilized if unilateral motion is restricted resulting in excessive tension. Horizontal incisions should be placed along the vermilion border or labiomental crease for best concealment and an M-plasty can be utilized to avoid extension of the vertical

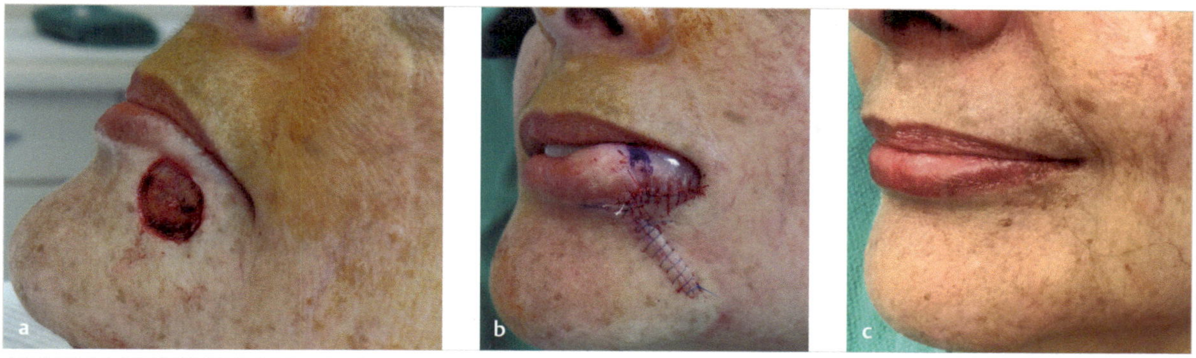

Fig. 8.29 Advancement flap. **(a)** Cutaneous lower lip defect bordering the vermilion-cutaneous junction. **(b)** Advancement flap sutured in place with inferior Burow's triangle incision along the radial relaxed skin tension lines (RSTLs). **(c)** Final result with incision lines well hidden along the RSTLs and vermilion border.

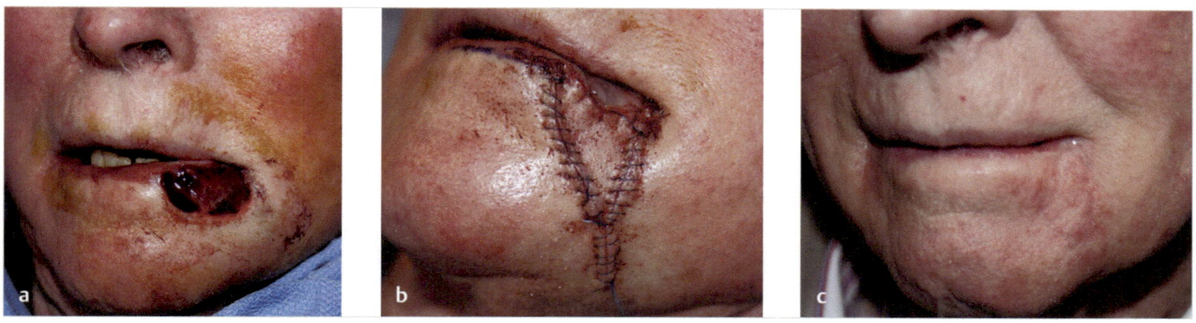

Fig. 8.30 V-Y advancement with partial mucosal advancement flap. **(a)** Cutaneous lower lip defect with vermilion involvement. **(b)** Inferiorly based V-Y advancement flap and partial mucosal advancement flap sutured into place with precise recreation of the vermilion-cutaneous junction. **(c)** Final result.

incisions onto the vermilion or through the labiomental crease.

Transposition flaps can also be utilized to repair large defects on the cutaneous lower lip.[40] The inferiorly based melolabial transposition flap is ideal for large defects involving the lateral cutaneous lower lip (and chin) that border the melolabial fold or marionette line (▶ Fig. 8.31). These flaps tap into tissue laxity of the medial cheek and allow for significant tissue mobility. The flap's medial edge extends superiorly from the defect along the melolabial fold where it meets its lateral edge at a 30-degree angle. The flap is incised and thoroughly undermined in the subcutaneous fat to allow a tension-free transposition over the oral commissure to the primary defect. A key suture is first placed to close the secondary defect. The inferior Burow's triangle is excised and the flap trimmed to match the defect edge. Dermal sutures are placed to secure the flap position, followed by epidermal sutures to appose skin edges. Careful thinning of the flap and thorough undermining help eliminate a bulky appearance to the flap, and the resulting incision lines of the secondary defect are well hidden in the melolabial fold. When utilizing this repair, one must consider the asymmetry of the cheeks and melolabial folds that may result. Additionally, the horizontal tension vectors of this repair may blunt the ipsilateral marionette line creating another point of asymmetry. Intradermal fillers can be utilized postoperatively to help mitigate this asymmetry.

A lip wedge repair is considered the standard method of reconstruction for deep partial or full-thickness defects and can be used for those involving up to one-third, or even one-half, of the width of the lower lip with minimal risk of microstomia or distortion of the subunit.[1] Although these guidelines are helpful, one must consider the inherent laxity of the skin on an individual basis to avoid undesirable outcomes. If the defect is small, limited removal of mucosa and muscle no further than the VCJ may be sufficient to reduce bulging at the free margin. In general, as the defect enlarges, the height of the full-thickness wedge may increase as necessary to the height of the gingival sulcus (▶ Fig. 8.32). A W-plasty can be incorporated into the lower lip wedge design in order to avoid extension below the labiomental crease. After composite resection of the mucosa-muscle-skin wedge, the three layers of tissue are approximated with four layers of sutures, as described for the upper lip wedge, without the

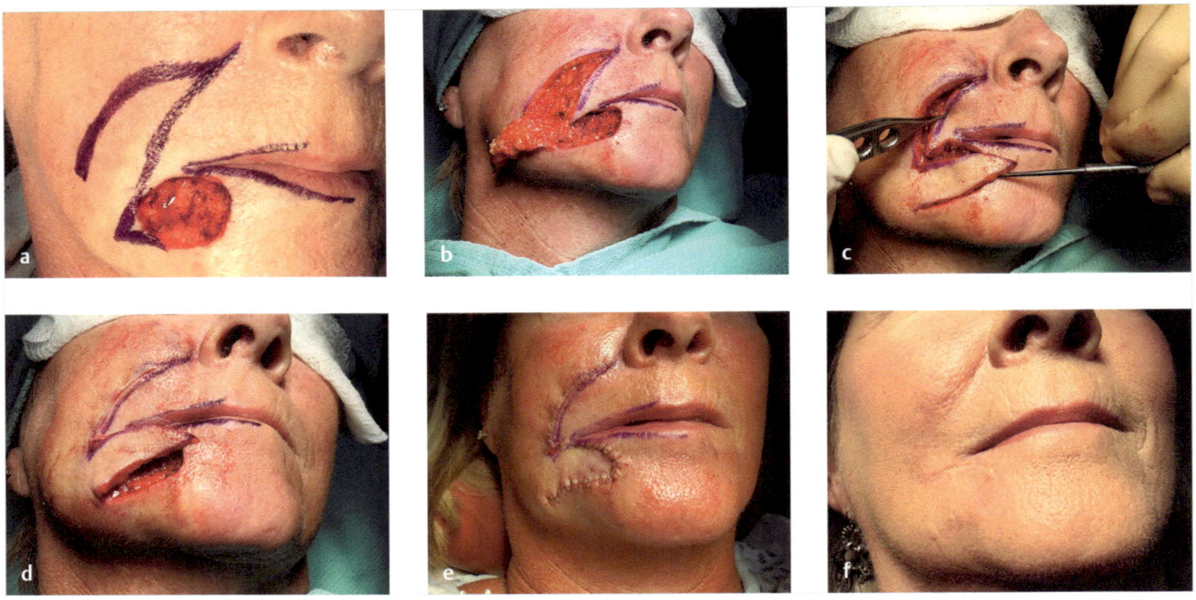

Fig. 8.31 Melolabial transposition flap. **(a)** Lateral cutaneous lower lip defect bordering the marionette line. Flap design marked with medial flap edge along the melolabial fold. **(b)** Flap incised, undermined, and elevated. Inferior Burow's triangle excised. **(c)** Flap transposed with minimal tension to cover primary defect. **(d)** Key suture in place closing secondary defect. **(e)** Flap completely sutured. **(f)** Final result. (These images are provided courtesy of Stanislav N. Tolkachjov, MD.)

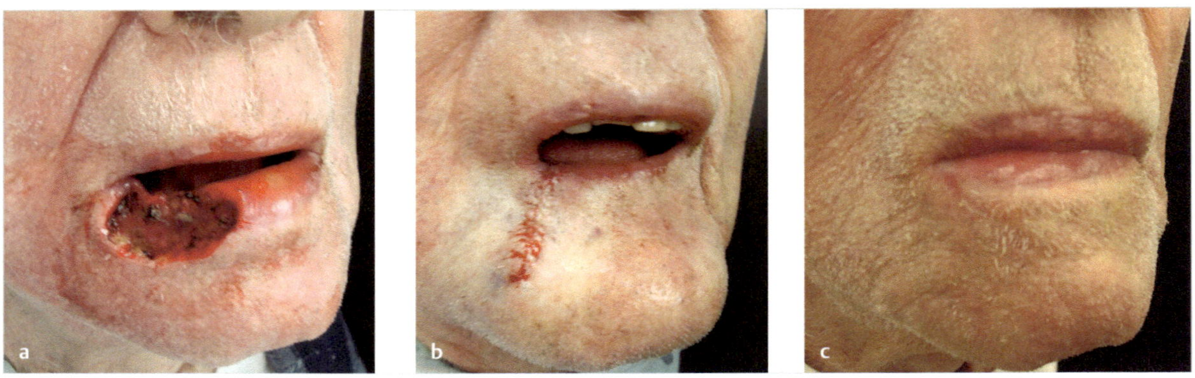

Fig. 8.32 Wedge repair. **(a)** Vermilion-cutaneous, full-thickness lower lip defect. **(b)** Wedge repair sutured in place with four-layer technique. **(c)** Final result. (These images are provided courtesy of John A. Zitelli, MD.)

need for undermining. Priority is placed on restoration of the orbicularis muscle sphincter as the ability to retain intraoral contents relies heavily on its function in the lower lip.[3] As always, precise realignment of the VCJ is crucial to ensure the best possible cosmetic outcome.

Full-thickness defects that involve more than one-third of the lower lip represent a considerable reconstructive challenge given the risk for microstomia and free margin distortion with the use of wedge repair or local cutaneous flaps. In these cases, circumoral, full-thickness rotation-advancement flaps can be utilized to transfer adequate amounts of tissue around the oral commissure as either single or bilateral opposing flaps and restore a functional muscle sphincter. The Karapandzic technique is ideal for centrally located defects and is typically based on two sliding rotation flaps formed by bilateral partial-thickness incisions extending from the inferior border of the defect along the labiomental crease and melolabial fold, creating flaps with a uniform width (▸ Fig. 8.33).[41,42,43] The incisions are made through the skin into the subcutaneous tissue and a separate, second incision through the mucosa on the deep surface of each flap can be reserved if additional movement is required.[1,13] For lateral defects, the contralateral flap can be made longer to avoid distortion of the central upper lip.[1] Key to this reconstruction is careful preservation of the neurovascular structures while separating the flap from the adjacent facial tissue. This allows for advancement of the myocutaneous flaps

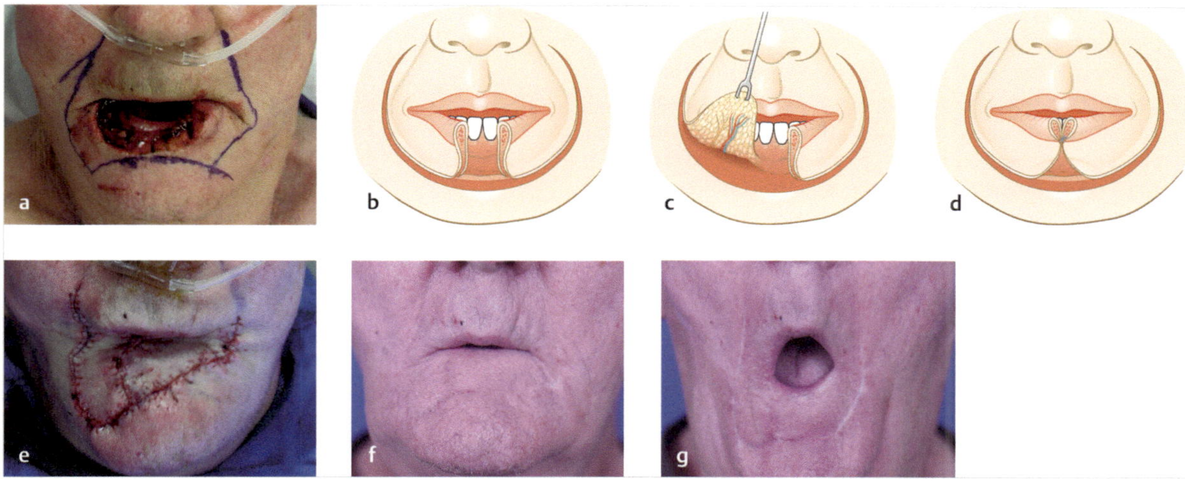

Fig. 8.33 Karapandzic flap. **(a)** Full-thickness defect of the lower lip with bilateral Karapandzic flaps marked in the labiomental crease and extending laterally to continue along the melolabial folds. **(b)** Flaps of uniform width incised to the subcutaneous tissue. **(c)** Myocutaneous flaps dissected with careful preservation of the neurovascular bundles. **(d)** Flaps advanced and approximated first at the anterior vermilion line. **(e)** Flaps fully sutured. **(f, g)** Follow-up at 3 months with notable microstomia. (These images are provided courtesy of Art J. Cox, MD.)

along with maximum vascular supply and optimal sensory and motor function. After medial advancement, the mucosa, muscle, and skin are closed in a four-layer fashion identical to that of the wedge repair. This reconstruction offers the unique advantage of preserving both the sensibility of the lips and motor function of the oral aperture. Additionally, the repair is performed in a single stage and suture lines are well placed in natural creases to optimize the aesthetic outcome. While in some patients the technique can be used for defects up to two-thirds the width of the lower lip, the variation in lip laxity among individuals, especially in relation to age, may result in limiting microstomia, proportional to the defect. A rounded distortion of the oral commissure and varying degrees of microstomia are major limitations of this reconstructive method. Altered sensation and tightness of the lip are the most commonly reported complications following the Karapandzic flap repair, and both have been shown to typically improve with time.[44] Additionally, the Karapandzic flaps are rarely utilized for full-thickness defects of the upper lip as flap advancement past midline results in unacceptable philtral distortion.

The Bernard–Burrow–Webster technique can be used for total or subtotal lip defects of the lower lip to avoid microstomia.[45,47] Two sliding flaps are formed by bilateral sets of horizontal, full-thickness incisions, both extending laterally about one-half the length of the defect, one from the commissure and one from the inferior border of the defect along the labiomental crease. The flaps are advanced medially and sutured in a layered fashion, as above, with Burow's triangles taken along the melolabial fold and the mucosa advanced to restore the vermilion. Although the oral aperture is preserved, this technique transects the orbicularis oris muscle and obliterates the majority of neurovascular structures, resulting in sensory loss and oral incontinence.

8.4 Complications and Revisions

Not unlike other areas of the face, bleeding, infection, and suboptimal scarring can complicate repairs of the perioral region. The abundant musculature and high mobility of the lip makes the perioral region especially vulnerable to postoperative bleeding and hematomas. The same factors can contribute to scar hypertrophy, inversion, or contraction leading to distortion of the free margin. Additionally, the proximity to the nose and oral mucosa increases the risk of bacterial contamination and infection. Systematic preoperative preparation, meticulous intraoperative hemostasis, and detailed postoperative instructions and wound care are essential to limit the incidence of these complications and maximize cosmetic results.

Prior to surgery, the face should be prepped with povidone–iodine solution. If the mucosal surface is breached during surgery, prophylactic antibiotics may be prescribed for 1 week starting the day of surgery. A secure pressure dressing is placed postoperatively and is left in place for 24 to 48 hours. Once removed, the patient is instructed to wash the area gently with soap and water and apply healing ointment (i.e., Aquaphor or petrolatum ointment) covered with a light dressing (i.e., Band-Aid) twice daily until suture removal at 1 week. For the first 48 hours, patients should be instructed to limit movement, including talking and chewing, of the perioral region and encouraged to have a liquid or soft food diet. Detailed instructions on postoperative care are provided in Chapter 12.

Particular limitations and potential complications of each reconstructive technique are reviewed in the corresponding sections. However, it is worth highlighting one complication that commonly plagues some repairs of the lip, pincushioning. As described earlier, this can be minimized at the time of repair with appropriate sizing and thinning of flaps and undermining of the skin surrounding the recipient site. Postoperatively, to help flatten the bulky tissue, intradermal steroid and 5-fluorouracil injections may be administered starting 4 to 6 weeks after surgery and continued until an acceptable cosmetic result is achieved.

References

[1] Baker SR. Local Flaps in Facial Reconstruction. 3rd ed. Philadelphia: Mosby Elsevier; 2014

[2] Salasche SJ, Bernstein G, Senkarik M. Classic systems of anatomy II: the facial nerve.in: Surgical Anatomy of the Skin. Norwalk, CT: Appleton & Lange;1988:108

[3] Langstein HN, Robb GL. Lip and perioral reconstruction. Clin Plast Surg. 2005; 32(3):431–445, viii

[4] Schulte DL, Sherris DA, Kasperbauer JL. The anatomical basis of the Abbé flap. Laryngoscope. 2001; 111(3):382–386

[5] Park C, Lineaweaver WC, Buncke HJ. New perioral arterial flaps: anatomic study and clinical application. Plast Reconstr Surg. 1994; 94 (2):268–276

[6] Al-Hoqail RA, Meguid EM. Anatomic dissection of the arterial supply of the lips: an anatomical and analytical approach. J Craniofac Surg. 2008; 19(3):785–794

[7] Pinar YA, Bilge O, Govsa F. Anatomic study of the blood supply of perioral region. Clin Anat. 2005; 18(5):330–339

[8] Zitelli JA, Brodland DG. A regional approach to reconstruction of the upper lip. J Dermatol Surg Oncol. 1991; 17(2):143–148

[9] Gloster HM , Jr. The use of second-intention healing for partial-thickness Mohs defects involving the vermilion and/or mucosal surfaces of the lip. J Am Acad Dermatol. 2002; 47(6):893–897

[10] Leonard AL, Hanke CW. Second intention healing for intermediate and large postsurgical defects of the lip. J Am Acad Dermatol. 2007; 57(5):832–835

[11] Zitelli JA. Wound healing by secondary intention. A cosmetic appraisal. J Am Acad Dermatol. 1983; 9(3):407–415

[12] Larrabee WJ, Sherris DA. Lips and chin.in: Sherris DA, Larrabee WJ, eds. Principles of Facial Reconstruction. Philadelphia, PA: Lippincott-Raven;1995:170

[13] Sobanko JF. Perioral reconstruction. In: Rohrer T, Cook J, Kaufman A, eds. Flaps and Grafts in Dermatologic Surgery. Philadelphia, PA: Elsevier;2018:258–287

[14] Mellette JR , Jr, Harrington AC. Applications of the crescentic advancement flap. J Dermatol Surg Oncol. 1991; 17(5):447–454

[15] Skouge JW. Upper lip repair-the subcutaneous island pedicle flap. J Dermatol Surg Oncol. 1990; 16(1):63–68

[16] Rustad TJ, Hartshorn DO, Clevens RA, Johnson TM, Baker SR. The subcutaneous pedicle flap in melolabial reconstruction. Arch Otolaryngol Head Neck Surg. 1998; 124(10):1163–1166

[17] Quatrano NA, Samie FH. Modification of Burow's advancement flap: avoiding the secondary triangle. JAMA Facial Plast Surg. 2014; 16 (5):364–366

[18] Salasche SJ, Jarchow R, Feldman BD, Devine-Rust MJ, Adnot J. The suspension suture. J Dermatol Surg Oncol. 1987; 13(9):973–978

[19] Zitelli JA. Tips for wound closure. Pearls for minimizing dog-ears and applications of periosteal sutures. Dermatol Clin. 1989; 7(1):123–128

[20] Roberts A, Leithauser L, Gloster HM , Jr. Combined vestibular mucosal advancement and island pedicle flaps for the repair of a defect involving the cutaneous and vermilion upper lip. Dermatol Surg. 2014; 40(5):580–583

[21] Spinowitz AL, Stegman SJ. Partial-thickness wedge and advancement flap for upper lip repair. J Dermatol Surg Oncol. 1991; 17(7):581–586

[22] Chapman JT, Mellette JR Jr. Perioral reconstruction. In: Rohrer TE, Cook JL, Nguyen TH, Mellette JR Jr, eds. Flaps and Grafts in Dermatologic Surgery. Philadelphia, PA: Saunders Elsevier;2007:217–233

[23] Godek CP, Weinzweig J, Bartlett SP. Lip reconstruction following Mohs' surgery: the role for composite resection and primary closure. Plast Reconstr Surg. 2000; 106(4):798–804

[24] Sabattini P. Cenno storico dell'origine e progressi della rinoplastica e cheiloplastica. Bologna: Belle Arti; 1838

[25] Mazzola RF, Lupo G. Evolving concepts in lip reconstruction. Clin Plast Surg. 1984; 11(4):583–617

[26] Abbe R. A new plastic operation for the relief of deformity due to double harelip. Plast Reconstr Surg. 1968; 42(5):481–483

[27] Estlander JA. Eine Methode aus der einen Lippe Substanzverluste der anderen zu ersetzen. [reprinted in English translation in Plast Reconstr Surg 42:361, 1968]. Arch Klin Chir. 1872; 14:622

[28] Smith JW. The anatomical and physiologic acclimatization of tissue transplanted by the lip switch technique. Plast Reconstr Surg Transplant Bull. 1960; 26:40–56

[29] Thompson N, Pollard AC. Motor function in Abbe flaps. A histochemical study of motor reinnervation in transplanted muscle tissue of the lips in man. Br J Plast Surg. 1961; 14:66–75

[30] Salasche SJ, Bernstein G, Senkarik M. Regional anatomy III: the lip. In Surgical Anatomy of the skin. Norwalk, CT: Appleton &Lange;1988:224–225

[31] Briedis J, Jackson IT. The anatomy of the philtrum: observations made on dissections in the normal lip. Br J Plast Surg. 1981; 34(2):128–132

[32] Paniker PU, Mellette JR. A simple technique for repair of Cupid's bow. Dermatol Surg. 2003; 29(6):636–640

[33] Davis JC, Bennett RG. A novel reconstruction to maintain Cupid's bow. Dermatol Surg. 2016; 42(11):1293–1296

[34] Kaufman AJ, Grekin RC. Repair of central upper lip (philtral) surgical defects with island pedicle flaps. Dermatol Surg. 1996; 22(12):1003–1007

[35] Srivastava S. Reconstruction of traumatic loss of vermilion and mucocutaneous junction of the lips. Br J Plast Surg. 1989; 42(5):526–529

[36] Garcés Gatnau JR, Ruiz-Salas V, Alegre Fernández M, Puig L. Reconstruction for defects at the base of the philtrum affecting the upper lip vermilion. Dermatol Surg. 2016; 42(5):677–680

[37] Brodland D. Flaps. In: Bolognia JL, Jorizzo JL,Rapini RP, eds. Dermatology.New York, NY: Elsevier Saunders; 2012

[38] Zitelli JA. Burow's grafts. J Am Acad Dermatol. 1987; 17(2, Pt 1):271–279

[39] McCarn KE, Park SS. Lip reconstruction. Facial Plast Surg Clin North Am. 2005; 13(2):301–314, vii

[40] Mu EW, Greenbaum SS. The transposition flap for the reconstruction of lower cutaneous lip defects. J Drugs Dermatol. 2017; 16(4):385–387

[41] Ethunandan M, Macpherson DW, Santhanam V. Karapandzic flap for reconstruction of lip defects. J Oral Maxillofac Surg. 2007; 65 (12):2512–2517

[42] Jabaley ME, Clement RL, Orcutt TW. Myocutaneous flaps in lip reconstruction. Applications of the Karapandzic principle. Plast Reconstr Surg. 1977; 59(5):680–688

[43] Karapandzic M. Reconstruction of lip defects by local arterial flaps. Br J Plast Surg. 1974; 27(1):93–97

[44] Teemul TA, Telfer A, Singh RP, Telfer MR. The versatility of the Karapandzic flap: a review of 65 cases with patient-reported outcomes. J Craniomaxillofac Surg. 2017; 45(2):325–329

[45] Bernard C. Cancer de la levre inferieure: restauratio a l'aide de lembeaux quadrilataires-lateraux querison. Scalpel (Brux). 1852; 5:162–164

[46] Konstantinović VS. Refinement of the Fries and Webster modifications of the Bernard repair of the lower lip. Br J Plast Surg. 1996; 49 (7):462–465

[47] Williams EF , III, Setzen G, Mulvaney MJ. Modified Bernard-Burow cheek advancement and cross-lip flap for total lip reconstruction. Arch Otolaryngol Head Neck Surg. 1996; 122(11):1253–1258

9 Chin Reconstruction

Christopher B. Harmon and Randall Proctor

Abstract

The chin is a midline cosmetic subunit in which cutaneous malignancies are common. Mohs micrographic surgery provides the highest cure rates and smallest defects after extirpation of these lesions. Preoperative assessment of the patient's normal anatomy is an important part of surgical planning. Delineation of any pronounced landmarks helps with designing reconstruction. Further, understanding resting skin tension lines along the convex chin can help the surgeon fashion a repair that is cosmetically pleasing. The baseline anatomy of the patient and suspected cosmetic outcomes should be discussed with the patient as much as possible. Curvilinear primary closures are a mainstay for reconstruction. For defects spanning a large portion of the chin, advancement and rotation flaps are excellent options and likely the most commonly used flaps. While larger defects may require transposition flaps harvested from adjacent submental neck or the skin of the jaw, care should be taken to take note of typical locations of the marginal mandibular nerve. Taking care to use sufficient undermining, release from the mentalis muscle near the wound edge and appropriate eversion of the wound edge will result in the best outcomes.

Keywords: chin, mental crease, labiomental crease, mental nerve block, marginal mandibular nerve

Capsule Summary and Pearls

- Delineate the labiomental crease and any mental cleft that is present prior to infiltration of local anesthetic.
- Assess thickness and mobility of the skin prior to infiltration of local anesthetic.
- Align linear closures to fit the convex contour of the chin when it is pronounced.
- Elongate Burow's triangles to account for a pronounced convex chin. This may include extending the removal of a standing cone to the submental neck.
- Avoid crossing the labiomental crease with suture lines to avoid upward displacement of the vermilion.
- With deeper defects, avoid crossing the mandible to prevent tethering of the scar to the underlying menton.
- Rich muscular anatomy and anastomosing blood supply allow for durable flaps if undermined in the appropriate plane on the chin.
- The marginal mandibular branch of the facial nerve lies lateral to the chin and should be avoided for larger reconstructions utilizing this tissue reservoir.

9.1 Relevant Anatomy

The chin is formed by a projection in the anterior-most portion of the mandible. It is bordered by the labiomental crease superiorly and the inferior extension of the nasolabial folds (or marionette lines) laterally (▸ Fig. 9.1). The nasolabial folds generally become more obvious in older patients with more pronounced skin laxity. The lack of significant nasolabial folds or marionette lines in younger patients makes the lateral borders of the chin more ambiguous. The inferior border of the chin is defined by the inferior border of the anterior mandible. The chin has a variably, but generally dense fibrous subcutaneous tissue mass with insertions of the *mentalis* muscle, which originates from the medial portion of the mandible at the lateral incisors. This muscle wrinkles the skin of the chin and helps protrude the lower lip. Other muscles in this area include the inferior portion of the *orbicularis oris* superiorly, the *depressor anguli oris*, and the *depressor labii inferioris* laterally. The inferior border of the chin includes the medial insertions of the *platysma* muscle.

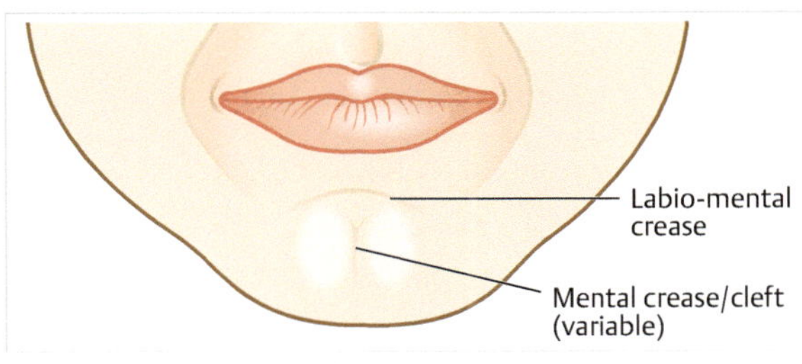

Fig. 9.1 Basic surface anatomy of the chin.

Resting skin tension lines follow a generally curvilinear or sickle-shaped course curving laterally along the rounded convex axis of the protruding mental prominence. The most obvious line of the lower face is often the labiomental crease, which should be identified prior to infiltration of local anesthetic. This line is of utmost importance in designing repairs of the chin. A natural surface anatomy feature of importance is the mental cleft, when present. This too should be identified with markings prior to infiltration of anesthetic. When linear closures and scars cross this line, an obvious and lasting deformity generally ensues, pushing the lower vermilion border upward and obliterating the labiomental crease. The lateral borders include a variable nasolabial fold or marionette line.

It is important to note the convexity of the chin, which varies with age. There is some structural loss of the mandibular prominence with bone resorption and aging as well as an increase in skin laxity, which can work to the advantage of the surgeon dealing with larger defects. While second intention healing is not classically advised on convex surfaces, the size and depth of the defect should be considered when approaching these wounds. If a Mohs layer can remove a tumor superficially in the presence of a bearded man, secondary intention healing can be the best option. Finally, this convexity leads to persistent standing cones when Burow's triangles are not long enough to account for the convexity.

Danger zones of the chin include the inferior labial arteries superiorly and the marginal mandibular nerve at the most lateral portion. These are unlikely to be encountered on the chin proper. It is also important to note that the labiomental crease is the inferior border of the lower cutaneous lip, which has variable thickness. The oral cavity can lie less than 1 cm from the skin at this point. When considering repairs for the chin, the lateral tissue reservoirs do contain the marginal mandibular nerve, and thus it should be identified by surface landmarks during design of reconstruction. On the chin proper, one may encounter the V3 branch of the trigeminal nerve (*mental nerve*), which provides sensory innervation to the chin and lower lip. The presence of this nerve root offers and easy solution to anesthesia via regional block of this area and can be utilized for patient comfort.

9.2 Aesthetic Subunits and Defects

Aesthetic subunits and defects are shown in detail in ▶ Fig. 9.2, ▶ Fig. 9.3, ▶ Fig. 9.4, ▶ Fig. 9.5, ▶ Fig. 9.6, ▶ Fig. 9.7.

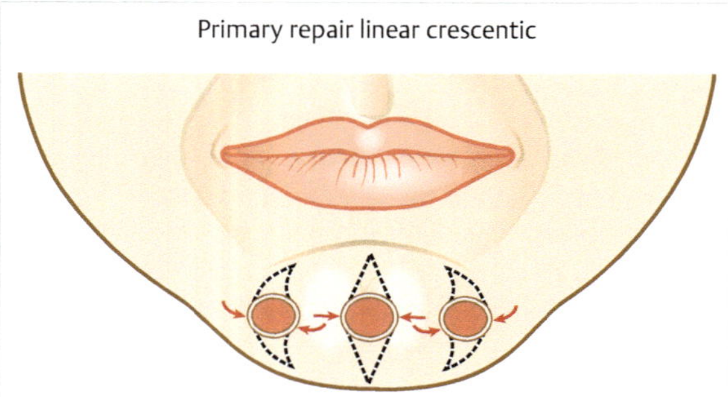

Fig. 9.2 Primary repair options. Midline defects with vertical closures. Lateral defects with curvilinear or crescentic closures.

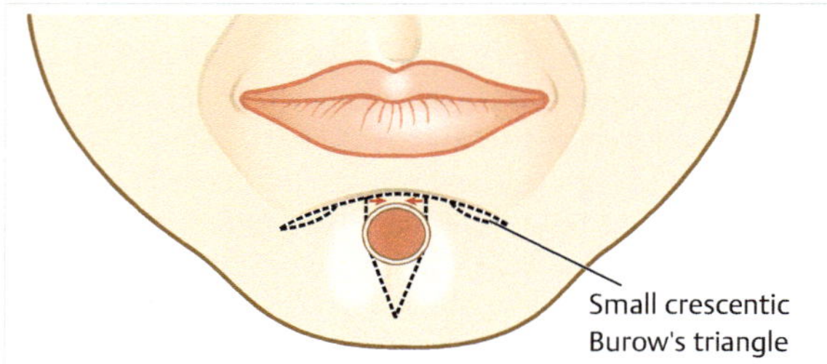

Fig. 9.3 O-T advancement flap. Note the small crescentic Burow's triangles along the sliding edges of the flap to eliminate length discrepancy and bunching of the standing edge. Note the desire to place the horizontal line along the labiomental crease.

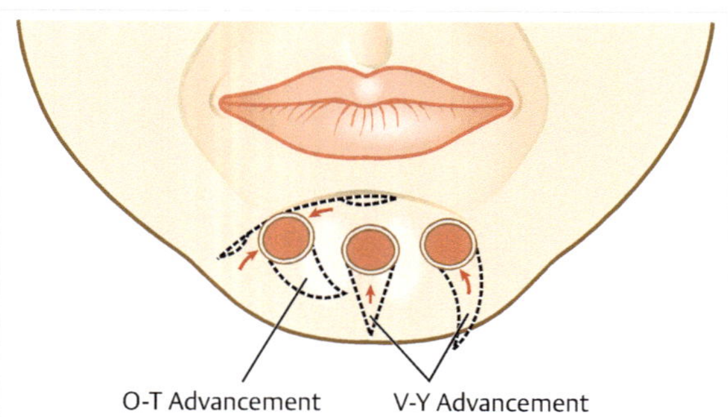

Fig. 9.4 V-Y advancement. Good option for midline defects and lateral defects. Note the curvilinear V used for the lateral defect designed toward midpoint of the chin. O-T advancement flap for defect lateral to midline.

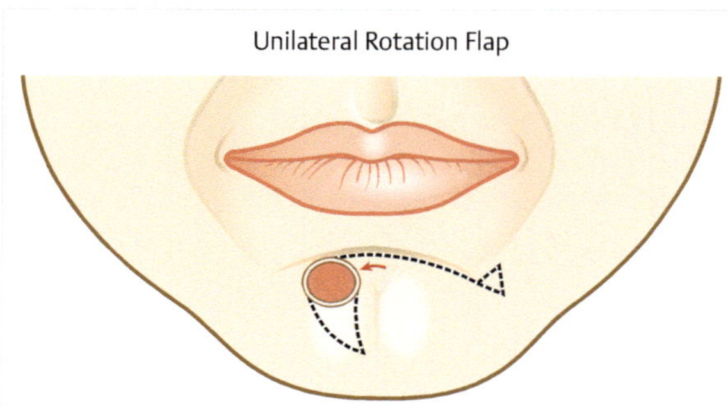

Fig. 9.5 Unilateral rotation flap. Note the arc extends along the labiomental crease and the standing cone is removed along the relaxed skin tension line of the lower lip or along the marionette line or from beneath the mandible if tissue is mobilized inferolateral to defect.

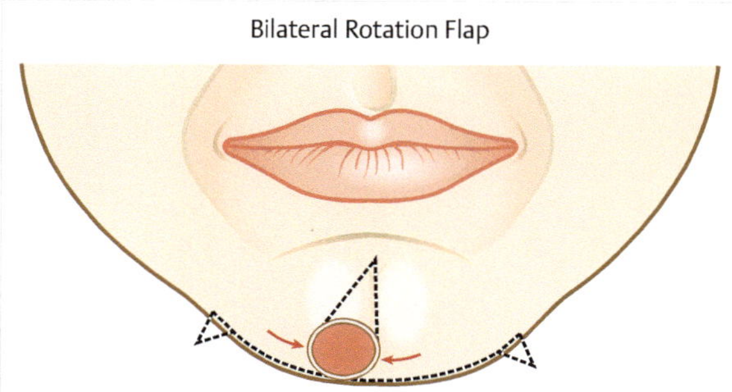

Fig. 9.6 Bilateral rotation flap. Standing cones removed from the area just inferior to the mandible at equal distances to maintain symmetry. This could also be considered an O-T advancement flap depending on the rotational or straight-line vector of tissue movement.

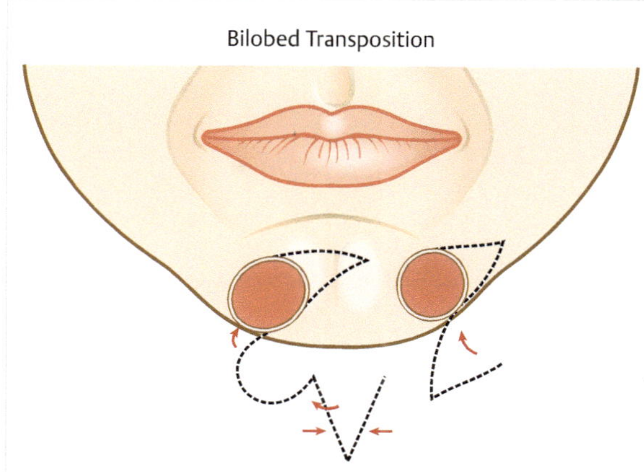

Fig. 9.7 Transposition flaps. Bilobed transposition offers the option of hiding secondary and tertiary defect scars on the submental area. A single lobe transposition can also be tailored to hide secondary defect scars in multiple locations below the mandible.

9.3 Reconstructive Options

9.3.1 Algorithm

- Second intention healing: This is reserved for superficial defects in men who normally grow beards or very broad defects where secondary intention is felt to appear superior to a full-thickness skin graft.
- Primary (side-to-side) closure: Primary closures should not cross the labiomental crease if at all possible. Upward distortion of the lower lip can occur when the labiomental crease is crossed.
- Bilateral advancement flap (O-T): Note this may have a component of rotation due to the convex nature of the chin and curved mental crease (this is a "go-to" flap for the chin).
- V-Y advancement/island pedicle flap.
- When there is lack of enough tissue laxity for above repairs:
  - Unilateral or bilateral rotation flap (bilateral is reserved for defects near the midline).
  - Inferiorly and laterally based transposition flap/ bilobed flap.
  - Full-thickness skin graft.

9.3.2 Healing by secondary intention

The chin can heal very well when defects are shallow and broad. This may be suitable for all shallow defects but is most practical for defects that are too broad for primary closures and are shallow. If the defect is partial thickness and present in a man that normally grows a beard, it may be the preferred option for this location. If the defect includes subcutaneous fat, or obliterates follicular structures, a closure is likely the better option. Delayed repair after secondary intention healing can be a consideration for defects smaller than 1 cm and no more than 3 to 5 mm in depth. By allowing healing, the patient and clinician can assess the appearance and decide if closure is preferred. Facial hair preferences can change; thus, scar appearance on a clean-shaven face should be considered.

9.3.3 Primary closure

Primary closures on the chin are a mainstay for many Mohs defects. Midline or near-midline defects are common, and primary linear closures are common. Lateral defects will often appear better with a curvilinear design when oriented in a vertical fashion. This is best facilitated with the use of two concave lines on the medial side and a longer convex line on the lateral side (see ▶ Fig. 9.2). It is important to have the inner curve equal the length of the outer/broader curve by creating two concave lines on either end of the defect. Otherwise, the curve will have two skin edges of unequal length, leading to redundancy on the longer side. Undermining widely through the fibrous attachments of the *mentalis* muscle will facilitate movement of the edges of the defect and reduce tension on the wound. Insufficient undermining may result in a dimpled or depressed scar in this location due to the muscular attachments into the dermis.

Primary closures should not cross the labiomental crease. If a primary closure will require crossing this crease, it should be altered in some way. This will generally make an O-T flap the best option. Similarly, if the primary closure will cross the mandibular prominence inferiorly, it may result in tethering of the scar at this prominence. A bilateral advancement flap with inferior incisions along the mandibular border will provide less likelihood of tethering at the bony prominence, which can cause an unappealing visible difference from the frontal view.

Some defects may lend themselves to closure horizontally, or slightly angled. These are generally an exception

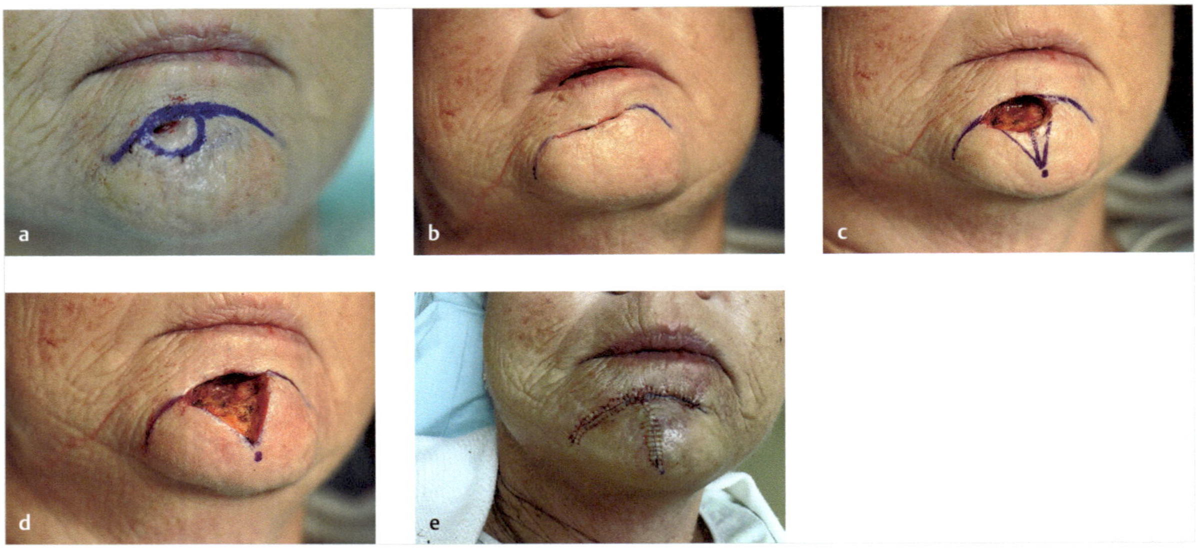

Fig. 9.8 **(a)** Preoperative marking of the tumor. Note delineation of the labiomental crease at this point prior to local infiltration. **(b)** A suture is temporarily placed showing the eclabium and displacement of mental crease produced by closing primarily in a horizontal manner. This is a poorly designed closure option for this defect. **(c)** Alternately, for the same defect a design of an O-T flap with the inferior standing cone and placement of suture lines along the labiomental crease. **(d)** Flap elevation at similar levels for each portion of the O-T flap. **(e)** Completed O-T demonstrating principle of standing cone taken out toward the midpoint of the chin and superior suture lines falling within the labiomental crease.

to the rule that primary closures oriented vertically have a better long-term outcome. However, patients can have differing facial contours, laxity, and defects. As with any primary closure, it is sometimes advantageous to undermine the circular defect in all directions and assess where the natural skin tension vectors "want" to close the defect. Burow's triangles should be long enough to account for the convexity of the chin. Otherwise, standing cone deformity is visible from many angles.

9.3.4 Bilateral Advancement (O-T flap)

The O-T flap (bilateral, single tangent flap) is a go-to flap for chin repairs (see ▶ Fig. 9.3, ▶ Fig. 9.8, and ▶ Fig. 9.9). Often, the convexity of the chin requires removal of longer dog-ears, and often, they will extend through the labiomental crease. Whenever the defect requires removal of a dog-ear that will cross the labiomental crease, the crease should be used as the line that defines the superior border (or the horizontal incision) for an O-T flap. This crossing arm of the "T" will often be curvilinear, following the crease. This at times will appear more consistent with a bilateral rotation flap. If a defect is closer to the inferior border of the chin, the O-T flap can be flipped so that the horizontal line of the T is along the inferior border of the mandible (see ▶ Fig. 9.6). The inferior dog-ear should ideally not cross the most inferior edge of the mandible. Crossing this prominence can lead to tethering of the scar to the bony prominence. A tethered appearance is not a certainty, and linear closures can often produce very acceptable outcomes. If a defect is sizable enough that an inferior dog-ear should cross onto the submental neck, and the superior dog-ear would cross the labiomental crease, one should consider a bilateral double tangent (O-H) flap. Horizontal lines can hide well within the labiomental crease and just under the chin on the submental neck. The O-T flap can be tailored to the site regardless of whether it is midline, or more laterally (see ▶ Fig. 9.4). The vertical arm of the T should be designed toward the central point of the chin, much like the spokes of a wheel radiating from the hub (chin midpoint) to the outer wheel (mental crease). When defects do not fall on midline, the dog-ear should follow the curvilinear shape of the relaxed skin tension lines on the chin. Again, this is generally a sickle shape curving laterally at the most convex point.

A key suture for this repair is the initial suture closing the defect side to side (near the superior end of the vertical suture line). It is helpful to avoid placing this key first stitch far enough away from the tips to avoid compromising blood supply. For very lax chins, the author prefers use of 5–0 Vicryl suture placed in a buried vertical mattress fashion. For deeper defects with thicker chins or a less mobile reservoir, 4–0 Vicryl suture is preferred. The crossing arm of the "T" will have a slightly shorter distance along the moving side of the flap. The disparate lengths require one to "sew out" the dog-ear or laxity that would need to be removed to avoid "bunching" of the nonmobile or standing wound edge. This is often necessary for rotation flaps if a Burow'striangle is not

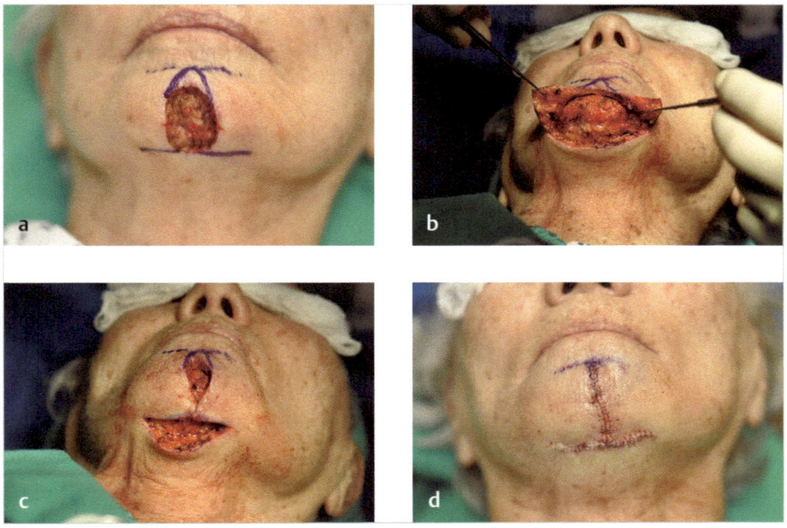

Fig. 9.9 (a) Defect on lower portion of chin with design utilizing incision along the chin and submental border. **(b)** Flap elevation with meticulous hemostasis. **(c)** Key suture placed at the broadest portion of defect near the meeting point of the "T." Note the sutures are not placed directly into the tips of the flaps to prevent tip necrosis. **(d)** Completed repair showing symmetry with suture line along the mental cleft and the chinsubmental border.

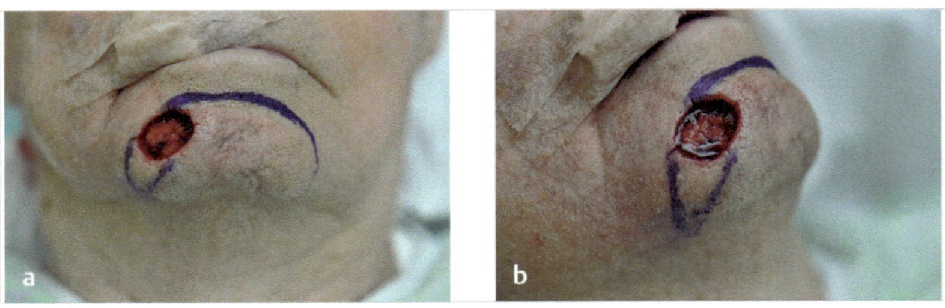

Fig. 9.10 (a, b) Design of V-Y flap recruited inferior and lateral to the defect to maintain curvilinear convex nature of the lateral chin. The superior edge of the V-Y flap will be a continuation of the labiomental crease.

removed at the end of the arc. The need to remove a Burow's triangle at either end can be overcome by sewing the edge with the "rule of halves" or by taking a crescentic Burow's, which lengthens the mobile ("sliding edge") of the flap to match the longer nonsliding edge of the flap and negate the need for Burow's removal.

9.3.5 V-Y Advancement Flap

The V-Y advancement utilizes a dog-ear-shaped piece of tissue to advance into the defect leaving the underlying vascular pedicle (see ▸ Fig. 9.4 and ▸ Fig. 9.10). This flap is used when there is overwhelming lateral tension for a bilateral advancement (O-T) or primary closure. This flap often works well when defects are in the midline of the chin or very laterally on the cosmetic subunit. The midline defect often has options that heal with better suture lines hidden in the crease (such as the O-T flap outlined earlier). However, if there is insufficient laxity laterally, sliding a V-Y flap from the inferior laxity can be helpful. A similar outcome occurs with the use of a Burow's triangle graft in this same manner. The defect should be sufficiently undermined in all directions prior to sliding the **V**-shaped flap into place. Sufficient undermining of the flap laterally as opposed to straight down will achieve movement while maintaining a sufficient vascular pedicle. Due to the usual rich muscular subcutis in this area, this flap is generally very robust. However, tension along the most superior edge of the flap should be minimized with deeper expansive undermining. After aligning the uppermost portion of the flap to the superior edge of the defect, the secondary defect is closed in a linear fashion. A first key suture is the one that aligns the leading edge of the flap to the superior border of the defect. A second key suture is the closure of the secondary defect. It is often helpful to perform these in this order. Next, sutures are placed to close the secondary defect in a linear fashion. Finally, sutures are placed along the sides of the **V**-shaped flap, taking special precaution to keep sutures placed in a way that does not compromise blood supply ("small bites"). It is important to "inset" the flap within the defect to avoid a pincushion appearance of the flap as the end result. Furthermore, appropriate undermining circumferentially around the defect prior to initiating flap elevation will help mitigate the risk of the trapdoor appearance.

The author finds this flap to be most helpful for midline defects on skin that has limited lateral laxity and more laxity inferiorly. Another suitable use of this flap is on laterally based defects where crescentic primary closure is anatomically distorting due to tension on the lower cutaneous lip or displacement of the mental crease. By utilizing laxity inferior to and lateral to the defect on a taut chin, a curvilinear shaped V flap can be slid upward and medially to achieve a cosmetically appealing closure. The superolateral border of the V-Y flap suture line can fall within the labiomental crease. The flap stays within the cosmetic subunit, or at worse extends inferiorly to the submental neck typically out of sight.

A drawback of this flap includes the number of suture lines and time of suturing required. Suture lines resting in the borders of the subunit are preferred. V-Y flaps typically will have at least one suture line that is not along the resting skin tension lines. Other drawbacks include the potential for a pincushion or trapdoor appearance, which can be mitigated with proper undermining and meticulous suturing technique.

9.3.6 Rotation flaps

When a defect is too broad for the options previously outlined, recruitment of lateral and inferior laxity is necessary. This tissue can be utilized with a unilateral rotation flap. Often, to maintain symmetry, a bilateral rotation should be utilized if a defect falls on both sides of the midline. Smaller defects can be readily repaired with unilateral rotation taking a Burow's triangle out in the marionette line opposite the side of the defect. For a larger defect, a curvilinear incision is placed along the mental crease and passes laterally to the inferior border of the mandible (see ▶ Fig. 9.5). This is elevated at the level of the dermis initially, but then diving deeper through and under the mentalis muscle working toward the submandibular neck. If undermining more than 2 cm lateral to the oral commissure, care should be taken to avoid the ascending facial artery and the marginal mandibular nerve.

The laterally based rotation flap does have limitations in movement. Also, there can be obliteration of the marionette lines or prejowl sulcus in a patient with more laxity and prominent jowls. An alternative takeoff point for the flap can be the inferior edge of the defect extending in a curvilinear fashion onto the submental neck and finishing laterally in the submandibular triangle of the neck (see ▶ Fig. 9.6). This inferior-based rotation flap may provide less cosmetic distortion of the prejowl sulcus. However, it is important to realize this flap will require extra length to overcome the convexity of a prominent mental protuberance to cover the most superior portion of the defect.

9.3.7 Transposition flaps

Transposition flaps will typically be reserved for larger defects or in patients who simply have insufficient laxity. A sizable central defect can be readily repaired with a bilobed or trilobed transposition flap, using the reservoir of the submental and/or submandibular neck. Design of this flap should attempt to hide suture lines from the secondary/tertiary defect on the submental neck. As with all chin closures, design of a bilobed flap should consider the convexity of the chin. The primary lobe should typically be slightly undersized for the defect, but should not have so much tension as to compromise blood supply. A design that does not consider the convexity may prove too short to provide coverage of the defect. This inability to "reach" will be most likely on thicker chins with a dense fibrous dermis and subcutis.

A key suture in the bilobed flap is first closing the tertiary defect. This is generally easier to achieve if an assistant transposes the secondary lobe of the flap in an upward fashion with a skin hook to allow placement of this key suture. A second key suture is the placement of the primary lobe into the defect, being sure to inset the flap within the defect. Appropriate undermining of the defect and elevation of the flap in the same plane is important for creating a broad area of contraction that is at the same level during wound healing. Otherwise, there is a risk of a pincushion or trapdoor appearance.

Laterally based transposition flaps that utilize medial cheek skin can provide good coverage of a broad defect when there is sufficient laxity of the cheek. The secondary defect suture lines can be placed along the marionette lines. These are typically reserved for lateral chin defects. Similarly, though less preferred, submandibular laxity can prove useful for larger defects on the lateral chin and jaw area. Special care should be taken to avoid the facial artery when elevating this flap as it crosses the mandible. Also, crossing the mandible with a transposition flap can produce less desirable tethered scarring across the mandible. Finally, asymmetry of the submental or submandibular neck laxity is a possibility. To overcome this asymmetry, bilateral transposition flaps can be utilized.

9.3.8 Full-Thickness Skin Grafts

Full-thickness skin grafting of the chin is considered a last resort for defect repair. One situation that is suitable and sometimes preferred over an advancement or rotation flap is the presence of a midline defect just inferior to the labiomental crease. A Burow's graft can be used here and provides very acceptable cosmesis. However, facial hair preferences should be taken into consideration. A skin graft is more suitable for patients with little or no terminal hair in the area (i.e., female patients). When defects are sizable enough to encompass the entire cosmetic subunit, full-thickness skin grafts can be acceptable cosmetically. Grafts can be harvested from the supraclavicular skin or the postauricular sulcus. However, secondary intention healing will likely provide a more cosmetically appealing appearance.

9.4 Complications and Revisions

A complication of dimpled or pebbled suture lines is not uncommon on a fibrous chin. Use of eversion can help mitigate this. Two to 4 months after closure, scars can be reliably treated with dermabrasion to have a smoother appearance. Areas of focal dehiscence can also be revised at a later date once a scar has matured. Thickened or hypertrophic scars readily respond to intralesional triamcinolone injection. The author prefers to use triamcinolone at a concentration of 20 mg/mL. Flaps with a thickened appearance can be injected 6 to 8 weeks after repair.

Suggested Readings

Benoit A, Leach BC, Cook J. Applications of Burow's grafts in the reconstruction of Mohs micrographic surgery defects. Dermatol Surg. 2017; 43 (4):512–520

Colville RJ, Patel R. The mental rotation flap. J Plast Reconstr Aesthet Surg. 2011; 64(3):e76–e77

Ibrahim AM, Rabie AN, Borud L, Tobias AM, Lee BT, Lin SJ. Common patterns of reconstruction for Mohs defects in the head and neck. J Craniofac Surg. 2014; 25(1):87–92

Larrabee YC, Moyer JS. Reconstruction of Mohs defects of the lips and chin. Facial Plast Surg Clin North Am. 2017; 25(3):427–442

10 Reconstruction of the Eyelids and Eyebrows

Gabriela M. Espinoza and Aleksandar L. Krunic

Abstract

Periocular cutaneous malignancies occur in up to 10% of all skin cancers, while approximately 14% of Mohs defects affect the lower forehead and the brow area. Hence, Mohs surgeons need to be familiar with this highly specialized area of the face. This chapter discusses a variety of techniques utilized for the reconstruction of eyelids, eyebrows, and the periorbital region after Mohs excision. After anatomical considerations of the eyelids and eyebrows, different reconstructive options are discussed and summarized in the algorithm for closure depending on the defect size, location, and thickness. A strict understanding of anatomic relationships and thorough knowledge of the principles of decision making when performing surgery in this area will enable the Mohs surgeon to achieve optimal cosmetic and functional results. Despite challenges that may require the assistance of oculoplastic surgeons, the majority of periocular repairs will have excellent results with proper globe protection and restoration of eyelid integrity.

Keywords: Eyelid anatomy, anterior lamella, posterior lamella, canaliculus, lacrimal system, medial canthus, lateral canthus, canthal tendon, primary closure, full-thickness skin graft, composite graft, wedge-excision, Tenzel semicircular flap, cross-eyelid flap, Hughes tarsoconjunctival flap, brow anatomy, brow reconstruction

Capsule Summary and Pearls

- Normal upper and lower eyelid structure is critical for globe protection and visual function.
- Restoration of eyelid integrity is critical for optimal functional and cosmetic reconstruction.
- The defects of the anterior and posterior lamella must be individually evaluated in order to choose the appropriate repair technique.
- If defects of medial canthi involve the lacrimal system, they may be assessed and repaired in consultation with an oculoplastic specialist.
- Brow reconstruction should consider aesthetic position of the brows, retention of brow symmetry, and the direction of the growth of the hair follicles.

10.1 Introduction

The eyes, eyebrows, and periocular area are the central aesthetic unit of the face. The functional and aesthetic importance of this region cannot be overestimated.

"The beauty of a woman must be seen from in her eyes, because that is the doorway to her heart, the place where the love resides."

—Audrey Hepburn, British Actress (1929–1993)

Reconstruction[1,2] of the eyelids is one of the most challenging areas in reconstructive surgery. No other region has such a delicate interaction of anatomy, function, and aesthetics. The primary goal in eyelid reconstruction is to restore a functional eyelid to protect the eye and permit normal vision. Proper eyelid function is required to maintain a normal tear film to avoid corneal irritation, desiccation, or perforation. The repaired eyelids should have normal appearance due to its critical importance in social relationships (secondary goal). Surgical objectives in the reconstructive process are[1,2,3,4]:

a) Align conjunctiva (nonkeratinized mucosal epithelium against the eye).
b) Provide support with firm connective tissue frame to appose the globe.
c) Enable adequate protractor muscle function and supple thin skin to facilitate and permit normal eyelid movements.
d) Obtain stable eyelid margin to prevent inappropriate turning of eyelids (ectropion, entropion, trichiasis) and irritation of the cornea and the globe.

The goal of this chapter is to present several reliably effective techniques that will address the majority of common defects to be encountered in the daily practice of Mohs surgery. Mohs micrographic surgery is ideal for skin cancer removal in the eyelid area as a cost effective, tissue-sparing procedure with the highest rate of cure.[2,3] Recent reports by Clark et al[5] showed that the safety profile of reconstruction after Mohs surgery performed under local anesthesia is comparable to ones performed by oculoplastic surgeons under general anesthesia.

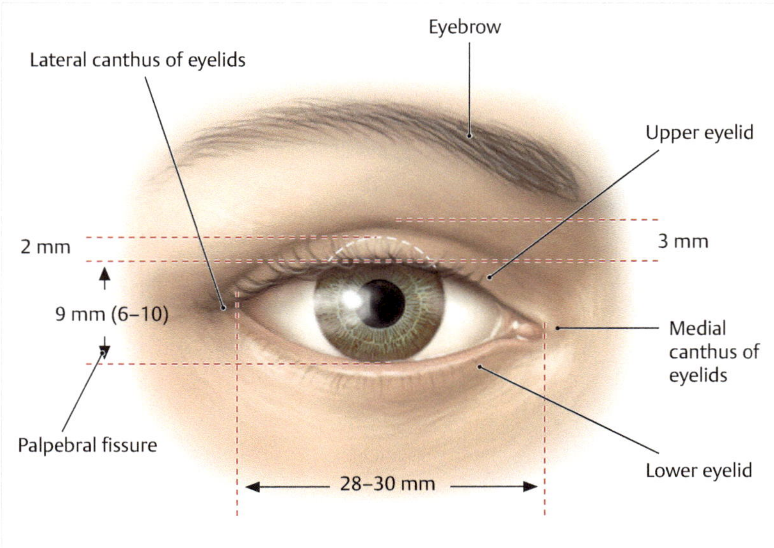

Fig. 10.1 Topography of the right eyelid. The highest point of the brow is at, or lateral to, the lateral limbus. The inferior edge of the brow is typically 10 mm superior to the supraorbital rim. Average palpebral height (10–12 mm), width (28–30 mm), and upper lid fold height (8–11 mm) vary with gender and racial differences. Note that the lateral canthus is 2 to 4 mm higher than the medial canthus. Intrapalpebral distance measures 10–12 mm. (Reproduced from Baker E, Lopez E, Schünke M, et al. Anatomy for Dental Medicine. Illustrations by M. Voll and K. Wesker. 3rd ed. New York: Thieme; 2020.)

10.2 Surgical Anatomy of the Eyelids and Eyebrows

The surgical anatomy of the eyelids and periocular area is one of the most complex parts of the head and neck.[6–8] Before one embarks on performing a variety of simple or more complicated reconstructive procedures in periocular area, thorough knowledge of surgical anatomy is mandatory. The purpose of this text is not just to reacquaint the leader with well-documented gross morphology of the eyelids and brows, but also to review newer concepts of eyelid anatomy relevant for clinical practice.

10.2.1 Superficial Topography of the Lids and Eyebrows (▸ Fig. 10.1)

The eyelids are complex lamellar structures responsible for globe protection and integrity of the ocular surface. The architecture of the eyelids must be respected to provide satisfactory repairs, both functionally and aesthetically.[9–12] The eyelids are for practical purposes divided into *anterior* (skin and muscle) and *posterior* (tarsus and conjunctiva) *lamella* (▸ Fig. 10.2). The orbital septum (OS) is considered a "middle lamella" by some authors due to its surgical and anatomic importance as a boundary between the preseptal soft tissues and postseptal content of the orbit. Of note, septum should not be repaired directly (aka "self-healing" layer), since it leads to tethering and lid retraction. For reconstruction purposes it is essential that at least one lamella have an intact blood supply.[8]

The eyebrows are approximately 4.5 to 5 cm long and slightly differ in female and male patients[8,13,14] (▸ Table 10.1). The female eyebrows are typically arched, with the highest point projecting at, or slightly lateral to the limbus, approximately 1 cm from the orbital rim, 1.5 cm and 2.5 cm from upper lid crease and pupil, respectively. The male eyebrow is less peaked and is positioned more closely to the orbital rim. The position of the brows is the result of opposing forces of brow elevator (frontalis muscle) and brow depressors (orbicularis oculi, procerus, and corrugators muscles). The soft tissue of the eyebrows consists of four layers[8,13]: (a) skin and subcutaneous tissue; (b) muscle; (c) retroorbicularis oculi fat (ROOF); and (d) periosteum. The lateral brow is firmly attached to temporalis fascia, which is also more prominent in males.[13]

The eyebrow hair is thinner in Asians, and thicker in Caucasians and comprises 200 to 400 follicular units (FU), each containing single hair shaft or rarely two, in contrast to the scalp hair, where four shafts can be found per FU.[8,14,15] In addition, the eyebrow hair follicle direction needs to be well understood and is of utmost importance when designing brow incisions, orienting flap repairs, or using hair transplant techniques or composite grafts to restore lost supercilia. Centrally (brow body) and laterally (brow tail) the hair follicles are directed inferiorly, while medially (brow head) hairs and ones on the lower brows are directed superiorly (see following text). Eyebrows' hair shafts lie quite flat on skin surface since they exit at very acute angle of 30 degrees. Eyebrow hair typically regrows within 6 months following plucking; however, repeated damage to eyebrow FU can result in traction alopecia and reduce growth over time. The three types of hair in the eyebrow are (a) fine, vellus hair; (b) the slightly larger and lightly pigmented hair; and (c) the large terminal hair, also known as the supercilia. The fine vellus hairs form an effective moisture barrier to keep sweat from running downward into the eye. The fluid flow is redirected medially and laterally, away from the eye.[8,15]

The eyelid skin is among the thinnest in the body and lacks underlying fat, which facilitates mobility but results

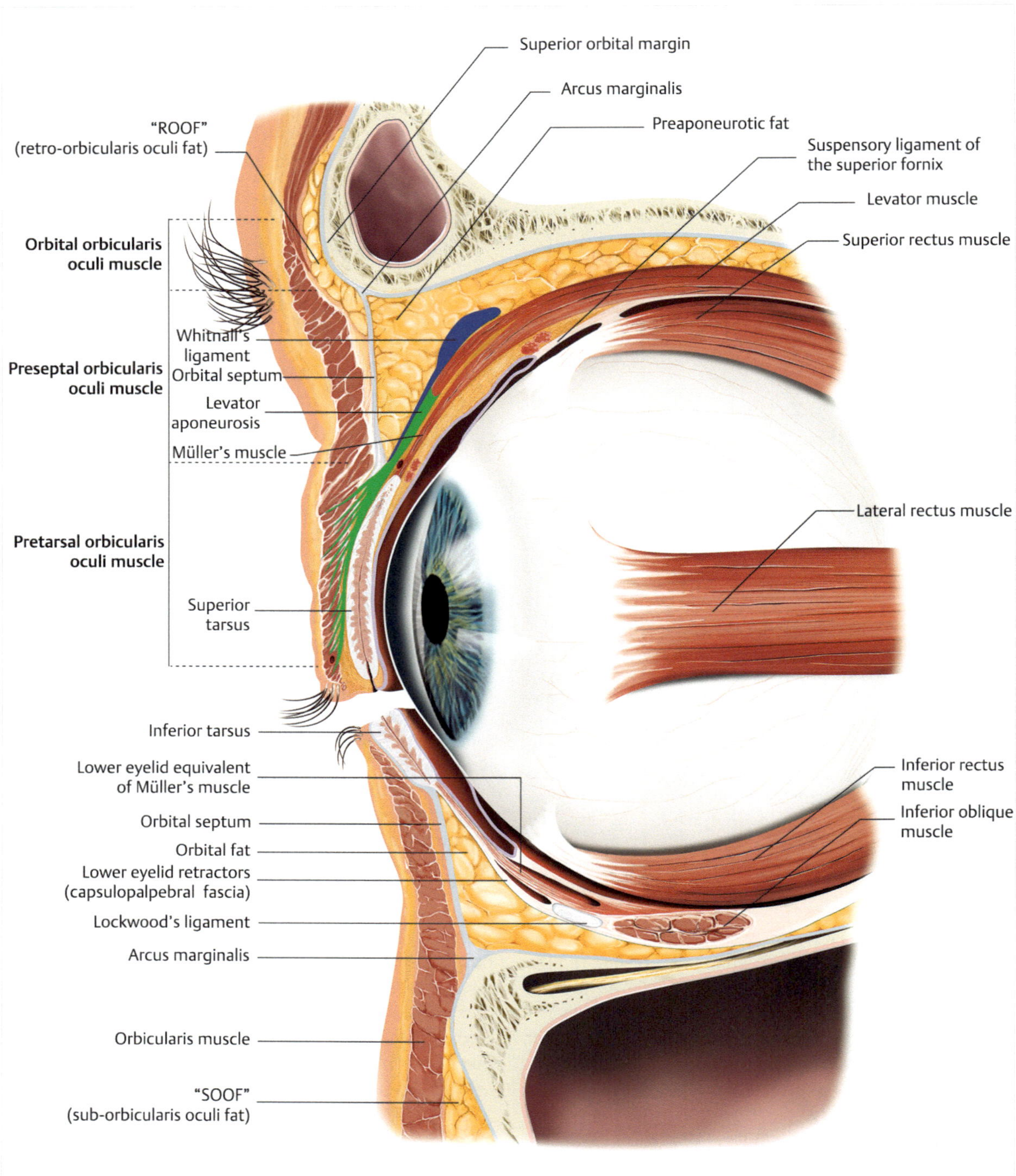

Fig. 10.2 Anterior and posterior lamella. The anterior lamella (*blue*) consists of skin, connective tissue, and orbicularis muscle, whereas the posterior lamella (*red*) consists of the tarsal plate and palpebral conjunctiva. (Reproduced from Leatherbarrow B. Oculoplastic Surgery. 3rd ed. New York: Thieme; 2019.)

Table 10.1 Anatomic and topographic differences of male vs. female upper face

	Male	Female
Forehead	>Width and height (avg. 6 cm)	<Width and height (avg. 5 cm)
Glabella	>Width and projection	<Width and projection
Orbit	Larger	Smaller and more oval
Orbit/skull ratio	Smaller	Larger
Brow	Thicker, positioned at the level of the rim, flat with none to minimal arching, no prominent peak or lateral tapering	Medially club shaped, positioned above the rim, ascend and arch laterally to its peak, tapers laterally
Upper eyelid	8–9 mm crease height, fuller with minimal pretarsal show	9–12 mm crease height, moderate pretarsal show
Lateral canthus	Neutral to slightly positive tilt	Neutral to positive tilt

in disproportionate redundancy with aging.[6,9] Relatively abrupt transition from thicker malar and brow skin renders the eyelids distinct and it should be respected when developing the reconstructive plan. Advancement and transposition flaps using lid skin provide the best color, thickness, and texture match. The adult *palpebral fissure* measures on average 10 to 12 mm vertically (midpupillary line) and 28 to 33 mm horizontally (horizontal palpebral aperture), with the upper eyelid covering upper limbus 1 to 2 mm, and the lower eyelid margin typically resting at the inferior limbus. The distance from the *lateral canthus* to the orbital rim is approximately 5 mm, and it is positioned approximately 2 to 4 mm higher than *medial canthus*. The upper and lower eyelid meet at an angle of ~60 degrees.[6,7,8,9] The highest point of the upper eyelid is just nasal to the midpupillary line, while the lowest point of the lower eyelid is lateral to the midpupillary line. The lateral canthus stabilizes the eyelid in direct apposition to the globe, while the medial canthus is more anteriorly located and is intimately associated with lacrimal sac.[6,9]

The *upper eyelid crease* (formed by the attachment of levator aponeurosis [LA] which interdigitates with orbicularis oculi at the superior tarsal margin) is typically 7 to 8 mm above the lid margin in men, and 10 to 12 mm in women. In Asians, the upper lid crease is much lower or absent due to lower insertion of the septum or lower or absent insertion of the LA (2–3 mm above the lid margin).[10,11] This anatomical arrangement allows the preaponeurotic fat to extend further into the eyelid. In the lower eyelid, septum fuses with capsulopalpebral fascia about 5 mm inferior to the tarsus forming the *lower eyelid crease* which is less visible and presents approximately 3 to 4 mm below the central and 5 to 6 mm below the lateral third of the lower lid margin, respectively.[8,9]

Interpalpebral distance of 10 to 12 mm can be further divided to margin-to-reflex distance (MRD) 1 (superior) and 2 (inferior) or MRD1 and MRD2. This is measured from the center of the pupil to the inferior edge of the upper eyelid, or superior edge of the lower eyelid, respectively. Its practical importance is the assessment of ptosis or eyelid retraction. Decreased intrapalpebral distance with a smaller MRD1 or MRD2 represents ptosis that can cause visual field obstruction. Increased interpalpebral distance with a higher MRD1 or MRD2 may mean eyelid retraction that causes exposure or ectropion.[8,9,16] The contour of the eyelid needs to be respected in any reconstructive procedure to ensure naturally appearing lid margins and optimal aesthetic result.

The eyelid margin, when closely inspected, has multiple linear structures including *lashes* (anteriorly), *Meibomian glands* (posteriorly), and the *gray line* (in-between).[6,8,9] Meibomian glands present the transition of anterior skin to orbital conjunctiva. Gray line is also known as the *muscle of Riolan*, which presents the most superficial extent of pretarsal orbicularis oculi muscle. This line presents important surgical landmark in tarsal strip procedure for reconstruction of the lateral canthus since it marks an anatomical separation of the anterior skin-muscle lamella from the posterior tarsus-conjunctiva lamella. The gray line also enables bloodless surgical dissection down to the septum and approach to the superior and inferior orbital margin.[6,9]

The most important differences between topography of the upper face in males vs. females are summarized in ▸ Table 10.1.

10.2.2 Orbicularis Oculi Muscle (OOM)[6,8,9] (▸ Fig. 10.3 and ▸ Fig. 10.4)

The *orbicularis oculi* is a contiguous muscle composed of *pars palpebralis* (pretarsal and preseptal) and *pars orbitalis*. This is the main eyelid protractor involved in blinking or voluntary winking (palpebral part) or forced eyelid closure (orbital part). The upper and lower pretarsal segment originate from deep and superficial heads of the medial canthal tendon (MCT) and then extend laterally over upper and lower tarsal plate in a horizontal fashion to form the lateral canthal tendon (LCT). Preseptal part originates from the borders of MCT and overlays OS in both upper and lower lid and ends near the lateral

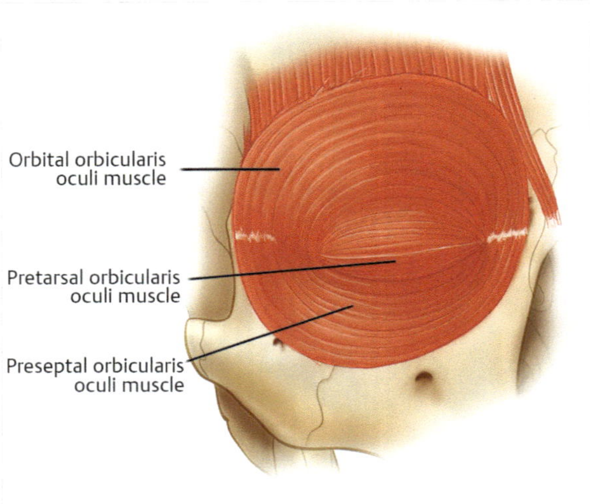

Fig. 10.3 Orbicularis oculi muscle. The muscle is traditionally divided into orbital and palpebral portions. The orbital portion arises from the anterior aspect of the MCT (medial canthal tendon) and the periosteum above and below it. The palpebral portion is further subdivided into pretarsal and preseptal portions, each lying over the tarsal plate or orbital septum, respectively. (Reproduced from Codner M, McCord C. Eyelid & Periorbital Surgery. 2nd ed. New York: Thieme; 2016.)

horizontal raphe. Apart from helping with blinking reflex (corneal reflex) pretarsal part assists the lacrimal pump (medial pretarsal portion of OOM, aka as tensor tarsi or "Horner's muscle"), maintains position of the canthal angle, and tightens the eyelid against the globe.

The orbital segment presents as concentric loops starting from maxillary and orbital processes of the frontal bone as well as MCT; the loops course along the orbital rim, extending superiorly into the forehead, up to 3 to 4 cm beyond the lateral canthus, and inferiorly to the variable distance on the cheek. They do not interrupt at the lateral commissure like the palpebral portion. The orbital part of OOM overlies frontalis muscle and corrugator supercilii, interdigitating with them along its superior border. Laterally the OOM covers the anterior temporalis fascia and inferiorly the origin of the lip elevators. It is innervated by zygomatic and temporal branches of the fascial nerve, which travel along its inferior surface.

Posterior to OOM and anterior to OS lies the *postorbicular fascial plane*, which provides avascular plane for easy dissection and identification of the OS in ocular reconstruction. In this plane, there is also adipose tissue known as *retroorbicularis oculi fat (ROOF)* and *suborbicularis oculi fat (SOOF)*. The ROOF is present beneath the ciliary portion of the brow and extends inferiorly under the orbital part of OOM. It contributes to eyebrow volume and helps mobility of lateral brow and eyelid. The SOOF continues inferiorly below the *orbitomalar ligament* which starts from arcus marginalis of bony orbit and inserts on the skin of the lower lid passing through fibers of OOM. The skin attachments of this ligament contribute to *nasojugal* and *malar folds*, respectively. Ptosis of the SOOF can lead to "malar bags" and contour deformities because the inferior orbital rim becomes exposed. In conjunction with the prolapse of the orbital fat (see following text), it can create characteristic "double contour" deformity of the lower eyelid. Hence, reposition of the SOOF is an important consideration in rejuvenation of the midface (▶ Fig. 10.4).[6,9]

10.2.3 Orbital Septum (OS) and Postseptal Fat Compartments (▶ Fig. 10.4 and ▶ Fig. 10.5)

The *orbital septum* is a thin sheet of fibrous multilayered connective tissue which arises circumferentially from the arcus marginalis of the orbital periosteum. It encircles the orbit as a continuation of the orbital fascial unit. The OS is very resistant to traction since it is firmly attached to arcus marginalis and as such can be easily identified during surgical procedure. In young patients it is relatively thick, while in older can be thin and dehiscent. Functionally, the OS acts as a barrier to infection and hemorrhage. In Caucasian upper lid, OS usually fuses with the LA approximately 3 to 5 mm above the tarsus, although it can vary from 0 to 15 mm from the superior tarsal edge. The fusion is more inferior or absent in Asian lids. In the lower lid OS fuses with capsulopalpebral fascia about 5 mm below the inferior tarsal plate.[8,9]

The *postseptal orbital fat compartments (preaponeurotic fat pads)* are divided in superior and inferior ones. *Superior compartments* comprise medial or nasal and central or preaponeurotic pads. The medial and central fat pads are separated by the trochlea, the tendon of superior oblique muscle and the median horn of the LA along with thin fascial strands of *Whitnall's ligament (superior transverse ligament)*, which further extends laterally over the *lacrimal gland* (located in the lateral upper eyelid postseptal compartment) to the superior edge of the rectus muscle. This ligament lies deep to the levator, forms a sleeve around levator palpebrae superioris, and acts as a pulley for this muscle. The medial fat pad is firmer and paler and is intimately adjacent to the medial palpebral artery and supratrochlear nerve. The preservation of the trochlea is of utmost importance in ptosis surgery, since its damage may result in superior oblique palsy or Brown's syndrome.[11,12]

The *inferior orbital fat pads* are divided into lateral, central, and medial pads. The inferior, central, and lateral compartments are continuous, separated anteriorly by *Lockwood's ligament (suspensory ligament of the eye)* (arcuate extension of capsulopalpebral fascia and inferior oblique muscle) while inferior, oblique muscle separates medial and central pads. The Lockwood's ligament is actually condensation of capsulopalpebral fascia (see following text) and serves as supportive sling for the globe. The lower eyelid medial fat pad is firmer and paler as the

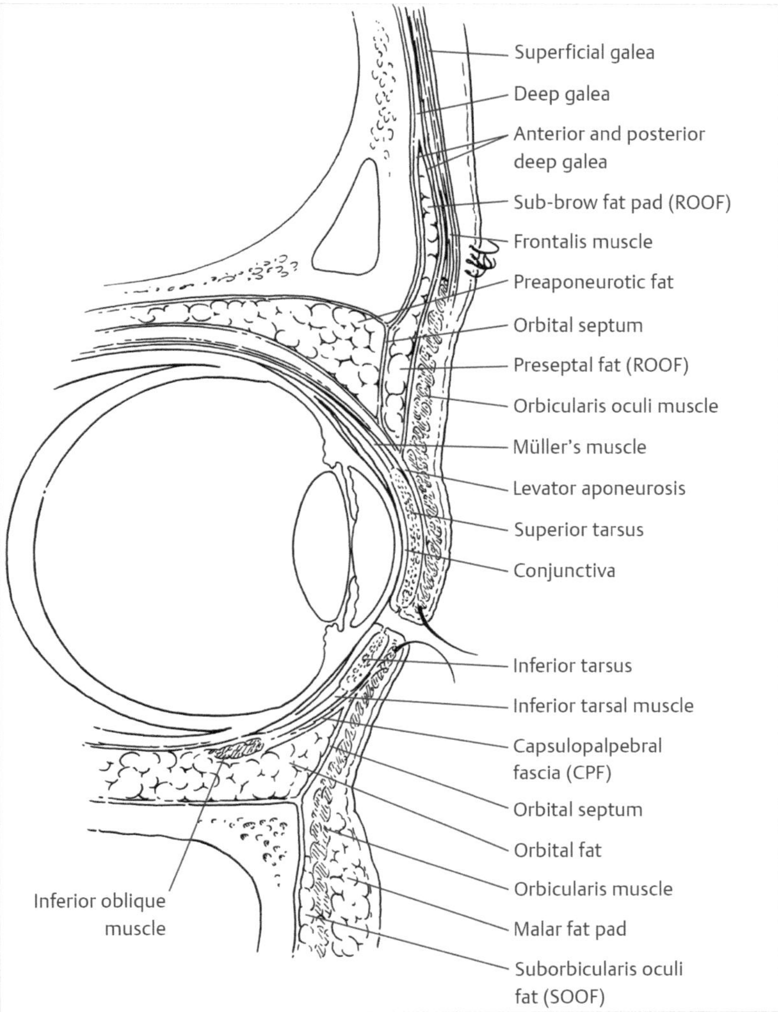

Fig. 10.4 Cross-sectional anatomy of the upper and lower lids and brows. The capsulopalpebral fascia and inferior tarsal muscle are retractors of the lower lid whereas Müller's muscle, the levator muscle, and its aponeurosis are retractors of the upper lid. Note the preseptal positioning of retroorbicularis oculi and suborbicularis oculi fat (ROOF and SOOF, respectively). The orbitomalar ligament arises from the arcus marginalis of the inferior orbital rim and inserts on skin of the lower lid, forming the nasojugal fold. (Reproduced from Papel I, Frodel J, Holt R, et al. Facial Plastic and Reconstructive Surgery. 4th ed. New York: Thieme; 2016.)

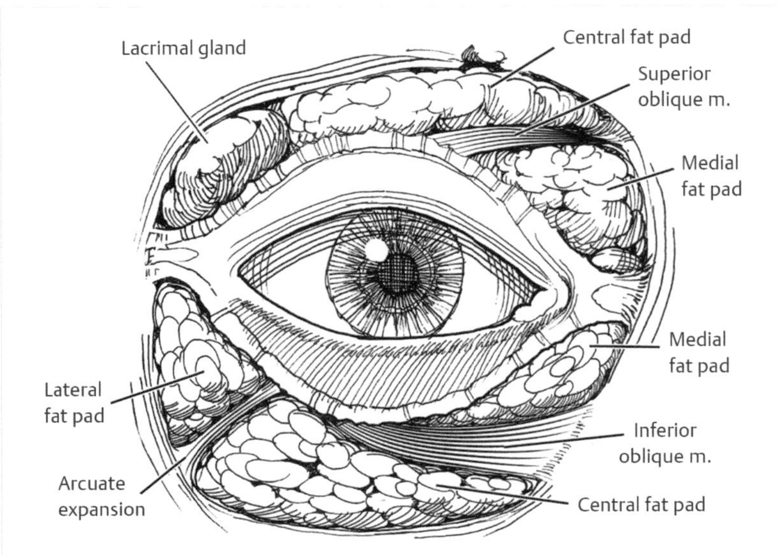

Fig. 10.5 Eyelid fat compartments. (Reproduced from Fedok F, Carniol P. Minimally Invasive and Office-Based Procedures in Facial Plastic Surgery. New York: Thieme; 2013.)

nasal one in the upper eyelid. It is important to avoid damage of the inferior oblique muscle when exploring or manipulating the medial fat pad, since that may result in diplopia and strabismus. Weakening of the OS can produce prolapse of postseptal fat anteriorly in both upper and lower eyelids; since the fat itself is intact these are called pseudoherniations. Prolapse of the lacrimal gland should not be mistaken for fat pad in the upper eyelid, and one should avoid excising it accidentally. The lacrimal gland can be differentiated from preaponeurotic fat by its firm, tan color, vascular, lobulated structure to avoid perioperative injury.[6,9]

Central preaponeurotic fat pads in both upper and lower eyelid are important surgical landmarks since they lie anterior to eyelid retractors and immediately posterior to OS. The lateral fat pad in the lower eyelid extends superiorly between the OS and the LCT and acts as a bursa during eyelid movements (Eisler's pocket).[9] The OS should not be sutured or repaired directly without traction of the eyelid in the opposite direction since there is a risk of significant eyelid retraction and lagophthalmos. Conversely, it is of utmost importance to identify eyelid retractors (levator aponeurosis or capsulopalpebral fascia) and separate it from OS before advancing one or the other in the eyelid reconstruction. Otherwise, significant shortening of the repaired eyelid may develop and result in lagophthalmos.[9]

10.2.4 Tarsoligamentous Sling (▶ Fig. 10.6)

Tarsal plates anatomically resemble cartilaginous structures but are actually made of dense fibrous tissue which is approximately 30 mm in length and 1 mm in thickness. Along with MCT and LCT they form a *tarsoligamentous sling* which provides support for the eyelids, as well as lattice for the insertion of the OS and muscles of eyelid retraction. The pretarsal skin is firmly attached to the underlying tarsal plate contrary to highly elastic preseptal skin, thereby allowing intense edematous response of preseptal eyelid at the postsurgical period. The superior tarsus is approximately 8 to 12 mm high, while the inferior eyelid tarsus is approximately one-third of its height (i.e., 4–5 mm). In Asian patients the tarsus measurements differ slightly with superior tarsus being up to 8 mm and inferior 5 mm high, respectively. The underside of each tarsus is aligned by densely adherent palpebral conjunctiva. Tarsal plates contain 20 to 30 vertically aligned multilobulated Meibomian glands which secrete important component of the tear film to prevent excessive tear evaporation and "dry eye" syndrome. The glands open on the posterior eyelid margin right behind the gray line.[6,8]

The *medial canthal tendon* (MCT; ▶ Fig. 10.6) is the centerpiece of medial canthal anatomy. It has an elastic lateral portion that supports lacrimal canaliculi and then splits in the anterior, superior, and posterior limbs, all of which then blend into the lacrimal sac fascia. The thicker anterior limb inserts on the orbital process of the maxillary bone (anterior to the lacrimal crest) and is formed by superficial head of the pretarsal orbicularis muscle. The thinner posterior limb is the extension of the fascia of deep head of the pretarsal orbicularis and inserts on the posterior lacrimal crest. The superior branch extends to lacrimal sac apex and covers it anteriorly and superiorly. These arrays of fibrous bands work as an isolated soft-tissue pump of the lacrimal drainage system and insert on the orbital process of the frontal bones. The posterior head of the preseptal OOM inserts here forming the soft tissue roof of the lacrimal sac fossa.[6,7,9]

The *lateral canthal tendon* (LCT) anchors the tarsal plates and lateral regions of pretarsal/preseptal orbicularis to orbital wall posteriorly and superolaterally to Whitnall's

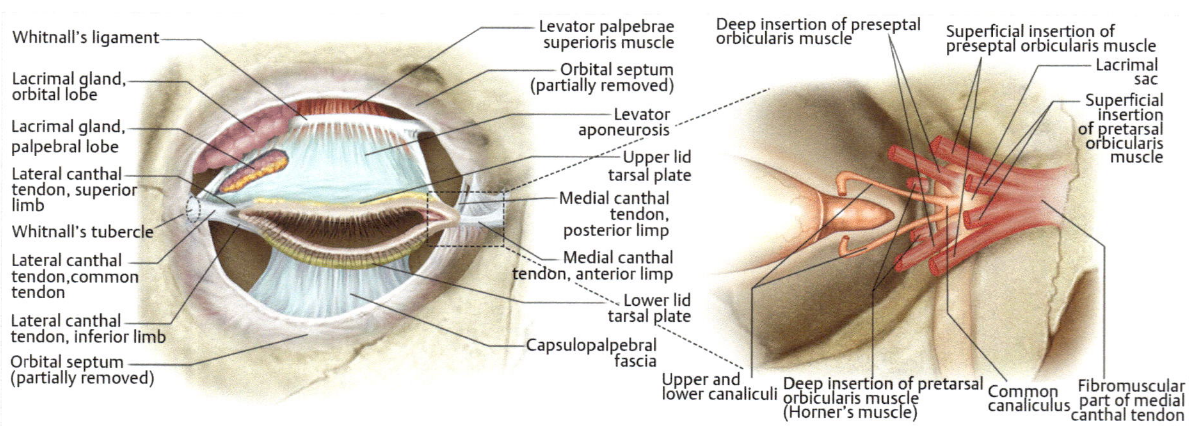

Fig. 10.6 Major retractors of the upper and lower eyelids (left) and medial canthal tendon structure (right): superior tarsal plate, lateral horn of levator aponeurosis, inferior tarsal plate, Lockwood's suspensory ligament, Whitnall's suspensory ligament, levator aponeurosis, medial horn of levator aponeurosis, and capsulopalpebral fascia. (Reproduced from Watanabe K, Shoja MM, Loukas M, Tubbs RS. Anatomy for Plastic Surgery of the Face, Head, and Neck. New York: Thieme; 2016.)

tubercle, 1.5 mm inside the lateral orbital margin. This unique anchoring system allows the lateral canthal angle to move in both vertical and lateral directions with the lateral gaze. Surgical manipulation of this structure is sometimes required to prevent unwanted ectropion and maintain lid globe apposition. The LCT measures 1 mm in thickness, 5 to 7 mm in length, and 3 mm in width at the point where superior and inferior crus unite. Then it broadens to 6 to 7 mm before its lateral insertion. At the superior edge, LCT blends with the lateral horn of the LA, inferolateral fibers of Whitnall's superior suspensory ligament, and lateral portion of Lockwood's inferior suspensory ligament (lateral retinaculum). The inferior crus of the LCT is divided in the lateral tarsal strip procedure (see following text) and for the tension release during canthotomy and cantholysis in the lower eyelid repair. The superior crus of LCT is divided for the tension release in the upper eyelid reconstruction (see following text). The intimate relationship with the lateral retinaculum (see earlier in the chapter) should be respected when performing division of the superior crus to avoid injury of this structure as well as palpebral part of the lacrimal gland.[1,2,8]

10.2.5 Eyelid Retractors (▶ Fig. 10.2 and ▶ Fig. 10.4)

The primary upper eyelid retractors are *levator palpebrae superioris* (innervated by oculomotor nerve) and *superior tarsal (Müller's) muscle* (innervated by sympathetic nervous system).[7,9] The proximal (muscle portion) of levator palpebrae arises from greater wing of sphenoid bone and is 40 mm long, while the distal aponeurotic portion is 14 to 20 mm long aka *levator aponeurosis (LA)*. This transition occurs at the region of Whitnall's ligament (see earlier in the chapter) where the central part inserts on the anterior tarsus while the lateral horns separate lacrimal gland in orbital and palpebral portion before they insert onto the LCT. Medial portion of the aponeurosis inserts on the posterior portion of the MCT. The LA comprises actually two layers: anterior (thicker with few muscle fibers) which fuses with OS few millimeters above the tarsus and posterior (thinner, more elastic) with the attachment the both the lower third of the tarsal plate and eyelids' subcutaneous tissue forming upper eyelid crease (see earlier in the chapter). With age, LA tends to elongate leading to involutional ptosis which can be usually corrected with the advancement of the aponeurotic attachment. Müller's muscle attaches to the anterior edge of the tarsal plate and is bordered anteriorly by LA and posteriorly by conjunctiva. It is responsible for 2- to 3-mm upper eyelid retraction and regulates the tension of the posterior lamella. The function of upper eyelid retractors is assessed by measuring the *upper eyelid excursion*, i.e., the movement of the upper eyelid from extreme downward gaze to extreme upward gaze with the eyebrow fixed by the digital pressure and is typically 10 to 15 mm.[6–8,11]

The primary retractor of the lower lid is *capsulopalpebral fascia (CPF)* and the *inferior tarsal muscle*, both of which ultimately attach to the lower tarsal plate. The CPF arises from rectus inferior muscle (capsulopalpebral head) as dense connective tissue expansion, wraps anteriorly around oblique inferior muscle, and contributes to Lockwood's ligament (see earlier in the chapter). At this point, the majority of fascia invests into the inferior border of the lower lid tarsal plate, with projections to the skin and the formation of the lower lid crease. It also fuses with OS several millimeters below the tarsal plate. The loss of attachments of CPF to tarsus can cause rotational instability of the lower eyelid and entropion. The inferior tarsal muscle is less developed than its superior counterpart and arises near the capsulopalpebral head, runs under the CPF, and inserts few millimeters below the inferior border of lower lid tarsus. Fortunately, disruption of this smooth muscle during surgery rarely results in eyelid malposition.[6,8,11]

10.2.6 Conjunctiva

The *conjunctiva* comprises a nonkeratinizing epithelium which lines the inner portion of the eyelid and is further divided into *bulbar* (covering large portion of the sclera to corneal limbus), *palpebral* (covering posterior tarsal surface and tarsal muscle), and *forniceal (superior and inferior)* covering apical interface of the eyelids and globe.[7–9] Conjunctival fornices have redundant tissue, permitting eyes to move freely. A healthy conjunctiva contains copious goblet cells which produce mucin for lubrication, as well as accessory lacrimal glands. Significant conjunctival loss can result in motility deficits, lid malposition, and ocular surface damage. Conjunctiva of the superior and inferior fornix, being redundant and freely movable, could also be advanced to substitute the loss of tarsal conjunctiva during periocular reconstruction. The superior fornix is stated to be about 10 mm above the superior corneal limbus, and the inferior fornix is about 8 mm below the inferior corneal limbus. They are supported by fine suspensory ligaments deriving from levator muscle and superior rectus (superior fornix) and Lockwood's ligament (inferior fornix). The medial canthus contains the caruncle which is modified skin with hair follicles, accessory lacrimal glands, sweat glands and sebaceous glands, and the plica semilunaris—a vertical fold lateral to the caruncle. The juncture between plica semilunaris and caruncle is surgically important as an access plane to the medial orbital wall.[9]

10.2.7 Lacrimal System (▶ Fig. 10.7)

The *lacrimal gland*[9] consists of two lobes (orbital and palpebral) divided by the LA. The adjacent palpebral lobe drains aqueous tears into the superolateral fornix, where significant scarring can result in xerophthalmia (dry eye). The "wiper-blade" action of OOM and tarsal plates moves

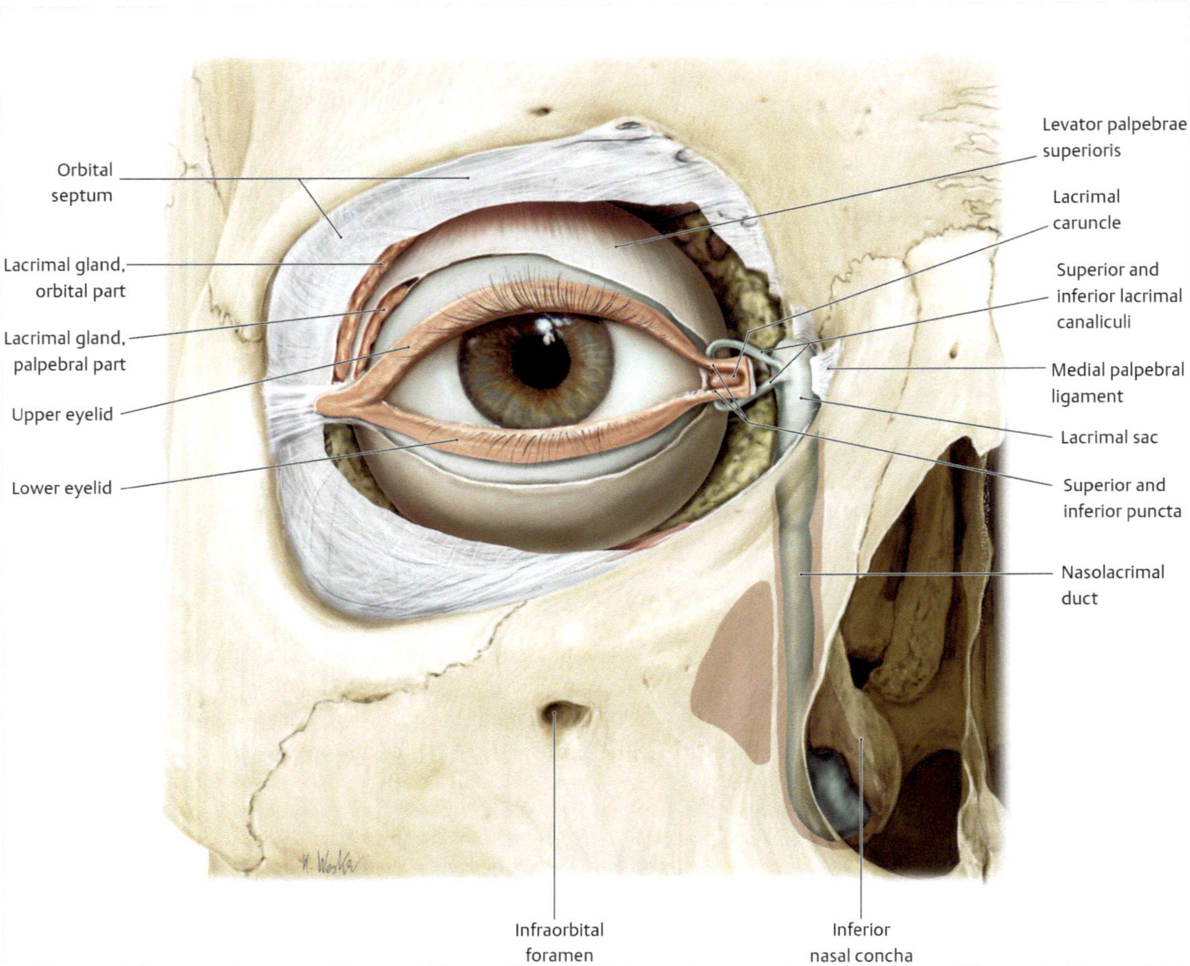

Fig. 10.7 Nasolacrimal drainage system. (Reproduced from Schuenke M, Schulte E, Schumacher U. Thieme Atlas of Anatomy: Head and Neuroanatomy. Illustrations by M. Voll and K. Wesker. 1st ed. Stuttgart: Thieme; 2010.)

tears from laterally to medially toward the *lacrimal puncta* located 5 to 7 mm lateral to the medial canthal angle. Blinking creates a pump function to drain the tears through the *superior and inferior canaliculus* to a common canaliculus (90% of the time), passing first through their vertical segment (2 mm) and then the horizontal one (8 mm). The inferior lacrimal punctum is placed 1 to 2 mm more laterally than the superior one.[6,9] The tears then drain into the *lacrimal sac*. The fundus of the lacrimal sac is approximately 5 mm above MCT and the body extends 10 mm inferiorly giving rise to nasolacrimal duct. The duct has intraosseous (proximal) portion and membranous (distal) portion before its termination into the nasal cavity. Canalicular disruption during eyelid surgery or punctal malposition after eyelid repair may result in epiphora. Obstruction of the lacrimal drainage system could be prevented by canaliculoplasty or silicone stent placement along with careful attention to the repair of the eyelid margin[8,9] (see following text).

10.2.8 Neurovascular and Lymphatic System of the Lids (▶ Fig. 10.8, ▶ Fig. 10.9, and ▶ Fig. 10.10a, b)

The main vascular supply of the lids comes from distal branches of internal and external carotid artery system.[6–9] The *ophthalmic artery* is the first branch of the *internal carotid system* supplying the globe, orbital soft tissues and overlying eyelids. It continues anteromedially from orbital apex and divides into *lacrimal* and *supraorbital artery*, and then distally becomes nasofrontal artery which divides into supratrochlear and dorsal nasal arteries behind the trochlea.

The branches of lacrimal artery laterally and dorsal nasal artery medially give rise to superior and inferior lateral and medial arteries, respectively, which anastomose over the eyelids forming the superior peripheral arcade located within Müller's muscle in the upper eyelid and the upper and lower eyelid marginal arcades. In addition,

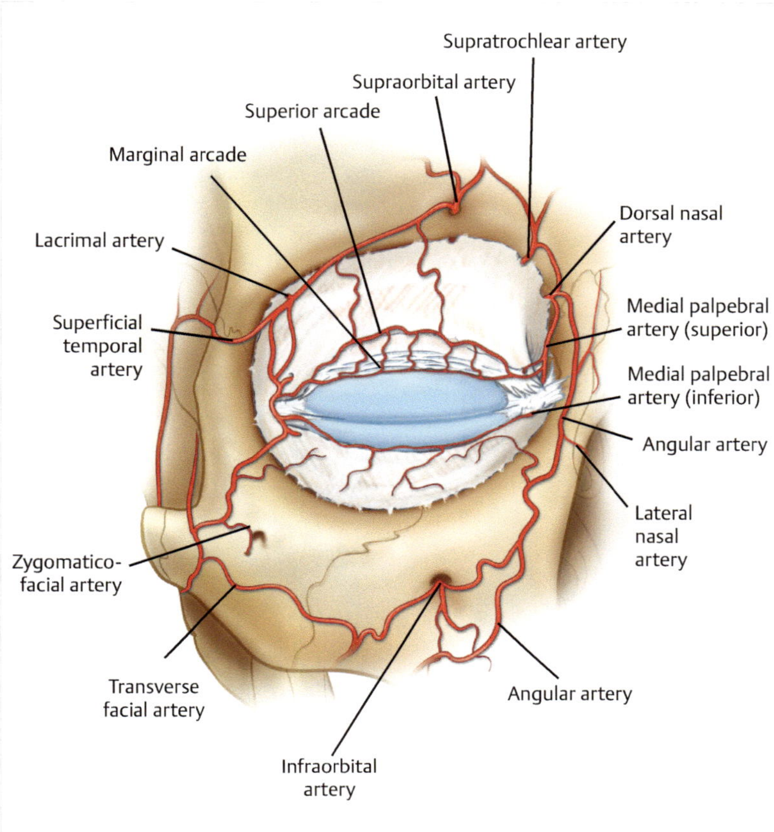

Fig. 10.8 Arterial supply to the eyelids. (Reproduced from Nahai F, Nahai F. The Art of Aesthetic Surgery: Principles & Techniques. 3rd ed. New York: Thieme; 2020.)

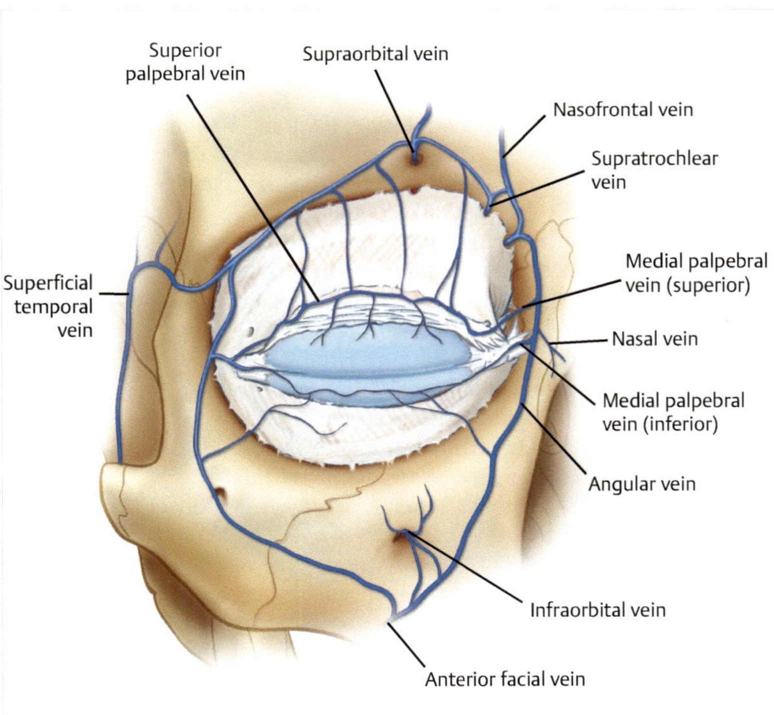

Fig. 10.9 Venous supply from the eyelids. (Reproduced from Nahai F, Nahai F. The Art of Aesthetic Surgery: Principles & Techniques. 3rd ed. New York: Thieme; 2020.)

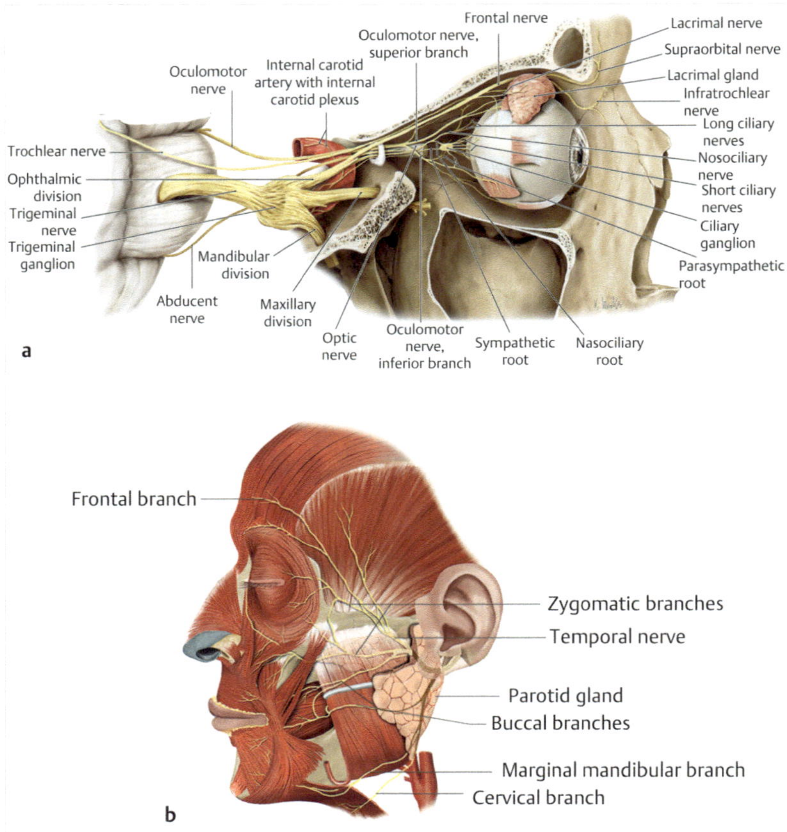

Fig. 10.10 (a) Sensory nerves from the eyelids via trigeminal nerve branches. (Reproduced from Schuenke M, Schulte E, Schumacher U. Thieme Atlas of Anatomy: Head and Neuroanatomy. Illustrations by M. Voll and K. Wesker. 1st ed. Stuttgart: Thieme; 2010.) **(b)** Motor innervation to the eyelid protractors from facial nerve branches. (Reproduced from Leatherbarrow B. Oculoplastic Surgery. 3rd ed. New York: Thieme; 2019.)

two other orbital margin arcades (deep and superficial) are formed in the superior orbit in-between the fibers of OOM (supratrochlear artery). Vascular contributions from the *external carotid system* are *temporal superficial artery*, *infraorbital artery*, and *angular artery* (terminal branch of facial artery). In 20% of cases, the lacrimal artery arises from the external carotid system.[6,9]

The venous system of the eyelids is developed mainly in the fornices and drains into both the *anterior facial veins* and veins of the intraorbital system via the *superior ophthalmic vein* and its tributaries (supratrochlear and supraorbital veins). Pretarsally, the angular vein drains the medial portion of the eyelid, and the superficial temporal vein drains the lateral portion of the eyelid. The superior and inferior ophthalmic veins, pterygoid plexus, and angular vein flow to the cavernous sinus and are involved in the venous drainage of postseptal structures. Another prominent structure is the supraorbital vein going along the brow's arch and is formed by confluence of supraorbital, supratrochlear, and angular vein tributaries.[6,7]

The lymphatics of the eyelids can be divided into a superficial (pretarsal) plexus and deep (posttarsal) plexus. Damage to this network during surgery can produce chemosis (conjunctival edema) postoperatively. Furthermore, primary drainage from the medial lids is into the *submandibular lymph nodes*, while lateral lids drain into the *preauricular (parotid) lymph nodes*. Recent studies in primates revealed that the entire upper lid, medial canthus, and lateral lower lid drain into parotid nodes, while the central lower lid drains into the submandibular network. This pattern suggests that central upper eyelid probably has dual lymphatic drainage.[2,7,8,9]

Lymphatic mapping is usually required to identify the primary pathway of drainage when evaluating patients with melanoma of the eyelid as there are frequent variations to the location of the sentinel lymph node.

The motor nerve supply of the eyelids derives from the *facial nerve (VII)* with the zygomatic branch being the main supply for OOM (eyelid protractor) and secondary innervation from the temporal branch. The main upper eyelid retractor—levator palpebrae superioris—is innervated by the *oculomotor nerve (III)*.[7,9]

The sensory supply of the eyelids derives from the *ophthalmic (V1)* and *maxillary (V2)* divisions of trigeminal nerve (V). The branches of the ophthalmic nerve which supply upper eyelid laterally to medially are *lacrimal*, *frontal* (supraorbital and supratrochlear), and *nasociliary* nerves. The branches of maxillary nerve which provide sensory innervation are *zygomaticotemporal* (lateral upper eyelid), *zygomaticofacial* (lateral lower eyelid), and *infraorbital* (central lower eyelid) nerve. The medial canthus is innervated by the *infratrochlear* nerve, i.e., terminal branch of the nasociliary nerve (V1). Sympathetic fibers innervate both upper and lower tarsal muscle.[2,8,9]

10.2.9 Orbit (▶ Fig. 10.6 and ▶ Fig. 10.10a)

The bony orbit consists of maxilla, zygoma, sphenoid, palatine bone, ethmoid bone, lacrimal bone, and frontal bones. The *lacrimal fossa* is positioned in the lateral orbit formed by the frontal bone. The *arcus marginalis* is the outline of the outside margin of the orbit where periosteum of the orbit is fused with OS and is also the location of the attachment of the orbitomalar ligament. On the lateral orbit wall there is *Whitnall's tubercule* which is the place of the attachment of the LCT.[7,9]

10.2.10 Eyebrow Anatomy

The eyebrow is comprised of the skin and soft tissue.[7,15] The anatomic boundaries of the brow are demarcated superiorly by the first forehead crease curing above the brow skin and inferiorly at the arcus marginalis where subciliary brow ends, at the superior orbital rim, transitioning into the upper eyelid skin. Eyebrow hair follicles have different and limited growth pattern than the ones on the scalp, and once lost may be difficult to be replaced in the reconstructive procedures[15] (▶ Fig. 10.11). Deep to the follicles is a paired *corrugator supercilii muscle* which originates at the superior orbital rim medially and runs laterally till the lateral third of the brow along the superior orbital rim and is responsible for vertical lines on the glabella. *Procerus muscle* is positioned more centrally, extending distally from the nasal root and creates horizontal lines in the central glabellar region. Apart from these strong depressors, OOM and *depressor supercilii* muscles also augment the brow depressing function against the principal brow elevator *frontalis muscle* (▶ Fig. 10.12). The vertical fibers of the frontalis muscle and the horizontal fibers of the orbicularis oculi muscles interdigitate at the eyebrow level; thus, the position of the eyebrow represents a dynamic interplay between elevating and depressing forces[9,13,15] (▶ Fig. 10.13).

The frontalis muscle is a part of the occipitofrontalis musculofascial complex of the scalp, which includes the occipitalis muscle, galea aponeurotica, and frontalis muscle. The vertically oriented fibers of frontalis muscle extend from the broad fibrous tissue of the galea aponeurotica just inferior to the hairline and insert into the supraorbital dermis. Contraction of the frontalis muscle can elevate the eyebrow more than 20 mm and also causes horizontal furrows across the forehead. These furrows do not extend to the temporal hairline because the frontalis muscle thins laterally and does not extend past the temporal fusion line to the tail of the brow. The lack of frontalis pull-over of the tail of the brow explains the common temporal brow ptosis seen so often in older adults. The frontal branch of the facial nerve innervates the frontalis muscle.[8,13,15]

The galea aponeurosis[13,15] joins the frontalis muscle anteriorly and splits around the frontalis muscle into a superficial and deep galea. The thinner superficial layer continues inferiorly as the anterior muscle sheath of the frontalis and orbicularis muscles, whereas the deep galea

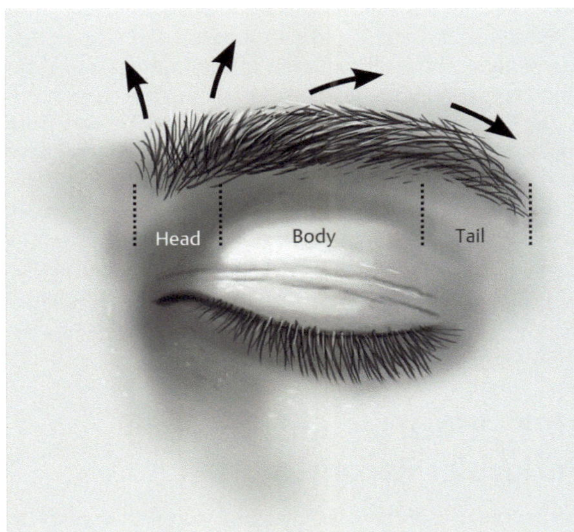

Fig. 10.11 Eyebrow segments (head, body, and tail) and multidirectional orientation of the hair growth.

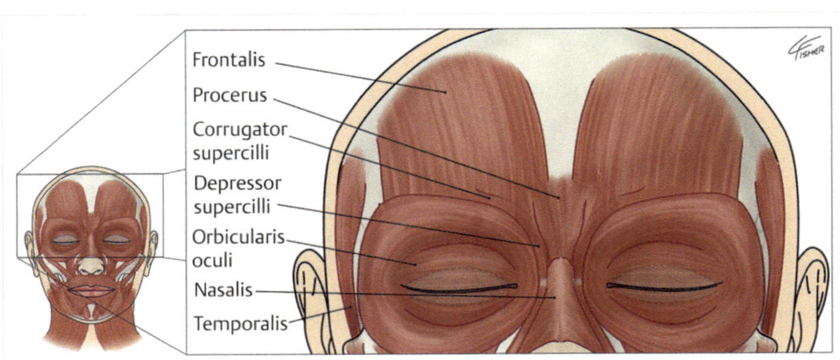

Fig. 10.12 Muscles of the forehead and temporal fossa. (Reproduced from Carniol P, Avram M, Brauer J. Complications in Minimally Invasive Facial Rejuvenation: Prevention and Management. New York: Thieme; 2020.)

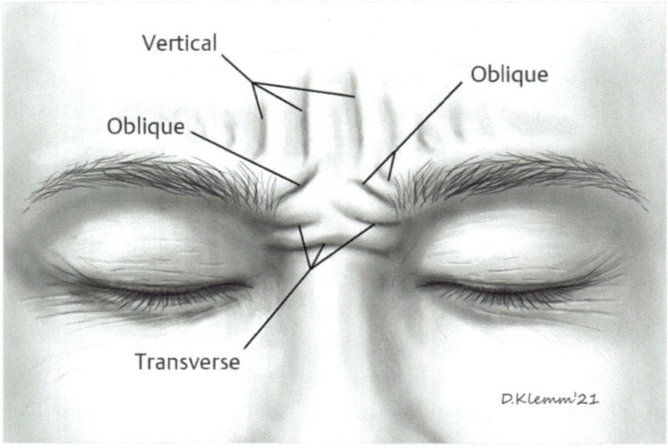

Fig. 10.13 Glabellar skin lines. Vertical skin lines are produced by action of the transverse heads of the corrugator supercilii muscles. Oblique skin lines are the result of action of three muscles: the oblique head of the corrugator supercilii, the depressor supercilii, and the medial head fibers of the orbicular oculi muscles. Action of the procerus muscle produces transverse skin line formation across the dorsum of the nose.

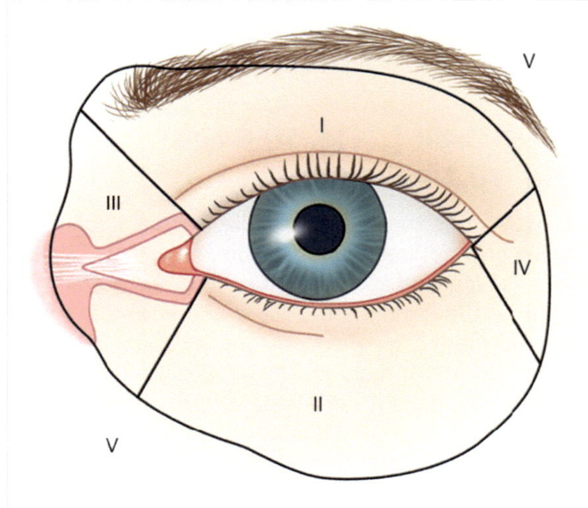

Fig. 10.14 The eyelids and periocular structures can be divided into five surgical zones. Almost 75% of skin cancers occur in zones II and III. (Reproduced from Woo A, Bhatt R. Plastic Surgery Case Review: Oral Board Study Guide. 2nd ed. New York: Thieme; 2020.)

becomes the posterior muscle sheath. This deep galea layer divides inferiorly and encompasses the fat pad that lies beneath the interdigitation of the frontalis and orbicularis muscles of the ROOF (see earlier in the chapter).

The sensory innervation of the eyebrows derives from supraorbital and supratrochlear nerves, which also have paired arteries and veins. The supratrochlear notch projects 17.5 mm from the midline, and both nerves are branches of the trigeminal nerve (ophthalmic nerve V1). The motor innervation of paired corrugators and procerus is from frontal branches of the facial nerve. Lymphatics generally follow the neurovascular bundles and travel laterally toward the orbital rim.[8]

10.3 Principles and Aims of Periocular Reconstruction

Dermatologic surgeons have many surgical options to choose from for the repair of eyelid defects after Mohs micrographic surgery. The choice of the repair depends on the size and location of the defect, skin texture and color match, surrounding tissue mobility, degree of vascular compromise, and extend of the lamellae loss. All reconstruction effort should attempt to maintain the integrity of reconstructed structures by following the rules of "like for like" approximation.[1] For extensive defects which require excessive mobilization of the tarsus, conjunctiva and skin consultation of experienced oculoplastic surgeon may be considered.

According to Spinelli,[17] periocular area is divided into five anatomic units: the upper eyelid is zone 1, the lower eyelid is zone 2, the medial canthus is zone 3, the lateral canthus is zone 4, and tissue outside these zones, but still related to them is zone 5 (▶ Fig. 10.14). According to Mutlu et al,[18] the majority of skin cancers involve zone II and III (75%), which may be helpful to guide novices in the field of periocular reconstruction how and where to begin their education in surgical techniques. The defects are also classified as *partial* (anterior lamella, i.e., skin and OOM) or *total* (anterior and posterior lamella—skin, OOM, tarsus, conjunctiva, eyelid retractors); *marginal* (ciliary margin involvement) or *nonmarginal*.[1,2] Furthermore, medial canthal involvement may require silicone stenting, repair of the lacrimal canaliculi, or lateral canthotomy if margin advancement is necessary. Finally, the reconstructed eyelid should match in height and shape the contralateral one, with medial and lateral canthi being positioned symmetrically on both sides.[2,3,4] Taking these things into consideration is necessary to maintain both function and aesthetics of the eyelid.

Relaxed skin tension lines (RSTL) are generally very useful for planning surgical incision and minimize scarring. In the periocular region, these lines are oriented horizontally in the upper and lower eyelid skin[3,4,8,11] (▶ Fig. 10.15). However, vertical tension created by closure of elliptical defects oriented along these lines has substantial risk to create iatrogenic cicatricial malposition, including lower eyelid retraction and ectropion. So, if there is not enough redundancy of skin for closure without vertical tension, conversion of the long axis of the ellipse to being perpendicular to the eyelid margin is preferable, even if the vertical approach may risk only minimal cicatricial retraction[1,2] (▶ Fig. 10.16). In contrast, excisions along RSTL will produce satisfactory outcomes at the glabellar region, medial or lateral canthi, and brows.[2,4,19,20]

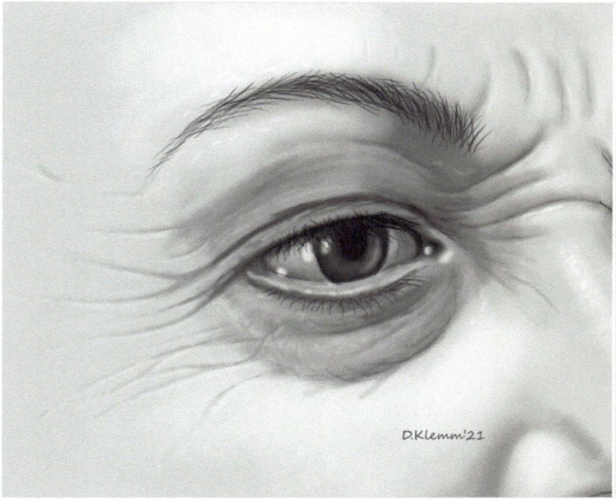

Fig. 10.15 Periocular wrinkles and relaxed skin tension lines (RSTL).

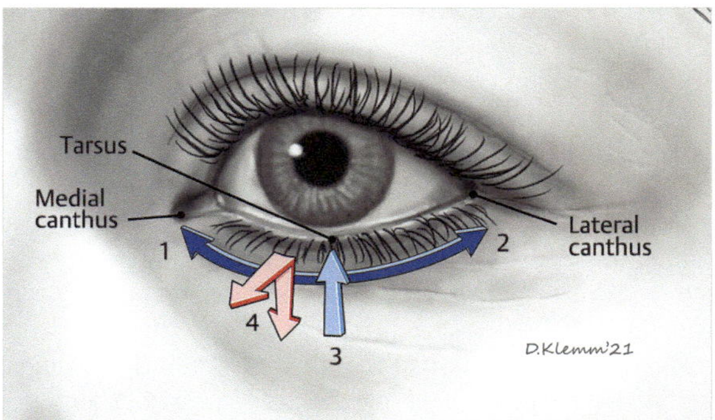

Fig. 10.17 Complex interplay of lower eyelid intrinsic support (*blue*): medial (1) and lateral (2) canthus, and tarsus (3) and distraction forces (*red*) which tend to displace periocular skin away (4).

Ineffective senescent or neuropathic orbicularis muscle tone may result in lower eyelid ectropion or upper eyelid lagophthalmos (▶ Fig. 10.17a, b).[17] Hence, valuable parts of pre-reconstruction exam are assessment of eyelid laxity, where the weakness of LCT and MCT is evaluated by doing *"pinch"* and *"snap back"* tests[19,20] (▶ Fig. 10.18a, b; ▶ Video 10.1). In the lid distraction test, aka "pinch test," the lower eyelid is outwardly displaced from the globe and if it can be distracted 7 to 8 mm, abnormal lid laxity is present. Greater than 3-mm distraction of the puncta from the medial or lateral canthus suggests abnormal laxity of canthal tendons. The eyelid is then released, and its return ("snap back") observed for slow return or one requiring multiple blinks indicative of poor lid tone. Excessive dermatochalasis of the upper eyelid which would otherwise require blepharoplasty may permit the use of the horizontally oriented ellipse in the upper lid in some individuals. This redundant skin can also be used as

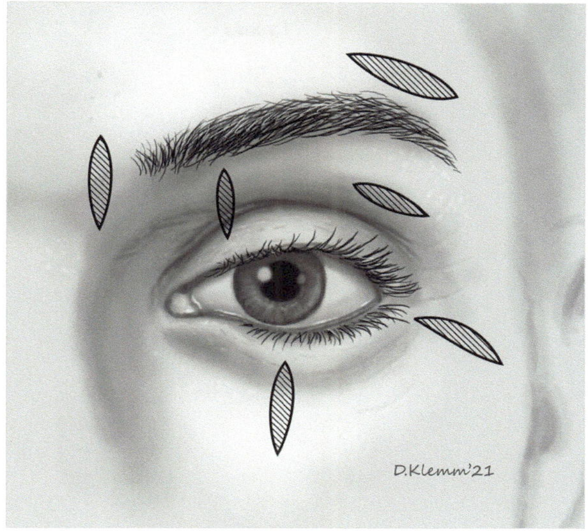

Fig. 10.16 Orientation and elliptical excision in the periorbital region to minimize wound closure tension and to prevent retraction of the upper or lower eyelid.

a good source for skin grafting for contralateral or ipsilateral lower eyelid when necessary.

10.4 Perioperative Surgical Tips, Instrumentations, and Sutures in Periocular Reconstruction

Before any surgical preparation, the ocular surface should be anesthetized using topical proparacaine 0.5% or topical tetracaine 1% to minimize discomfort and stinging of the eyes. Surgical preparation needs to be safe if the solution comes to the contact with the eye and the use of Betadine 5% sterile ophthalmic prep solution (povidone-iodine ophthalmic solution, which has 0.5% available iodine) is safer than using an alcohol-based preparation which can injure the epithelium of the cornea.[21,22]

Local anesthesia should be placed with 25- to 30-gauge needles for any injections in the eyelids. Subconjunctival injection is less painful than subcutaneous injections and should be used for repairs involving the margin. The use of a topical anesthetic prior to injection is very effective in providing comfort to the patient. Corneal shields with eye lubricant should be used to prevent drying of cornea, photophobia, or abrasion during the procedure. Alternatively, an assistant can hold a shoehorn protector (Jaeger lid plate) (▶ Fig. 10.19) just inside the eyelid when working in the proximity of the globe.

When suturing the eyelid margin, it is recommended using 5–0 silk suture on semicircular cutting needle through the Meibomian gland orifices, in a vertical mattress fashion to provide good eversion and leave the long tails to be incorporated later in skin sutures at the front,

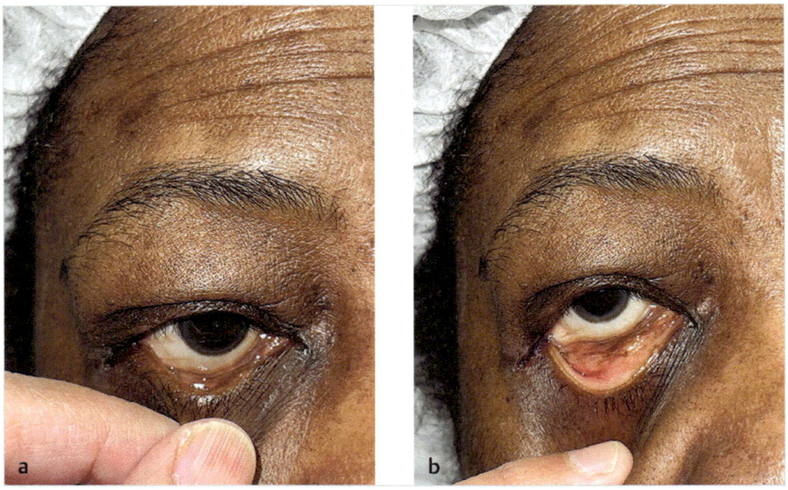

Fig. 10.18 **(a)** The snap test. The lower eyelid is displaced inferiorly and then released. A slow return to normal position reflects poor tone. **(b)** The distraction test. The lower eyelid is grasped gently and pulled anteriorly. If the distance of distraction exceeds 6 to 8 mm, lid laxity is present.

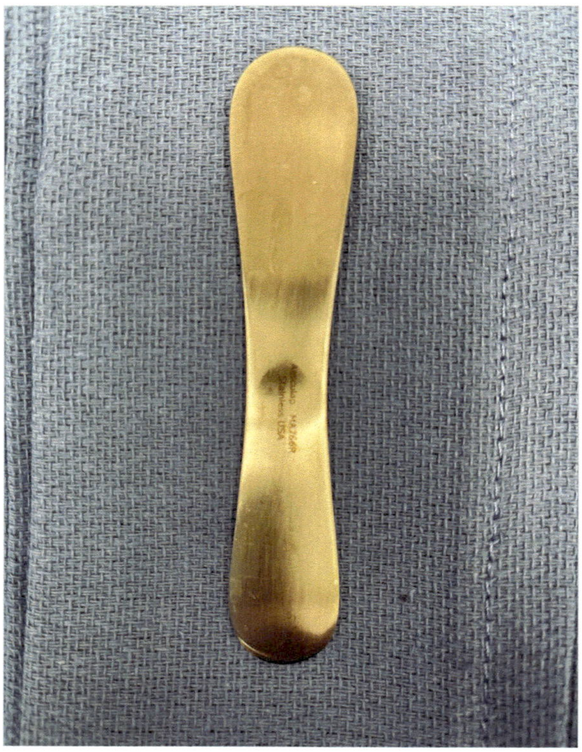

Fig. 10.19 Jaeger lid plate (shoehorn protector).

in order to avoid corneal abrasion. Absorbable sutures utilized for eyelid defects should be 6–0 or 5–0 multifilament polyglactin 910 or monofilament polyglecaprone 25, while nonabsorbable sutures should be 6–0 polypropylene or nylon for brows, nose, and glabella, and 7–0 for eyelid skin. The eyelid tissue should be handled gently during the procedure by using 0.3-toothed forceps for skin, and 0.12-toothed forceps for the tarsus, conjunctiva, or punctum. During retraction and dissection, it is better to grasp more OOM than the skin to avoid tearing of the thin tissue and consider using small double-pronged skin hooks when manipulating the anterior lamella.[1,2,21,22]

Hemostasis should be meticulous to reduce postoperative bruising and hemorrhagic complications. Bleeding from palpebral arcades, if transected, could be particularly brisk, but controllable with gentle pressure and gentle applications of bipolar electrocautery.

After surgery, patients are asked to avoid activity that would increase their heart rate or blood pressure and use ice packs to the affected lids to reduce swelling and bruising.

Occasionally an eye pad is applied for the first 24 hours as an occlusive dressing. An ophthalmic antibiotic ointment is given to be used on the stitches to decrease any risk of infection. Sutures are removed in 5 to 7 days. Marginal eversion sutures usually stay longer and are removed after 3 weeks.

Among common surgical needles (▶ Fig. 10.20a–d), *side-cutting (spatula) needles* are also an important part of ophthalmic surgery armamentarium. They are flat on the top and bottom surfaces to allow maximum ease of penetration and control as they pass between and through tissue layers to maintain the proper tissue plane and avoid exposure of the suture on the inner surface of the eyelid against the eye. The most used spatula needle is an S-14, which is especially useful for anchoring tarsus to canthal tendons or periosteal flaps since it is designed to cut on the sides and do not tear through the tissue[1,2,20] (▶ Fig. 10.20c).

10.5 Surgical Assessment of the Periocular Defect and Reconstruction Guidelines[1,2,3,4,19,20]

Every reconstruction effort in the periocular area needs to be evaluated by using fundamental guidelines. Partial

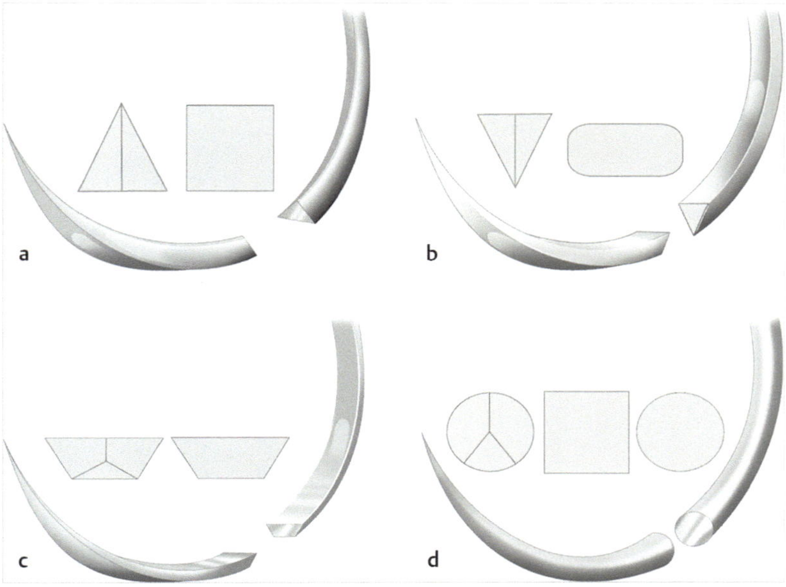

Fig. 10.20 The differences between surgical needles: **(a)** conventional cutting, **(b)** reverse cutting, **(c)** spatulated, and **(d)** taper needle. (Reproduced from Leatherbarrow B. Oculoplastic Surgery. 3rd ed. New York: Thieme; 2019.)

thickness defects involve skin and OOM whereas full-thickness defects extend from the skin to involve tarsus, eyelid retractors, and conjunctiva. Each lamella needs to be addressed and repaired separately during eyelid reconstruction. When using a free graft, a vascular source must be provided by either the anterior or posterior lamella. The anterior and posterior lamella cannot be simultaneously replaced within one defect unless an orbicularis advancement flap can be interposed in-between the two to enable proper blood supply to the grafted tissue. Posterior lamellar defects can be restored using grafts from upper tarsus (free or pedicle based), ear cartilage, nasal chondromucosa, or hard palate. The anterior lamella is best repaired by transferring the neighboring tissue or using full-thickness skin grafts (FTSGs) if the adjacent tissue reservoir is not sufficient. The best donor sites are redundant skin from contralateral or ipsilateral upper eyelid, then retroauricular, inner arm, or supraclavicular skin. Lid sharing procedures like Cutler-Beard flap or Hughes flap should be avoided in individuals where the affected eye is the only functional eye, since they will not be able to tolerate prolonged (2–3 wk) eye occlusion, and alternative options should be considered. Whenever the skin graft is considered, it should be properly anchored in place to avoid any postoperative malposition.

When evaluating eyelid margin defects, it is important to assess the amount of the loss of the horizontal lid. If the defect involves up to 25% of upper or lower lid margin (20% in younger and 30% in older individuals) it can be closed primarily. Extra length can be obtained by canthotomy and cantholysis. Defects which comprise 25 to 50% of the upper and lower margin can be repaired by a Tenzel semicircular flap. Defects longer than 50% of the upper eyelid margin will require Cutler-Beard pedicle or Leone flap. Defects longer than 50% of the lower eyelid margin will require Hughes tarsoconjunctival flap or Mustarde cheek rotational flap with posterior lamellar graft. The reconstructive ladder for periocular defects is summarized in ▶ Fig. 10.21.

Reconstruction of the upper eyelid is more intricate since preservation of function and contour is more demanding to achieve than in the lower eyelid. The levator muscle's function has to be respected; an inadequate dynamic function can compromise the visual axis of the patient. Furthermore, good eyelid closure is necessary to prevent exposure keratopathy due to lagophthalmos. For maintenance of corneal integrity and clear vision, upper eyelid must have minimally 5 to 10 mm of movement and blink.[1–4,19,23–25]

10.6 Secondary Intention Healing[1,2,26]

Granulation is an excellent option for superficial (shallow) surgical defects of the anterior lamella < 10 mm in diameter especially in concave regions of the eyelid like medial canthus, particularly if the defect is centered between the upper and lower eyelid. The tarsal plate's semirigid fibroskeleton serves as ideal scaffold for skin re-epithelization and helps prevent the unwanted contractures. Individuals with excessive sun damage, prior history of radiation, or ones who are poor surgical candidates can also be considered for second intention healing for small defects. Another possible situation is use of delayed skin grafting after the wound is allowed to granulate to enable better take of the graft. The size of the defect can also be decreased with partial closure by using the purse-string suture and hence reduce granulation time, resulting in faster healing with even tension on the wound edges. Second intention healing is also a good practical way to monitor tumor recurrence, especially

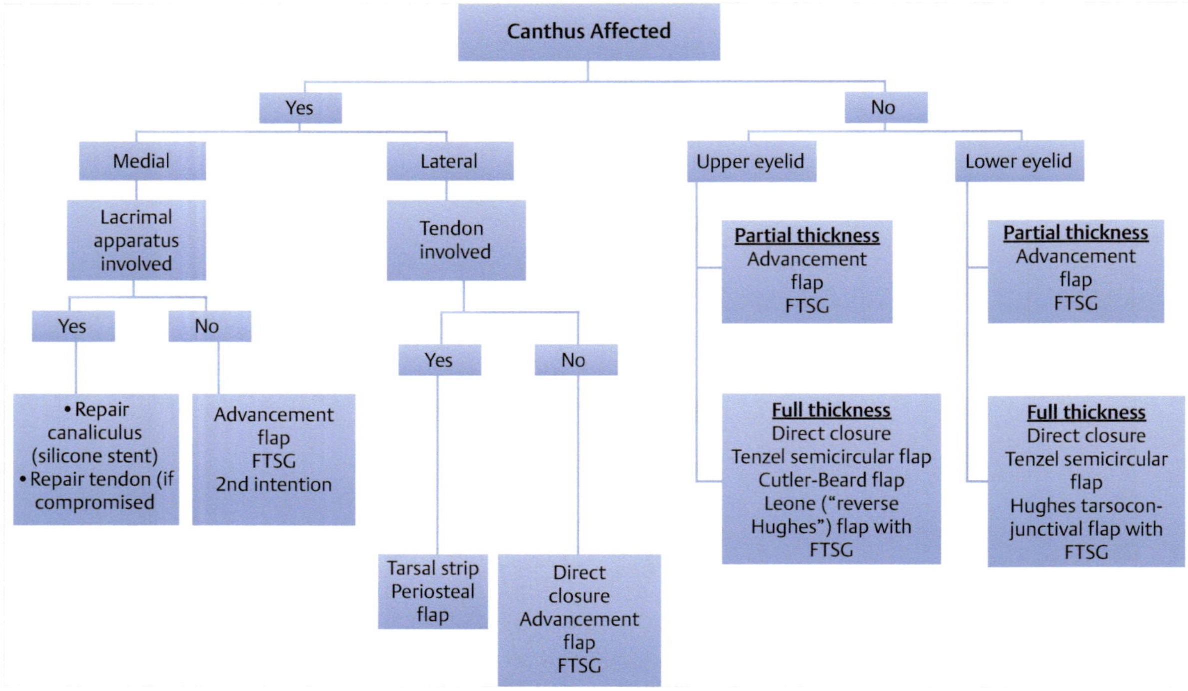

Fig. 10.21 Algorithm for closure of periocular defects. FTSG; full-thickness skin graft.

when tumors are larger, have aggressive histology, or are associated with perineural invasion.

10.7 Grafts in Periocular Reconstruction[1,2,19,20,24]

In eyelid reconstruction, the most commonly used grafts are FTSGs. Split-thickness skin grafts contract significantly and generally should be avoided in periocular reconstruction. Allografts and xenografts are derived from cadaveric or porcine skin, respectively. They are used often as temporary coverage for big defects until autograft can be placed at the later date. Patients with hypersensitivity to porcine byproducts should avoid xenografts.

FTSGs are ideal for pretarsal defects limited to the anterior lamella where secondary intention or primary closure is not possible. The best match is the donor site from contralateral upper eyelid. Alternative sites are hairless preauricular or postauricular area, supraclavicular area, or inner arm (► Fig. 10.22 and ► Video 10.2). The graft needs to be completely defatted, before its placement to enable good adherence for the recipient site. In addition, when covering preseptal eyelid skin, the graft needs to be approximately 30% oversized to prevent contracture, lagophthalmos, or ectropion. When positioning FTSG over the pretarsal subunit, there is no need to create bigger graft, since the fibroskeleton of the tarsus provides good support for its healing and prevents contraction. To enable better take of the graft, the tie-over bolster should be applied using 6–0 silk or prolene on medial, lateral, and inferior border.

Tarsoconjunctival grafts (► Fig. 10.23) are excellent choice for the repair of posterior lamella following the principle "replace 'like-with-like'." They contain conjunctiva and tarsus and are harvested from the ipsilateral or sometimes contralateral upper eyelid leaving at least 4 mm of the marginal tarsus intact to avoid upper eyelid distortion. The donor site is left to heal by secondary intention. Tarsoconjunctival grafts can be used to repair up to 75% of the length of the eyelid. For bigger defects, posterior lamella can be reconstructed using mucoperiosteal grafts from hard palate, and rarely nasal chondromucosa, auricular cartilage, or even buccal mucosa. Despite reliable results, some of them may be associated with significant donor- and recipient-site morbidity.

Tarsoconjunctival grafts are usually designed slightly smaller than the original defects so that adequate horizontal tension can be achieved in the reconstructed lower eyelid. Replacing the posterior lamella avoids LCT relaxation used in a Tenzel semicircular flap, and therefore, the risk of lateral canthal angle deformity.

The tarsoconjunctival graft is harvested from the most central part of the everted upper eyelid (where the tarsus is the highest) with the help of cotton tip applicator or Desmarres retractor (► Fig. 10.24). It is important to place the graft at or slightly above the reconstructed eyelid margin and extend extra conjunctiva (harvested from the

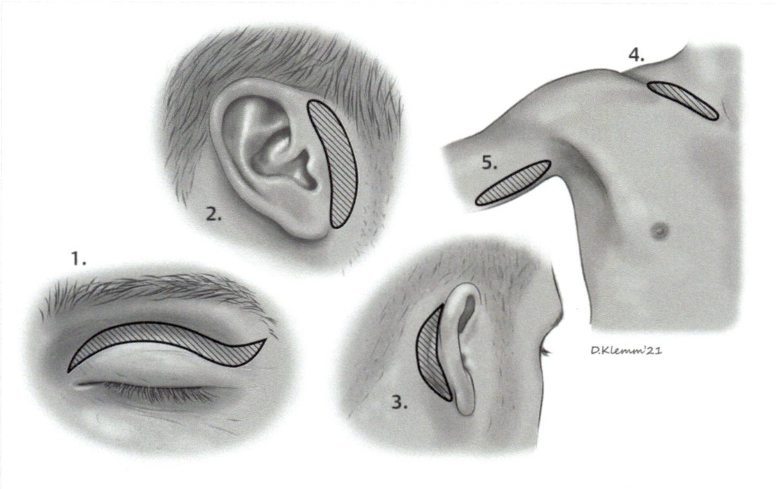

Fig. 10.22 Donor sites for full-thickness skin grafting in order of preference: upper eyelid, preauricular, postauricular, supraclavicular, and upper inner arm.

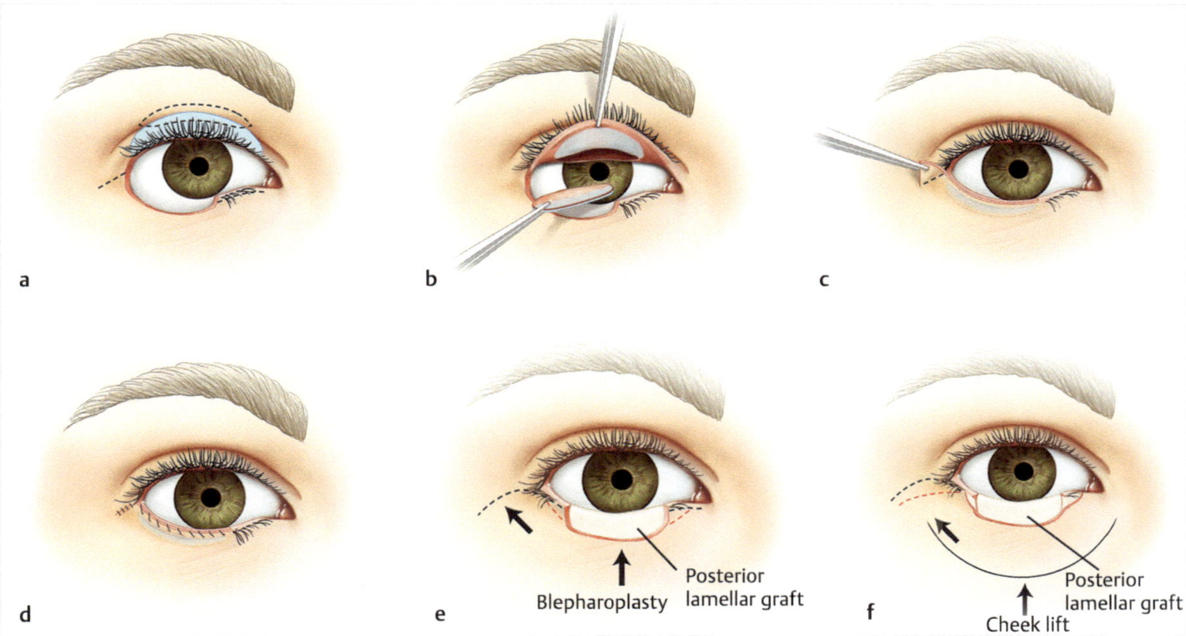

Fig. 10.23 (a–f) Free tarsoconjunctival graft harvested from the upper lid placed on the full-thickness lower eyelid defect. (Reproduced from Codner M, McCord C. Eyelid & Periorbital Surgery. 2nd ed. New York: Thieme; 2016.)

donor site) over the eyelid margin to avoid excavation of the reconstructed eyelid in the area of the graft. The lower aspect of the graft should join the lower lid retractors and conjunctiva unless the lid defect extends to inferior fornix, when only conjunctiva should be connected and capsulopalpebral fascia left recessed to avoid graft retraction. A 6–0 plain gut is used to connect tarsoconjunctival graft with the anterior lamella, be it repaired with a myocutaneous flap or FTSG with interposed OOM flap. Another advantage of tarsoconjunctival grafts in the repair of the posterior lamella is avoidance of eye occlusion as seen with Hughes transposition flap.

Composite grafts (CG) (▸ Fig. 10.25) consist of skin, cartilage (tarsus), and conjunctiva. They are used for full-thickness defects of the eyelid which involve both anterior and posterior lamella. Composite grafts are most often harvested from contralateral upper or lower eyelid. Donor site defect is repaired by direct closure (see following text). When the lower eyelid full-thickness defect is not deep (5–10 mm in height), and if concomitant skin laxity does not allow flap closure for anterior lamella defect, a full-thickness pentagon could be excised from the contralateral upper or lower eyelid, and the muscle has to be removed. The graft obtains its vascular supply at

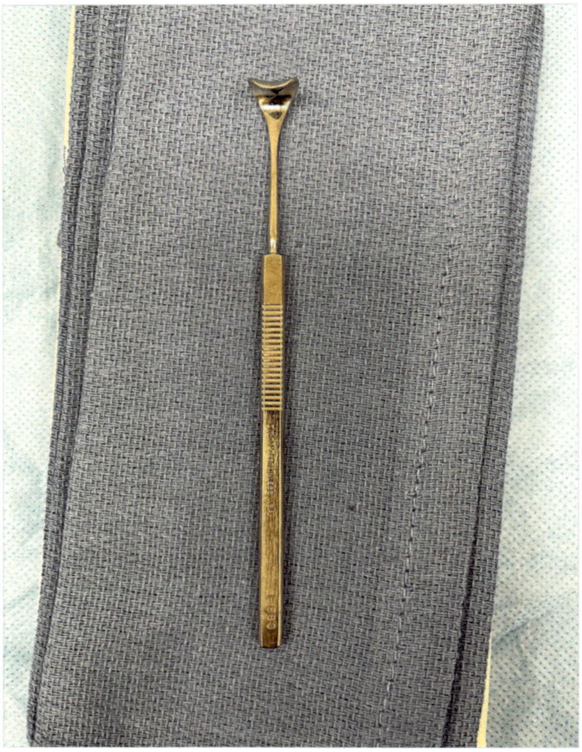

Fig. 10.24 Desmarres lid retractor designed to pull the lid away from the cornea and other structures during the eye surgery procedure.

the recipient site from OOM which is undermined and sutured into the space left by divided muscle. The drawback of this repair is the donor site morbidity. If the anterior lamella is repaired by skin graft, and posterior lamella by tarsoconjunctival graft, the peripheral OOM needs to be interposed in-between the two to enable good vascularization and graft survival. CGs are ideal for patients who are anxious or cannot tolerate temporary eyelid closure (see following text—flaps in periocular repair).

10.8 Repair of Superficial Nonmarginal Eyelid Defects[1–4,19,20,24,25,27,28]

In periocular reconstruction and evaluation of the defect, it is of utmost importance to provide separate attention to posterior and anterior lamellae, canthal ligament support, retractor function, and mucocutaneous margin. Meticulous repair of each of these structures, if affected, is essential. The elimination of all vertical tension is necessary to prevent any malposition that can interfere with eyelid closure.

Whenever possible *primary closure* of nonmarginal defects should be considered. To release tension, it is important to generously undermine subcutaneous edges of the defect. Incision lines should be parallel to RSTL (▸ Fig. 10.15 and ▸ Fig. 10.26); however, in the area of lower eyelid where downward traction could result in scleral show and frank ectropion, all tension should be

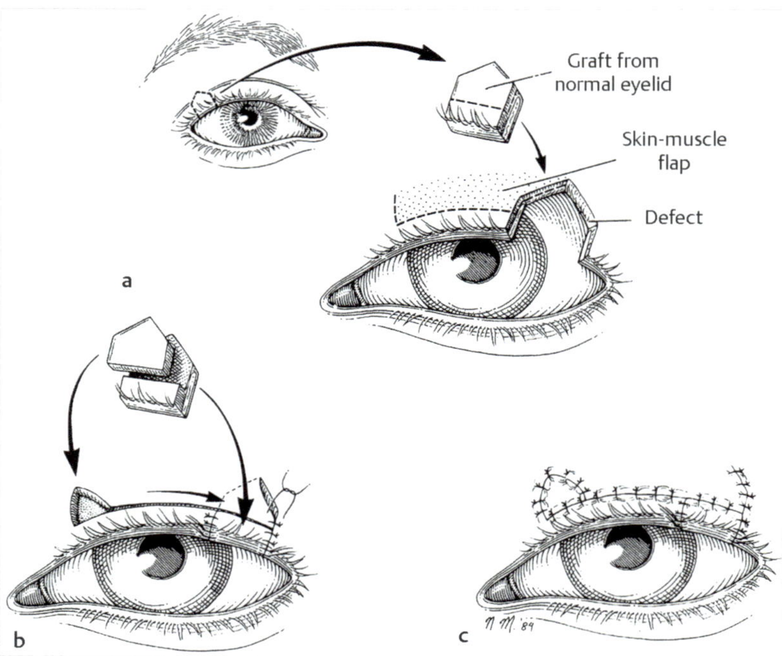

Fig. 10.25 (a–c) Modified composite graft (skin, lashes, tarsus, and conjunctiva) harvested from the contralateral lower eyelid. (Reproduced from Chen W. Oculoplastic Surgery: The Essentials. New York: Thieme; 2001.)

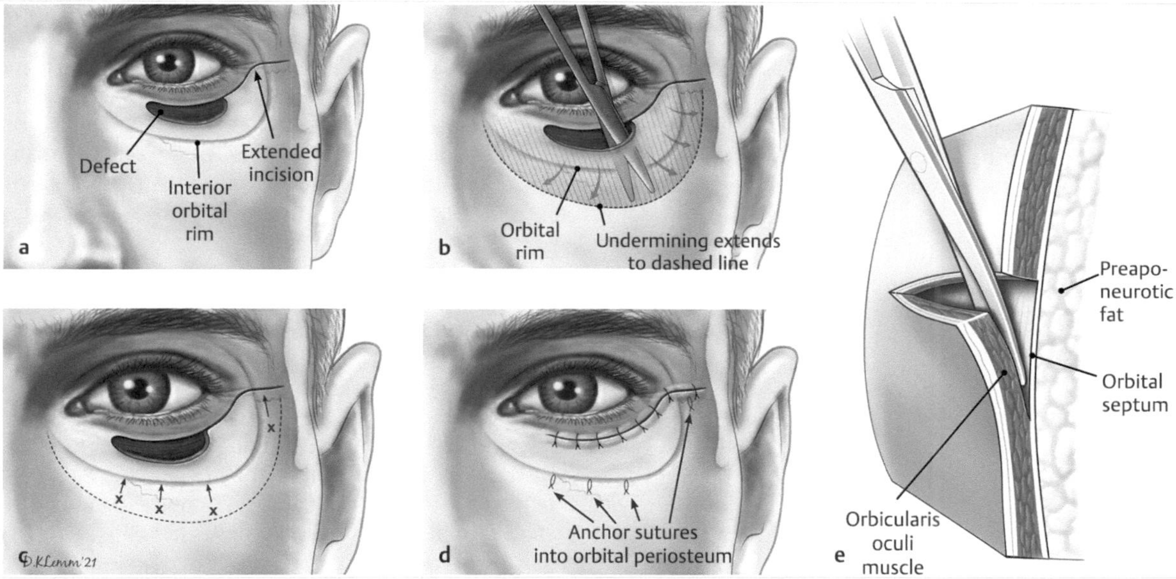

Fig. 10.26 Lower eyelid defect repaired with anchoring sutures. **(a)** Lower eyelid defect. **(b)** Undermine and advance cheek superiorly. Extend the incision laterally into a laugh line at the lateral canthus. **(c,d)** Use anchoring sutures into the inferior rim periosteum and lateral canthus temporalis fascia to support the tissues and take the vertical tension off the eyelid. In some patients, you may want to support the posterior lamella with a lateral tarsal strip as well. **(e)** Level of undermining below the orbicularis oculi muscle (OOM) and above the orbital septum (OS).

nearly as horizontal as possible, so that vertical or oblique incision lines are preferable (▶ Fig. 10.16). For defects close to lid margin, periosteal pecking sutures can be used to stabilize the flap and avoid pull of the eyelid margin (▶ Fig. 10.26). M-plasty and S-plasty variations of side-closure can be utilized to shorten the overall closure length or conceal better the incision line along RSTL, respectively (▶ Fig. 10.27).

When direct closure is not possible due to excessive loss of tissue, *local flaps* present a great option for surrounding tissue mobilization and tension-free closure. Flaps offer superior aesthetic result than FTSG due to better color and texture match, as well as less scar depression. Further, the ample vascular supply of this region permits the myocutaneous flaps to be used as a great support site for free grafts for reconstruction of the posterior lamella.

Advancement flaps used for the repair of the anterior, lamellar, nonmarginal defects include *unipedicle* and *bipedicle* (▶ Fig. 10.28a,b) flaps, as well as *V-Y flap* (island pedicle) flap. Rectangular-shaped, unipedicle, advancement flaps are excellent options for cutaneous defects of the anterior lamella of the medial upper or lower eyelid as well as brows. The incision lines and resulting scar will be parallel or fall into lid crease without malposition of the lid margin. In younger individuals where skin is less elastic, bilateral advancement can be considered and the skin mobilized from both sides of the defects resulting in H- or T-shaped scar. The pedicles do not need to be identical but mobilized based on laxity obtained after undermining on each side. These flaps can repair the defects up to 25 cm^2 in size. V-Y flaps can be designed in vertical or horizontal direction for the defects on the upper or lower lids. They provide ideal color match, texture cover, and robust blood supply from underlying OOM. With respect to their design it is important that the widest portion of the flap be placed in the area of redundant or more lax skin to avoid unwanted ectropion. It can also be tacked for underlying periosteum to minimize eyelid distortion. The flap design should ensure that maximal vertical or horizontal dimension of the flap is equivalent to the width of the defect, depending on the orientation.

Glabellar flap (▶ Fig. 10.29a–d) is also a quick reconstructive option for medial canthal defects, where "inverted-V" is created adjacent to medial canthal defect and is subsequently converted to "Y" after the flap is transferred to cover the defect. The main disadvantage of this flap is that it narrows the space between the eyebrows and could potentially create a bulky nasal bridge and loss of medial canthal concavity. This can be avoided if the area of the flap placed in the medial canthus is thinned adequately to match the thickness of the surrounding canthal skin. *V-Y flaps* can also be used to lengthen palpebral fissure, close the donor sites, or manage scar contractures and epicanthal folds.

Rotational flaps are used in situations when it is desirable to move adjacent skin sideways into the eyelid defect without the tension. The small secondary defect is repaired with direct closure or skin graft if there is enough laxity. The *A(O) to T flap* is a good technique for medial canthal defects, where perpendicular T-shaped incision is made at the medial edge of the wound. The redundant skin cone is removed centrally, and the skin edges everted sutured. This flap can also be used in the

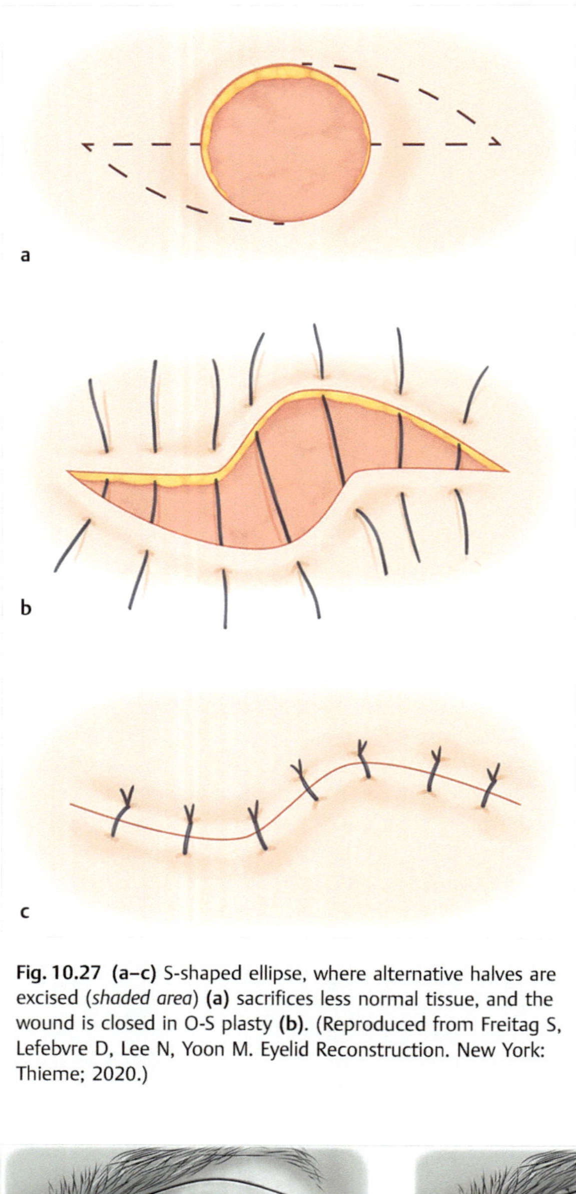

Fig. 10.27 (a–c) S-shaped ellipse, where alternative halves are excised (*shaded area*) **(a)** sacrifices less normal tissue, and the wound is closed in O-S plasty **(b)**. (Reproduced from Freitag S, Lefebvre D, Lee N, Yoon M. Eyelid Reconstruction. New York: Thieme; 2020.)

hairline and brow. *Upper eyelid rotational flap*[27] (▶ Fig. 10.30a–d) presents a useful option for lateral (**c, d**) and medial (**a, b**) canthal defects less than 1.5 cm in diameter which do not involve lacrimal system. This flap has the advantage of being recruited from contiguous cosmetic subunit, where the upper eyelid skin is rotated inferomedially and redundant skin cones removed along the bridge of the nose in the RSTL. The *Mustardé flap* (▶ Fig. 10.31) (aka cheek rotational flap) is used to repair nonmarginal and marginal (see following text) lower eyelid and medial cheek defects where vertical dimension is longer than the horizontal one. This semicircular flap is designed from the lateral canthus just anterior to the ear. The secondary donor area mobilizes the skin that is three to four times the size of primary defect. The incision is directed curvilinearly upward above the lateral canthus to minimize ectropion development by converting lateral/vertical tension vector to horizontal direction. After extensive and deep undermining, the flap is rotated medially to cover the defect. Several retaining sutures can be placed along the flap to hold it in the position and decrease the risk of ectropion. In addition, a *frost suture* (▶ Fig. 10.32)[28] can be placed by passing 4–0 nylon through the inferior tarsus and taping to the forehead to secure the position of the lower eyelid and keep the upward support. They are usually removed in 3 to 5 days. The needle is passed twice through the inferior tarsus entering and exiting through the openings of Meibomian glands. The posterior lamella is then examined to secure that there was no conjunctival violation (i.e., passing of the tarsal suture through conjunctiva) and all four resulting strands are tied as described above.

Transpositions flaps are used when appropriate skin is not available adjacent to the primary defect, so that distant skin can be mobilized to cover the defect. Since the flap is often transposed through the 90 degrees angle, proper preservation of vascular flow must be ensured by deep undermining and gentle tissue manipulation. The design of the flap needs to be carefully planned perioperatively to avoid any vertical traction on the eyelid margin, eyelid crease, or eyebrow. On the contrary, vertical tension is desirable in the medial or lateral canthal area, provided that the canthal position is not changed. A *rhombic transposition flap* is very useful in the periocular area, and most common flap designs are shown in ▶ Fig. 10.33 where scars can be nicely camouflaged in the glabellar folds, the eyelid crease or medial and

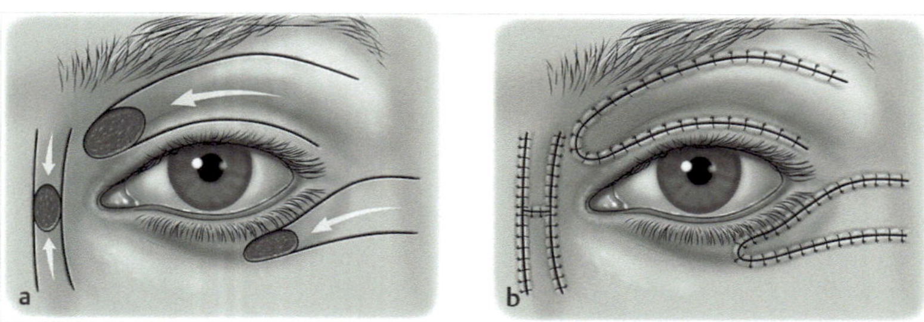

Fig. 10.28 Advancement flaps for the eyelid repair design **(a)** and repair **(b)** for medial canthus, upper and lower eyelid.

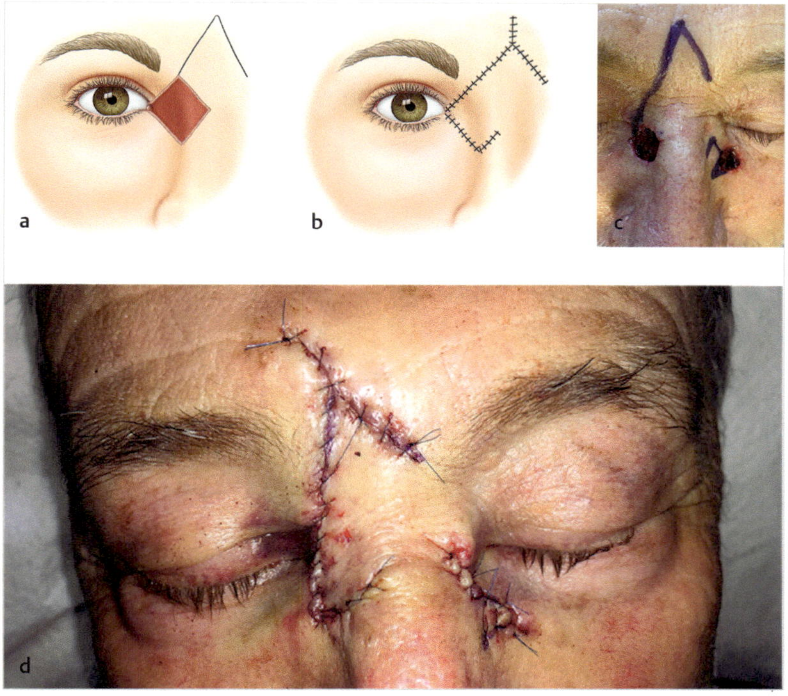

Fig. 10.29 Glabellar transposition flap medial canthal anterior lamella design: defect **(a,c)** and execution **(b,d)**. The left medial lower eyelid defect is repaired by rhombic transposition flap. (See ▶ Fig. 10.33 for design.) (**a, b**: Reproduced from Codner M, McCord C. Eyelid & Periorbital Surgery. 2nd ed. New York: Thieme; 2016.)

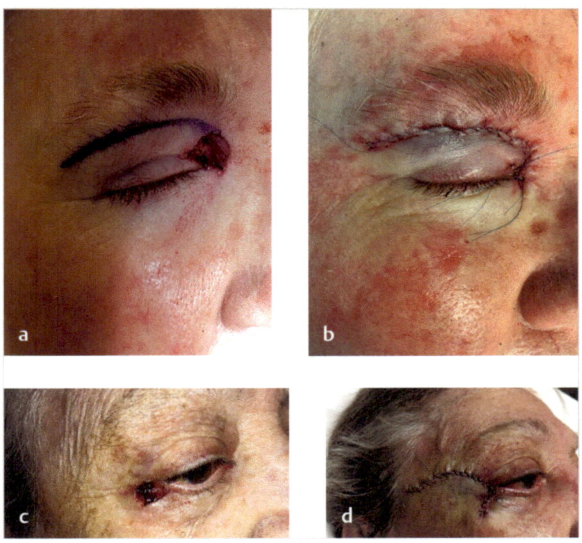

Fig. 10.30 Rotational flap for medial **(a,b)** and lateral **(c,d)** canthal defect.

lateral canthal angles. The *bilobed flap* is a two-lobe transposition flap that has been used successfully to repair defects of the lower eyelid, medial canthus, and nasojugal fold. Most flaps employ Zitelli's modification where total arc of rotation is limited to 90 to 100 degrees, with each lobe around 45 degrees each. This modification reduces wound tension and minimizes tissue distortion, which is so crucial in periocular area. *Switch flap or banner transposition flap* (▶ Fig. 10.34a–f) is an excellent option for lower eyelid anterior lamella defects, when sufficient skin is present on the ipsilateral upper eyelid. After the blepharoplasty incision is made, with the lower edge connecting to the lateral point of the lower eyelid defect and upper edge extending to maintain the vascularize base, the medial aspect is tapered, and the length customized to match the defect size. A myocutaneous flap (skin-OOM) is then elevated from the underlying septum, swung to the defect, and anchored with 7–0 prolene sutures. Hemostasis needs to be gentle, to avoid compromise of the vascular pedicle. *Z-plasty* (▶ Fig. 10.35) can be utilized for the defects where lengthening of the wound bed is indicated, for reduction of tension, redirection of stress or reposition of the canthal angle. The creation and transposition of two triangular flaps under the angles of 30–45–60 degrees can provide elongation of the residual closure to 25–50–75%, respectively.

10.9 Reconstruction of the Full-Thickness Eyelid Defects

10.9.1 Primary Closure of the Full-Thickness Defects of the Eyelids[1–4,19,20,24,25]

Small full-thickness marginal defects can be closed by direct layered closure depending on the laxity of the eyelid (▶ Fig. 10.36). In the upper eyelid, marginal defects up to 25 to 30% of eyelid length can be repaired primarily. In older individuals up to 40% of the upper eyelid can be closed directly. Excessive horizontal tension is less critical in the lower eyelid, so defects up to 30 to 40% of the lower eyelid margin can be closed primarily. Defects over 30 to

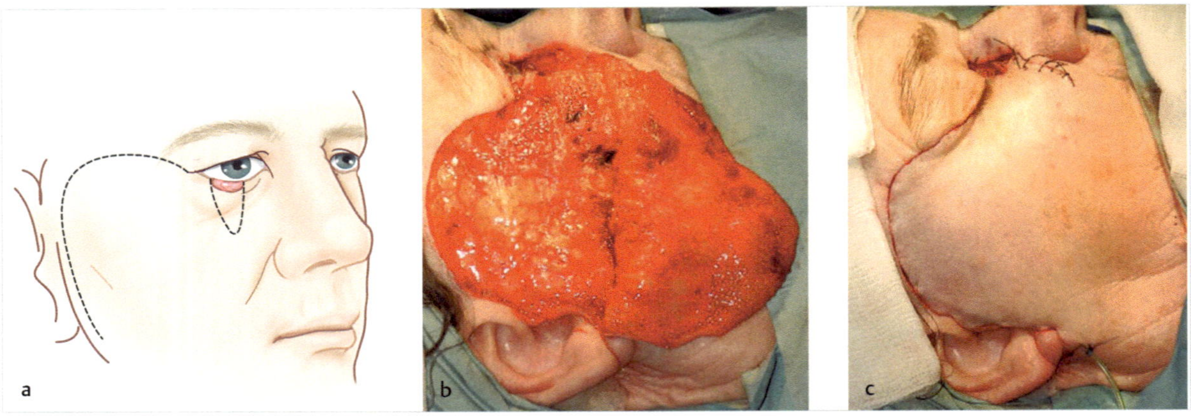

Fig. 10.31 Mustardé myocutaneous cheek rotational flap: design **(a)**, level of undermining **(b)**, and final closure **(c)**. (**a**: Reproduced from Woo A, Bhatt R. Plastic surgery case review: oral board study guide. 2nd ed. New York: Thieme; 2020; **b, c**: Reproduced from Leatherbarrow B. Oculoplastic Surgery. 3rd ed. New York: Thieme; 2019.)

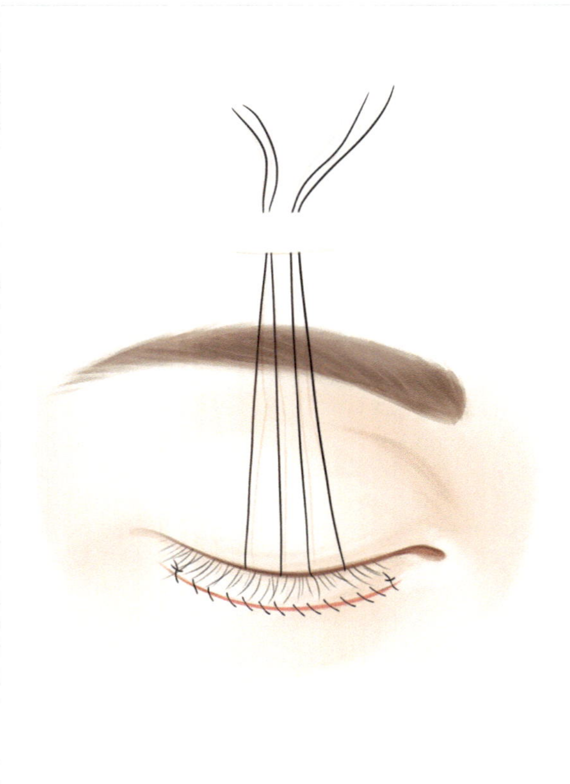

Fig. 10.32 Frost gray line suspension suture. It is passed once or twice through the inferior tarsus entering and exiting the orifices of Meibomian glands. (Reproduced from Freitag S, Lefebvre D, Lee N, Yoon M. Ophthalmic Plastic Surgery: Tricks of the Trade. New York: Thieme; 2019.)

40% may require canthotomy and cantholysis, i.e., LCT release to provide few additional millimeters of margin elongation (see ▶ Fig. 10.38). When performed properly,

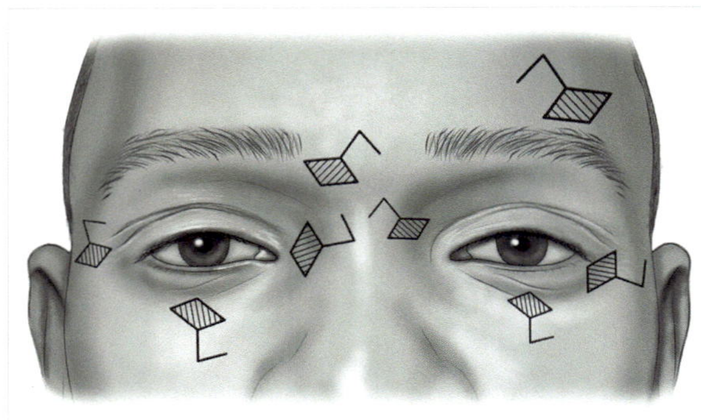

Fig. 10.33 Common designs for rhombic transposition flap in the periocular region.

the primary closure has best cosmetic results leaving an intact eyelid margin and full lash line in a single-stage procedure. As mentioned previously, “like-for-like” lamellar reapproximation must be performed to optimize the final functional and cosmetic result.

When performing direct closure, meticulous approximation of the eyelid margin is of utmost importance. Direct closure recreates smooth margin contour and reconstitutes the lash line and the tarsal plate. If edges of the defect cannot be brought together without the tension or hammocking of the lid under the globe, canthotomy and cantholysis should be performed with or without the frost suture. If the defect involves only partial thickness of the tarsus, a *pentagonal excision* (▶ Fig. 10.37a) design is preferred to avoid standing cutaneous deformities. The incisions are performed perpendicularly to excise rectangle of the tarsus to the upper eyelid crease. From there, pointed incision toward the conjunctival fornix is carried only in the anterior lamella, completing the tip of the pentagon. Next, it is important to align and evert the lash line, which will prevent

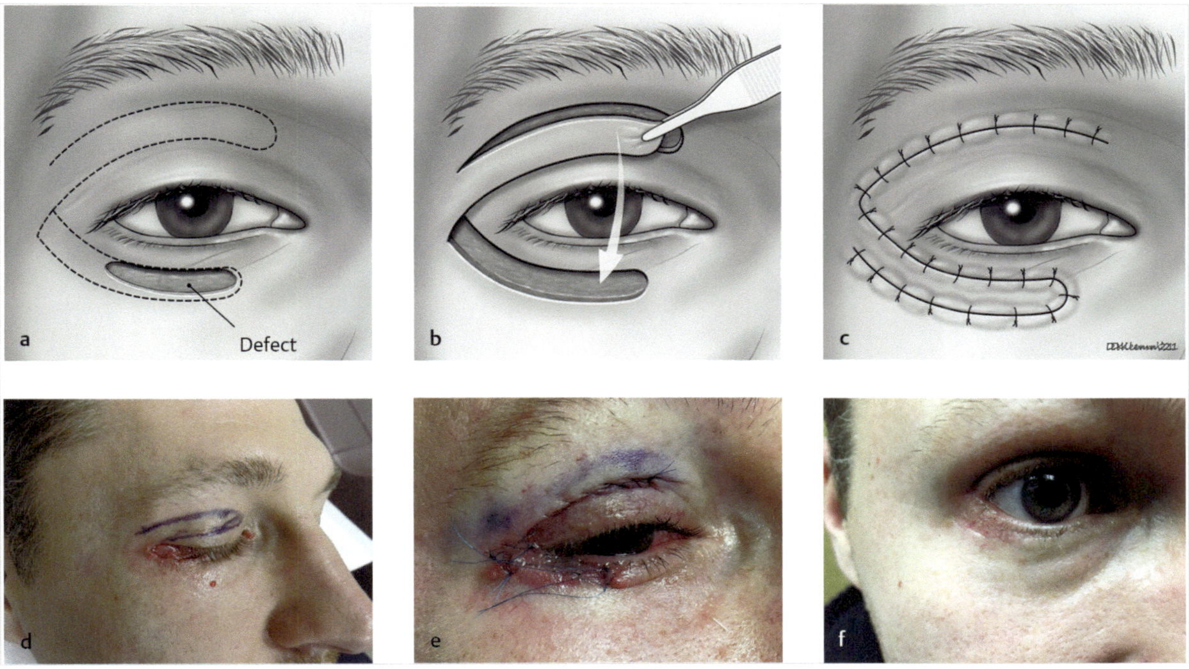

Fig. 10.34 Cross eyelid switch flap (banner transposition flap). Defect and flap design **(a,d)**. Flap execution **(b)** and suturing **(c,e)** and 6-months follow-up **(f)**.

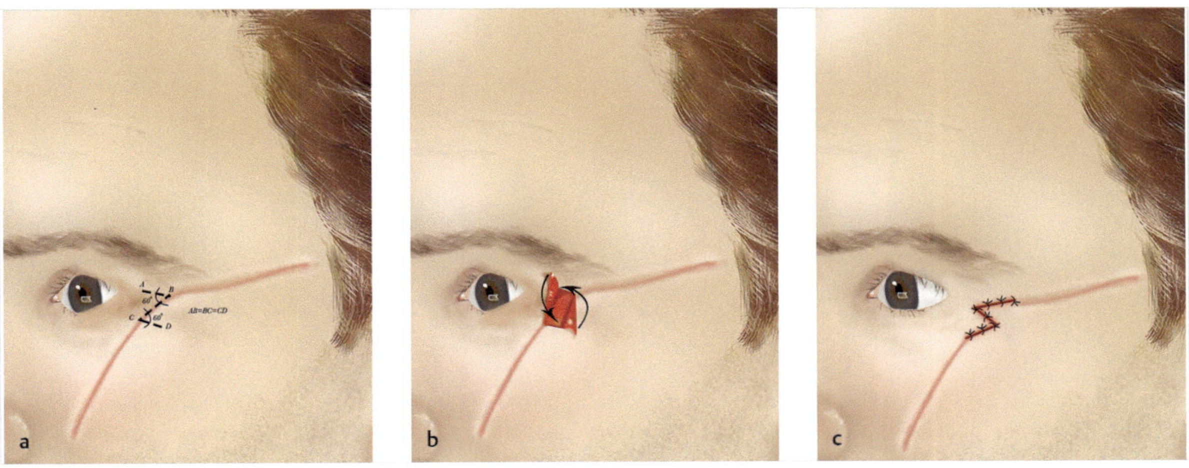

Fig. 10.35 **(a–c)** Z-plasty. Multiple triangular flaps used to correct scar contracture-induced ectropion of the lower lid. (Reproduced from Thornton J, Carboy J. Facial Reconstruction after Mohs Surgery. New York: Thieme; 2018.)

notching or step-off appearance. This is usually achieved by placing 6–0 prolene or silk *vertical mattress suture though the gray line (Meibomian gland orifices) in a far-far near-near* fashion. This will evert the wound edges and re-establish good alignment of the eyelid margin. The tarsus needs now to be reapproximated using 6–0 polyglactin sutures, placing in a partial thickness to avoid corneal abrasion and discomfort from exposed sutures. The upper eyelid usually requires four to five and lower two to three tarsal and subcutaneous sutures. To facilitate suture passage 2 to 3 mm of OOM should be dissected from the tarsal edges. The margin suture is then tied and left long so the ends can be incorporated in the skin closures, which are tied in the final stage with 7–0 prolene suture resulting in vertically oriented scar. The correct vs. incorrect designs of the pentagon are shown in ▶ Fig. 10.37b.

Lateral canthotomy (▶ Fig. 10.38a, b) is performed by cutting horizontally through the canthus to the lateral orbital

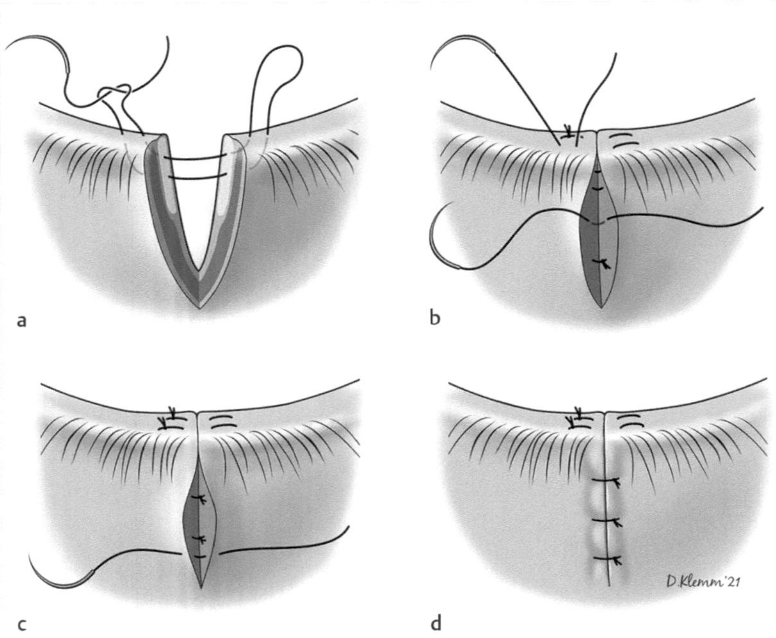

Fig. 10.36 Direct closure of the lower eyelid marginal defect. **(a)** 6–0 prolene or silk is used to align and evert the lash line, by placing vertical mattress suture in a far-far near-near fashion. **(b)** The tarsus is reapproximated using 6–0 polyglactin sutures which are placed **(c)** partial thickness to avoid corneal abrasion. **(d)** The marginal stitch is then tied and left long so the ends can be incorporated in the skin closures, with the rest of the skin approximated with 7–0 prolene suture resulting in vertically oriented suture line.

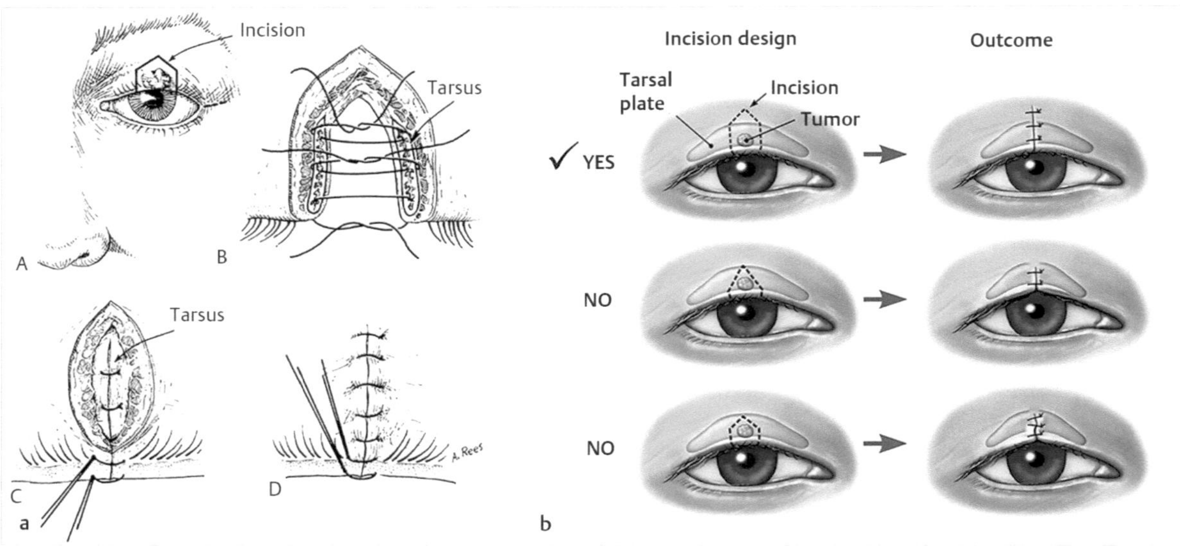

Fig. 10.37 **(a)** Direct closure of the marginal defect after conversion to pentagonal design. **(A)** Establish clean tarsal edges to avoid notching, extend the skin incision to form the triangular tip of pentagon above the horizontal lid margin (superior tarsal edge); **(B)** sutures passed through anterior two-third of the tarsal plate to avoid corneal irritation and eyelid retractors (levator aponeurosis or capsulopalpebral fascia); **(C)** vertical mattress sutures are used to approximate precisely the eyelid margin; and is **(D)** incorporated in the skin closure to avoid corneal irritation. **(b)** Correct vs. incorrect design of pentagonal wedge excision. The superior triangle has to be based above the tarsus to avoid eyelid margin notching or kinking. (**a:** Reproduced from Chen W. Oculoplastic Surgery: The Essentials. New York: Thieme; 2001.)

rim using Stevens tenotomy scissors. This splits the tendon in the inferior and superior components. *Cantholysis* is then performed by grasping the inferolateral eyelid (lower eyelid defects) or superolateral eyelid (upper eyelid defects) and pulling superiorly or inferiorly for the release of inferior crus (lower eyelid repair) or superior crus (upper eyelid repair). The canthotomy incision is typically left unclosed or can be sutured with 7–0 prolene in continuous manner.

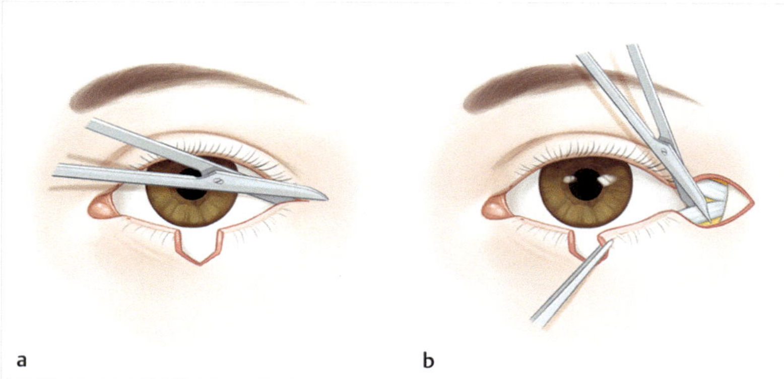

Fig. 10.38 (a,b) Lateral canthotomy and cantholysis of the inferior crus of the lateral canthal tendon (LCT) (*above*) incorporated in pentagonal design of the direct lower lid margin closure to release lateral tension (*below*). (Reproduced from Freitag S, Lefebvre D, Lee N, Yoon M. Eyelid Reconstruction. New York: Thieme; 2020.)

10.9.2 Semicircular Flap (Tenzel)[1,4,19,20,24,25]

Initially described by Tenzel in 1978, the semicircular myocutaneous flap remains a valuable technique for closing defects occupying up to two-thirds of the lower eyelid (33–75%) (▶ Fig. 10.39a–d, h–j; ▶ Video 10.3) and upper eyelid (30–66%) (▶ Fig. 10.39e–g, k–m). This flap is used when canthotomy and cantholysis do not provide sufficient mobilization to permit tension-free primary closure. The Tenzel flap is most successful when there is adequate lateral, canthal skin laxity and availability of at least a small segment of full-thickness eyelid on the lateral side of the defect. In cases where there is no tarsus on the lateral side of the wound, it is advisable to perform periosteal flap or posterior lamella graft for optimal results (see following text). With Tenzel flap, the canthotomy incision needs to be angled upward and outward starting following the curve of the opened lower eyelid margin below the lateral extent of the eyebrow approximately 2 to 3 cm lateral to the canthal angle. The design for the upper eyelid repairs is the mirror image of the one for the lower lids, and the curve follows the opened upper eyelid margin, and continues downward and laterally at the point 2 to 3 cm below the lateral extent of the brow. As with the primary closure the tarsal edges need to be smoothened vertically, and lateral canthotomy and cantholysis is performed. The flap is undermined and advanced medially to cover the defect. Lid margin sutures and tarsal sutures are placed in similar manner as with direct closure, to avoid conjunctiva penetration and globe irritation. The skin is closed with 7–0 prolene (eyelid) or 6–0 prolene (periocular skin and temple) as described before.

Lateral sagging of the eyelid can be prevented by fixation of the lateral flap tissue for superolateral orbital rim periosteum with 4–0 polyglactin suture. If there is need to improve lower eyelid contour, additional support may be necessary by performing *periosteal flap* (▶ Fig. 10.40). The base of the flap is designed high at the arcus marginalis (midpupillary level), extending laterally at the 45-degree angle, approximately 8 to 10 mm wide to the length corresponding to the distance from the remaining tarsus to lateral orbital rim. This maneuver will recreate tight lower eyelid with proper posterior contour. Larger defects, without any tarsus left at the wound edge, would require stronger backing of the repaired anterior lamella by using auricular cartilage, hard palate mucosa, nasal chondromucosa, or tarsoconjunctival graft from the upper eyelid. With the periosteal flap, a mucosal graft or conjunctival advancement is not necessary. Mobilization from the inferior fornix should be performed and sutured to the superior skin margin of a myocutaneous flap with 7–0 chromic gut or polyglactin sutures. Reconstruction of the canthal ligaments is less important with the upper eyelid procedures because the effects of gravity enhance upper lid position rather than opposing it as with lower lid. As with direct repair, meticulous reconstruction of the eyelid margin is critical to exclude keratinized epithelium, and prevent notching and trichiasis.

10.9.3 Tarsoconjunctival Flap for Lower Eyelid Reconstruction (Hughes Flap)[2,3,19,20]

This pedicle flap described by William Hughes in 1937 is considered for large lower eyelid defects encompassing two-thirds to total lower eyelid loss (▶ Fig. 10.41a–h). Vascular autogenous tarsus lined with conjunctiva is relatively ideal replacement for loss posterior lamella. The anterior lamella can be reconstructed with a myocutaneous flap or FTSG. The drawback of this repair technique is temporary obstruction of the vision for 7 to 45 days, i.e., until the second-stage procedure with pedicle division is performed. Nevertheless, it continues to be a highly effective and popular technique for reconstruction of large eyelid defects. The flap is harvested from the ipsilateral upper eyelid, always leaving 4 mm of the marginal tarsus intact. After retracting the upper eyelid over a Desmarres retractor, a caliper is used to mark the 4 mm of tarsus to remain attached to the lid margin. The caliper may then be used to measure the width of tarsus needed to reconstruct the lower eyelid, designed to be slightly less than the width of the defect on the lower eyelid and using the

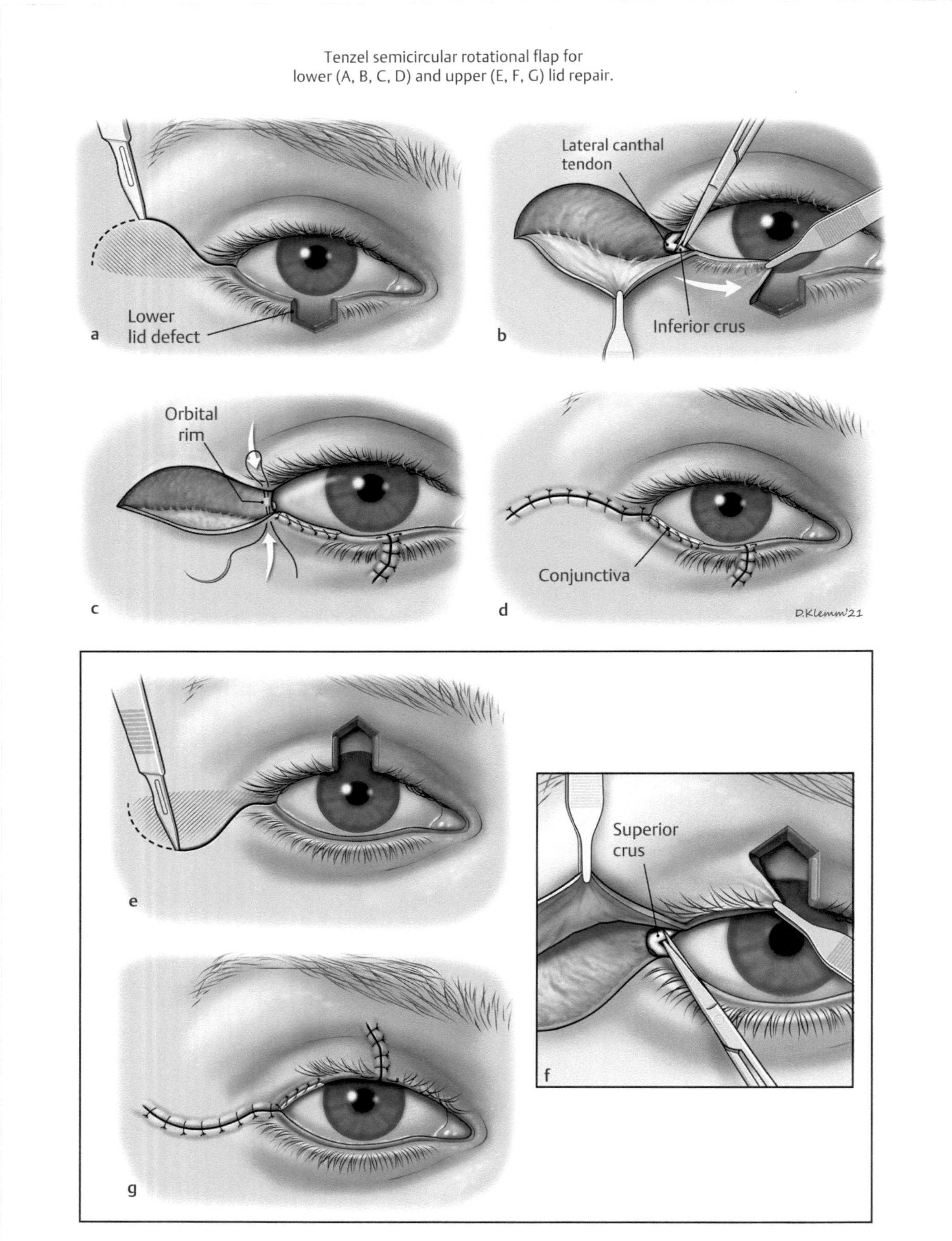

Fig. 10.39 Tenzel semicircular rotational flap design for lower **(a–d)** and upper **(e–g)** eyelid full-thickness marginal defects with cantholysis of the lower **(b)** and upper crus **(f)** of lateral canthal tendon.

(Continued)

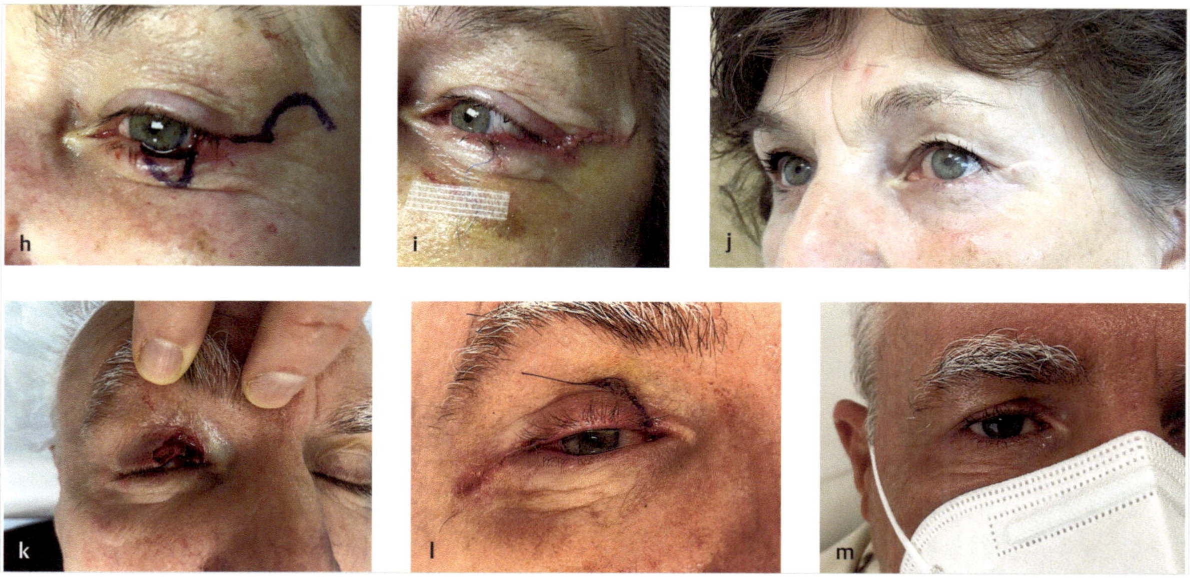

Fig. 10.39 (*Continued*) Fully executed Tenzel flap for post Mohs surgery defect after removal of left lower eyelid basal cell carcinoma **(h, i)** and right upper eyelid squamous cell carcinoma **(k, l)**, with six-month follow-ups **(j, m)**.

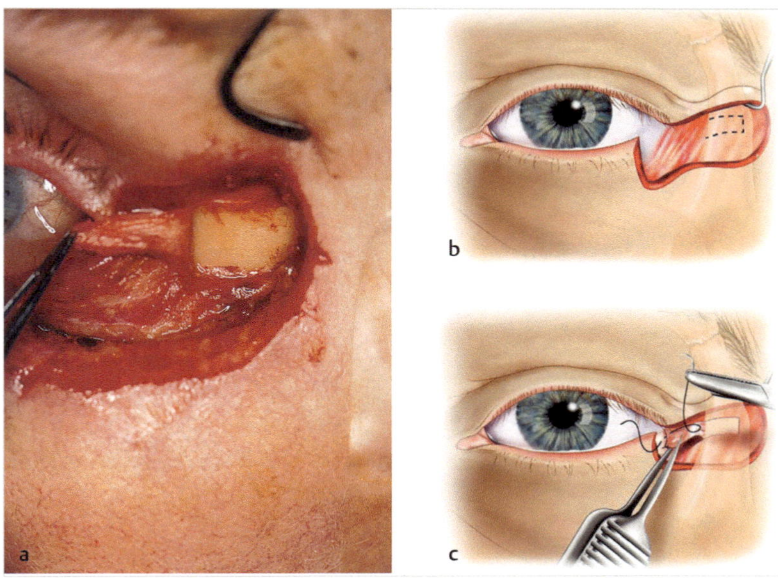

Fig. 10.40 (a–c) Periosteal inversion flap for the posterior lamella reconstruction of the temporal lower eyelid. The flap is angled 45 degrees so that the lower eyelid contour is maintained after the strip is reflected inferomedially. (Reproduced from Leatherbarrow B. Oculoplastic Surgery. 3rd ed. New York: Thieme; 2019.)

maximum height of the tarsus available. A 15c blade can be used to create the full-thickness tarsal incision, leaving the superior conjunctiva attached to the tarsus. The dissection then goes at the anterior side of the tarsus until the superior tarsal margin using blunt scissors. Then the scissors should be directed more posteriorly, i.e., behind the Müller's muscle and anterior to conjunctiva to avoid incorporation of the muscle into the flap. The visualization of the plane of dissection can be facilitated by infiltration of local anesthetic. Care should also be taken to avoid injuring the vascular arcade at the superior tarsal border. The dissection continues until the conjunctival pedicle can be advanced inferiorly without the tension and sutured in the lower eyelid defect by using 6–0 polyglactin suture. Relaxing incisions can be made vertically at the medial and lateral conjunctival edges of the flap. Conjunctiva and retractors are advanced from the inferior fornix and secured for the lower border of the tarsoconjunctival flap. The superior tarsal border of newly reconstructed posterior lamella should approximate the presurgical eyelid margin. At this point the cornea will be covered and protected by conjunctival pedicle of the flap and the upper eyelid will rest roughly at midpupillary height. With the total lower eyelid loss, the Hughes flap will be secured with lateral or medial (or both) periosteal grafts which will replace lost LCT or MCT. The anterior lamellar replacement may be fixated to the superior edge of the tarsus using a 7–0 polyglactin suture in a horizontal mattress fashion.

Postoperatively, patient is instructed to use ophthalmic eye drops four times a day (gentamicin, ciprofloxacin). Because peripheral vision is obviously reduced, use of a metal eye shield is helpful to prevent inadvertent injury of the flap, graft, and eye itself from blunt trauma. Chromic sutures are left to dissolve, while silk or prolene nonabsorbable sutures must be removed in 1 week.

Second-stage reconstruction of the tarsoconjunctival flap is performed at 2 to 4 weeks. A narrow malleable retractor is inserted under the flap to protect cornea. The flap is separated at the intended position of the new lower eyelid margin where mucocutaneous margin is ideally placed anteriorly to the apex of the reconstructed eyelid. The transected edges can be left to heal by secondary intent at this point.

10.9.4 Tarsal Transposition Flap for Lateral Upper Eyelid Reconstruction[2–4,25]

Tarsal transposition flap (▸ Fig. 10.42a–c), described by Kersten in 1986, is a good option for defects involving lateral upper eyelid. It is an alternative to Tenzel flap, composite graft, and even Cutler-Beard flap (see ▸ Fig. 10.42) when the defect is predominantly lateral. It is a single-stage procedure, using local vascularized eyelid tissue rather than creating additional comorbidity from the donor site of the contralateral upper eyelid as a donor site for composite graft, or other options of replacing posterior lamella with chondromucosal graft, or ear cartilage. The remaining ipsilateral tarsus presents the source for the reconstruction of lost upper eyelid posterior lamella in this case. The anterior lamella can then be repaired with FTSG or myocutaneous flap. The flap is designed from superior,

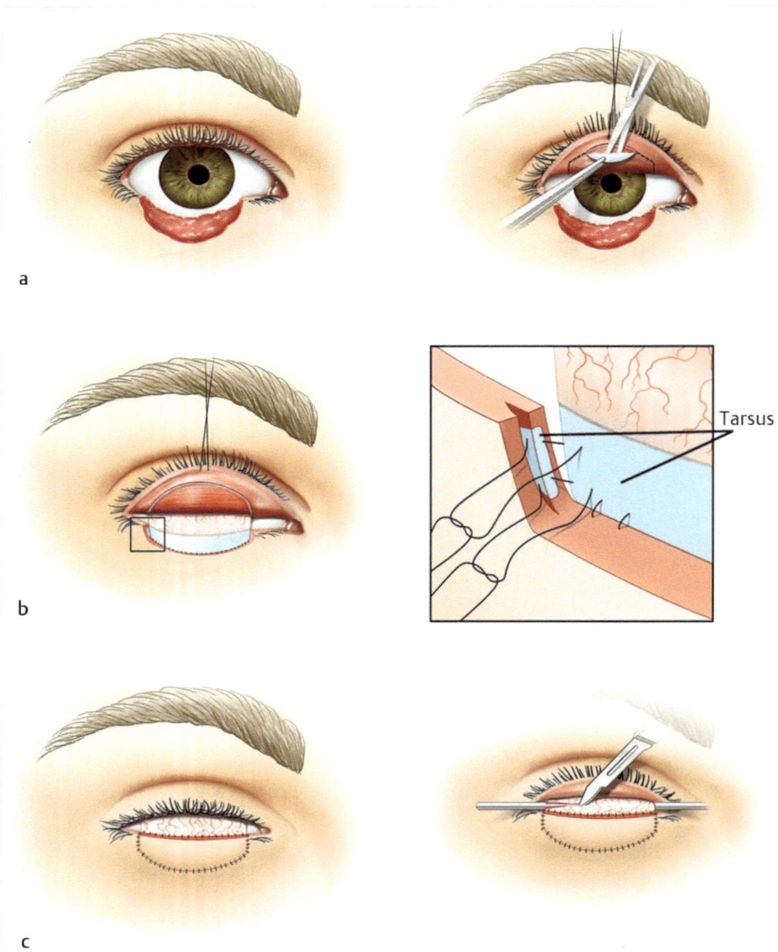

Fig. 10.41 (a–h) Hughes tarsoconjunctival flap for lower eyelid reconstruction. Full-thickness defect of the medial lower eyelid with the flap harvested leaving at least 4 mm distance superior to posterior upper lid margin **(a)**; upper border of the tarsus in the flap aligned with the lower eyelid margin and sutured to remaining tarsus on the sides of the loser eyelid **(b)**; anterior lamella reconstructed with full-thickness skin graft (FTSG) with the superior border of the conjunctiva sutures 1 to 2 mm above the border of the tarsus and pedicle divided after 2 to 4 weeks **(c)**.

(Continued)

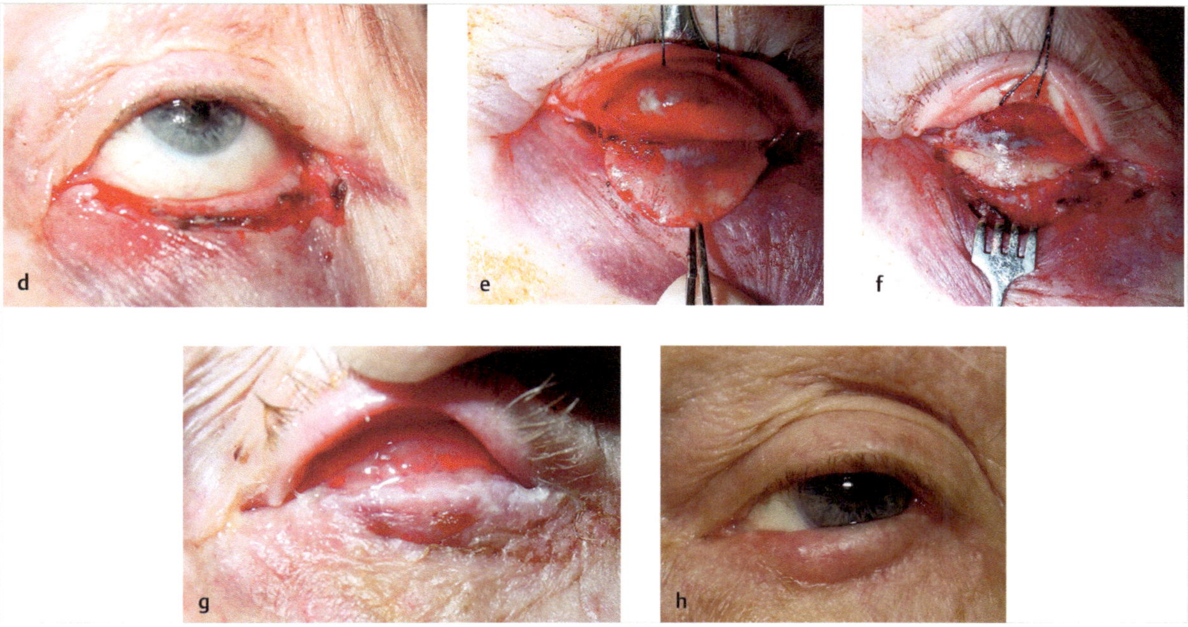

Fig. 10.41 (*Continued*) Hughes flap planning and execution **(d–f)** with pedicle division and final result **(g–h)**. (**a–c:** Reproduced from Codner M, McCord C. Eyelid & Periorbital Surgery. 2nd ed. New York: Thieme; 2016.)

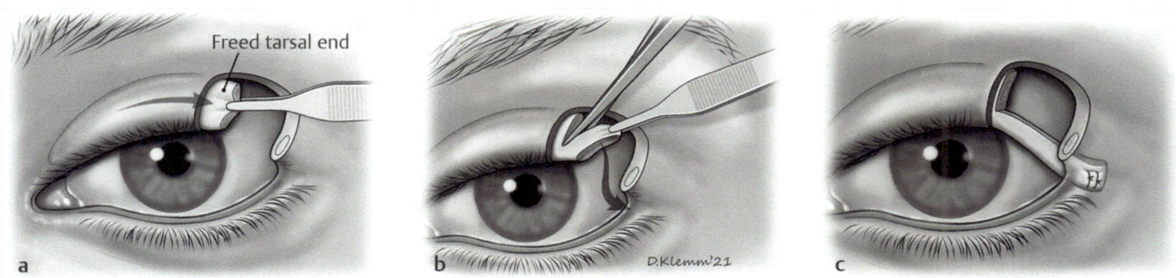

Fig. 10.42 Tarsal transposition flap. Superior border of the tarsus incised horizontally **(a)** followed by vertical tarsal incision creating inferiorly based transposition flap **(b)** which is then fixed to lateral canthal tendon (LCT) or lateral orbital rim **(c)**.

placing the incision from superior tarsus, at the 3 to 4 mm width, down to 1 to 2 mm above the upper lid margin. The flap is divided from OOM, and then pivoted 90 degrees and attached to LCT, or periosteal flap, whichever was the method used to reconstruct lateral canthal angle, with 5–0 polyglactin suture on S-14 spatula needle using the "cross-sword" technique. Conjunctiva can now be advanced from superior fornix and be approximated to the flap with 7–0 chromic gut. The manipulation of the levator is not necessary since the existing attachments to medial part of the tarsus are adequate for proper eyelid elevation.

Horizontal tarsoconjunctival transposition flap (▶ Fig. 10.43a–e) is a way to mobilize more ipsilateral tarsus for lateral upper eyelid defects and is harvested by placing horizontal conjunctival incision parallel and approximately 3 to 4 mm from the eyelid margin. The width of the flap corresponds to the size of the defect, and the wound should be closed under mild tension. Incision is continued toward the fornix, LA is cut as well as the Müller's muscle, and the incision completed further in the subconjunctival plane. Then, the flap is transposed horizontally into the defect and sutured to the tarsal edge of the remaining eyelid with interrupted 6–0 polyglactin stitches, without compromising the conjunctiva as explained before. The opposite side should be sutured for the remnant of lateral canthal ligament or periosteal flap as discussed above. The LA has to be engaged and advanced to be sutured to the superior part of the transposed tarsal flap. It is essential that the LA be advanced without retraction of the eyelid. If that is not possible, the aponeurosis should be allowed to retract and sutured to the conjunctiva above the tarsus. The patient should be asked to look up, so that appropriate height of the eyelid margin is confirmed. The anterior lamella can then be repaired as already explained above.

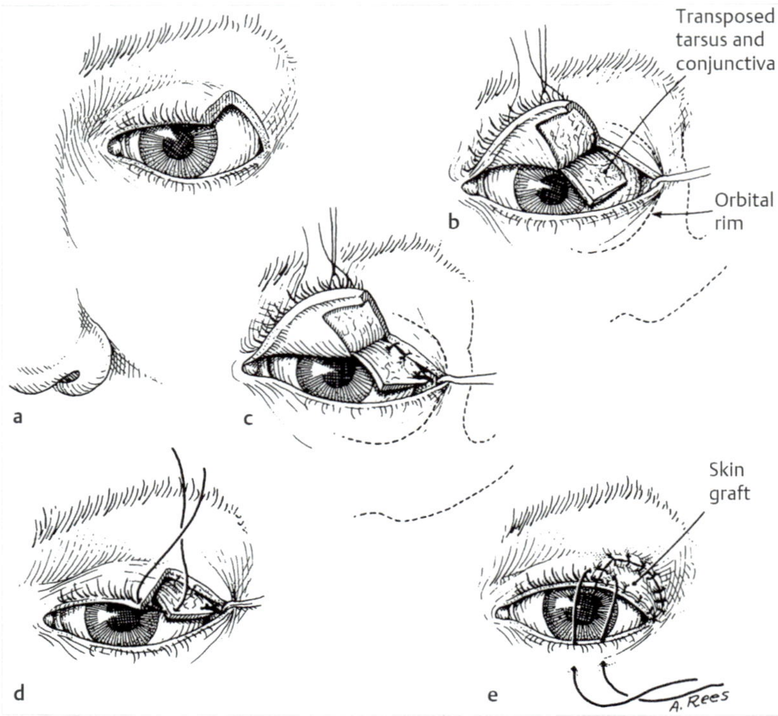

Fig. 10.43 Horizontal tarsoconjunctival transposition flap. **(a–c)** Flap harvested with the conjunctival incision 3 to 4 mm away and parallel to eyelid margin **(a)**, separated from Müller's muscle **(b)**, transposed and sutured to medial tarsal border **(c)**. Lateral side of the flap connected to remaining lateral canthal tendon (LCT) **(d)** and anterior lamella repaired with full thickness skin grafts (FTSG) **(e)**. (Reproduced from Chen W. Oculoplastic Surgery: The Essentials. New York: Thieme; 2001.)

10.9.5 Cutler-Beard Flap for Complete Upper Eyelid Reconstruction[1,2,24,25,29]

The reconstruction of the large defects of the upper eyelid is very challenging and no single operation can achieve all goals satisfactorily. Cutler-Beard flap is one of the best available techniques for total upper eyelid reconstruction (▶ Fig. 10.44a–e). As already emphasized for the maintenance of corneal integrity, crisp vision, and patient comfort, the upper eyelid must have a 5- to 10-mm range of movement and dynamic blink. This flap does not provide rigid posterior lamella which may result in instability of the reconstructed eyelid margin over time. Hence, free tarsoconjunctival graft or free hard palate mucosal grafts, auricular cartilage, or donor sclera can be used for the support. The flap is designed on the lower eyelid along the inferior tarsal border and extended laterally to correspond the defect on the upper eyelid, which should be reshaped in the rectangular fashion. The flap is then extended inferiorly 15 to 20 mm toward the inferior conjunctival fornix, with the lid pulled superiorly over the Jaeger plate or similar lid guard to protect the cornea. After full-thickness blepharotomy is performed, the composite flap is now brought below the lower eyelid margin bridge and sutured to the defect of the upper eyelid. This composite flap consists of skin, OOM, lower lid retractors, and conjunctiva. First the conjunctival flap should be approximated using 6–0 plain gut. Then the posterior lamella replacement, i.e., auricular cartilage, should be placed and sutured with remnants of tarsus or canthal ligaments on each side of the upper eyelid defect. LA should be advanced and attached to the upper edge of the graft using 6–0 polyglactin suture. Finally, the skin muscle flap which was already separated from the conjunctiva should be attached to the anterior side of the graft, replacing anterior lamella.

Inset of the flap can be performed in 2 to 4 weeks with the division cut about 2 mm below the desired upper eyelid margin. Upon resection, the longer piece on the conjunctival side is draped and sutured to the skin with 7–0 chromic gut suture, ensuring that the new upper eyelid margin is not keratinized. The inferior edge of the lower eyelid bridge is then freshened, and the bases of the lower eyelid flap sutured to the bridge in a layered fashion using 6–0 polyglactin for conjunctiva and retractors and 6–0 polypropylene for the skin. If there is a risk of lower eyelid ectropion, the skin and orbicularis may need to be undermined and any horizontal laxity should be repaired with lateral tarsal strip procedure (see following text).

In 1983, Leone published a procedure similar to Hughes flap ("reverse Hughes flap") but designed for the upper eyelid reconstruction up to the size of 70% of the margin. Here, the tarsoconjunctival flap is harvested from the lower eyelid posterior lamella, approximately 1.5 mm below the margin of the lower lid. Upon the flap release from retractors, *tarsoconjunctival advancement flap* (▶ Fig. 10.45a–d) is brought upward and sutured to remaining tarsus of the upper eyelid, while inferior tarsal margin of the lower lid flap will become the lid margin of the upper eyelid. The anterior lamella is repaired by FTSG

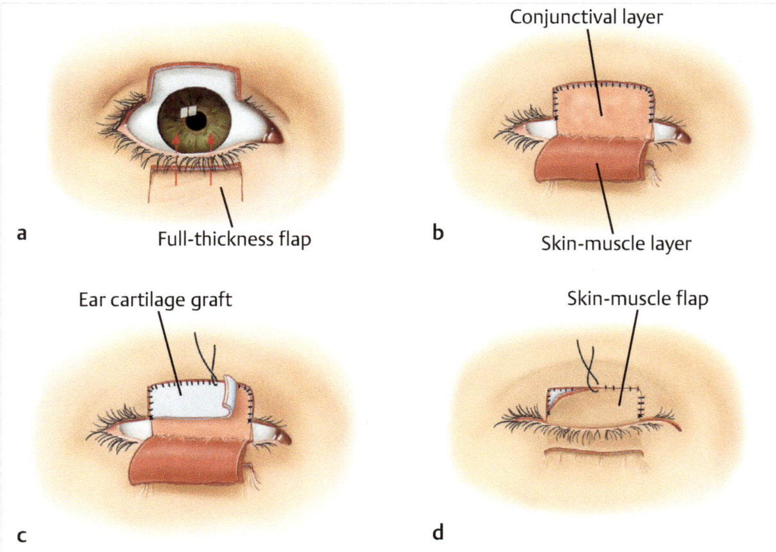

Fig. 10.44 Cutler-Beard flap—full-thickness incision on the lower lid **(a)**, anterior and posterior lamella separated with conjunctiva sutured to upper lid defect **(b)**; ear cartilage graft in place **(c)** and skin-muscle part attached **(d)**. The division with recreation of the upper lid margin occurs in 2 to 4 weeks. (Reproduced from Codner M, McCord C. Eyelid & Periorbital Surgery. 2nd ed. New York: Thieme; 2016.)

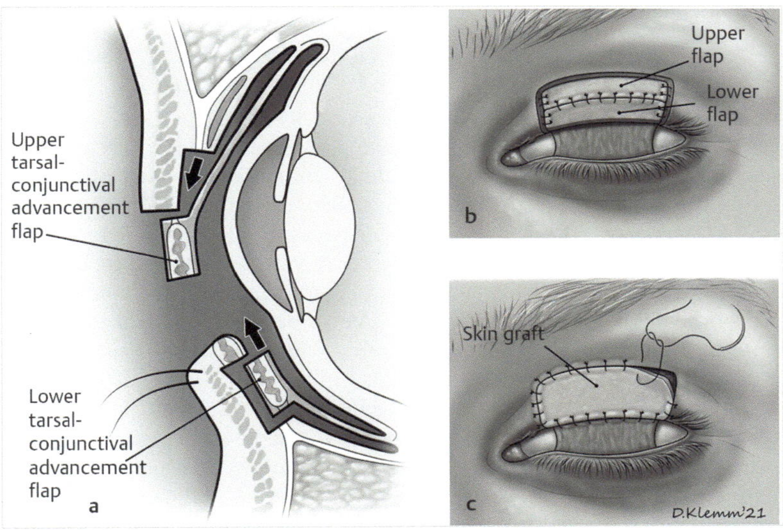

Fig. 10.45 Leone tarsal-conjunctival advancement flap. Incision made 1.5 mm from the posterior lid margin **(a)**; flap is brought upward and sutured to remaining lid margin **(b)** and defect repaired with full-thickness skin grafts (FTSG) **(c)** donor site postauricular skin (not shown).

(postauricular skin) which adheres firmly to the tarsus, preventing the skin from overhanging against the globe. The advantage of this flap compared to Cutler-Beard flap is that it requires only tarsal/conjunctival portion and not full thickness of the lower eyelid for bridging the defect on the upper lid. Hence, 1.5 mm of remaining tarsal height on the lower lid should be enough to prevent ectropion more commonly seen with Cutler-Beard technique. The tarsal flap, regardless of being only several millimeters, provides enough stability to upper eyelid to keep the skin from rolling inward. It also eliminates the need for harvesting donor tissue for eyelid support like nasal chondromucosal graft or ear cartilage, as already described with Cutler-Beard technique. The division of the pedicle is planned in 2 to 4 weeks as with Cutler-Beard flap.

10.10 Lower Lid Tightening Procedures[30–32]

We have already emphasized that lower eyelid laxity can be present upon removal of skin cancer and if not properly addressed can result in ectropion and dry eye syndrome. One of the most common procedures used to tighten lower lid is *lateral tarsal strip* (▶ Fig. 10.46a–g). A lateral canthotomy and cantholysis of the lower crus of LCT is performed as explained before. A free tarsal strip is created from the lateral edge of the lower eyelid by splitting it at the gray line for the distance of 5 to 10 mm (depending on the amount needed for lid shortening) and denuding it from superior and anterior skin and OOM, and posteriorly from the conjunctiva and retractors. If excessive eyelid laxity is noticed, extra 2 to 4 mm of tarsus may be removed; otherwise the

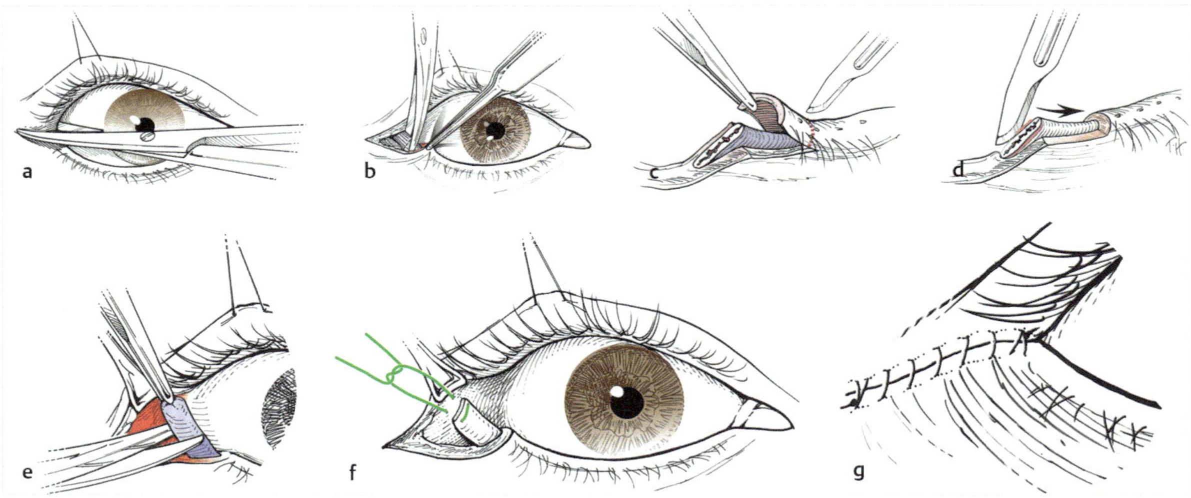

Fig. 10.46 The lateral tarsal strip procedure. After canthotomy **(a)** and cantholysis **(b)** are performed the lateral tarsal strip is created by dividing anterior and posterior lamella at the gray line removing the skin and conjunctive **(c–e)**; lateral tarsal strip attached to the periosteum of the lateral orbital rim. **(f)** Lateral canthal angle recreated with interrupted absorbable suture through the gray line with the skin closed with nonabsorbable interrupted sutures **(g)**. (Reproduced from Cheney M, Hadlock T. Facial Surgery: Plastic and Reconstructive. New York: Thieme; 2014.)

tarsus length should be left intact, since in most situations its attachment to inner lateral orbital wall is sufficient to produce desired amount of eyelid tightening. A 6–0 polydioxanone (PDS), polypropylene or nylon is passed first through the superior aspect of the tarsus, then LCT remnant and continued to grasp periosteum (approximately 2 mm inside at the superior position of the lateral orbital rim) and finished by going through the inferior aspect of the tarsal strip. Before tying it, use 6–0 chromic gut through the gray line of the lateral upper and lower eyelid to prevent blunting and recreating the lateral canthal angle. After this the skin incision can be closed as described before.

After any surgical procedure on the lower eyelid, it is also important to assess medial canthal laxity by laterally displacing the lacrimal punctum. If the punctum lacrimale moves beyond medial limbus, there is a risk of disruption of normal lacrimal drainage and subsequent epiphora. Hence, the laxity of medial canthus needs to be addressed and patient referred for prophylactic canthopexy of medial eyelid.

10.11 Wound Dressing and Postoperative Care in Periocular Surgery Patients

Wound dressing[1,2,3,4,20,24] consists of erythromycin or gentamicin ophthalmic ointment. Cotton gauze is not necessary but if used it should be in the form of an eye pad and carefully applied over the closed eyelid to avoid risk of corneal abrasion. It may help prevent hematoma and should be removed in 1 to 2 days. The frequent application of the icepacks for 20 minutes several times a day in the first few postoperative days may decrease bruising and swelling. Antibiotic ointment should be applied twice daily at the incision site and in the eye at the bedtime until suture removal in 5 to 7 days. Most patients do not tolerate application of the ointments during the day since it blurs the vision. The use of artificial tears three to six times a day may be needed. Contact lenses cannot be worn while ointment is used during daytime hours.

Current ocular medications[20,24] such as glaucoma eye drops should be applied in the preoperative and postoperative periods prior to application of the ointments. Frost sutures are usually removed in 3 to 5 days, and the vertical mattress eyelid margin suture in 2 to 3 weeks. If FTSG is covered with a bolster dressing, the sutures are never affixed to eyelid tissue but instead at the brows, nose, or arcus marginalis. The bolster is removed in one week as in the other areas. After suture removal, ophthalmic antibiotic ointment is applied for additional 3 to 7 days. Patients should avoid strenuous physical activity for the first 2 weeks after the procedure.[1,2,20,24]

10.12 Lacrimal Canalicular System Assessment and Reconstruction [1–3,20,26]

Defects in the medial upper and lower eyelid and medial canthus may frequently involve the lacrimal drainage system, especially puncta and canaliculi. Primary reconstruction of these structures will usually prevent epiphora and the need for more extensive procedures like *conjunctivodacryocystorhinostomy* with Jones tube.

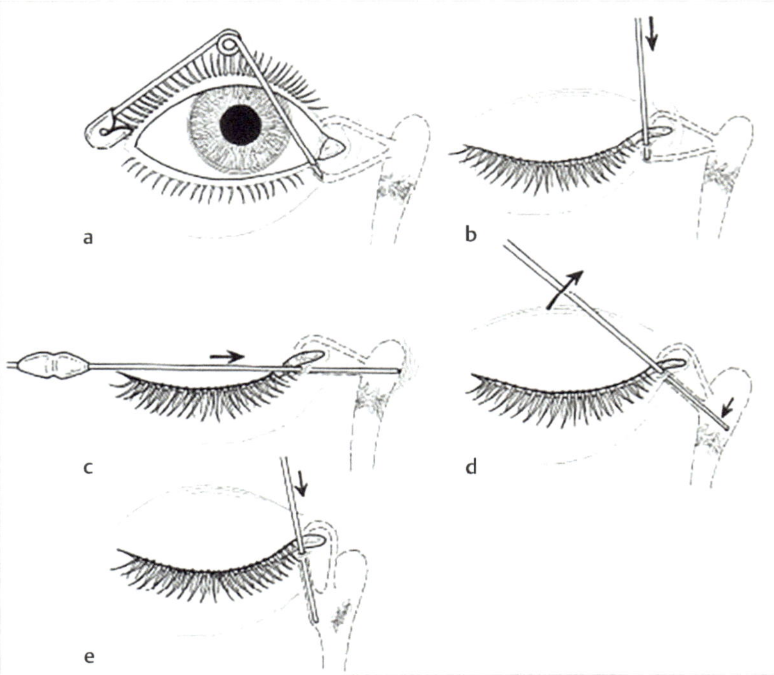

Fig. 10.47 (a–e) Technique of Bowman lacrimal probe insertion. Punca dilated with sterile safety pin **(a)** and lubricated Bowman probe inserted first vertically—J form **(b)** and then horizontally and medially **(c)** until reaching the end of lacrimal sac **(d)**. Probe is then engaged downward and 15 degrees posteriorly for additional 15 to 20 mm until it reaches nasal cavity **(e)**. (Reproduced from Gallin P. Pediatric Ophthalmology: A Clinical Guide. New York: Thieme; 2000.)

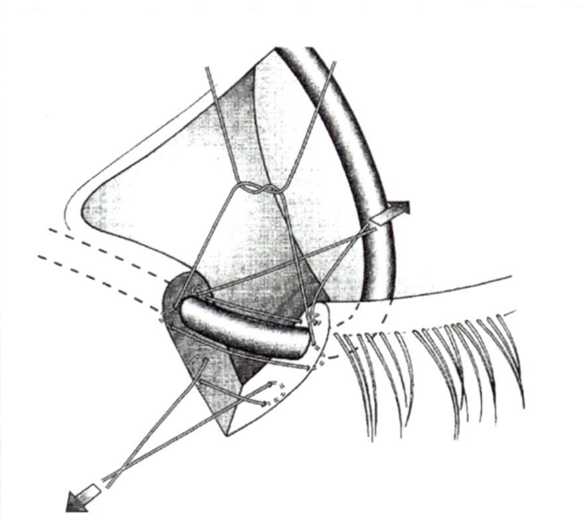

Fig. 10.48 5–0 Vicryl pericanalicular sutures (anterior and posterior) ensure repair of the medial canthal tendon, as the canaliculi run through the middle of it. (Reproduced from Chen W. Oculoplastic Surgery: The Essentials. New York: Thieme; 2001.)

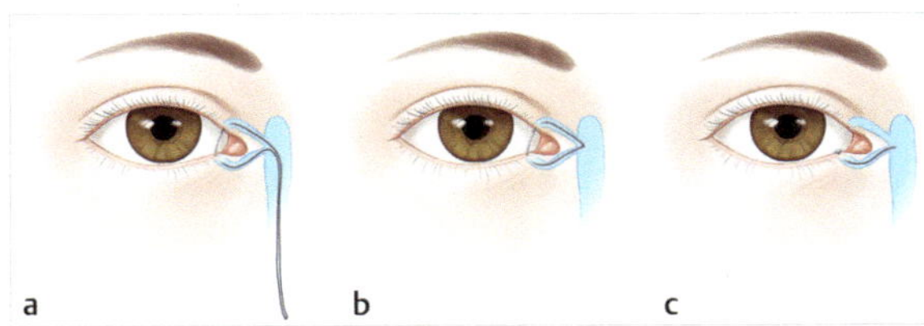

Fig. 10.49 Bicanalicular **(a,b)** and monocanalicular stents **(c)**. (Reproduced from Freitag S, Lefebvre D, Lee N, Yoon M. Ophthalmic Plastic Surgery: Tricks of the Trade. New York: Thieme; 2019.)

First it is important to determine if the punctum or the canaliculus have been violated. After punctum dilation a *Bowman probe* (▶ Fig. 10.47a–e) is inserted in the punctum and ampulla perpendicular to the eyelid margin for a distance of 2 mm. Then it is rotated 90 degrees medially so that it is parallel with the eyelid margin. Gentle lateral tension is now applied to the eyelid and probe smoothly directed toward the nasal sidewall ("hard stop"). If the probe is not visible, and reaches the nasal sidewall and slides easily without tension or force, the canaliculus and lacrimal system are intact.

The canaliculi run through MCT (see ocular anatomy earlier in the chapter) which provides an anchor and horizontal support for the medial eyelids. If violated, MCT needs to be approximated to allow proper eyelid function by placement of the pericanalicular sutures (▶ Fig. 10.48).

If there is partial damage of one or both canaliculi, *mono or bicanalicular silicone stenting* (▶ Fig. 10.49a, b) with a Crawford stent needs to be performed. Once the probe is passed through vertical and horizontal parts of the canaliculus (see earlier in the chapter), it is directed toward lacrimal bone; once the bone is reached, medially, the probe is redirected inferomedially until it passes into the inferior nasal meatus. Finally, the probe is retrieved with Crawford hook or any other clamp and cut from the silicone, with two silicone ends being tied together so

Table 10.2 Complications of eyelid reconstruction

Eyelid retraction
Cicatricial ectropion or entropion
Ptosis
Lagophthalmos
Dry eye
Trichiasis
Infection
Graft failure
Scarring
Dyschromia (hyperpigmentation, hypopigmentation)

that there is neither tension on the nostril nor on the medial canthus. The probes are left for 3 to 6 months and pulled out after the securing sutures are cut. If more extensive damage of the canaliculi and lacrimal system is anticipated or evaluated, consultation with an oculoplastic surgeon and subsequent conjunctivodacryocystorhinostomy with Jones tube is required. One should bear in mind that epiphora is not as common in individuals more than 60 years old as well as in cases where the lower canalicular system is intact.

10.13 Complications of Eyelid Reconstructions[1–4,20,24,33,34] (▶ Table 10.2)

One of the most common complications of periorbital surgery is lower eyelid ectropion and eyelid retraction. It occurs as a result of anterior lamellar shortening, vertical tension from the flap, and medial punctal ectropion. Common errors that lead to this outcome are poor fixation of the lateral canthal ligament to the lateral wall of the orbit, improper fixation of the posterior portion of the medial canthal ligament, undersized graft or flap, or improper deep fixation of a flap. The shortening of anterior lamella is usually remedied by complete scar lysis and its replacement by full-thickness skin graft. It is essential to ensure sufficient graft size and provide vertical support to lower eyelid margin by applying a "frost suture" (see earlier in the chapter). In addition to the skin graft, it is important to assess lateral and medial canthal angle laxity and consider lateral canthal tightening (tarsal strip) or fixation of the medial canthal ligament if cicatricial ectropion is more pronounced medially.

Other common complications to be avoided when operating in the periorbital area are corneal abrasion, lagophthalmos, and trichiasis. When using upper eyelid skin as a donor site for the FTSG, at least 20 mm of the skin (from eyelid margin to the brow) should be left in place to have proper closing of the eyelids and avoid postoperative lagophthalmos.

Plastic corneal eye shields are often used during periorbital procedures to prevent corneal and scleral abrasion, severing of extraocular muscles and corneal or globe perforation. Many Mohs surgeons (81.8%) report the use of internal eye shields in their practices. Apart from preventing operative injuries, corneal eye shields help patient relax by preventing the patients from seeing the operation itself and facilitate the take of the eyelids skin incision by tautening the skin.

Before insertion, cornea is anesthetized by 0.5% proparacine and lubricant applied over concave surface of the eye shield. The eye shield is inserted in the superior fornix with the patient positioning the eyes in the downward gaze. The removal follows the steps of the insertion in the reverse and with the use of suction cup unless the corneal shield has built in handle (▶ Video 10.4).[34]

10.14 Aims and Principles of Eyebrow Reconstruction[8,9,15,35,36]

The most important goals for eyebrow reconstruction are to achieve (a) shape, hair direction, and thickness appropriate to race and gender; (b) closure within the same cosmetic units; (c) hide incisions parallelly above and below the brows; (d) maximize preservation of the hair follicles; (e) avoid notching/elevation/ptosis; (f) preserve symmetry by having height of the reconstructed and contralateral eyebrow within 3 to 5 mm of each other.

The medial brow is far more aesthetically significant than the lateral brow. In general, one should move tissue more from lateral to medial, and avoid lateral displacement of the medial brow. During reconstruction, follicular transection should be avoided by creating beveled incisions parallel to the hair direction and also undermine the flaps in the subcutaneous fat to protect dermal papillae. Rotation flaps should generally be avoided, since they produce brow distortion. The use of local flaps is preferred over hair-bearing grafts, since there is about 25 to 50% of hair follicle loss in the latter.

For smaller defects options include primary closure, advancement flaps, transposition flaps, and subcutaneous pedicle flaps. For larger defects besides using the grafts and flaps there is net loss of follicular tissues. These can be addressed with follicular unit transplantation, tattooing, or make-up. Alternatively, hair-bearing skin can be recruited by using flaps from the scalp, contralateral brow, or by harvesting composite skin-hair grafts from the scalp depending on the size of the defect.

In the cosmetic subdivision of the forehead, brow is labeled as zone 4 (▶ Fig. 10.50).

10.14.1 Primary Closure of Brow Defects[14,15,35]

Horizontal ellipse can nicely match the curvature of the brows, immediately below and above the brows. However, the risk of brow elevation does exist. This can be assessed by pulling inferior and superior border of the defect together using the skin hooks. Using vertical closure, the risk of brow elevation can be avoided

(▶ Fig. 10.15 and ▶ Fig. 10.51a–e). This approach is recommended for defects affecting one-fifth to one-fourth of the eyebrow length.

10.14.2 Advancement Flaps[15,35]

A variety of the advancement flaps can be utilized for the brow reconstruction like unilateral (O-L) (▶ Fig. 10.53a–c), bilateral (A-T, O-T, or O-Z) (▶ Fig. 10.52 and ▶ Fig. 10.54a, b), unipedicle (O-U) or bipedicle (O-H) closures (▶ Fig. 10.55a, b). The design of the flap depends on the location and should be executed in such a way as to not disturb the position of the brow. For small- to medium-sized defects the scar can be very well hidden at, below, or above the brows. Horizontal incisions are drawn immediately beneath, above, or in the eyebrow itself from inferolateral border of the defect. Superiorly located standing cones can be removed after the approximation of the flap edges. Unilateral advancement flaps are generally preferred over bilateral since they involve less movement of the skin from medial to lateral.

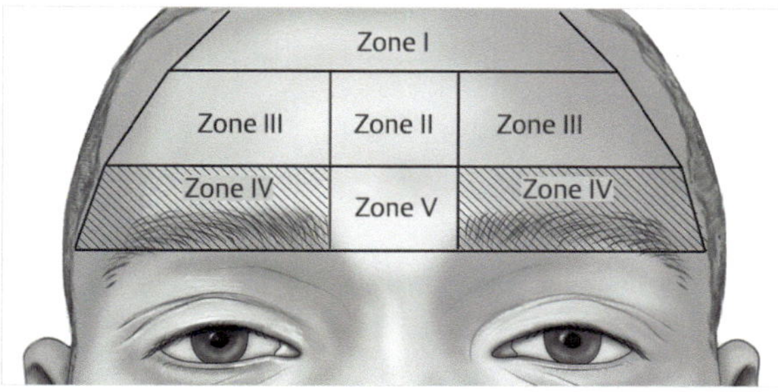

Fig. 10.50 Eyebrows are considered Zone IV of the cosmetic subdivisions of the forehead.

10.14.3 Island-Pedicle Flaps[35,37]

The subcutaneous island pedicle flap or V-Y flaps (▶ Fig. 10.56a–e) may be used for lateral, central, or medial defects. For medial defects, the flap can be designed to include the whole brow as reported by Bakkour et al,[37] where the flap is moved medially and positioned for symmetry with contralateral eyebrow. Lateral displacement of the brow is less likely since glabellar skin is not that lax and moves less. To reduce lateral displacement tacking suture to the frontal bone periosteum may be considered. For larger defects affecting up to half of the brow the flap should be based on the preparation of the deep pedicle based on superficial temporal artery for medial locations or supratrochlear artery for lateral brow, respectively.

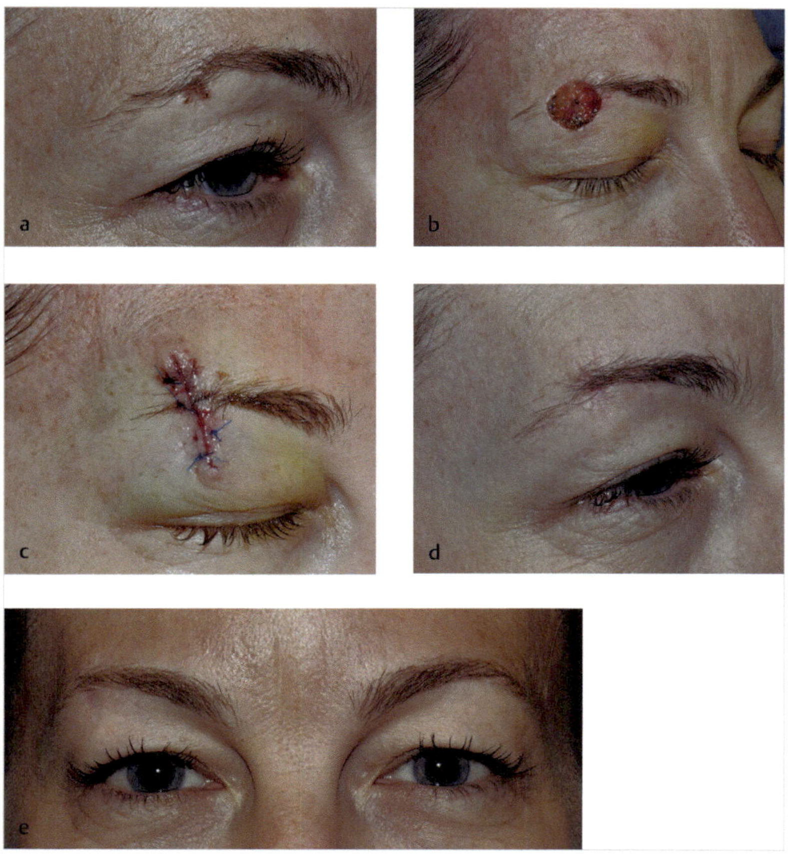

Fig. 10.51 Direct vertical closure suitable for defects 1/5 to ¼ of the brow length. Vertical orientation eliminates brow malposition and shortening. Melanoma in situ of the R brow with corresponding defect after excision **(a,b)**. Closure with vertical orientation **(c)** and subsequent cosmetic result 4 and 11 months after the procedure **(d,e)**. (Reproduced from Freitag S, Lefebvre D, Lee N, Yoon M. Eyelid Reconstruction. New York: Thieme; 2020.)

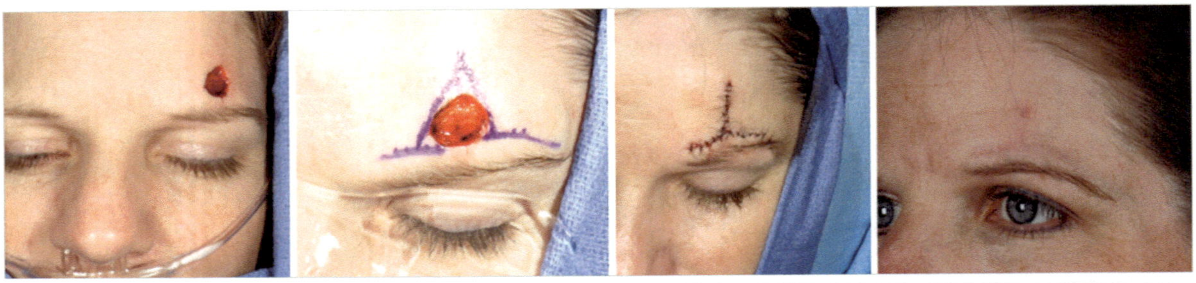

Fig. 10.52 A-T closure (defect, design, flap sutured in place and cosmetic result in 1 month). (Reproduced from Thornton J, Carboy J. Facial Reconstruction after Mohs Surgery. New York: Thieme; 2018.)

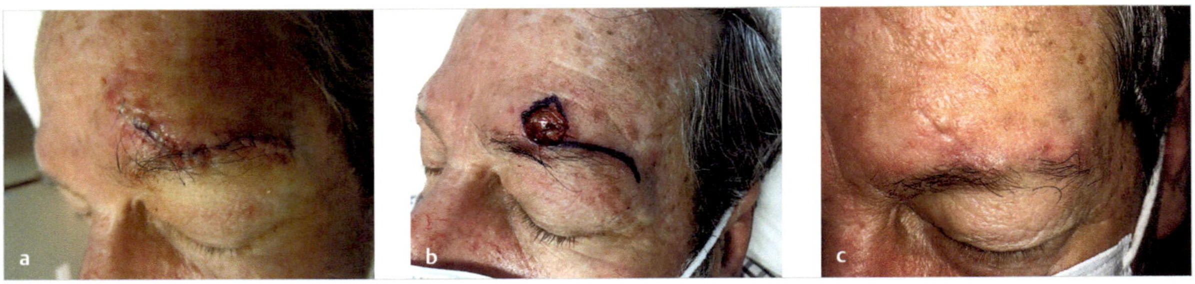

Fig. 10.53 O-L closure: defect and design **(a)**, flap in place **(b)** and one-month cosmetic result without eyebrow malposition **(c)**.

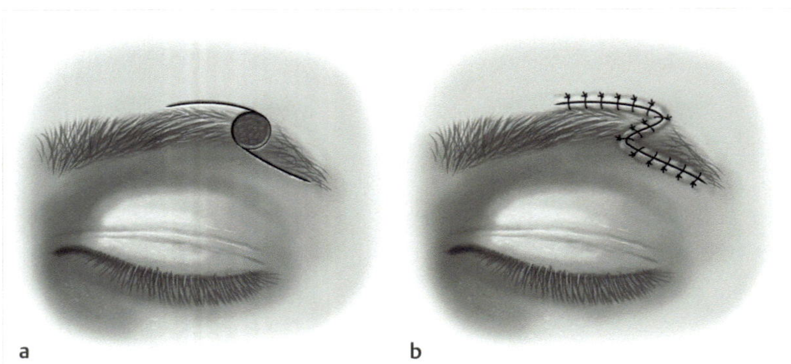

Fig. 10.54 (a,b) O-Z closure: flap design **(a)** and flap in place **(b)**.

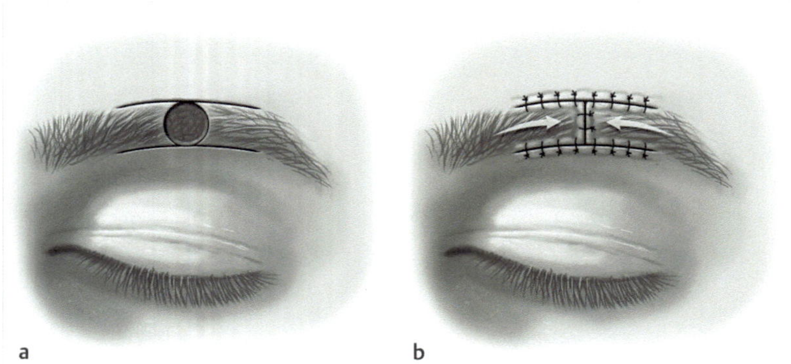

Fig. 10.55 (a,b) Bilateral advancement flap (H-plasty).

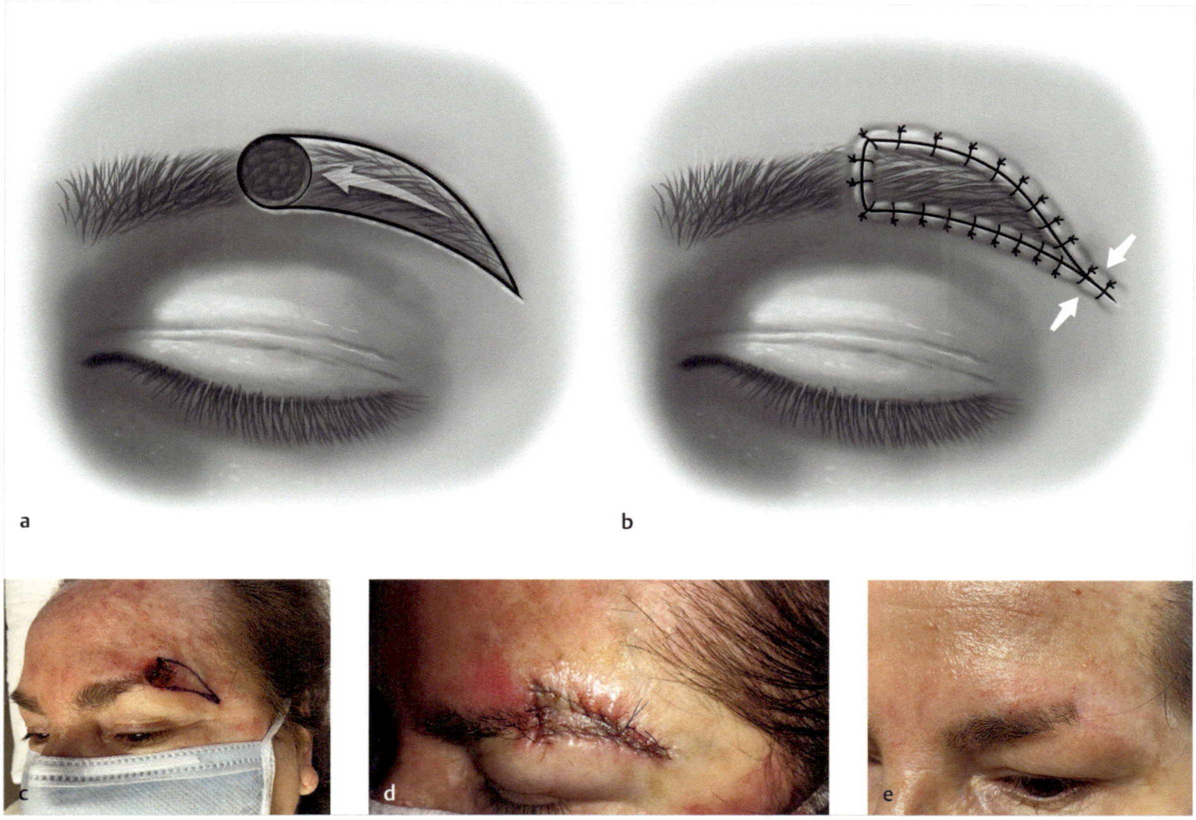

Fig. 10.56 Island pedicle flap. Flap design **(a,c)**; flap sutured in place **(b,d)** and 6 months cosmetic result **(e)**.

10.14.4 Transposition Flaps[38]

Double Z-plasty (▶ Fig. 10.57a–c) described by Cedar[38] can close midbrow defects horizontally like accordion, and may hide scars within the brow. However, it can be used only for smaller defects in the central location. Otherwise, the whole contour of the brow may be compromised.

10.14.5 Pedicle Flaps[15,35] (▶ Fig. 10.58a, b and ▶ Fig. 10.59a–d)

For isolated lateral or medial defects, as well as for the total brow defects, sometimes pedicle flaps from contralateral eyebrow, or adjacent scalp can be considered. However, there are the risks of ischemia, venous stasis, and thrombosis, in cases where pedicle is designed too narrow and the perfusion pressure is not adequate.

Pedicle flap from contralateral brow (▶ Fig. 10.58a, b) is designed on the glabellar pedicle and is used for medial brow defects. The flap is split longitudinally and transposed to fill the medial defect on the contralateral brow. The flap should be designed approximately 30% larger to compensate for the shrinkage and follicle lose on the edges.

Temporal flap is designed from temporal scalp, must extend to the midline for adequate blood supply, and is used for reconstruction of the lateral part of the brow. The pedicle inset occurs after 3 weeks, and the donor site is closed primarily. Distal end of the new brow may be at risk for ischemia due to lower perfusion pressure.

Temporal flap based on superficial temporal artery (▶ Fig. 10.59a–d) can be designed as cutaneous flap (requires pedicle division in 3 wk) or tunneled flap through the subcutaneous space of the upper forehead, beneath the zygomatic branch of the facial nerve and OOM. Besides carefully creating subcutaneous vascular pedicle, one should be meticulous about choosing the suitable scalp donor site and the establishment of the correct orientation of the hair shafts at the donor site.

Other free flap options include secondary vascularized hair-bearing island flaps based on ipsilateral retroauricular hair (for female brows) or free supraorbital artery pedicled flap from contralateral midbrow. Scalp donor site can be improved by tissue expanders, hence reducing the follicle density to match the recipient skin at the brow defect.

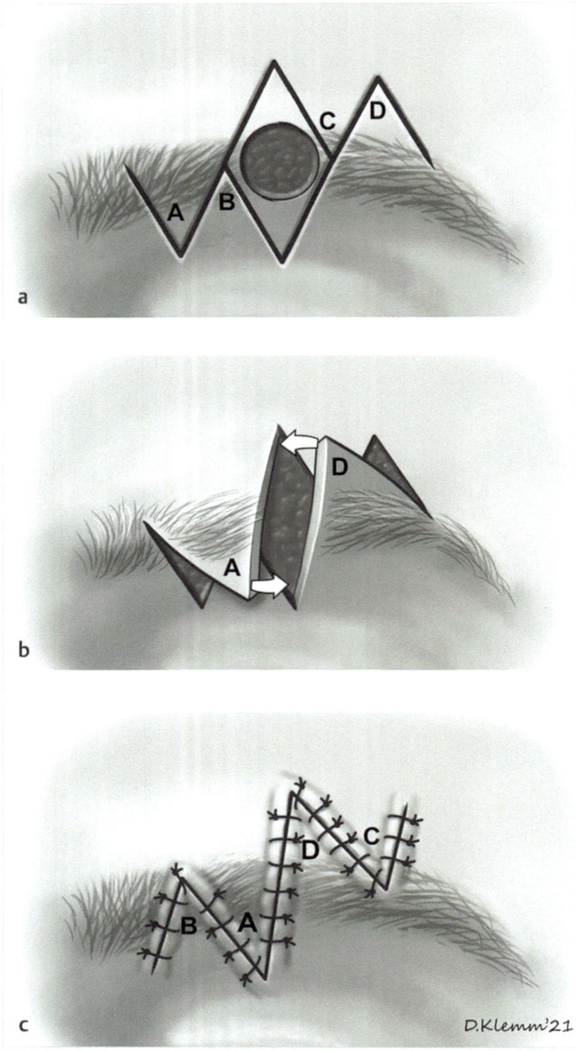

Fig. 10.57 Double-Z rhombic flap. The rhombus is excised **(a)**, and additional excisions are made and transposed **(b)** and flap sutured in place as demonstrated **(c)**.

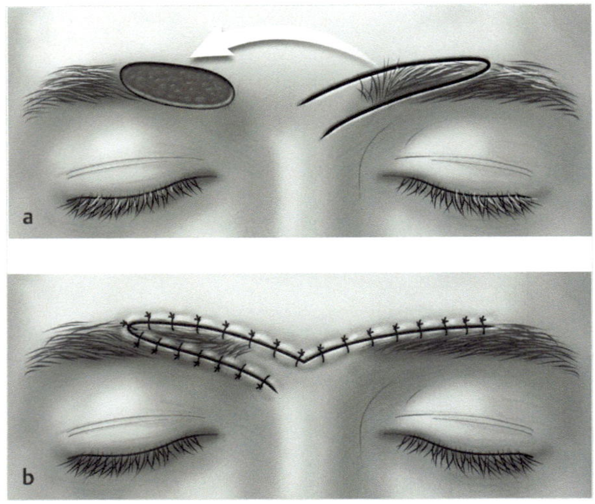

Fig. 10.58 Pedicled sharing flap from contralateral eyebrow design **(a)** and execution **(b)** for medial brow defect reconstruction.

10.14.6 Free Hair-Bearing Grafts (Composite Grafts—Skin and Hair)[15] (▶ Fig. 10.60)

These composite grafts are usually harvested form postauricular temporoparietal region. The graft at the donor site is designed with the vertical long axis so that the hairs have superolateral orientation when transferred to the eyebrow. Incisions are made at the subcutaneous level just above the galea to ensure that hair follicles are obtained. Recipient skin is excised down to the frontalis and OOM. Recipient bed hemostasis is critical for graft survival. Original hair falls from the graft in the first 2 weeks, and if successfully transplanted, new hair will grow in the next several months. Satisfactory results can be seen at 6 months.

The summary of different types of brow reconstruction based on the size of the defect is presented in ▶ Fig. 10.61.

10.15 Conclusion

The function of the eyelids and brows is critical for ocular health, vision, and cosmesis. Mohs micrographic surgery is ideal for the cancer removal in these delicate regions where tissue conservation is of utmost importance. The prerequisites of successful functional and aesthetic outcomes of the reconstruction in these delicate areas depend on surgeon's knowledge of the eyelid and brow anatomy and his or her ability to assess repair requirements and execute appropriate procedures from the plethora of different reconstructive techniques available. Constant education with improvement of the experience and techniques through studying, performance, and collaboration with other surgical specialties will ensure that our patients receive optimal outcomes, restore the function of their eyelids, and obtain best aesthetic results.

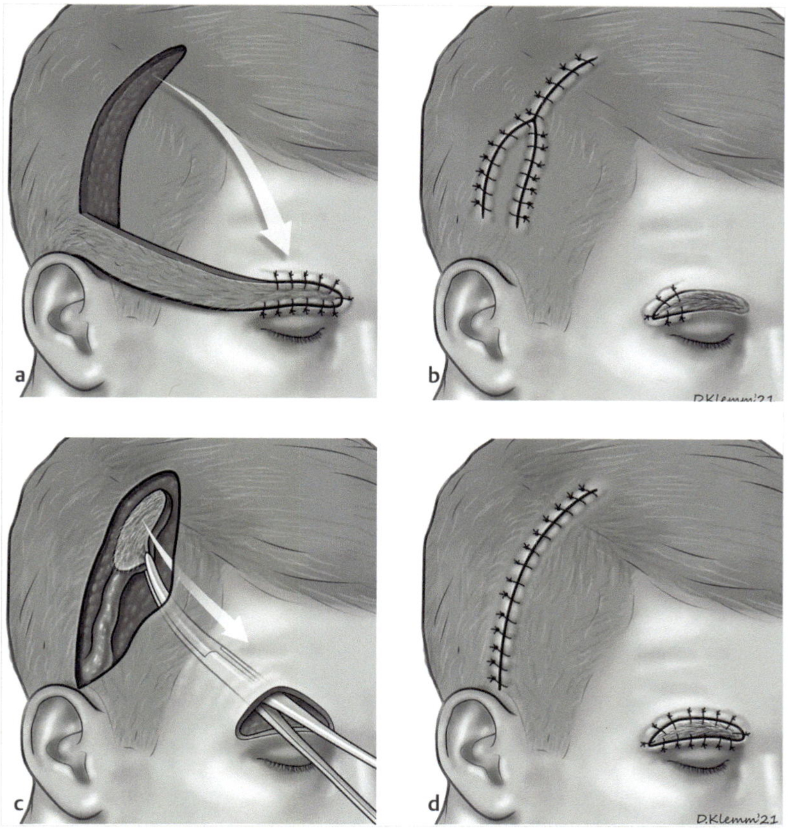

Fig. 10.59 Superficial temporal artery-based flaps: cutaneous pedicle transposition flap **(a,b)** and tunneled pedicle transposition flap **(c,d)**.

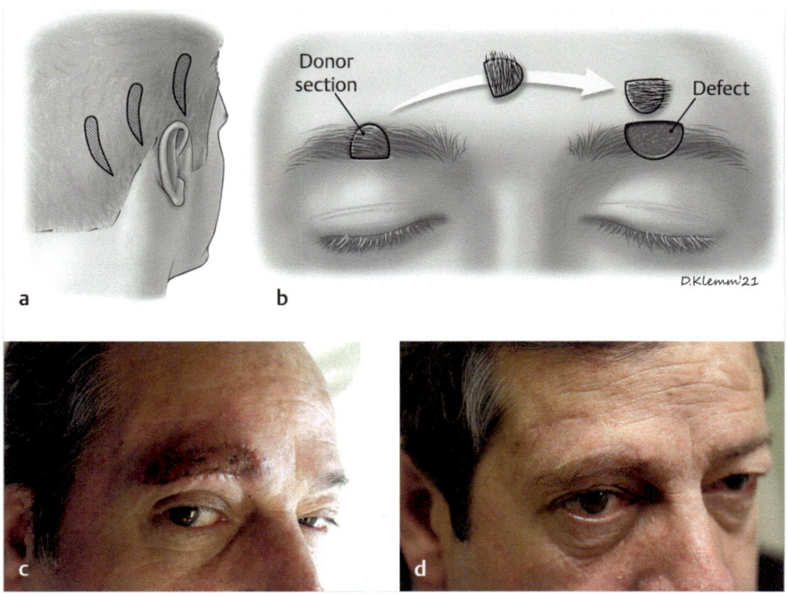

Fig. 10.60 Orientation of donor strips from the scalp **(a)** and from contralateral eyebrow for composite skin-hair grafts for brow repair **(b)**. Graft in place **(c)** and 6 months follow-up **(d)**.

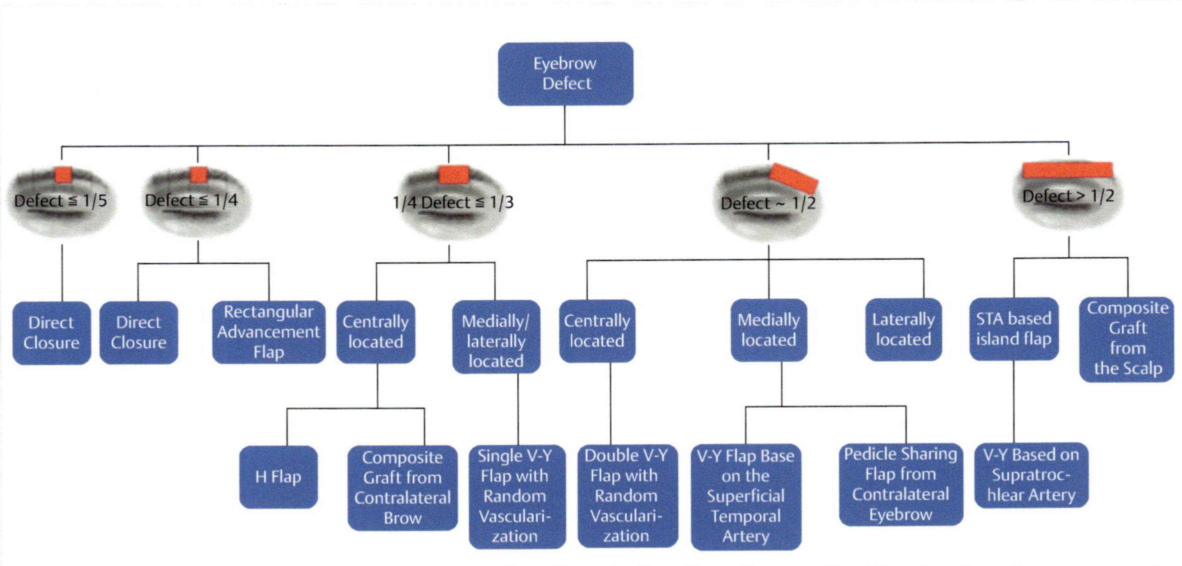

Fig. 10.61 Eyebrow reconstruction algorithm.

References

[1] Segal KL, Nelson CC. Periocular reconstruction. Facial Plast Surg Clin North Am. 2019; 27(1):105–118

[2] Harvey DT, Taylor RS, Itani KM, Loewinger RJ. Mohs micrographic surgery of the eyelid: an overview of anatomy, pathophysiology, and reconstruction options. Dermatol Surg. 2013; 39(5):673–697

[3] Patel SY, Itani K. Review of eyelid reconstruction techniques after Mohs surgery. Semin Plast Surg. 2018; 32(2):95–102

[4] Lee WW, Erickson BP, Ko MJ, Liao SD, Neff A. Advanced single-stage eyelid reconstruction: anatomy and techniques. Dermatol Surg. 2014; 40 Suppl 9:S103–S112

[5] Clark ML, Kneiber D, Neal D, Etzkorn J, Maher IA. Safety of periocular Mohs reconstruction: a two-center retrospective study. Dermatol Surg. 2020; 46(4):521–524

[6] Most SP, Mobley SR, Larrabee WF , Jr. Anatomy of the eyelids. Facial Plast Surg Clin North Am. 2005; 13(4):487–492, v

[7] Sand JP, Zhu BZ, Desai SC. Surgical anatomy of the eyelids. Facial Plast Surg Clin North Am. 2016; 24(2):89–95

[8] Branham G, Holds JB. Brow/Upper lid anatomy, aging and aesthetic analysis. Facial Plast Surg Clin North Am. 2015; 23(2):117–127

[9] Shams PN, Ortiz-Pérez S, Joshi N. Clinical anatomy of the periocular region. Facial Plast Surg. 2013; 29(4):255–263

[10] Ridgway JM, Larrabee WF. Anatomy for blepharoplasty and brow-lift. Facial Plast Surg. 2010; 26(3):177–185

[11] Neimkin MG, Holds JB. Evaluation of eyelid function and aesthetics. Facial Plast Surg Clin North Am. 2016; 24(2):97–106

[12] Becker DG, Kim S, Kallman JE. Aesthetic implications of surgical anatomy in blepharoplasty. Facial Plast Surg. 1999; 15(3):165–171

[13] Garritano FG, Quatela VC. Surgical anatomy of the upper face and forehead. Facial Plast Surg. 2018; 34(2):109–113

[14] Sedgh J. The aesthetics of the upper face and brow: male and female differences. Facial Plast Surg. 2018; 34(2):114–118

[15] Figueira E, Wasserbauer S, Wu A, Huilgol SC, Marzola M, Selva D. Eyebrow reconstruction. Orbit. 2017; 36(5):273–284

[16] Mancini R. Nonsurgical considerations for addressing periocular aesthetics: a conceptual dimensional approach. JAMA Facial Plast Surg. 2014; 16(6):451–456

[17] Spinelli HM, Jelks GW. Periocular reconstruction: a systematic approach. Plast Reconstr Surg. 1993; 91(6):1017–1024, discussion 1025–1026

[18] Özkaya Mutlu Ö, Egemen O, Dilber A, Üsçetin I. Aesthetic unit-based reconstruction of periorbital defects. J Craniofac Surg. 2016; 27 (2):429–432

[19] Hayano SM, Whipple KM, Korn BS, Kikkawa DO. Principles of periocular reconstruction following excision of cutaneous malignancy. J Skin Cancer. 2012; 2012:438502

[20] Holds JB. Lower eyelid reconstruction. Facial Plast Surg Clin North Am. 2016; 24(2):183–191

[21] Ghosh YK, Ahluwalia H, Beamer J. Povidone-iodine antisepsis before ophthalmic surgery. Anaesthesia. 2006; 61(11):1128–1129

[22] Mehta S, Belliveau MJ, Oestreicher JH. Oculoplastic surgery. Clin Plast Surg. 2013; 40(4):631–651

[23] Lo Torto F, Losco L, Bernardini N, Greco M, Scuderi G, Ribuffo D. Surgical treatment with locoregional flaps for the eyelid: a review. BioMed Res Int. 2017; 2017:6742537

[24] Espinoza GM, Prost AM. Upper eyelid reconstruction. Facial Plast Surg Clin North Am. 2016; 24(2):173–182

[25] Morley AMS, deSousa J-L, Selva D, Malhotra R. Techniques of upper eyelid reconstruction. Surv Ophthalmol. 2010; 55(3):256–271

[26] Humphreys TR. Repair of the medial canthus following Mohs micrographic surgery. Dermatol Surg. 2014; 40 Suppl 9:S96–S102

[27] Behroozan DS, Goldberg LH. Upper eyelid rotation flap for reconstruction of medial canthal defects. J Am Acad Dermatol. 2005; 53 (4):635–638

[28] Connolly KL, Albertini JG, Miller CJ, Ozog DM. The suspension (Frost) suture: experience and applications. Dermatol Surg. 2015; 41 (3):406–410

[29] Leone CR , Jr. Tarsal-conjunctival advancement flaps for upper eyelid reconstruction. Arch Ophthalmol. 1983; 101(6):945–948

[30] Jordan DR, Anderson RL. The lateral tarsal strip revisited. The enhanced tarsal strip. Arch Ophthalmol. 1989; 107(4):604–606

[31] Hsuan J, Selva D, Franzco F. The use of a polyglactin suture in the lateral tarsal strip procedure. Am J Ophthalmol. 2004; 138(4):588–591

[32] Triana RJ , Jr, Larrabee WF , Jr. Lower eyelid blepharoplasty: the aging eyelid. Facial Plast Surg. 1999; 15(3):203–212

[33] Shin S, Khachemoune A. Use of eye shields for Mohs micrographic surgery of the eyelids and periorbital area. Dermatol Surg. 2019; 45 (2):210–215

[34] Ogle CA, Goodwin JA, Shim EK. Use of the eye shields and eye lubricants among oculoplastic and Mohs surgeons: A survey. J Drug Dermatol. 2009; 8(9):855–860

[35] Silapunt S, Goldberg LH, Peterson SR, Gardner ES. Eyebrow reconstruction: options for reconstruction of cutaneous defects of the eyebrow. Dermatol Surg. 2004; 30(4 Pt 1):530–535, discussion 535
[36] Quatrano NA, Dawli TB, Park AJ, Samie FH. Simplifying forehead reconstruction: a review of more than 200 cases. Facial Plast Surg. 2016; 32(3):309–314
[37] Bakkour W, Ghura V. Medial eyebrow defects: reconstruction with whole eyebrow subcutaneous island pedicle. Ophthal Plast Reconstr Surg. 2013; 29(4):330–332
[38] Cedars MG. Reconstruction of the localized eyebrow defect. Plast Reconstr Surg. 1997; 100(3):685–689

11 Combination Reconstruction

Stanislav N. Tolkachjov

Abstract

Reconstructive surgery blends the knowledge of proper techniques, a framework of when these techniques should be used, execution, foresight of the healing process, as well as vision, creativity, and the art in medicine. Planning out a proper reconstruction involves evaluating the defect, cosmetic subunits involved, tissue properties (thickness, actinic damage, appearance of pores, presence or absence of hair), anatomic landmarks and danger zones, tissue reservoir, and free margins. With experience and proper evaluation of tumors and patient selection, a potential defect and reconstructive options may be planned prior to surgery. The majority of this book has focused on an algorithm and framework for reconstruction; however, large defects, defects involving multiple subunits, and multiple defects in the same patient may require a combination of reconstructive techniques and creativity.

This chapter focuses on using reconstructive techniques like combinations of primary closures, full-thickness skin grafts and Burow's grafts, and flaps to reconstruct large or difficult, multisubunit defects and multiple defects on patients on the same surgical day. Keys to the evaluation and management of these defects are discussed, and pearls on how to best execute these reconstructions are highlighted. A case-based approach is used to illustrate these concepts. The "Combo-Z" flap is introduced to close two defects in close proximity using a combination of flap movements. The "West by East-West" flap combination is also introduced for large or multi-subunit nasal defects including the tip, supratip, and nasal sidewall. Mastering these key principles allows for a comfort level and confidence in approaching any defect(s) and broadening the reconstructive armamentarium of early career and seasoned surgeons.

Keywords: Combination reconstruction, multiple defects, flap, graft, subunit reconstruction

Capsule Summary and Pearls

Pearls for combination reconstruction:

- Reconstruction may confirm tissue tumor clearance.
  - Removing a standing tissue cone at the edge of previous positivity or inflammation.
  - Taking a deeper base to help clear tumor stroma or inflammation.
- Combinations of flaps, grafts, linear repairs, and second intention healing allow for preservation of cosmetic subunits and decreasing tension of improperly designed reconstructions.
  - Periocular full-thickness skin graft (FTSG) to avoid ectropion or eyelid tension.
  - FTSG after cheek advancement flap for large nasal sidewall defects (see ▶ Fig. 11.5a–c).
  - Second intention healing or mucosal advancement flap for mucosal lip combined with reconstruction of the cutaneous lip defect (see ▶ Fig. 11.11a–c).
- Determine if one reconstructive option may repair multiple defects while sparing normal tissue.
  - Consider the "Combo-Z" flap (see ▶ Fig. 11.15a, b).
- Repair larger of multiple defects first (see ▶ Fig. 11.9a–e).
  - See how tissue moves when larger defect is repaired.
  - Determine the direction and repair type of remaining adjacent tissue.
  - Alternating orientations of primary repairs avoids tissue pull in the same direction.
- Determine if a planned repair may remove or reorient previously displeasing scars or lesions.
  - Make sure to obtain informed consent, and discuss the removal of adjacent lesions prior to doing so.
- Consider using another flap or "back-graft" to close a secondary or tertiary defect (see ▶ Fig. 11.2a–n; ▶ Fig. 11.7a–c).
  - FTSG or O-T advancement flap for a secondary defect created by a forehead flap.
- Keep standing tissue cones or any excised tissue (may be used as Burow's grafts).
- Don't repair an area from which a graft may be taken until you determine the size of the graft needed (see ▶ Fig. 11.2c, j; ▶ Fig. 11.15f, g).

- Determine the direction of where a standing tissue cone is best removed.
  - Extending a longer incision inferiorly on a cheek or preauricular area may help prevent pucker.
  - Allows for reaching a tissue reservoir.
- Determine donor site properties for proper tissue match.
  - Hair-bearing versus non-hair-bearing area.
    - Forehead flap, cheek advancement flap, cheek rotation flap, FTSG.
  - Actinic damage and pore density (preauricular vs. retroauricular vs. conchal bowl):
    - Conchal bowl pore density matches the distal nose and alae.
    - Retroauricular sulcus skin has less actinic damage than preauricular.
    - Thin retroauricular sulcus tissue matches superficial helical or canthal defects.
    - Non-hair-bearing preauricular skin matches the actinic damage and thickness of the nasal dorsum or sidewall.
  - Supraclavicular skin and the inner upper arm allow for large reservoirs of free tissue.
    - Supraclavicular skin typically has more actinic damage than inner arm.
- When harvesting an FTSG, trim tissue to the desired depth accounting for atrophy and metabolic demand.
  - Even mild sloughing after incomplete FTSG thinning may allow a better long-term outcome than extensive immediate thinning causing a "skeletonized" appearance of the nose.
  - Dermabrasion, intralesional corticosteroids, serial excisions, or scar revision can be done at a later time to improve aesthetic outcome.
- Suturing considerations.
  - Create extra eversion when sewing from flap to flap (see ▶ Fig. 11.9d).
  - Consider pulley sutures for key tight areas that can later be removed or left.
  - Epidermal (top) pulley sutures may be used to bring adjacent tissue together over an FTSG allowing basting of the FTSG and gradual guiding contraction of the adjacent tissues (tie-over sutures) (see ▶ Fig. 11.17c, d).
  - "*Set in*" graft or flap to surrounding tissue or base, respectively, to account for pincushioning.
    - Sew *from* graft or flap to surrounding tissue.
    - Take a more superficial bite of graft or flap and a deeper bite of the target tissue.
    - Exiting the needle at the base farther from the graft allows for a better inset of the graft (especially for FTSG of the nasal ala).

11.1 Introduction

Patients with cutaneous malignancies often have multiple lesions requiring treatment. Single-site surgery is most common; however, the following reasons may lead to treatment of several tumors in a single day: patient preference, difficulty traveling for treatment, and multiple tumors in one cosmetic subunit or anatomic area which would encroach on a potential reconstruction. Treating more than one tumor at a surgical visit allows "cleaning up" the tumor burden on a patient analogous to field therapy treating actinic keratoses. To spare normal tissue, a combination reconstruction or using one reconstruction for multiple defects may be chosen.[1,2,3]

Inaccurate estimation of tissue laxity and reservoir can hinder a planned reconstruction and create aesthetically or functionally unsuitable results. This is often seen when overestimating the mobility of inherently tight forehead tissue, working in a scar, or approaching a free margin. Sometimes, a well-designed flap fails to close the defect. Even seasoned surgeons have elevated a large flap and realized it just won't reach. In these cases, a comfort level with combination reconstructive techniques may improve outcomes.

11.2 Combination of Primary and Graft Reconstruction

As primary or linear repairs are commonly used reconstructive options, they should be the first reconstructive consideration after second intention. While the 3:1 length-to-width ratio of elliptical excisions with 30-degree angles of the standing tissue cones is frequently used, certain anatomic sites allow for lengthening or shortening of this ratio and widening or "cheating" the vertex angle of the standing tissue cones. For example, the hairless triangle of the lip, the medial canthus, and the back often allows for shortening of the excision and widening the vertex angle. However, ellipses on the nasal dorsum and columella, the scalp, the vermilion lip, and the helical rim are often extended past the 3:1 ratio, with angles that are even more acute, in order to lengthen the incision over a curved surface for a smooth transition and avoid a pucker.

In combination reconstruction, this extension of an ellipse allows for harvesting a graft without creating a new incision. Burow's grafts are full-thickness skin grafts (FTSG) obtained from adjacent tissue from a standing cone of a primary repair, allowing for a better color, thickness, and texture match when used for adjacent tissue reconstruction.[4–7] Traditionally, they are used on the nasal dorsum or tip with the proximal nose closed primarily providing the grafted tissue distally.[8,9] However, they can be used in almost any location. In addition, FTSG from other locations can be used in combination with primary repairs.

The *key points* of using Burow's grafts or FTSG in combination with primary reconstructions are:

1. Determine the appropriate tissue properties for the graft site.
2. Determine if the reservoir available in the standing tissue cone is sufficient for the defect after accounting for partial closure of the defect with a primary reconstruction.
3. If a unilateral or bilateral Burow's grafts do not allow for sufficient tissue, FTSG may be harvested from a matching tissue reservoir (retroauricular, preauricular, conchal bowl, supraclavicular, inner arm, and femoral canal) depending on the amount of tissue needed.
4. Don't discard tissue until the reconstruction is finished.
5. Don't harvest the graft until you determine the area needed to be grafted.
6. Extend the primary repair from which a Burow's graft may be harvested where an extended incision may best heal (inferior curvature of the cheek as opposed to zygoma, proximal nasal dorsum as opposed to distal nose).[8,9]
7. Consider tissue match (thickness, color, texture, hair density, pore density).
8. Suturing from graft to the surrounding base and "setting in" the graft helps limit pincushioning.

Anatomic examples will be discussed in the following text.

11.2.1 Arm/Hand

The dorsal hand or large forearm defects are great for FTSG/primary repair combinations. While granulation, purse string repairs, single arm rotation flaps, O-Z double rotation flaps, and the "Mercedes" flap are used in these locations, Burow's grafts offer an acceptable reconstruction, especially on tight and often atrophic skin.[10] If the defect is too large to use a Burow's graft without significant tension, it may be prudent to repair much of the defect primarily and use a supraclavicular or axillary upper arm FTSG to close the remaining part of the defect.

11.2.2 Temple

Horizontally and vertically oriented primary repairs, rotation flaps, and advancement flaps are typically used to reconstruct the temple. While FTSG of the forehead often lead to an atrophic appearance, Burow's grafts of the temple and lateral suprabrow offer an acceptable repair option (▶ Fig. 11.1a–c).

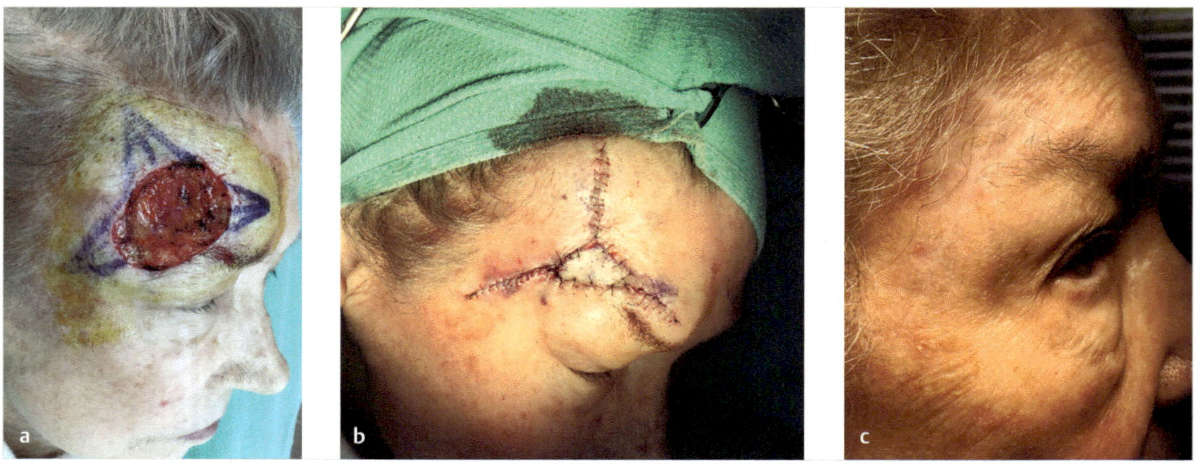

Fig. 11.1 Combinations of full-thickness skin graft (FTSG) and primary linear repairs of the forehead/temple. **(a)** Defect involving the lateral eyebrow, lateral forehead, and lower temple. **(b)** Burow's graft and primary repairs bilaterally and superiorly causing slight elevation of the brow. This is often called a "Mercedes" flap when a Burow's graft isn't used. The brow elevation settles back to baseline within weeks to months of the repair. **(c)** Four-month follow-up with settling of the eyebrow and continued fading of the FTSG.

11.2.3 Cheek

Primary curvilinear reconstruction or flaps are used on the cheek. In instances when a primary repair may not close the defect without significant tension on the oral commissure or a flap is unnecessary, a Burow's graft may be used.

11.3 Combination of Flap and Graft Reconstruction

As we approach defects with regard to subunits involved and wound tension, a flap may be the reconstructive choice. If the flap is unable to appropriately repair the entire defect, a graft may be used in combination. Donor sites for grafts are discussed in other chapters and earlier in this chapter. Below are some specific examples of flap and graft combination reconstruction.

11.3.1 Lateral Infraocular Cheek

The bilobed transposition and rotation flaps, such as the Mustarde cheek rotation flap, are used to close large infraocular defects. However, this cheek rotation flap is difficult to execute with the goal of avoiding any tension on the lower eyelid and preventing an ectropion. Keys to this flap include oversizing the flap (especially in the temple area), tacking the flap superolaterally from the lateral canthus with sutures to the taught temporal skin in the vertical vector or the orbital rim, and tacking the anterior edge of the flap in a horizontal direction to the medial portion of the defect or the nasal sidewall in order to avoid tension to the eyelid itself. However, if the cheek defect is large and too lateral to allow the secondary defect of the flap to be sewn out, other modifications must be made (▶ Fig. 11.2a). Even with a maximum amount of tissue rotated starting immediately preauricularly and stretching superiorly to the lateral temple, the secondary defect may be too large. An FTSG may be taken out inferiorly from the flap standing tissue cone and purposely sized to close the secondary defect. The keys to the flap are similar to those previously discussed; however, an inferior tissue cone should not be removed until the secondary defect is maximally closed without giving too much pull to the flap or the lower eyelid. Subsequently, a template may be made of the remaining secondary defect and used to outline the area of the inferior standing tissue cone (▶ Fig. 11.2b). This can then be sewn in to close the secondary defect without greatly changing the tissue vectors of the flap (▶ Fig. 11.2c–e). In the case of medial or extremely large defects, a wider rotational arc maximizing the preauricular cheek availability and additional FTSGs may be needed (▶ Fig. 11.2f–n).

11.3.2 Periauricular Cheek/Ear

Large defects in the preauricular area lend themselves to a cheek advancement flap. However, the involvement of the tragus or crura of the helix may require additional closure with an FTSG. This may come from the excised infra-auricular skin needed to pull up the cheek advancement flap, the anteriorly excised standing tissue cone, or from a separate retroauricular FTSG. For a larger residual defect, a supraclavicular FTSG may be used.

In addition, if the postauricular area is involved along with the proximal superior ear, and a single-stage reconstruction is desired, the scalp and preauricular skin can be used in combination. Combinations of rotation from the postauricular scalp and transposition flaps from either the preauricular or postauricular skin are good sources of tissue (▶ Fig. 11.3a–f). Preauricular rotation is not ideal, as the rotated edge may blunt the superior crus of the helix.

11.3.3 Upper Cutaneous Lip/Philtrum/ Alar Sill

When an upper cutaneous lip defect also involves the nasal ala, hairless triangle, and the alar sill, a combination of an advancement or rotation flap and FTSG may be used. The crescent excised to freely move the flap is an obvious reservoir for the nasal portion of the defect (▶ Fig. 11.4a, b). Attention must be paid to the possible need for cartilaginous support, and meticulous suturing and appropriate basting must be used as FTSGs on the columella or the distal nasal ala have a high risk of failure. In the case of graft failure, this may become the patient's best "biologic bandage," but additional revision may be needed if a significant step-off is created.

If the philtrum is involved, the subunit approach is important to consider. While Karapandzic, bilateral crescentic advancement, and Abbe flaps are designed to repair large defects involving multiple subunits of the upper or lower lips, an FTSG from adjacent skin such as the excised crescent or marionette standing cone may be combined with the crescentic advancement flap to cover similar defects when muscle is preserved (▶ Fig. 11.4c–h).

11.3.4 Medial Cheek/Nasal Sidewall

Advancing or rotating the cheek to partially close a commonly seen defect involving the medial cheek and lateral nasal sidewall allows an FTSG to be placed on the lateral nasal sidewall portion (▶ Fig. 11.5a–c). Attention must be paid to tacking the cheek portion to the nasal periosteum to avoid tenting and blunting of the nasofacial sulcus. However, a slight malar curve recreates the natural appearance depending on the age of the patient and the level of the malar fat pad loss. Tacking of the FTSG to the nasal sidewall and possible nasalis muscle hinge or sling may be needed for the FTSG to survive. The reservoir for this may be the superiorly excised standing tissue cone on the nasal sidewall, the standing tissue cone from the rotated cheek, or a combination of both.

11.3.5 Forehead/Temple

While FTSG on the forehead may have aesthetically displeasing results, the immobile nature of forehead skin may require a combination repair.[11,12] For a large defect, an O-T advancement flap may be chosen. However, if the defect is located laterally on the forehead, one must be careful in undermining to avoid branches of the temporal nerve and arteries, and therefore, potentially limiting mobility. The defect may be partially closed with the bilateral advancement motion and the closure of the superiorly based standing tissue cone. The standing cone tissue can then be used to graft the central portion of the defect (▶ Fig. 11.6a, b).

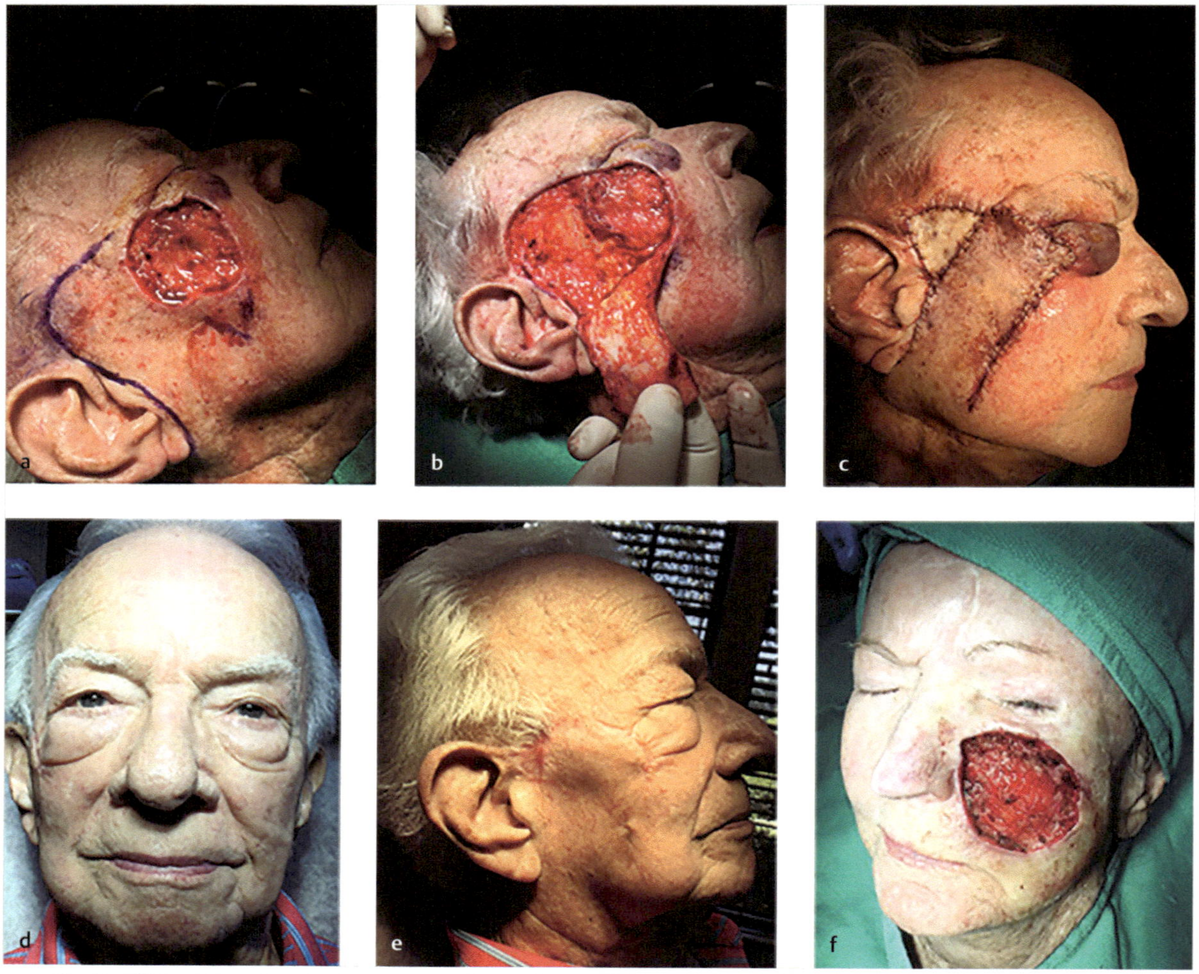

Fig. 11.2 Combination of a cheek rotation flap and a back graft. **(a)** Medium-to-large defect after a melanoma resection involving the infraocular cheek. This defect poses difficulty as the defect is wider than the preauricular cheek reservoir, the area of undermining is at risk for damaging the temporal and zygomatic branches of the facial nerve, and the proximity to the lax lower eyelid puts the patient at high risk for an ectropion. **(b)** Cheek rotation flap fully undermined bluntly in the mid fat in order to avoid the temporal branch of the facial nerve. A bilobed flap from the retroauricular area may also be used transposing tissue over the ear. **(c)** Combination of a cheek rotation flap and a full-thickness skin graft (FTSG) (back graft) from the inferior standing tissue cone. Periocular swelling is expected due to numbing and oozing in the thin eyelid skin. The patient was also on an anticoagulant. Drains may be placed in large cheek rotation flaps to allow drainage. Some authors advocate tacking sutures of the cheek flap to prevent hematomas by avoiding dead space; however, this must be done with caution in order to avoid cutting off any blood supply of the flap or collaterals. **(d)** Anterior view of the patient 4 months from surgery. No ectropion is noted and the eyelid swelling is back to his contralateral baseline. **(e)** Lateral view at 4 months. Note contraction of the graft site as well as anterior and inferior edges of the flap. An infection caused some unwanted eschar to develop, leaving some areas to granulate. **(f)** Larger melanoma defect involving the medical buccal and infraocular cheek. Of note, the patient has had a previous Mustarde cheek rotation flap after a melanoma resection by an oculoplastic surgeon with significant scarring at the eyelid causing lid retraction and mild ectropion.

(Continued)

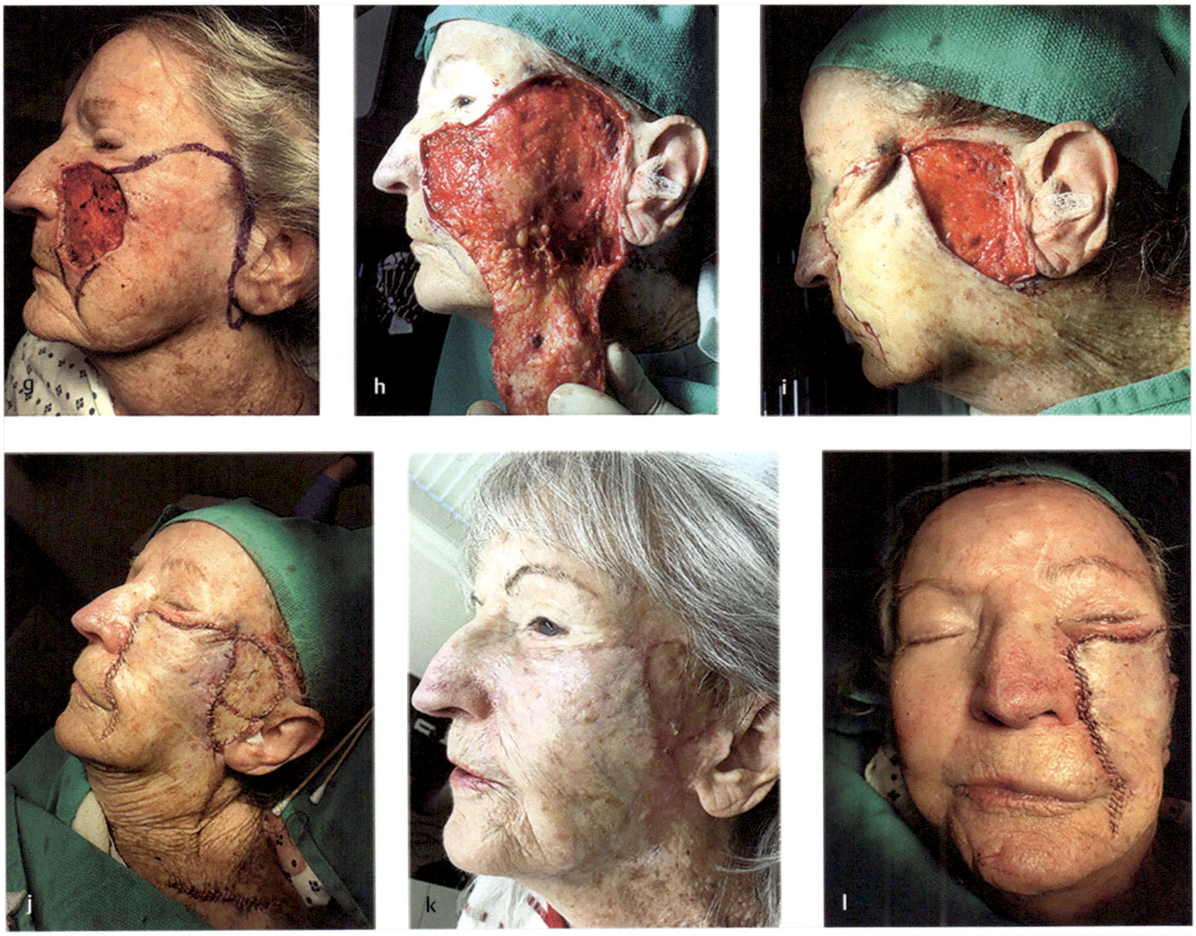

Fig. 11.2 (*Continued*) **(g)** Cheek rotation flap planned. Note the inferomedial standing cone designed in the melolabial fold and the marionette lines. The superior temporal arc is designed higher than the eyelid margin in order to avoid excessive tension and the previous scar. **(h)** Flap undermined down to the superior platysmal bands with great care taken to avoid injury to the marginal mandibular nerve, parotid duct, or other facial nerve branches. Of note, when prior surgery has been done, it's important to be extra careful as normal anatomy may be distorted. **(i)** Key stitches are placed superiorly to the taught temporal skin creating a vertical vector prior to involving the eyelid skin. Tacking to the orbital rim was not done in this case and rarely done by the author. The second set of key sutures is toward the medial portion of the defect with a slight raise to the horizontal vector allowing the eyelid skin to be free of tension and creating a buttress holding up the lower lid. In her case, the left lateral canthal scar was extremely thick, and caution was taken to avoid causing any extra damage. **(j)** Lateral view of the final repair showing suture lines placed in the nasofacial sulcus extending down to the melolabial fold and the marionette line. A back graft from the inferior standing tissue cone is used; however, a supraclavicular graft was also harvested to close the secondary defect. Dissolving tacking sutures were used at the depth of the grafts. The author prefers to use nylon top sutures in larger facial flaps. No drains were used in this case. **(k)** Two-month follow-up comparison showing improvement of her previous ectropion. Scar lines are expected to fade over time, especially further out from the contraction phase of the scars. **(l)** Frontal view of the final repair showing placement of the final suture lines. Note the left oral commissure is drooping due to the lidocaine. **(m)** Frontal view at 2 months for comparison demonstrating preservation of the melolabial fold, nasal symmetry, and the oral commissure. Slight ectropion from previous surgeries is present; however, the patient thought it was improved from her baseline. **(n)** Closer view at 2 months demonstrating scar fading and lower lid margin preservation.

(*Continued*)

11.3.6 Large Nasal Defects

For certain nasal defects, the bilobed flap is a "workhorse." However, when the flap is pushed for larger defects or inappropriately designed, there may be too much elevation of the alar rim, significant pull on the medial canthus, or inability to close the tertiary defect. While we often say hindsight is "20/20," when a preventable complication occurs or a flap doesn't move as predicted, and a trilobed transposition or another flap altogether should have been used, a "back graft" may be a good option, especially if the defect is greater than 2 centimeters (▶ Fig. 11.7a–c). The reservoir for this graft may

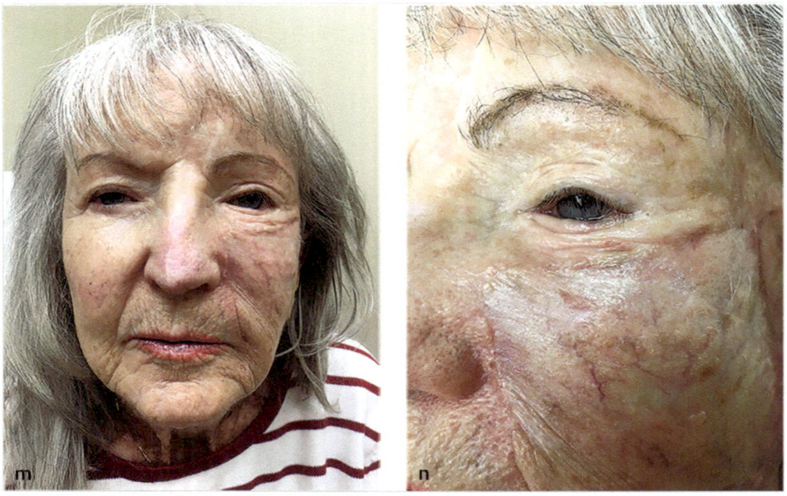

Fig. 11.2 (*Continued*) **(m)** Frontal view at 2 months for comparison demonstrating preservation of the melolabial fold, nasal symmetry, and the oral commissure. Slight ectropion from previous surgeries is present; however, the patient thought it was improved from her baseline. **(n)** Closer view at 2 months demonstrating scar fading and lower lid margin preservation.

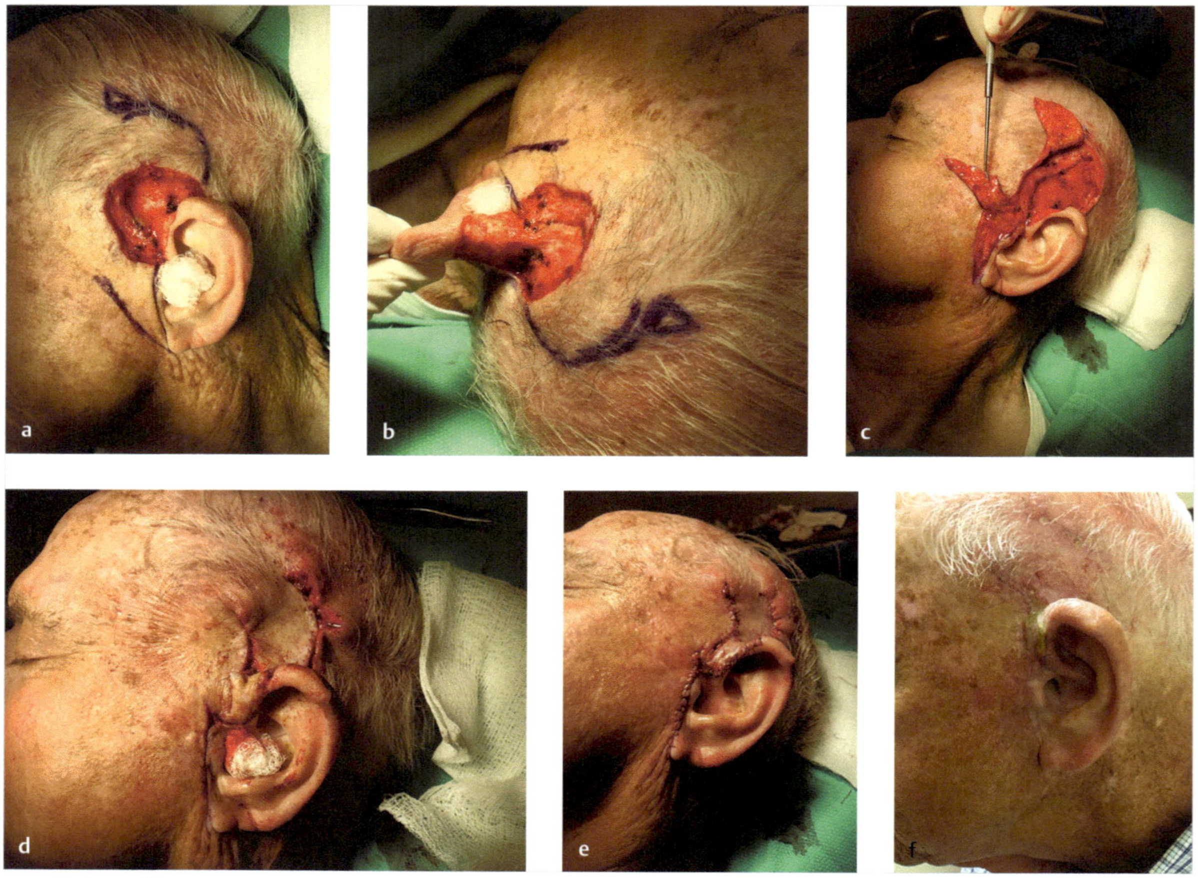

Fig. 11.3 Combination auricular reconstruction with a superiorly based scalp rotation flap and a preauricular transposition flap. **(a)** Defect involving the proximal helical crus and superolateral temple/scalp. **(b)** Superior view of the defect. **(c)** Flap undermining done at the mid fat anteriorly and under the hair follicle bulbs posteriorly. Note the course of a temporal vessel branch that is avoided in undermining. **(d)** Key deep sutures placed to close the majority of the defect. Care must be taken to evert the helical rim edges. The preauricular transposition flap should be folded to recreate the normal rolled contour without compromising flap vascularity. **(e)** Final repair. **(f)** Three-week follow-up. Slight sloughing is noted at the transposition flap surface; however, the distal flap survival avoided any step-off.

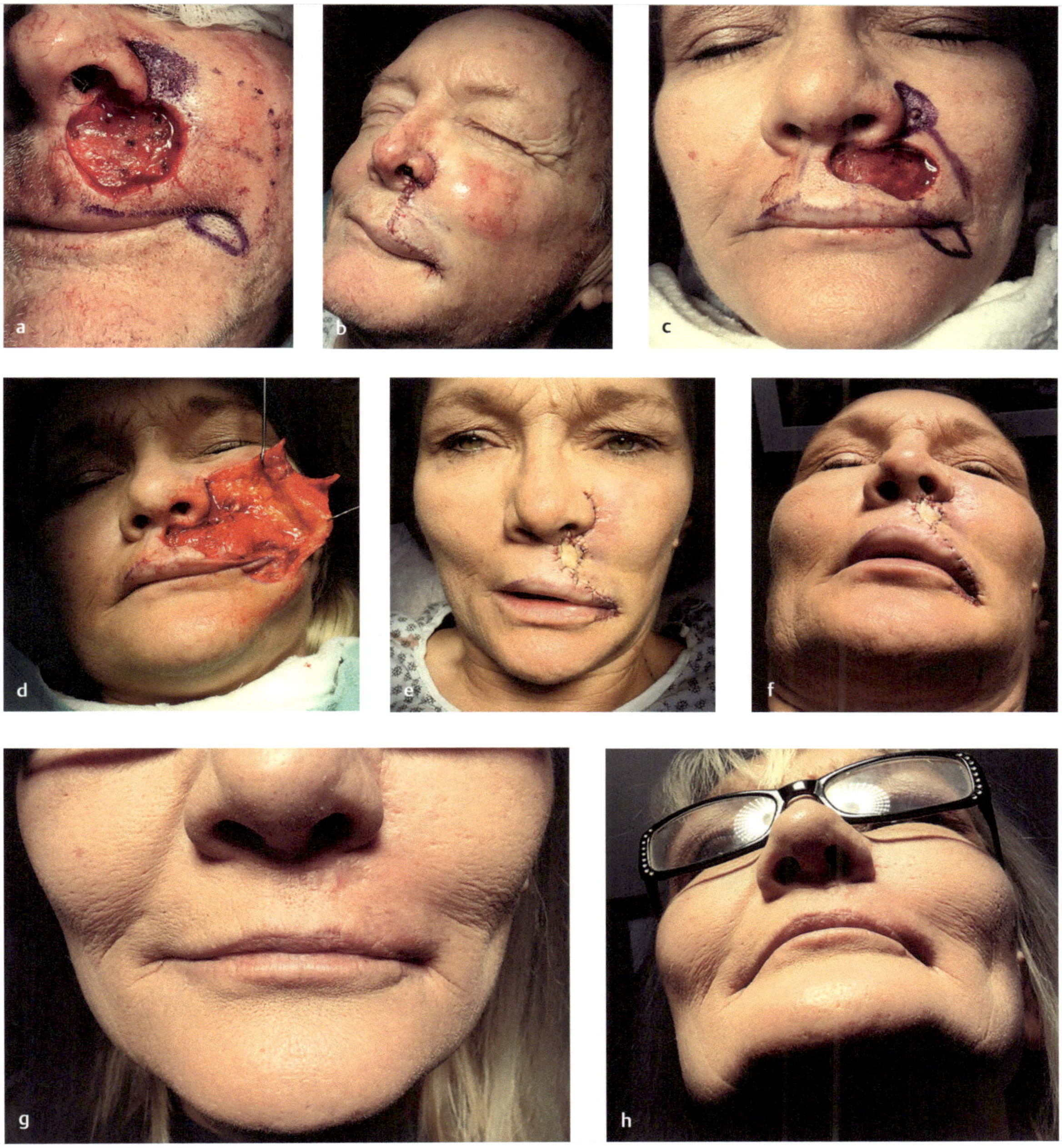

Fig. 11.4 Combination reconstruction with a paranasal crescentic advancement flap (CAF) and full-thickness skin graft (FTSG). **(a)** Large defect involving the upper cutaneous lip, nasal sill, and the inferolateral nasal ala. Note the inferior standing tissue cone of the CAF is drawn as a triangle under the lateral portion of the vermilion at the oral commissure in order to better hide the scar. Original designs of the flap use a large triangle standing tissue cone in the marionette lines. **(b)** Combination reconstruction with a paranasal CAF and an FTSG taken from the standing tissue cone of the hairless triangle of the upper cutaneous lip. The suture lines are well hidden in the natural subunit junctions, and the FTSG is firmly tacked to buttress the nasal ala and tacked down to the nasal sill to replace the junction of the mucosal and cutaneous lining of the alar sill. Swelling and lateral oral commissure drooping is normal due to local anesthetic infiltration. **(c)** Similar large defect of the upper lip of a cosmetically sensitive patient. Note the involvement of the philtrum. **(d)** Flap elevated after crescents removed by the ala and the inferior lip corner. Undermining done above the muscle on the lip, and the superficial-to-mid fat on the cheek portion of the flap, while taking care to avoid lacerating labial artery branches. **(e)** Final repair demonstrating significant nasal shift, lip drooping, and the placement of the graft. Note that the lines drawn preoperatively allowed appropriate placement of the graft when normal anatomy is shifted. **(f)** Worm's eye view of the repair demonstrating nasal shift. **(g)** Four-month follow-up with nasal symmetry preserved. FTSG outline is noted but may be treated with laser ablation. **(h)** Worm's eye view at 4 months.

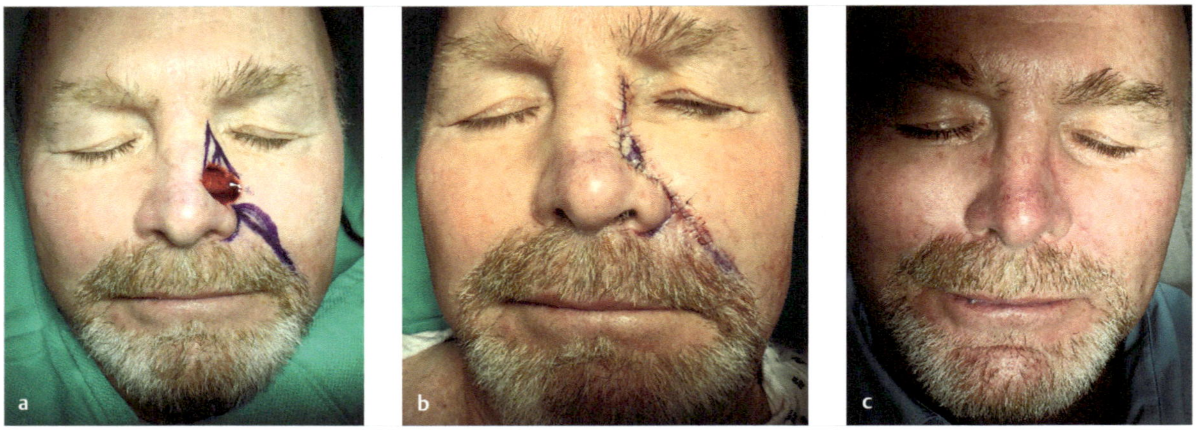

Fig. 11.5 Combination reconstruction with a laterally based cheek crescentic advancement flap (CAF) and a full-thickness skin graft (FTSG). **(a)** Frontal view of the defect. Note the design of the flap allows for potentially closing the entire defect with a single flap; however, surgeons with a purely cosmetic subunit approach would argue against solely using this flap for this defect. **(b)** Frontal view of the reconstruction showing mild nasal ala pull. **(c)** One-month follow-up demonstrating return of the nasal ala to its original position and nice camouflaging of the scar lines in the cosmetic subunit junctions of the melolabial fold, alar groove, and the nasofacial sulcus.

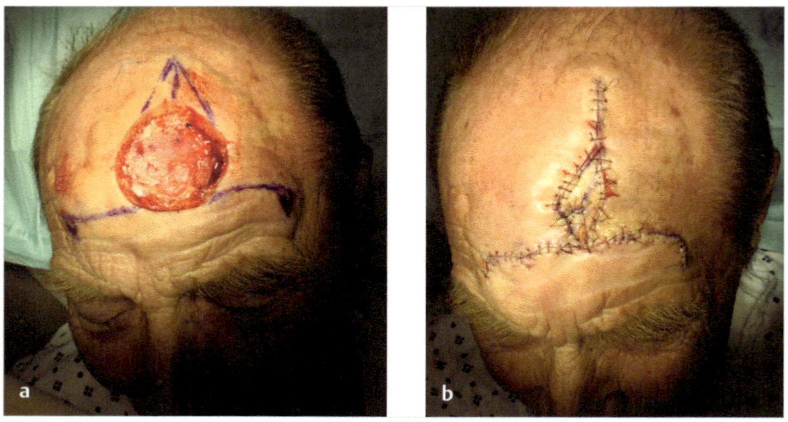

Fig. 11.6 Combination reconstruction of an O-T advancement flap and a full-thickness skin graft (FTSG). **(a)** Wide defect of the central superior forehead. **(b)** Combination repair with an O-T advancement flap and an FTSG from the superior standing tissue cone. Of note, some authors would design the "T" superiorly in an arciform fashion and take an extended inferior tissue cone. Wide defects of the forehead are sometimes tricky due to the underestimation of the rigidity of the medial forehead skin.

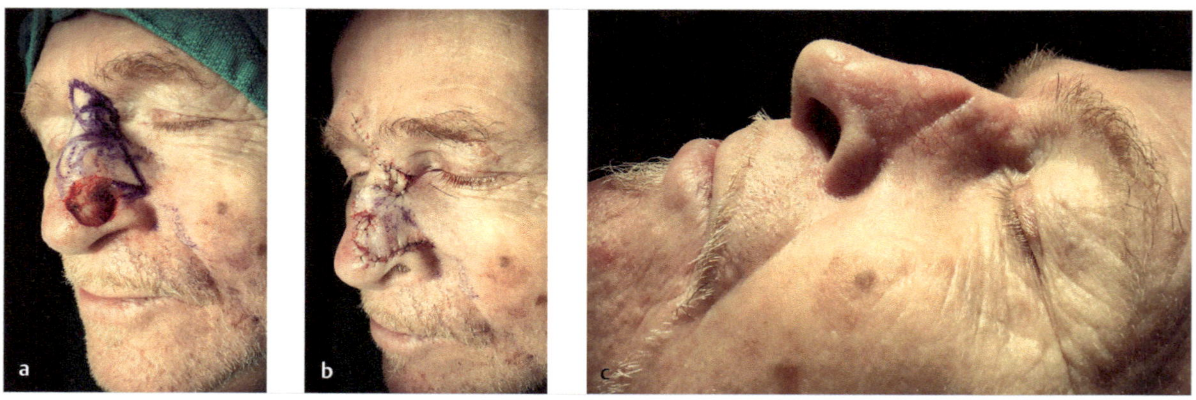

Fig. 11.7 Combination reconstruction of a bilobed transposition flap and a back graft. **(a)** Defect greater than 2 centimeters involving the nasal ala approaching the alar rim, nasal alar groove, and inferior nasal sidewall. **(b)** Combination reconstruction of a bilobed transposition flap and an FTSG (back graft) to avoid excess pulling on the medial canthus and too much alar rim elevation. Graft reservoirs may be the trimmed tissue from the secondary lobe or the tissue cone of the primary defect. The author removed this tissue cone first to see the full movement of the bilobed flap. Mild alar rim elevation tends to resolve, and the alar groove often re-forms naturally or may be guided with tacking suture to the nasal valve or sidewall, depending on the defect depth. **(c)** Three-month follow-up demonstrating normal alar rim position, appropriate graft appearance, and reformation of the nasal alar groove and nasofacial sulcus.

be the trimmed tissue from the secondary lobe or other tissue previously discussed to match the nose. Similarly, a graft to "buttress" the alar rim may be used with meticulous attention paid to suturing and basting. Dermabrasion or carbon dioxide (CO_2) laser may be needed for postoperative finessing at long-term follow-up.

In a similar manner, the dorsal nasal rotation flap may be used to repair a large portion of the nasal tip and dorsum; however, some defects with large lateral portions require additional tissue transfer in the form of a cheek-based flap (▶ Fig. 11.8a–d) or an FTSG.

11.4 Combination of Flaps for Reconstruction of Single and Multiple Defects

11.4.1 Large Nasal Defects

The nose is a common site where a combination repair is needed. While FTSG often serve to close a portion of the defect with a flap, a secondary flap may be used instead. The common flap reservoirs for nasal tissue are adjacent nasal tissue, forehead/glabella, and cheeks.

A dorsal nasal rotation flap (previously described) can be used in combination with a bilateral or unilateral cheek advancement flap(s) (▶ Fig. 11.8a–g) and a glabellar transposition flap (▶ Fig. 11.9a–e).

If two large defects are present on the same nose, the aforementioned rule of closing the larger defect first should apply. ▶ Fig. 11.10a–k illustrates a case of two defects on the opposite sides of the nose that are repaired with a combination of flaps. A laterally based rotation flap (also known as crescentic cheek advancement flap) can be used to repair the large nasal sidewall defect, which then clearly shows the size and complexity of the contralateral alar defect. To close a full-thickness alar defect with structural loss, a cartilage strut can be sewn in to lift the remaining mucosa and the cheek can be slightly advanced and tacked down to create a base for a nasal-alar groove. A melolabial interpolation flap can then be used to repair the alar defect. Sometimes, a batten graft can be used in isolation to give structure and healing deep alar defects with granulation of the alar groove; however, the author does not utilize this option.[13]

To illustrate the principle of subunit reconstruction, which is crucial on the nose, a combination of melolabial interpolation flaps (MLIF), cheek advancement and rotation flaps, and V-Y advancement flaps has been described.[14] In the case of defects involving portions of the ala, the nasal sidewall, and the cheek, an MLIF or even an FTSG can be used once the other cosmetics subunits are repaired. The superiorly-based V-Y advancement flap is used when the defect is wider than it is tall. The laterally based rotation (crescentic cheek advancement) flap is used when the defect is taller than it is wide (▶ Fig. 11.10q).

In the case of a forehead flap, the secondary defect is often granulated or closed linearly; however, if a large defect is left and granulation is not preferred, an O-T advancement flap or a W-plasty may be used to close the secondary defect.

11.4.2 Lip

Defects involving the inferior cutaneous and mucosal lip may pose difficulty. A bilateral V-Y advancement flap may be used; however, for large asymmetric defects, a transposition or a rotation flap from the cheek or chin can repair the cutaneous portion and a mucosal advancement may then repair the mucosal defect (▶ Fig. 11.11a–c). A Burow's advancement flap with a mucosal extension or partial mucosal advancement to the vermilion border allows for closure of large and difficult defects while hiding scars in the melolabial fold, Marionette lines, and the vermilion border.[15]

11.5 Reconstruction of Multiple Defects

Some patients may come from long distances and present with multiple tumors. It is not uncommon to treat several tumors on the same day. Sometimes, a second tumor is found in the adjacent tissue planned to repair a primary defect. In such cases, a repair may be designed to reconstruct multiple defects together or use redundant tissue from one repair to close a second defect.

11.5.1 Multiple Defects Repaired as One

If a primary linear or curvilinear repair can close multiple defects, this is often preferred, given it does not cross multiple subunits that should otherwise be respected. The addition of an FTSG to a linear repair has previously been discussed.

11.5.2 "West by East-West"

A bilateral advancement flap such as the Burow's advancement flap or the "East-West" flap (EWF) can be designed to close two defects; in a similar manner it is used to shift the standing tissue cone deformity as described in nasal reconstruction.[11–14] This concept is not unique to the nose and may be applied to any anatomic site.

The author described another take on the nasal EWF.[16] When the defect involves a large part of the lateral sidewall, nasal tip, and/or dorsum, and multiple adjacent defects are involved, a crescentic advancement flap (CAF) is combined with the EWF to create the "West by East-West" (WEW) flap (▶ Fig. 11.12a–f).

The key steps to the WEW flap are as follows:

1. Design the flap standing cone to include the entire defect or the combined multiple defects.
2. Design the CAF portion to include enough laxity to at least close half of the defect while removing enough of a crescent

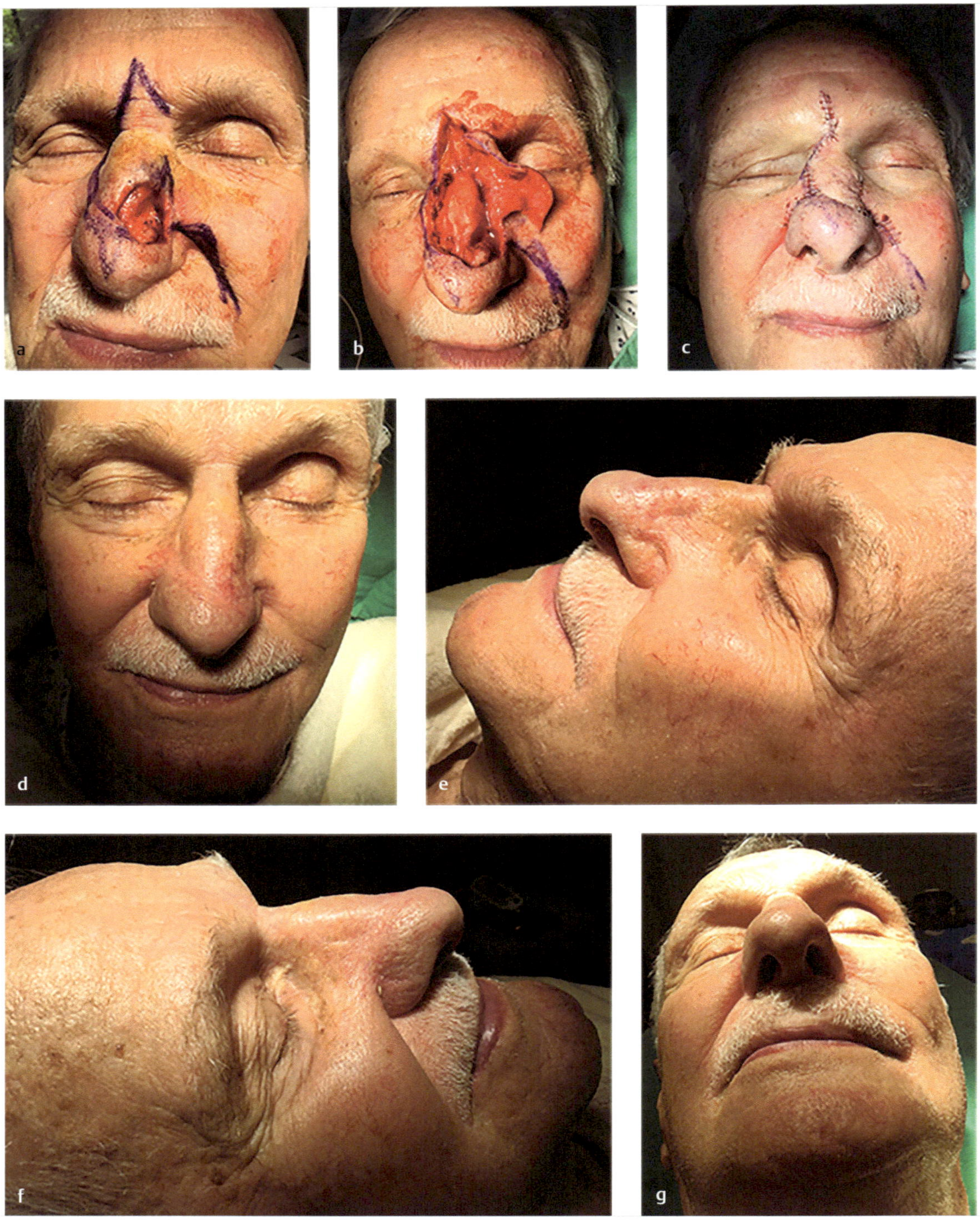

Fig. 11.8 Combination of a dorsal nasal rotation flap (DNRF) and bilateral laterally based cheek crescentic advancement flap (CAF). **(a)** Deep and tall defect involving the lateral nasal sidewall, dorsum, and nasal tip subunits in a sebaceous nose. The laterality and height of the defect make a purely DNRF difficult. **(b)** Undermining of the DNRF to the perichondrium allowing for maximum rotation. Note that in combination single-stage reconstruction, it is critical to close the large defect first, or in case of one defect involving multiple subunits, the larger reconstructive portion will often be done first. If a second stage is planned, the order of reconstruction may differ. **(c)** Combination reconstruction using the DNRF and bilateral laterally based CAF. Mild but symmetric nasal tip elevation is noted. **(d)** Four-month follow-up with some telangiectasias on the sebaceous nose. Dermabrasion was done at 2 months. **(e)** Left lateral view. **(f)** Right lateral view. **(g)** Worm's eye view.

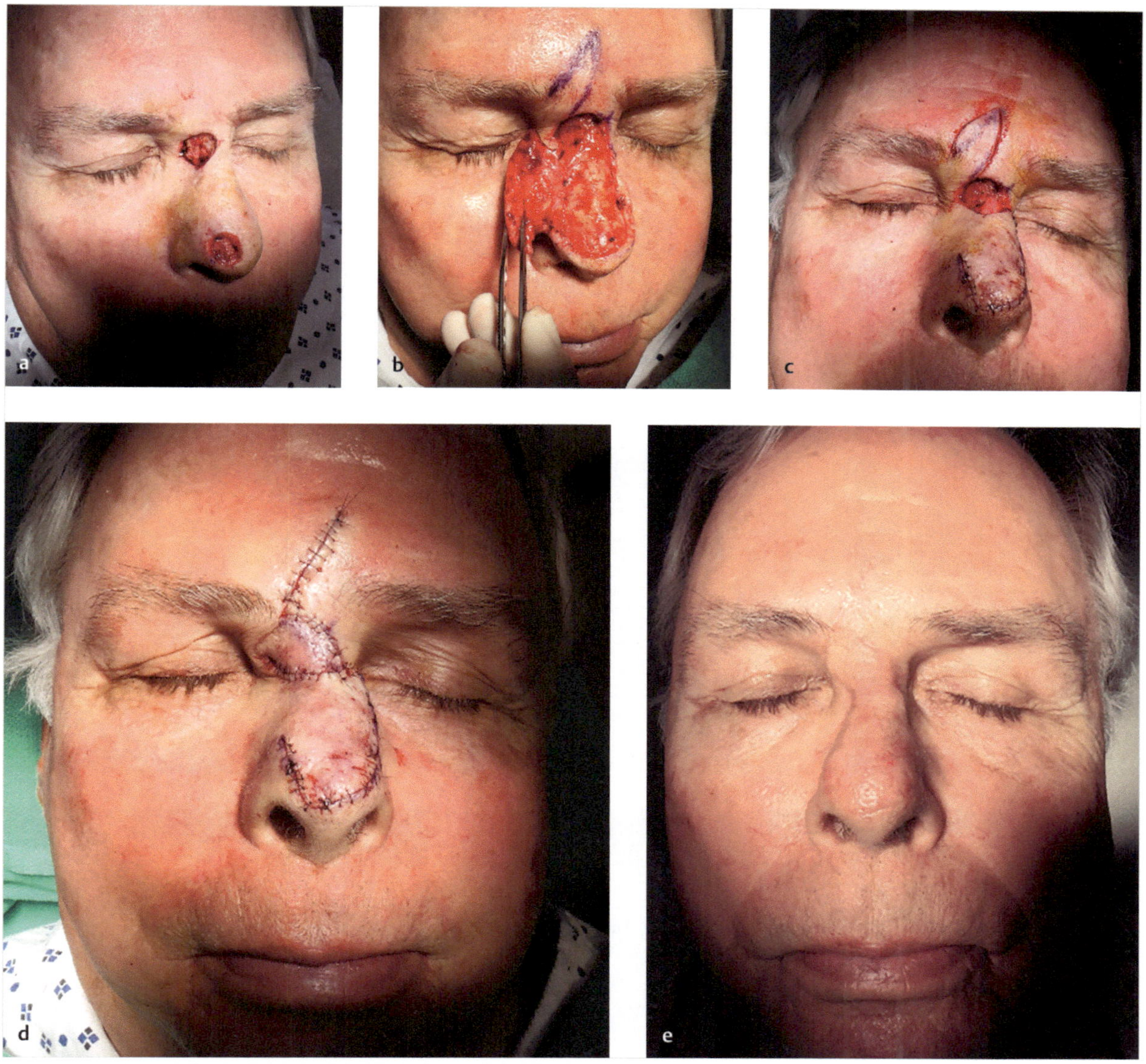

Fig. 11.9 Combination reconstruction with dorsal nasal rotation flap (DNRF) and glabellar transposition flap (GTF). **(a)** Two deep defects involving the nasal root and nasal tip, respectively. **(b)** Flap elevation of the DNRF to the perichondrium with wide undermining. Note the GTF outlined superiorly to match the initial defect of the nasal root. **(c)** DNRF positioned which widens the secondary defect of the nasal root. Note the increased width of the incised GTF highlighting the importance of closing the larger defect first in single-stage reconstructions. **(d)** Combination repair with a DNRF and a GTF with mild nasal tip elevation. **(e)** Two-month follow-up with appropriate ptosis of the nasal tip (anterior view). Note the slight curvature of the nasal root which was present prior to surgery due to a previous nasal fracture and deviated septum.

to avoid blunting the nasofacial sulcus or nasal groove and possibly getting enough of a pivotal rotational motion after the advancement to close some of the nasal tip.

3. Design the EW portion to close the medial half of the defect without "beaking" the nasal tip or columella.
4. Remove the standing tissue cone and undermine above the perichondrium on the nose medially and in the mid cheek fat laterally.
5. Excise and close the columellar defect first, followed by the standing tissue cone of the nasal dorsum to align the flap edges.
6. Close the crescent of the CAF taking meticulous care to preserve the nasal groove, avoid pushing down on the ala, and preserve nasal valve patency.
7. As always, preserve the standing tissue cones in case an FTSG is needed.

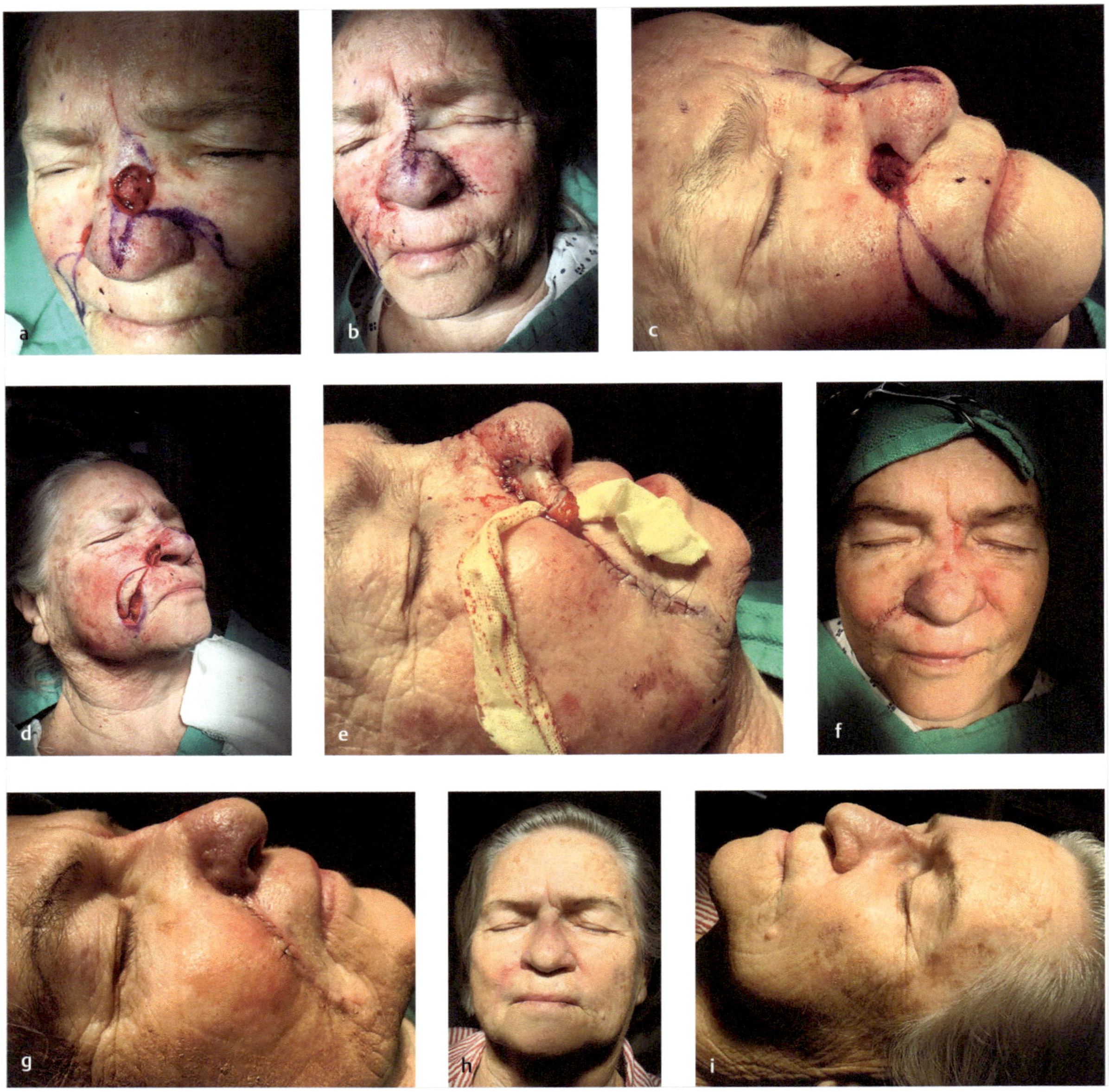

Fig. 11.10 Combination reconstruction with crescentic advancement flap (CAF), cartilage graft, and a melolabial interpolation flap (MIF). **(a)** Large defect of the left nasal sidewall. **(b)** CAF. Note the mild nasal tip elevation. Compression of the ala is avoided by removing the crescent superiorly to the melolabial fold. **(c)** Full-thickness defect of the right nasal ala, medial cheek, and alar rim. **(d)** Cartilage graft from the contralateral ear antihelix in place and MIF incised prior to de-epithelialization. **(e)** MIF sewn in tightly with just enough space to pass a petrolatum-impregnated gauze. We often change these dressings for patients weekly until flap takedown. **(f)** Immediately after MIF separation and thinning at 3 weeks. Note the healing of the left nasal sidewall defect. **(g)** Lateral view of the thinned MIF immediately after takedown. The author uses a midline incision (note sutures on the ala) through the thinned flap to remove a standing cone in order to make sure the rounded share of the ala is preserved when setting in the divided tubed pedicle. **(h)** Two-week follow-up after tubed pedicle takedown (frontal view). **(i)** Left lateral view.

(*Continued*)

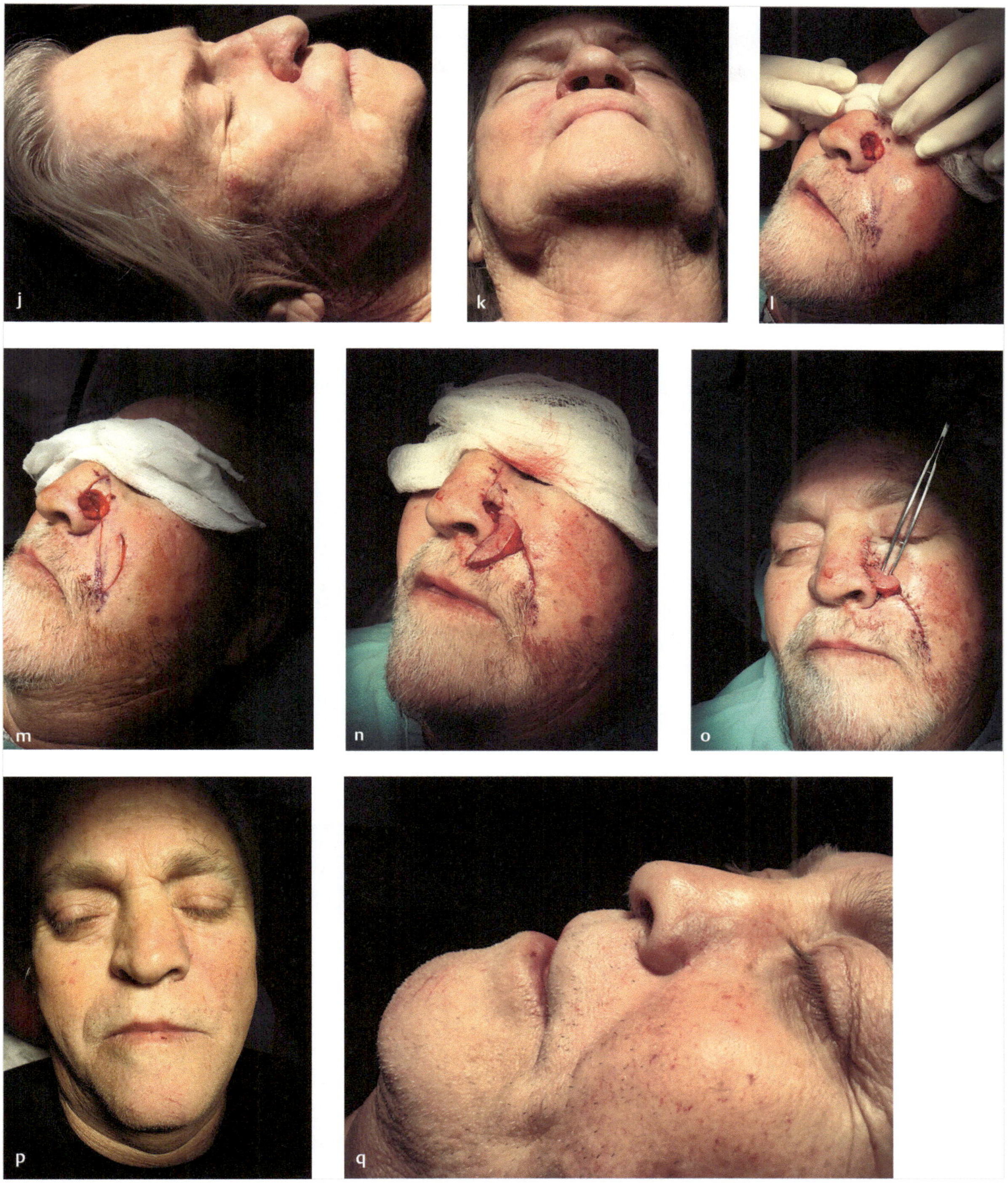

Fig. 11.10 (*Continued*) **(j)** Right lateral view. **(k)** Worm's eye view (note that no additional thinning of the flap or cartilage is necessary). **(l)** Another defect involving the lateral nasal sidewall, nasal ala, and a small portion of the cheek. **(m)** Superiorly based V-Y advancement flap and MIF incised. **(n)** V-Y advanced to close the small nasal sidewall defect to avoid blunting of the nasal-alar groove if a single flap closed the entire defect. The cheek is rotated medially to isolate the alar defect. MIF is shown thinned to the defect at the tip with full-thickness preservation at the pedicle base. **(o)** Combination reconstruction with a tight space (shown by forceps) for petrolatum-impregnated gauze to pass. **(p)** Two-month follow-up. The patient had a flattened anterior projection of the nasal tip at baseline due to trauma and surgery as a child. **(q)** Lateral view at 2 months showing slight pincushioning that resolved with massage and time. The patient did not want to consider dermabrasion or intralesional corticosteroid injections.

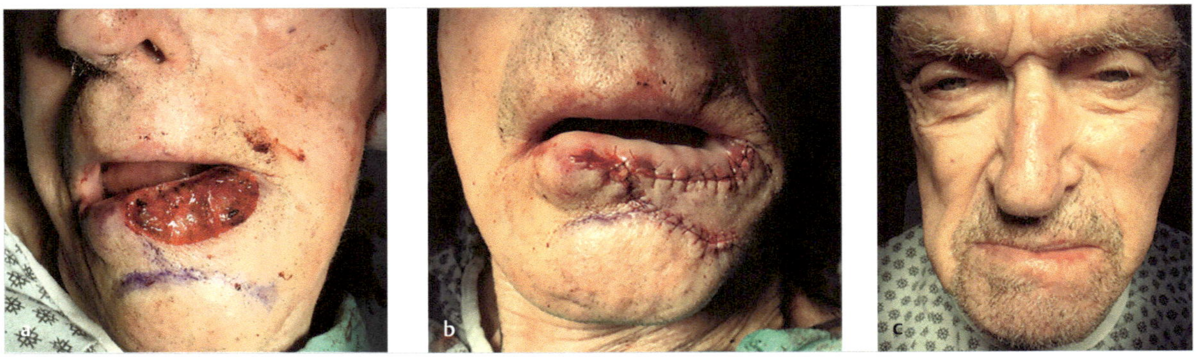

Fig. 11.11 Combination reconstruction with a chin rotation flap and a mucosal advancement flap (MAF). **(a)** Deep defect involving more than half of the lower vermilion and cutaneous lip extending almost down to the mental crease. **(b)** Combination repair of a chin rotation flap placing the inferior scar line in the mental crease with a laterally extended MAF. **(c)** One-month follow-up demonstrating appropriate appearance of the lip margin at baseline with closed lips. Note, hair regrowth of the chin rotation portion was noted on later follow-up visits.

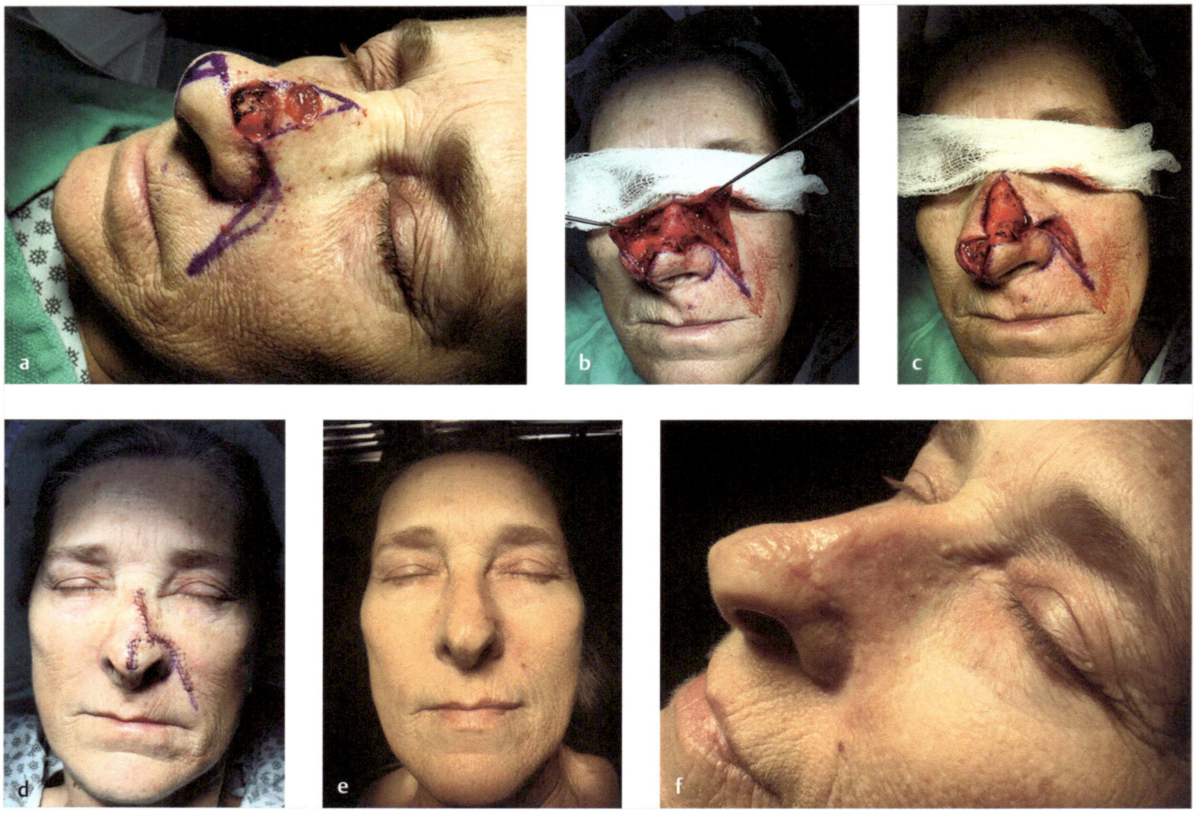

Fig. 11.12 "West by East-West" (WEW) combination flap for large or multiple lateral nasal defects. **(a)** Two defects involving the proximal nasal tip/ala, lateral nasal dorsum, and nasal sidewall. Note the design combining the standing cones from both flaps to encompass both defects. Burow's advancement flap ("East-West" flap) is drawn medially and the crescentic advancement flap (CAF) is drawn laterally. **(b)** Undermining done at the level of the perichondrium on the nose and mid cheek fat laterally. **(c)** Flap undermined. **(d)** WEW flap repair. **(e)** Frontal view at 2 months. **(f)** Closer lateral view at 2 months demonstrating nasal-alar groove preservation and fading of the scar line.

11.5.3 O-T Advancement Flap, Scalp/Forehead Rotation Flap, and Paramedian Forehead Flap

The O-T advancement flap also demonstrates versatility for repairs of multiple defects.

When used for multiple nasal defects, the O-T advancement flap may cause significant elevation of the nasal tip and possible depression of the nasal dorsum; however, the nasal tip elevation improves over time with natural age-related ptosis and settling of the scar tissue.

In a similar manner, multiple or large scalp defects may lend themselves well to advancement or rotation flaps. The scalp rotation flap is useful for tapping into a reservoir of mobile occipital or parietal scalp skin to close large scalp or forehead defects.

The key steps to a scalp rotation flap (SRF) are as follows:

1. Design the arc of an SRF at least double to four times the size of the defect and laterally enough for the leading edge to cover the entire defect to rotate comfortably without flap blood flow compromise once the standing tissue cone is removed anteriorly and contralaterally from the flap leading edge (▶ Fig. 11.13a, b).
2. In order to spare needle sticks and avoid lidocaine toxicity, numbing can be done with lidocaine and epinephrine in the areas of the defect, around the flap incision design, and the proposed standing tissue cones anterolaterally and posteriorly. The bulk of the flap does not need numbing as undermining will be done in the bloodless and "mostly" painless subgaleal plane. Touch-ups are sometimes needed intraoperatively if the galea is stuck to the periosteum due to previous surgery or radiation, as this can be extra sensitive. Tumescent anesthesia can also help avoid excessive bleeding expected with scalp flaps.
3. The flap is incised all the way to the subgaleal plane, and the flap should be undermined in this plane to minimize bleeding and freely and quickly undermine. This should be done efficiently, as bleeding from the flap edges can be significant, and heavy cautery is expected for actively bleeding vessels. Cautery of the entire edge is not needed as the small oozing vessels will stop once pressure from flap inset and sewing create a tamponade effect.
4. After undermining and elevating, the flap should be rotated into the desired direction and key sutures placed. The author uses 3–0 polyglactin 910 or deep sutures is appropriate to close the defect with the leading flap edge.[17] Pulley sutures may be needed if the defect is large or the flap is undersized (▶ Fig. 11.13c, d).
5. The rotated incised edge of the flap is then sewn out with the rule of halves balancing tension out over the entire flap arc. Again, top, deep, or a combination of both sutures may be used (▶ Fig. 11.13e).
6. If the flap is insufficient to cover the entire defect without compromising its viability, an additional incision and flap can be made to meet the leading edge of the initial flap or an FTSG can be taken from the standing tissue cone (▶ Fig. 11.13f, g).

In the case of multiple deep or large defects on the nose, a paramedian or paramidline forehead flap may be used after removing adjacent tissue and extending both defects in a similar manner as extending the nasal defect to the size of the entire subunit to allow forehead flap reconstruction while hiding the flap lines in natural subunit junctions.

11.5.4 "Combo-Z" Flap

One of my favorite reconstructions of two adjacent defects is a bilateral motion flap, something I like to call the "Combo-Z" flap.[18] While the Burow's advancement flap uses an advancing motion to shift the direction of a standing tissue cone, when applied to multiple defects, a central diagonal incision may be made, and the entire surrounding tissue may be undermined to elevate flap edges. Once the flap tissue is elevated, skin hooks may be used to displace tissue with different motion types to estimate the optimal outcome. The flap edges may be advanced to slide into both defects; they may be rotated in the direction of the diagonal incision or may be transposed across each other to close the defects while shifting the direction of the standing tissue cones to adjust for surrounding free margins (▶ Fig. 11.14).

These movements are analogous to the Burow's advancement flap if horizontally advanced and the Z-plasty, if transposed.[19–26] However, the key differences of the "Combo-Z" with these flaps are the utility of this flap with multiple defects, the ability to not remove standing tissue cones until the desired direction/movement is achieved after undermining and flap elevation, and the ability to utilize multiple aforementioned flap movements to create the desired direction. The desired direction itself is determined by any free margin (such as the eyelid) (▶ Fig. 11.15a, b) (▶ Video 11.1 and ▶ Video 11.2), the natural movement of the elevated tissue, and the skin lines which would best camouflage the scar.

Another option to closing two defects in close proximity, if there is at least a separation area of similar size to one of the defects, is to use this area of separation as a rhombic flap transposed into one of the defects and closing the other defect primarily.

11.5.5 Multiple Defects Repaired with Burow's Grafts

When defects are not in close proximity due to multiple surgeries being performed on the same day, the creativity and

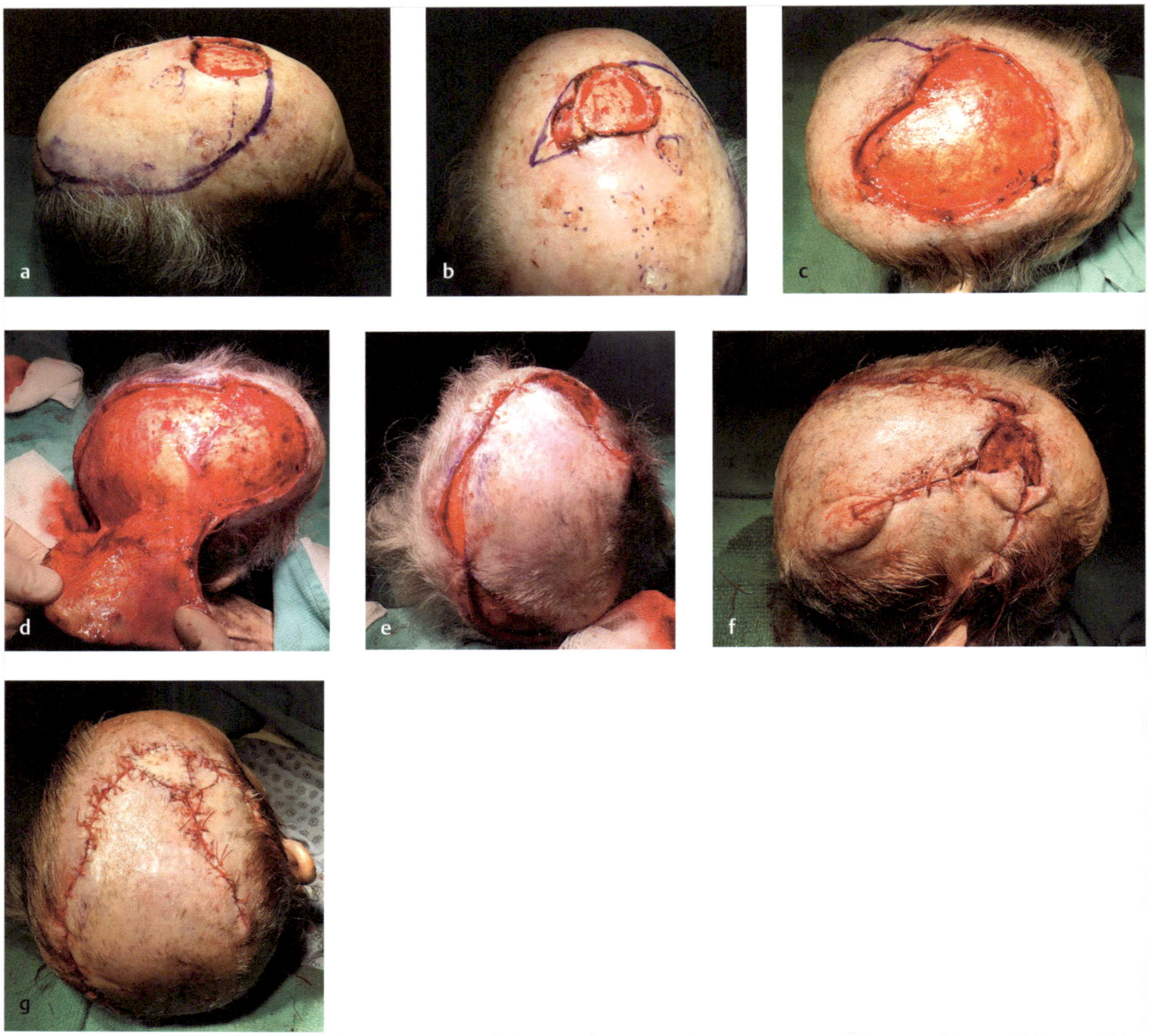

Fig. 11.13 Scalp rotation flap and combinations to repair large or multiple scalp defects. **(a)** Medium-to-large scalp defect with flap drawn into the hairline to tap into mobile occipital scalp tissue. **(b)** Planned standing tissue cone. **(c)** Large defect involving the majority of the superior scalp. **(d)** Flap undermining at the subgaleal level exposing the calvarium. **(e)** Key sutures typically closing the frontal portion of the defect. Due to the extreme defect size, only a portion of the defect was closed anteriorly. Pulley sutures are placed to distribute tension in the midportion of the flap edge. **(f)** A secondary flap is rotated medially to meet the planned scalp rotation flap. **(g)** A full-thickness skin graft (FTSG) from hair-bearing standing-tissue cone is used to close the remaining defect.

vision at the onset of surgery will allow one to look at the surgical sites and find a way to avoid wasting tissue and close all defects with minimal extra surgery. Burow's grafts, previously discussed in this chapter, are the easiest way to achieve these goals. Frequently, a patient presents with a tumor on the ear as well as another site. If a full-thickness epidermal/dermal repair is needed on the ear, the second site's standing tissue cone may serve as the donor for an FTSG to the ear.

In a similar manner, patients with multiple defects on the nose or those presenting with a tumor on the nose and another site may be good candidates for FTSG. As previously discussed, FTSG are good reconstructive options for the lateral alae, soft triangle, and the columella. If a primary linear reconstruction is done on a dorsal nose defect, the remaining standing tissue cones can be used to close the alar defects (▶ Fig. 11.16a–h). Similarly, if a flap is needed to close one of the defects, any redundant tissue that may be created with flap movement can be used as an FTSG.

The nose and ear are not the only anatomic sites in which Burow's grafts may be used.[6] This concept may be used on several defects which may not be closed as separate simple reconstructions or using one reconstruction for defects.

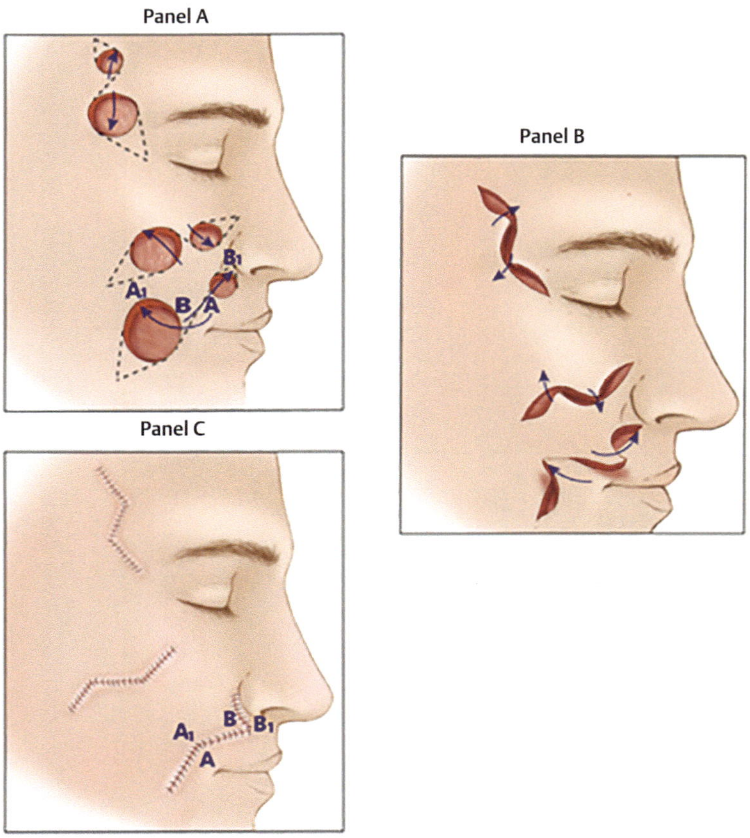

Fig. 11.14 The "Combo-Z" variable tissue movement flap for repair of multiple adjacent defects. Panel (A): Variably-sized defects in the periocular, buccal cheek, and upper cutaneous lip areas. The arrows demonstrate potential flap movement. Note the transposition movement demonstrated in the inferior defects as flap tip "A" is transposed over flap tip "B" to join "A_1" and "B_1" respectively. Panel (B): Superior; rotational motion of the "Combo-Z". Middle; Advancement motion, similar to the Burow's advancement flap, of the "Combo-Z". Inferior; Transposition motion of the "Combo-Z" to hide the scars in the melolabial fold, nasal sulcus, and under the nasal sill. Panel (C): Scar-line orientations after "Combo-Z" repairs of the demonstrated defects. (Reproduced with permission from Tolkachjov SN. The "Combo-Z" variable tissue movement flap for repair of multiple adjacent defects. Int J Dermatol 2020;59(3):e58–e60.)

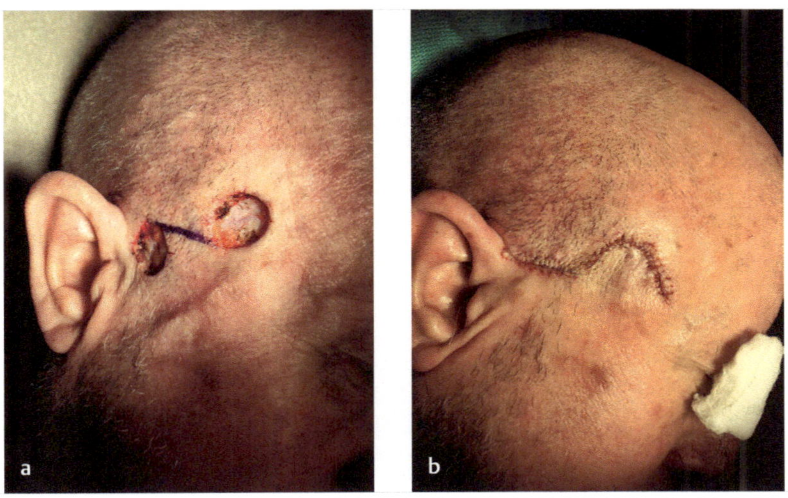

Fig. 11.15 "Combo-Z" flap for two adjacent defects. **(a)** Two adjacent temporal defects. **(b)** "Combo-Z" reconstruction with a transposition motion. An advancement motion could also be done in this case; however, the natural skin laxity at the time of undermining was deemed better for transposition, allowing the tension to be toward the eye rather than away. A diagonal line is incised between the adjacent defects, and the entire area around the defects is undermined. As the flaps are elevated, skin hooks can be used to advance or transpose the flap edges in the desired direction. This is often guided by the natural tissue movement or the desire to avoid displacement of a free margin. The advancement motion is that of a Burow's advancement flap while the transposition motion is similar to a Z-plasty with the flap edges transposed over one another prior to trimming the standing tissue cones. The accompanying videos allow for the visualization of the various movements of the versatile "Combo-Z" (Videos 11.1 and 11.2).

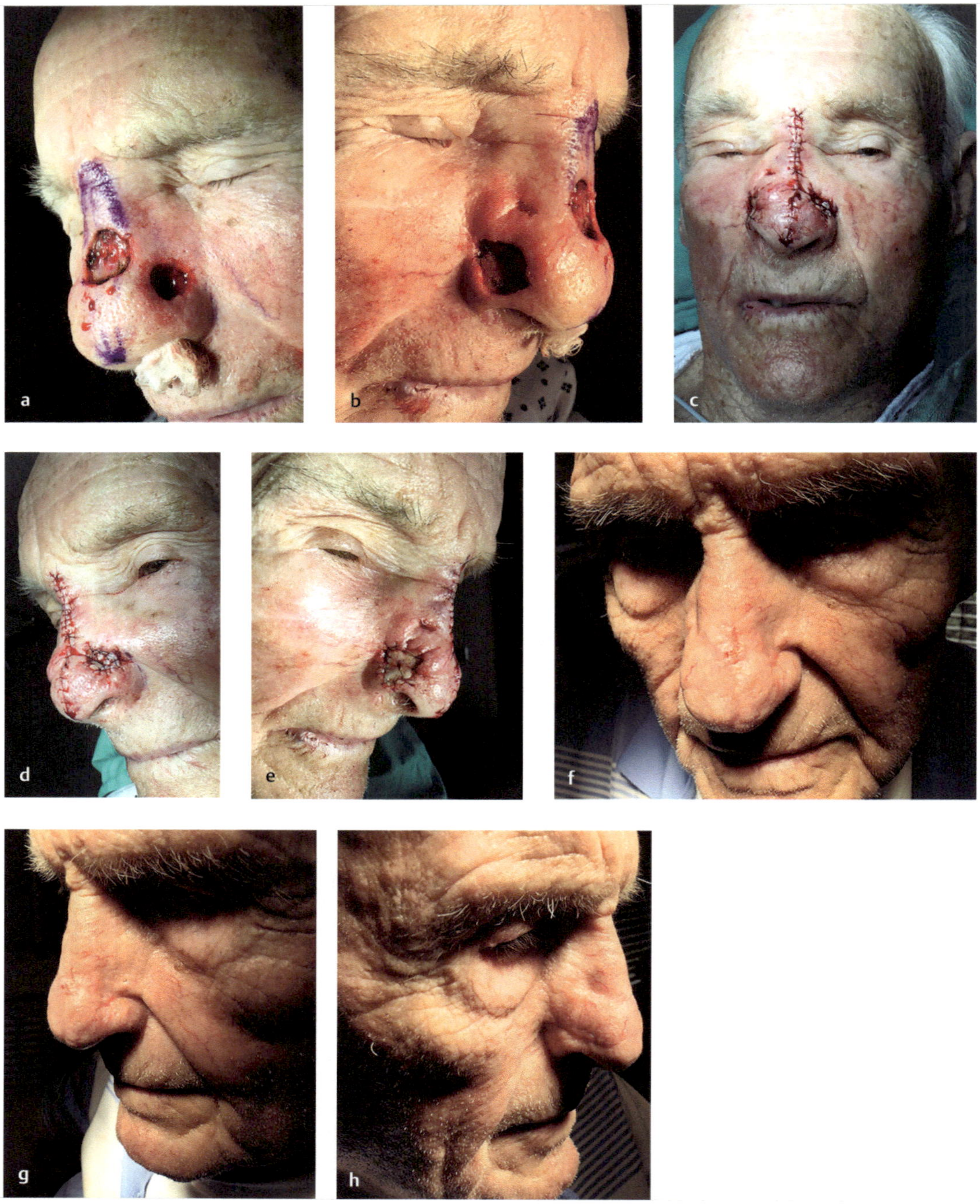

Fig. 11.16 Combination reconstruction of three nasal defects in an elderly patient. **(a)** Left lateral view of two deep defects in a patient on anticoagulants. **(b)** Right lateral view of two deep defects. Note that the right ala has had previous work with flap reconstruction. The small defect is a scouting biopsy site prior to Mohs micrographic surgery. **(c)** Combination reconstruction of three nasal defects using each end of the primary repair as a full-thickness skin graft (FTSG) for the alar defects. A template of each alar defect can be made prior to primary reconstruction of the nasal dorsum. One must take into account the widening of the alar defects when undermining and repair are done of the nasal dorsum. **(d)** Left lateral view. **(e)** Right lateral view. Note the "setting-in" of the FTSG by taking superficial bites of the graft and inserting deep while coming out distally on the base. This technique helps control pincushioning, and in the author's opinion allows for a better blood supply. **(f)** One-month follow-up with appropriate healing of the nasal dorsum. The papule in the center of the scar was biopsied to rule out a recurrence but showed an inflamed sebaceous gland and resolved with the biopsy alone. **(g)** Left lateral view. Appropriate appearance of the FTSG and contour of the nasal dorsum profile. **(h)** Right lateral view. The patient's previous flap at an outside facility is present; however, the deep alar defect has healed well with FTSG repair.

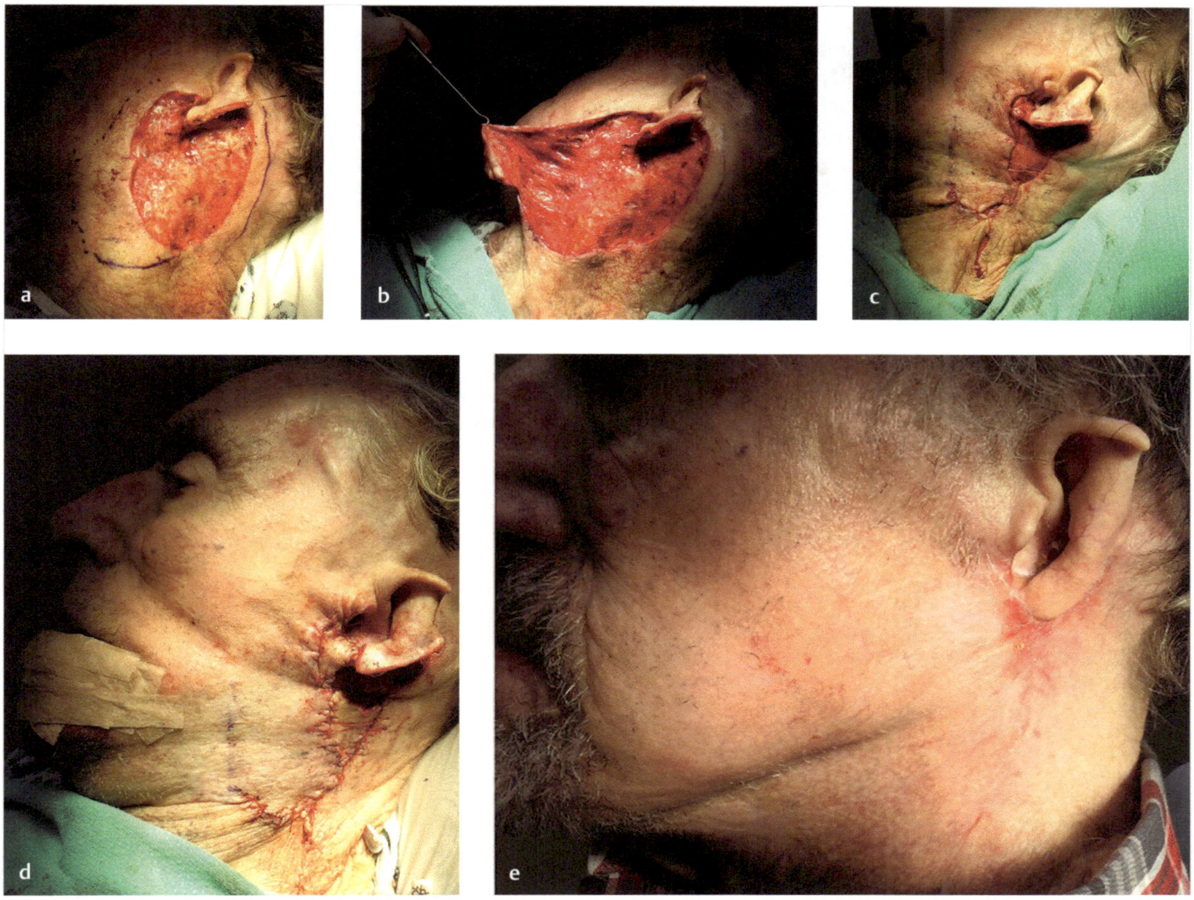

Fig. 11.17 Combination reconstruction including second-intention healing (granulation). **(a)** Large defect of a recurrent squamous cell carcinoma (SCC) involving the entire inferior ear and canal, preauricular cheek, and neck. A previous surgeon elected not to reconstruct the superior helix. **(b)** A rotation flap is elevated to close the majority of the infra-auricular defect. **(c)** Rotation flap is set in place with guiding pulley sutures and an inferior primary repair closed a portion of the defect. **(d)** Two full-thickness skin grafts from the inferior primary repair is used for a partial Burow's graft and grafting of the ear canal defect. The remainder of the infra-auricular neck and ear are left to granulate. An interpolation flap was offered to reconstruct the new and previous helical rim defects; however, the patient declined. **(e)** Two-month follow-up with tightening of the jawline skin but appropriate healing.

11.5.6 The "Kitchen Sink": When Combination Reconstruction and Granulation Gets Us Out of a Jam

In this chapter, combination reconstruction has been introduced with combinations of primary repairs, grafts, and flaps. Some defects require that extra creativity allowing a surgeon to use baseline knowledge of combination repairs and apply it while pushing the limits of local reconstructive options. Concepts of flap and graft combinations, Burow's grafts from primary repair standing tissue cones, pulley tie-over sutures, and granulation (second intention healing) can be used in conjunction. As granulation of wounds was once the primary "reconstructive" method after Mohs micrographic surgery, one must not forget to think of granulation as a viable primary or an adjunct option for combination reconstruction (▶ Fig. 11.17a–e).

11.6 Summary

Combination reconstruction may be used when multiple defects are created, when one defect may be too large for one reconstructive option or encompasses multiple cosmetic subunits, or when a repair may not be properly planned or executed. In other words, a combination reconstruction may help a surgeon to get out of a jam and still create functionally and cosmetically appropriate results for the patient. This chapter uses select cases and anatomic examples of combination reconstructions to demonstrate key principles when approaching such defects and situations. Combinations of primary linear reconstructions, FTSG, and multiple flap types are discussed. The "West by East-West" combination flap is introduced to close large or multiple lateral nasal defects. The "Combo-Z" flap is also introduced to close two defects in close proximity using a combination of flap movements. Mastering these key principles allows for a comfort level and confidence in approaching any defect(s) and broadening the reconstructive armamentarium of early career and seasoned surgeons.

References

[1] Bain EE , III, Carucci J. Repair of adjacent ocular defects. Dermatol Surg. 2015; 41(6):741–743
[2] Jackson Cullison SR, Maher IA. Repair of two adjacent defects of the lateral nasal tip and ala. Dermatol Surg. 2017; 43(8):1087–1090
[3] Sobanko JF, Miller CJ. Midface composite defect: laterally based bilobed flap as a platform for a 3-stage folded paramedian forehead flap. Dermatol Surg. 2014; 40(3):327–332
[4] Zitelli JA. Burow's grafts. J Am Acad Dermatol. 1987; 17(2 Pt 1):271–279
[5] Chester EC , Jr. Surgical gem. The use of dog-ears as grafts. J Dermatol Surg Oncol. 1981; 7(12):956–959
[6] Benoit A, Leach BC, Cook J. Applications of Burow's grafts in the reconstruction of Mohs micrographic surgery defects. Dermatol Surg. 2017; 43(4):512–520
[7] Cabeza-Martínez R, Leis V, Campos M, de la Cueva P, Suárez R, Lázaro P. Burow's grafts in the facial region. J Eur Acad Dermatol Venereol. 2006; 20(10):1266–1270
[8] Behroozan DS, Goldberg LH. Combined linear closure and Burow's graft for a dorsal nasal defect. Dermatol Surg. 2006; 32(1):107–111
[9] Lee KK, Mehrany K, Swanson NA. Fusiform elliptical Burow's graft: a simple and practical esthetic approach for nasal tip reconstruction. Dermatol Surg. 2006; 32(1):91–95
[10] Neill BC, Roberts E, Tolkachjov SN. Reconstructive options for cutaneous dorsal hand defects. Int J Dermatol. 2021; 60(9):1131–1134
[11] Salmon PJM. Forehead defect with periosteal loss. Dermatol Surg. 2018; 44(1):115–119
[12] Hankinson A, Holmes T. Repair of defects of the central forehead with a modified banner transposition flap. Dermatol Surg. 2018; 44(3):459–462
[13] Rotunda AM, Cabral ES. Free cartilage batten graft with second intention healing to repair a full-thickness alar wound. Dermatol Surg. 2014; 40(9):1038–1041
[14] Patel PM, Greenberg JN, Kreicher KL, Burkemper NM, Bordeaux JS, Maher IA. Combination of melolabial interpolation flap and nasal sidewall and cheek advancement flaps allows for repair of complex compound defects. Dermatol Surg. 2018; 44(6):785–795
[15] Neill BC, Tolkachjov SN. Reconstruction of a Large Oral Commissure Defect. Dermatol Surg. 2021; 47(12):1623–1625
[16] King BJ, Tolkachjov SN. "West by East-West": combination repair of wide or multiple distal nasal defects. Int J Dermatol. 2020; 59(10):1270–1272
[17] Jibbe A, Tolkachjov SN. An efficient single-layer suture technique for large scalp flaps. J Am Acad Dermatol. 2020; 83(6):e395–e396
[18] Tolkachjov SN. The "Combo-Z" variable tissue movement flap for repair of multiple adjacent defects. Int J Dermatol. 2020; 59(3):e58–e60
[19] Ascari-Raccagni A, Dondas A, Righini M, Trevisan G. The east-west advancement flap (horizontal advancement flap) to repair a defect on the nose ala. J Eur Acad Dermatol Venereol. 2010; 24(8):926–929
[20] Bugatti L, Filosa G. "East-west" advancement flap for nasal reconstruction. Clin Exp Dermatol. 2008; 33(4):498–499
[21] Geist DE, Maloney ME. The "east-west" advancement flap for nasal defects: reexamined and extended. Dermatol Surg. 2012; 38(9):1529–1534
[22] Hale EK, Robins P. "East-west" flap defined. J Am Acad Dermatol. 2005; 52(1):181–182
[23] Goldberg LH, Alam M. Horizontal advancement flap for symmetric reconstruction of small to medium-sized cutaneous defects of the lateral nasal supratip. J Am Acad Dermatol. 2003; 49(4):685–689
[24] Lambert RW, Dzubow LM. A dorsal nasal advancement flap for off-midline defects. J Am Acad Dermatol. 2004; 50(3):380–383
[25] Barreiros H, Goulão J. Z-Plasty: useful uses in dermatologic surgery. An Bras Dermatol. 2014; 89(1):187–188
[26] Dzubow LM. Z-plasty mechanics. J Dermatol Surg Oncol. 1994; 20(2):108

12 Perioperative Management and Wound Care

Jason R. Castillo, Jennifer L. Hanson, and Randall K. Roenigk

Abstract

Structured perioperative management and wound care is essential to successful surgical outcomes during Mohs micrographic surgery (MMS). At the authors' institution, these structured protocols focusing on perioperative antibiotics, anticoagulation, conscious sedation/analgesia, and implantable cardioverter-defibrillators (ICD)/implantable devices are closely followed to ensure patient safety. A discussion of these protocols in a step-wise fashion with a review of the current literature is included in the following chapter to help the dermatologic surgeon use evidence-based medicine to support their decision-making process. Furthermore, an in-depth focus is provided on the management of dressings based on the following closure or procedural types: second intention wound healing, porcine xenografts, biologic dressings, dermabrasion, primary closure, postflap care, and postgraft care. These step-by-step dressing recommendations will help to provide a framework on the management of wounds following MMS. Even in the most skilled dermatologic surgeon's hands, complications can arise including hematoma, infection, and postprocedural pain. A brief discussion on these postoperative complications with management recommendations is included.

Keywords: Antibiotic prophylaxis, anticoagulants, conscious sedation/analgesia, pacemakers/defibrillators, postdermabrasion care, postprimary closure care, postflap care, postgraft care, hematoma, infection, pain management

Capsule Summary and Pearls

- Highlight preoperative and postoperative considerations during Mohs micrographic surgery.
- Management of perioperative antibiotics, anticoagulation, conscious sedation/analgesia, and ICD/implantable devices.
- Management of dressings based on closure type.
  - Second intention/granulation.
  - Dermabrasion.
  - Porcine xenografts and biologic dressings.
  - Primary closure.
  - Postflap care.
  - Postgraft care.
- Approach to postoperative complications including hematoma and infection.
- Postoperative pain management.

12.1 Preoperative Considerations

12.1.1 Antibiotic Prophylaxis

Antibiotic prophylaxis, utilized to prevent surgical site infection (SSI), infective endocarditis (IE), and hematogenous total joint infection, is an important consideration in Mohs micrographic surgery (MMS). The low rates of SSI, hematogenous total joint infection, and IE seen with MMS have led to guidelines that recommend against the routine use of prophylactic antibiotics. Despite the 2007 guidelines from the American Heart Association on the prevention of IE,[1] the 2008 Journal of the Academy of Dermatology (JAAD) advisory statement on prophylactic antibiotics in dermatologic surgery,[2] and the clinical practice guideline from the American Academy of Orthopaedic Surgeons-American Dental Association,[3] studies show that antibiotics are used more than are recommended, which translates to an increased risk of adverse side effects and antimicrobial resistance.[4] According to the JAAD advisory statement, the ultimate decision on the use of prophylactic antibiotics should be tailored to each individual patient's clinical scenario; however, the following four factors should be considered[2]:

1. Skin condition (infected vs. noninfected).
2. Anatomic site (high risk vs. low risk of SSI).
3. Type of procedure.
4. High-risk cardiac conditions or high risk of prosthetic joint infection.

Bacteremia, the predisposing factor for IE and hematogenous total joint infection, can occur via two ways in dermatologic surgery. Bacteria can be introduced intravascularly during a perforating procedure or can spread into the vasculature from an infected surgical site. Perforating dermatologic procedures are defined by invasion or immediate destruction of the epidermis or mucosa and include MMS, excision, biopsy, ablative laser, incision and drainage, and electrodessication and curettage. Nonperforating procedures include cryotherapy and nonablative laser. Pooled studies have shown a low rate of bacteremia of 1.9% during dermatologic procedures on clinically noninfected, eroded, or intact skin.[2] This low risk of bacteremia is comparable to the rate of bacteremia during daily activities and therefore argues in favor of reduced routine utilization of prophylactic antibiotics.[1,2] Cutaneous infection has been attributed as the likely cause of cases of IE and as many as 50% of late onset hematogenous total joint infections, highlighting the importance of assessing the risk for SSI and prompt, aggressive treatment of cutaneous infection, especially in patients with high-risk features for IE and prosthetic joint infection.[2] Procedures involving infected skin should be postponed until the infection has been treated. If surgery on infected skin is necessary, the patient should be covered by empiric antibiotics.

In addition to minimizing the risk of bacteremia to prevent IE and prosthetic joint infection, antibiotic prophylaxis should also be utilized for areas and cases in which an SSI may result in adverse outcomes, such as graft or flap failure on the nasal tip resulting in poor cosmesis. Antibiotic prophylaxis should also be considered in prolonged procedures as studies have demonstrated an increased infection rate in this setting.[5]

We will discuss the indications for prophylactic antibiotics in MMS and provide recommendations on antibiotic selection and administration.

Prevention of Infective Endocarditis

According to the 2008 JAAD advisory statement on antibiotic prophylaxis in dermatologic surgery, antibiotic prophylaxis is recommended in three circumstances to prevent IE and nonvalvular cardiovascular device-related infection:

1. Procedures on infected skin.
2. Any breach of the oral mucosa in the setting of high-risk cardiac conditions.
3. For sites that are at a high risk for SSI.[2]

High-risk cardiac conditions as defined by the American Heart Association Guidelines are outlined in ▶ Table 12.1,[1,2] and surgical sites or techniques with a high risk of SSI are shown in ▶ Table 12.2.[2,6,7]

Devices and prosthetics that do not warrant antibiotic prophylaxis include: pacemakers, defibrillators, peripheral vascular stents, coronary artery stents, central nervous system shunts, breast implants, and penile prostheses.[2]

Table 12.1 High-risk cardiac conditions that warrant prophylactic antibiotics in perforating dermatologic surgery involving the oral mucosa or infected skin

History of infective endocarditis
Prosthetic valve or prosthetic material for valve repair
Cardiac transplant patients with valvulopathy
Unrepaired cyanotic CHD
First 6 months following repaired CHD with prosthetic material or device
Residual defects in repaired CHD at site or adjacent to site of prosthetic patch or device
Abbreviation: CHD, congenital heart disease.

Based on the American Heart Association Guidelines on Prevention of Infective Endocarditis and Wright et al.[2,8]

Table 12.2 High-risk locations and techniques for surgical site infection that warrant prophylactic antibiotics in dermatologic surgery

Groin
Lower leg
Widespread inflammatory dermatosis
Nasal flaps
Skin grafts
Wedge excision of the lip or ear
Prolonged procedure, multiple sites

Based on Wright et al, Dixon et al, and Maragh and Brown.[2,6,7]

Table 12.3 High-risk features in patients with prosthetic joints that warrant prophylactic antibiotics to prevent prosthetic joint infection in dermatologic surgery

Within 2 years of joint replacement
History of prior prosthetic joint infection
Immunosuppression due to medication, radiation, inflammatory disease
Type 1 diabetes
Hemophilia
HIV/AIDs
Malignancy
Malnourished state

Based on Wright et al, American Dental Association and American Academy of Orthopaedic Surgeons guidelines on prevention of prosthetic joint infection.[2,3]

Prevention of Hematogenous Total Joint Infection

Based on guidelines from the American Dental Association and American Academy of Orthopaedic Surgeons, the American Heart Association, and the 2008 JAAD advisory statement on antibiotic prophylaxis in dermatologic surgery, antibiotic prophylaxis should be used in the following three instances to prevent hematogenous total joint infection:

1. Procedures that breach the oral mucosa in high-risk orthopaedic patients as defined in ▶ Table 12.3.[2,3]
2. When the procedure involves infected skin.
3. With a technique or for area at high risk for SSI (▶ Table 12.2).[2,6,7]

Guidelines do not recommend antibiotic prophylaxis in dermatologic surgeries on nonmucosal or noninfected skin, or locations or techniques that are not at a high risk for SSI. Orthopaedic pins, plates, or screws do not warrant prophylactic antibiotics.[1–3]

Surgical Site Infection

SSI is defined as postoperative infection at the operative site. ▶ Table 12.2 shows procedure locations and techniques which have been found to have a high risk for SSI and therefore warrant prophylactic antibiotics to prevent potential local complications and bacteremia from infection.[2,6,7] These sites are thought to be at high risk for SSI due to increased microbial burden.[9] These high-risk locations were determined from large studies that evaluated reported overall cutaneous surgical infection rates, which generally range from 0.7 to 8.7% of cases.[7,9,10,11,12,13] A prospective study by Maragh and Brown found an overall low rate of SSI of 0.7% for Mohs surgery.[7] Of these infections, a large percentage occurred on the nose. The ear has also been found to have a high infection rate.[14] Studies have shown that SSIs were more likely in patients with immunosuppression, diabetes, widespread inflammatory disease due to colonization with *Staphylococcus aureus*, hematoma formation, in malignant vs. benign lesions, procedures in the groin or lower extremity, and flap or graft reconstruction.[2,10,12,13] In the editor's experience, in the case of lower extremity SSI or threatened dehiscence, it may be useful to use a tetracycline-based antibiotic-like doxycycline, along with wound care and compression.[15]

It is believed that endogenous flora are responsible for the majority of SSIs.[16] Colonization with *S. aureus* and the increasing incidence of methicillin-resistant Staphylococcus aureus (MRSA) are a known cause of SSI.[17] Evaluation for *S. aureus* nasal carriage can help to predict those at an increased risk for postoperative wound infection. Approximately 37% of the population is a carrier of *S. aureus*.[18] While the anterior nares are easily accessible and are typically the highest colonized site, extranasal reservoirs include the pharynx, axilla, and groin.[16] Studies showed that carriers of *S. aureus* who underwent topical decolonization including topical mupirocin and chlorhexidine gluconate wash for 5 days had fewer SSIs when compared with patients who received perioperative antibiotics or no treatment.[16,18] In the setting of an overall low infection rate, the individual practitioner will have to determine whether the preoperative testing and treatment of *S. aureus* are cost effective and feasible given the time and labor involved.

Prophylactic antibiotics can be delivered pre-, intra-, and postoperatively; however, it is ideal to have the antibiotic present in the bloodstream at the procedure site prior to incision as it is believed that antibiotics delivered preoperatively are more effective as they are incorporated into the wound, which does not occur with postoperative administration.[5]

Topical antibiotics have been studied for the prevention of SSI, given the ability to deliver high levels of drug directly to the operative site while avoiding the adverse effects of systemic antibiotics. Their ointment base also provides a moist wound environment, which promotes healing. Studies have shown no statistically significant difference in SSI with the use of petrolatum compared to topical antibiotics.[19,20,21] Topical antibiotics are also associated with adverse effects including contact dermatitis, anaphylaxis, and drug reactions. In addition, their use adds an unnecessary cost and promotes antimicrobial resistance.[19–21] Therefore, the use of petrolatum is recommended on postoperative dermatologic wounds.

Perioperative Antibiotic Prophylaxis Summary

The guidelines discussed above have been summarized into a chart adapted from Mayo Clinic's Division of Dermatologic Surgery (▶ Fig. 12.1).[2,22] Ultimately the decision regarding the use of antimicrobial prophylaxis should be individualized, weighing the risks and benefits of antibiotic use specific to each patient's clinical scenario.

12.1.2 Anticoagulants

Patients undergoing MMS often have medical comorbidities that necessitate the use of antithrombotics. Antithrombotics are divided into two classes, anticoagulants, which inhibit thrombin generation and fibrin formation, and antiplatelets, which block platelet activation and aggregation.[23] Knowledge of these agents is important as many patients undergoing MMS are on one or multiple antithrombotic agents concomitantly and novel anticoagulants are continually being developed. Given an estimated 46% of patients undergoing cutaneous surgery are on at least one anticoagulant or antiplatelet agent, the proper perioperative management of these medications is critical to prevent adverse outcomes and even death.[24]

The decision of whether to stop antithrombotic agents in the perioperative period requires assessment of the risk benefit ratio of developing potential thrombotic events such as stroke, myocardial infarction, and pulmonary embolism, while minimizing intra- and postoperative hemorrhage. Blinded observers of cutaneous surgeries demonstrated that visual inspection of intraoperative oozing was not predictive of antithrombotic status.[25] Studies evaluating perioperative antithrombotic use in cutaneous surgery have shown only minor bleeding complications when antithrombotics were continued, while many cases of thrombotic events were reported with antithrombotic cessation, even for a short duration.[23,26–28] The thromboembolic risk for those in whom warfarin has been stopped is estimated to be approximately one in 6,219 patients and the risk in those with aspirin cessation is one in 21,448.[26] In addition to the complications arising from antithrombotic cessation, the blood work and

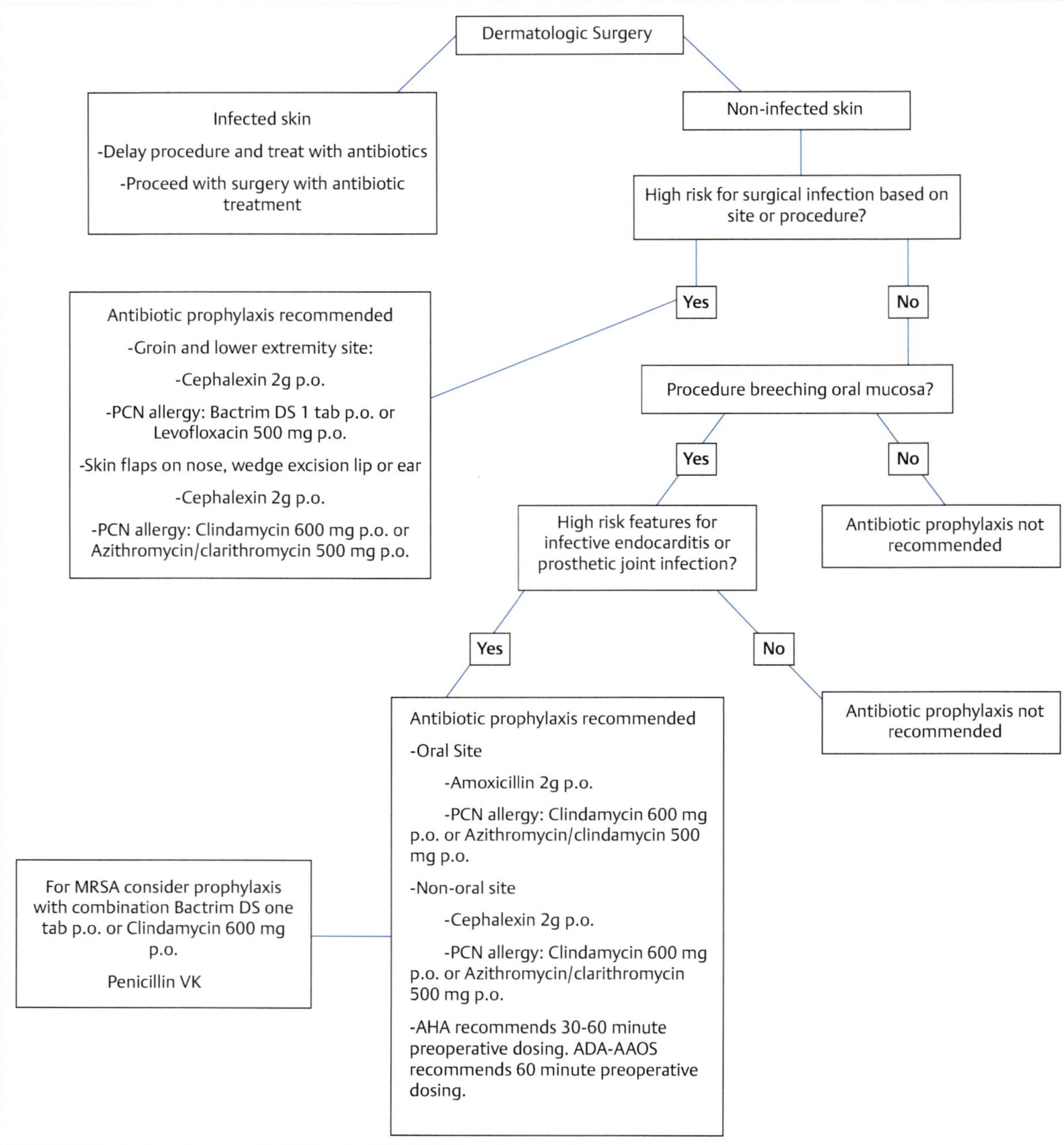

Fig. 12.1 Approach to antibiotic prophylaxis. Consider a longer duration of antibiotic treatment (7–10 days) in addition to the preoperative dose in high-risk situations. Based on Wright et al.[2]

testing required upon medication reinitiation adds additional cost.[29]

Brief interruption of antithrombotic therapy, typically 3 to 14 days prior to surgery depending on the agent, is a common method to attempt to balance potential perioperative bleeding and thrombotic events. In a study by Otley et al, only 1.6% of patients who underwent MMS or excision while on warfarin or platelet inhibitors developed severe complications.[30] This was comparable to that seen in the control group who were not on antithrombotics.[30] In addition, those who had their antithrombotic held perioperatively did not experience a statistically significant reduction in the rate of severe complications.[30] Several other studies found similar results with antithrombotic continuation and did not see a significant increase in complications such as hematoma formation with associated necrosis, dehiscence, or infection.[29,31,32,33,43]

Although some studies have demonstrated an increase in severe hemorrhagic complications in patients taking warfarin or clopidogrel, these complications were non-life-threatening.[35,36,37] As expected, those taking more than one antithrombotic agent are at an increased risk of postoperative bleeding.[38] Cutaneous surgery is often postponed when an international normalized ratio (INR), typically checked within 24 hours of surgery for patients on warfarin, is greater than 3.5. If the INR is supratherapeutic, then the dermatologic surgeon should have a discussion with the patient regarding the trends of his/her INR in order to determine the need for close follow-up with the patient's primary care provider.

Consideration has been given to the use of unfractionated heparin as a bridge during the temporary interruption of anticoagulant therapy in order to shorten the duration of thromboembolic risk. No reduction in hemorrhagic complications was seen with this approach. Instead, this led to hospitalizations and increased blood work.[33] The low-molecular-weight heparins have a more predictable biologic response when compared to unfractionated heparin and therefore do not require laboratory monitoring; however, their safety during cutaneous surgery has not been well characterized.[39]

Chang et al also studied patients undergoing cutaneous surgery who were taking the novel oral anticoagulants (nOAC) Rivaroxaban and Dabigatran and found no severe hemorrhagic complications in patients on these agents.[40] Novel anticoagulants have been reported to have an increased risk of postoperative hemorrhagic complications compared to all other anticoagulants combined; however, these complications were mild in severity.[24] Therefore, despite a possible increased risk for postoperative bleeding, it is recommended that patients be maintained on their nOAC when undergoing MMS. A recent study reviewing a complication rate at one institution suggested that perioperatively interrupting nOAC may be safe and efficacious. They also briefly reviewed nondermatologic literature and guidelines, where a similar interruption to nOAC was recommended.[41]

In addition to a review of antithrombotics, attention should be given to the use of supplements, such as vitamin E and fish oil, which can possess intrinsic anticoagulant properties and may increase blood pressure, thereby contributing to bleeding.[40,42] Given that evidence-based studies regarding the management of these supplements are lacking, the decision regarding their perioperative use is at the discretion of the individual provider.[27]

Discontinuation of antithrombotics can be associated with patient discomfort in the case of nonsteroidal anti-inflammatory drugs (NSAIDs) utilized for pain. In these cases, acetaminophen, in the appropriate clinical context, may be substituted for pain control. At the authors' institution, we currently advise against using NSAIDs during the first 72 hours, given the increased risk of postprocedural bleeding in comparison to that of acetaminophen. Given that there is newer emerging evidence to suggest that better pain control is achieved when adding NSAIDs to acetaminophen in the postoperative period, the dermatologic surgeon must consider the utility of adding NSAIDs in the postprocedural period at the theoretical risk of increasing bleeding on a case-by-case basis.

As a result of numerous studies which demonstrate potential life-threatening thrombotic events with discontinuation of antithrombotics and the relative lack of major complications with antithrombotic continuation during cutaneous surgery, we strongly recommend that cutaneous surgeons maintain patients on their current antithrombotics, which is the practice at the authors' institution. If taken for preventative purposes, aspirin and aspirin-containing products can be discontinued 7 to 10 days before surgery.[23,29,43]

It is important to recognize that certain techniques predispose a patient to a higher risk of bleeding. In comparison to linear closures, flaps and full-thickness skin grafts have a higher hemorrhagic complication rate even when factors including age, sex, postoperative size, and anticoagulation status are controlled. Extensive undermining is thought to account for the increased bleeding and hematoma formation.[24] Therefore, use of plication sutures and other techniques to minimize cutting tissue should be considered. To prevent postoperative bleeding, emphasis should be placed on careful intraoperative hemostasis, the application of proper pressure dressings, patient education on minimizing physical activity in the postoperative period, and management of postoperative bleeding.

Recent guideline updates in 2017 from the American Academy of Cardiology have suggested holding direct oral anticoagulants (DOACs), such as apixaban, dabigatran, and rivaroxaban, 24 hours prior to procedures with low risks of bleeding.[44] Siscos et al performed a retrospective chart review over a 4-year time period at a single center where they found that among their 750 Mohs micrographic surgery procedures, 1 patient experienced a transient ischemic attack (TIA) and 2 patients experienced a hematoma and minor bleeding in the 30-day postoperative period when holding their DOACs for surgery.[45] The DOACs were held 24 hours prior to their Mohs micrographic surgery and resumed 1 day after surgery with only three minor complications.[45] Randomized controlled trials and further studies are needed to determine the appropriateness of holding DOACs in the perioperative period for Mohs micrographic surgery.

12.1.3 Conscious Sedation/Analgesia

Conscious Sedation

Given that the majority of MMS cases are performed on the face with a case length typically exceeding 2 hours, dermatologic surgeons are faced with the challenge of reducing patients' anxiety. The advantage of local anesthesia becomes increasingly evident with the number of comorbidities for the typical patient undergoing MMS. At the authors' institution, the administration of oral midazolam as an anxiolytic and sedative has helped maintain the focus on patient-centered care during surgery without the distraction of an overly anxious patient. Midazolam, a benzodiazepine, acts on the benzodiazepine receptor located on the postsynaptic GABA neurons of the central nervous system.[46] The focused targeting of the GABA-A receptors in the central nervous system has allowed for numerous providers across specialties to use this medication as a tool for anxiolysis, antegrade amnesia, and light sedation.[47] In comparison to diazepam, midazolam has a quicker onset of action and a shorter half-life.[48] In a meta-analysis from nine trials involving 587 patients, only 58 of the 296 patients who received midazolam could recall the procedure while 140 of 291 patients who received diazepam had recollection of the procedure (RR 0.45, 95% CI 0.30–0.66).[49] The onset of action for midazolam is typically 10 to 20 minutes with a peak effect at 30 to 60 minutes after administration.[46] Although hepatic and renal disease may impede excretion of the medication leading to increased sedation, the half-life is typically 3 hours. Midazolam has often been utilized by gastroenterologists as an anxiolytic during flexible sigmoidoscopies; however, it does not reduce actual pain. As was seen by Kuganeswaran et al, in comparison to placebo, patients' anxiety, and perceived comfort was significantly lower with 7.5-mg midazolam PO thought to be due to the amnestic effect of benzodiazepines.[50] There are limited randomized controlled studies on MMS using oral midazolam; however, Beer et al[51] in a randomized, double-blind prospective study during facial procedures under local anesthesia compared the patient reduction in anxiety when administered clonidine, midazolam, morphine, or placebo.[48] Although a small sample size of 150 patients were in the study, midazolam and clonidine were found to reduce anxiety during facial plastic procedures performed under local anesthesia.[48] The patients treated with midazolam had increased risk of respiratory depression.[48] In Otley et al, they found during 11 episodes of conscious sedation while treating 8 pediatric patients undergoing excision or pulsed dye laser (PDL) therapy that the combination of oral benzodiazepine with inhaled nitrous oxide (35–50%) with oxygen via nasal cannula resulted in an adequate level of sedation while performing the procedures.[52] As was mentioned in their study, minimal side effects of nausea were experienced; however, the use of conscious sedation must be performed in a closely monitored procedural setting with practitioners who are certified with basic and advanced cardiopulmonary life support, access to a crash cart, and training in case respiratory or cardiac depression occurs.[52] During our cases we do not routinely use nitrous oxide, given that the adult population responds well to monotherapy with midazolam to ease their anxiety. The advantage of oral midazolam with or without inhaled nitrous oxide is the swift ease of onset and lack of needing intravenous access.

Given the known risk of respiratory depression with benzodiazepine use, a strict protocol is followed during all MMS cases performed at the authors' institution. Following rooming of the patient, review of the patient's preoperative questionnaire, and vital signs, the Mohs surgeon assesses the possible need for anxiolysis. If the patient meets criterion for midazolam, the surgeon confirms the dosage with the nurse (typical starting dose ranges from 5 to 10 mg). Factors taken into account to decide on an appropriate starting dose include: history of pulmonary disease (i.e., COPD), sleep apnea, supplemental oxygen dependence, renal and hepatic disease given excretion of the medication, age of patient, low body weight, fall risk, and medication list. In these high-risk patients, a lower dose by half or one-third is safer and may require longer onset of action than higher doses. If a patient does not have a family member or friend present on the day of surgery, midazolam will not be administered for patient safety. Given that the risk of respiratory depression and level of sedation are increased if the patient is also on opioid-based medications, we typically do not administer benzodiazepines in this case. Although unlikely in light sedation if ventilation was compromised, the benefit of midazolam and other benzodiazepines is that flumazenil may be administered to improve spontaneous ventilation. If hypoxia does occur, it is recommended based on the guidelines to (1) encourage the patient to take deep breaths, (2) start the patient on supplemental oxygen, (3) administer positive pressure ventilation, and (4) observe the patient following reversal with flumazenil.[53]

The baseline vital signs are obtained including blood pressure, pulse, and oxygen saturation. Patients either have a nurse or a family member in the room while the tissue is processing to ensure that the patient is never unattended. Repeat vital signs are obtained after every dose administration and prior to discharge from the clinic. The Richmond Agitation-Sedation Score (RASS) is calculated by the nurse prior to departure with a goal of 0 to −1. All providers and nurses are trained and certified in basic and advanced cardiac lift support and have access to a crash cart in the clinic. Patients are advised to not drive, operate heavy machinery, or take any sedating medications or alcohol for at least 24 hours to reduce the risk of central nervous or respiratory depression. In our experience, midazolam is a useful tool for eyelid or large central facial cases.

The editors follow the same guidelines and use of midazolam as described above in the outpatient/office setting. However, in the past 12 months we have begun utilizing certified registered nurse anesthetist (CRNA) services in the office with even greater patient satisfaction, in our opinion. An IV hep-lock is used to allow greater bioavailability of midazolam and a more rapid onset with lower total dosages, yet the same reduction in anxiety and the desired amnesic effect. The addition of low-dose fentanyl also provides a beneficial analgesic effect. For ocular cases involving tumors of the medial canthus in which the lacrimal duct is compromised and probing is required for the placement of Crawford tubes or a Jones tube, we have found that propofol is necessary to keep these patients comfortable. We used propofol in the setting of a fully equipped ambulatory surgery center where there is the capability of end tidal CO2 monitoring along with the other monitoring equipment mentioned above.

Analgesia

Adequate control of a patient's discomfort during and after surgery is considered a high priority during MMS. As part of the preoperative questionnaire given to patients on the day of surgery, the presence of pre-existing pain and the patient's postprocedural pain threshold are reviewed. If the patient highlights that they have pre-existing pain or a low pain threshold, this is further addressed in depth with the nurse and surgeon. During the informed consent, the provider discusses with the patient that we recommend acetaminophen for postprocedural pain for the first 48 to 72 hours. As is standard for the majority of Mohs surgeons, we infiltrate the marked surgical site in the superficial subcutaneous tissue with a 30-gauge syringe with lidocaine 1% with epinephrine (1:200,000). Pertinent guidelines for the use of local anesthetics in dermatologic surgery are summarized in ▶ Table 12.4.[52] The nurse pays special care to not go through the clinically evident tumor to avoid floaters during tissue removal. Following removal of the first and every subsequent stage, the nurse provides additional local anesthesia with subcutaneous infiltration of lidocaine 1%, bupivacaine 0.25%, and epinephrine (1:200,000) in a 2-mL syringe to allow for better pain control during tissue processing. Benzodiazepines increase the seizure threshold and allow large doses of lidocaine to be given safely without toxicity symptoms. The extended time period over which the local is administered between Mohs layers and before reconstruction also reduces toxicity risks. Cardiac monitoring should also be provided with large doses of bupivacaine. For very large cases such as dermatofibroma sarcoma protuberans or melanoma excisions, we often utilize tumescent anesthesia based on the components as seen in ▶ Table 12.5. As recommended ways to reduce pain during tumescent administration, inject slowly and injecting room-temperature or slightly warmed solution is helpful. Furthermore, buffering the acidic solution with bicarbonate also reduces the burning sensation experienced during administration.[53]

Following the procedure, based on the presence of large facial flaps or surgical defects in which the patient has a low pain threshold, a typical prescription given to patients is tramadol 50-mg tablets one to two tablets every 6 hours with a total number of six pills. Based on the increasing misuse and dependence on opiate-based narcotic pain medications, we do not routinely prescribe alternative controlled substances which are beyond the scope of this chapter. Patients are provided the call number for the resident and surgical fellow on call in case pain is not controlled following normal business hours.

Table 12.4 Pertinent extracted recommendations based on AAD guidelines for Mohs micrographic surgery

Local anesthesia type	Maximum amount to use (adult)
Lidocaine without epinephrine	4.5 mg/kg
Lidocaine with epinephrine	7 mg/kg
Tumescent anesthesia	55 mg/kg
Multistage procedure such as MMS	Do not exceed 500-mg lidocaine

Abbreviation: MMS, Mohs micrographic surgery.
Based on Kouba et al.[52]

12.1.4 Implantable Devices

Pacemakers/Defibrillators

Prior to and throughout surgery, the provider must ensure adequate work-up and management of implanted devices including cardiac, deep brain stimulator, and cochlear implants to ensure that no harm comes to the patient or their device. Implantable cardioverter-defibrillators (ICD) are devices that have revolutionized medicine to terminate ventricular tachycardia (VT) and ventricular fibrillation (VF).[54] Sustained VT and VF can lead to sudden cardiac death; thus, it is imperative that cauterization methods used during surgery do not interfere with the ICD function. A pacemaker can electrically stimulate or pace the heart with the newer models having the option

Table 12.5 Formula of tumescent we use for larger cases such as DFSP or deeper tumors

Ingredient in tumescent mixture	Quantity in tumescent mixture
1% Lidocaine	1,000 mg
Epinephrine	1 mg
Sodium bicarbonate	12.5 mEq
Normal saline (0.9%)	1,000 mL

Abbreviation: DFSP, dermatofibrosarcoma protuberans.

Table 12.6 Characteristics affecting electromagnetic interference (EMI) during dermatologic surgery

Proximity of electrosurgical device to implantable device
Length of pulse delivery of electrosurgical device
Lead placement (left-sided unipolar are at higher risk of sensing EMI)
Noise protection algorithms
ICD has increased sensitivity during pacing onset when there are absent sensed complexes in order to detect fine VF
Patient's level of dependence on pacemaker

Abbreviations: EMI, electromagnetic interference; ICD, implantable cardioverter-defibrillators; VF, ventricular fibrillation.
Based on Pinski SL, Trohman RG.[56]

to detect intrinsic cardiac activity.[55] The indications of ICD/pacemaker placement is beyond the scope of this chapter; however, certain characteristics increase the risk for electromagnetic interference (EMI) as seen in ▶ Table 12.6.[56]

Newer ICDs have protective fields in which nonphysiologic EMI leads to asynchronous pacing.[55] Sustained asynchronous pacing has the increased risk of producing tachyarrhythmias.[55] Similarly, newer cardiac devices have an insulated, sealed stainless steel or titanium case that reduces the distance between the electrodes.[57] The guidelines by the Heart Rhythm Society (HRS) and the American Society of Anesthesiologists (ASA) recommend the following: patients who are pacemaker dependent with a pacemaker, patients with an ICD and pacemaker dependent, or patients with an ICD and not pacemaker dependent, use short electrosurgical bursts less than 5 seconds with magnet placement for procedures above the umbilicus and cardiac monitoring during the procedure.[58] For nondependent patients with a pacemaker the magnet may not be required. Across dermatologic surgery there are various approaches to managing patients with ICDs and pacemakers. Per a survey administered to American College of Mohs Micrographic Surgery and Cutaneous Oncology (ACMMSCO) members, common practices of 166 members included using short bursts less than 5 seconds duration (71%), individual present with ACLS certification (68%), use of minimal power (61%), avoid use around device (57%), place grounding plate away from path of heart (37%), use bipolar forceps (19%), deactivate ICD (15%), and obtain a cardiac consultation (11%).[59] Given the diverse responses, it becomes evident that there is no clear consensus among dermatologic surgeons. Common side effects from EMI during dermatologic surgery results include altered mental status, palpitations, syncope, and hemodynamic instability.[59] Given the complexity and diversity of devices, the recommendation at our institution is to have the device interrogated either prior to or on the morning of surgery. Since 2000, when Mohs surgery orders are placed into our electronic medical record system, it automatically sends the pacemaker clinic (a part of the cardiovascular medicine division) notification that a device will need further investigation. Depending on the specifics of the device and the procedure, anatomic location and duration, the pacemaker clinic will make recommendations based on the telephone interrogation (or rarely in person) from their evaluation of the device. Continuous cardiac monitoring is performed by a registered nurse who is ACLS trained with appropriate postprocedural analysis of the device. Based on recommendations from the HRS and ASA, it is recommended that for elective procedures that the patient have had their pacemaker interrogated within the last 12 months and their ICD (if applicable) within the last 6 months.[58] If in the unlikely event the EMI results in the need for defibrillation, it is advised to place the paddles 15 cm away from the device and place them in an anterior-posterior manner so that the electric field created with the shock is perpendicular to the leads of the implantable cardiac device.[60]

Five main types of electrosurgery are encountered in dermatologic surgery including electrodesiccation, electrofulguration, electrocoagulation, electrosection, and electrocautery. Electrodesiccation and electrofulguration are high frequency and low ampere methods to achieve hemostasis during surgery. Electrodesiccation involves direct contact with the electrode tip and the tissue whereas electrofulguration involves holding the electrode tip approximately 1 to 3 mm from the area being treated resulting in a visible spark. Advantages for these two methods of monoterminal electrosurgery include that the current is lower so there is both less tissue destruction and the patient acts as a ground. Contrastingly, electrocoagulation and electrosection have higher ampere and lower voltage resulting in increased tissue destruction and requiring the patient to be grounded. In order to reduce the likelihood of EMI, it is recommended to ground the patient to avoid having the device in the path. For example, if surgery were to be performed on the right arm, it would be recommended to ground the patient on the right lower extremity rather than the contralateral arm or leg. True electrocautery with a hot wire tip is not commonly used in dermatologic surgery, given the need for hemostasis for larger caliber vessels, but this method is less likely to cause interference, given that it uses thermal energy instead of electrical. Per a retrospective chart review at Mayo Clinic for the years 2001 to 2004, 173 patients with pacemakers and 13 with ICDs who underwent dermatologic surgery had no complications related to electrosurgery.[61] Although the authors' institution has the benefit of a pacemaker clinic allowing for pre- or postprocedural device interrogation, this study supports the use of bipolar cautery to reduce the risk of EMI during dermatologic surgery. Based on this study and general recommendations made by Dawes et al we recommend the following: (1) Ensure appropriate work-up investigation regarding the device type including if patient is pacemaker dependent. (2) Cardiac monitoring and O2 saturation during the procedure by ACLS trained provider and staff. (3) Use bipolar forceps if possible. (4) Use short bursts less than 5 seconds in duration. (5) Discuss if use of magnet is appropriate during use of electrocautery. (6) Place the grounding plate in an anatomic position to the electrocautery tip to limit the flow of current in the path of the device. (7) Have access to a crash cart. (8) Ensure that device is investigated postprocedurally and do not take off monitoring until device is restored to its original settings.[61,62]

Deep Brain Stimulators

With the aging patient population, deep brain stimulators are also increasingly encountered in patients undergoing MMS. Given that some of the main features of Parkinson's disease include a resting tremor, muscular rigidity, and slower movements, a deep brain stimulator has helped to control the symptoms for patients who have Parkinson's and other movement disorders.[63] The deep brain stimulator is an implantable device with four electrodes implanted in the brain (specifically thalamus) and the neurostimulator located to the chest wall connected via a coiled wire. Settings are adjustable including the amplitude, width, and frequency of the pulse to reduce the motor symptoms in these neurologic conditions. Patients are able to turn the device on and off by using an external magnet to be placed over the neurostimulator implanted in the chest wall. Martinelli et al describe a case report of a patient with a deep brain stimulator for Parkinson's undergoing MMS on the left ear for a squamous cell carcinoma in which no complications occurred with use of a battery-operated electrocautery device.[64] Contrastingly, Weaver et al described a patient with a deep brain stimulator undergoing MMS for a basal cell carcinoma on the left cheek in which hemostasis was achieved with a hyfrecator (electrofulguration).[65] With the use of the hyfrecator, the patient experienced the sensation of "electric shocks" on the ipsilateral arm and leg.[65] Given the sensation, the surgeon switched to ophthalmic handheld battery-operated cautery which did not result in the symptoms that the patient had previously experienced with electrofulguration.[65] Both of these case reports highlight the importance of screening for the presence of deep brain stimulators prior to surgery or use a magnet to turn the device off. If the underlying movement disorder would impede surgery with the device turned off, then the surgeon should consider using a battery handheld form of cautery that relies on thermal energy or bipolar forceps.

12.2 Postoperative Care

Following MMS, postoperative care varies based on the closure type. For all cases, photographs are obtained following the closure, and wound care is reviewed with the surgeon, nurse, and patient. As seen in ▶ Fig. 12.2, our standard tray to create a pressure dressing includes: normal saline, petrolatum jelly, cotton-tip-based application sticks, Telfa nonadherent dressing (Medtronic, Minneapolis, MN), 4 × 4 gauze, paper tape or Hypafix dressing (BSN Medical, Hamburg, Germany), and scissors. Patients are provided an educational pamphlet with the following instructions for daily wound care:

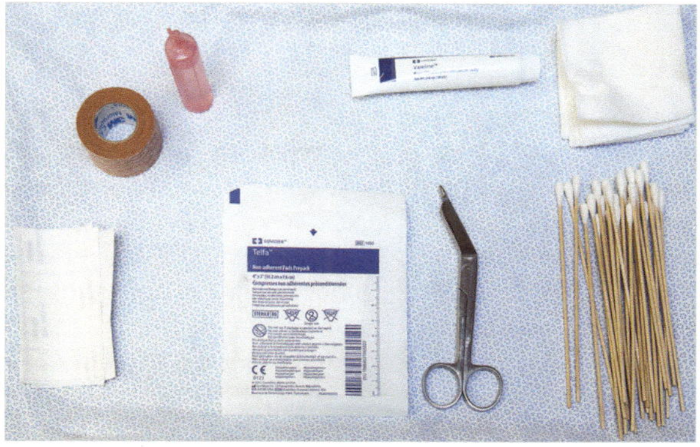

Fig. 12.2 Standard surgical tray with dressing supplies to form a pressure dressing including normal saline, petrolatum jelly, cotton tip-based application sticks, Telfa nonadherent dressing (Medtronic, Minneapolis, MN), 4 × 4 gauze, paper tape or Hypafix dressing (BSN Medical, Hamburg, Germany), and scissors.

1. Gently remove the pressure bandage the morning after surgery.
2. Change the dressing twice daily or if the bandage becomes saturated.
3. Wash hands with soap and water prior to cleaning the surgical site with cotton-tipped swabs or gauze moist with soap and water.
4. Gently remove any adherent crust or petroleum jelly from the previous application.
5. If the crust is adherent, soak the surgical site with wet gauze for 20 minutes.
6. Gently pat dry the affected area.
7. Reapply a new layer of petroleum jelly using a cotton-tipped swab.
8. Cover the petroleum with a nonstick dressing followed by clean gauze and paper tape.
9. Repeat the previous steps until stitches are removed or until advised by the surgeon.[66]
10. In the editors' experience, dilute white vinegar soaks help with antibacterial properties while not damaging normal tissue as can be seen with peroxide. They recommend a dilution of 1 tablespoon of white vinegar to 2 cups of warm water, or 1 "capful" to 1 cupful of white vinegar to warm water, respectively, with a clean cloth or gauze for 15 minutes daily prior to reapplication of dressings.

12.2.1 Granulation/Second-Intention Healing

The previously described postoperative wound care steps are used in all of our closure types; however, there are some minor modifications dependent on the anatomic location and size of the repair. Second-intention wound healing often is utilized with concave surfaces, superficial defects, for patients who cannot tolerate a larger closure, or areas of high tension where primary closure is not an option (i.e., lower legs or portions of scalp). As described by Zitelli, defects in the NEET facial regions (concavities of the Nose, Eye, Ear, and Temple) typically leads to minimally noticeable scarring whereas defects located in the NOCH regions of the face (convexities of the Nose, Oral lip, Cheek and Chin, Helix of ear) often leads to more noticeable scarring.[67] Following tumor clearance and adequate hemostasis, in order to promote reepithelialization of the defect, petrolatum jelly under occlusion is advised. It is also recommended to avoid hydrogen peroxide and antiseptic solutions to allow for granulation tissue formation.[68] For defects on the ear that are allowed to heal with second intention, we recommend applying Gelfoam (Pfizer Inc., New York, NY) in the defect prior to application of the pressure dressing to reduce the risk of postprocedural bleeding as seen in ▶ Fig. 12.3a–c. At the authors' institution, for eyelid repairs referred to oculoplastics, patients are typically advised to apply erythromycin 0.5% ointment to the wound instead of petrolatum jelly in the initial healing phase.

12.2.2 Porcine Xenografts and Biologic Dressings

For second-intention wound healing in deeper defects, we often will recommend the use of porcine xenografts, as seen in ▶ Fig. 12.4a–c, to both promote granulation at the MMS defect and protect underlying structures during healing. Per a retrospective chart review for 128 Mohs and excision surgical defect sites, the use of a porcine xenograft to promote second-intention wound healing was associated with a low rate of infection, improved

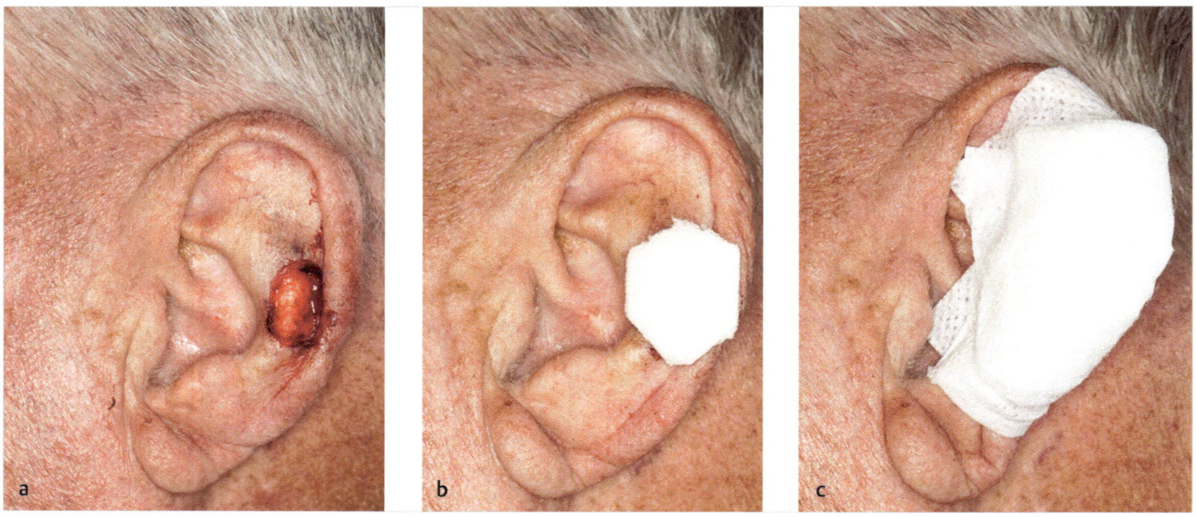

Fig. 12.3 (a) Postoperative Mohs micrographic surgery (MMS) defect on the ear allowed to heal with second intention. **(b)** Placement of Gelfoam (Pfizer Inc., New York, NY) at base of defect prior to applying standard pressure dressing. **(c)** Ear defect following placement of pressure dressing.

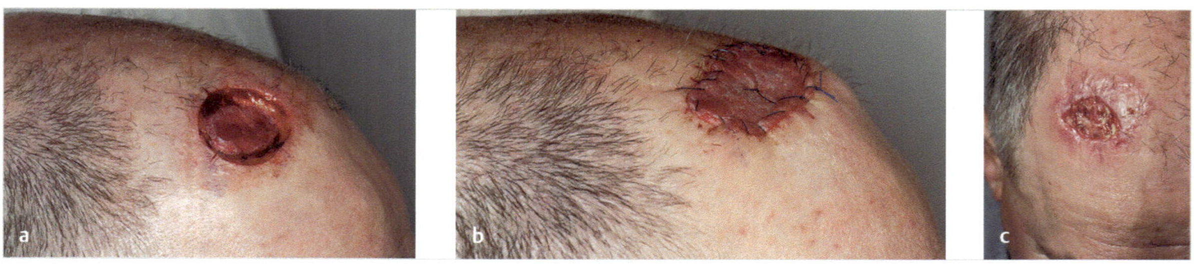

Fig. 12.4 (a) Postoperative Mohs micrographic surgery (MMS) on scalp, note the deep surgical defect. **(b)** Following placement of porcine xenograft. **(c)** Two weeks following porcine xenograft placement, note granulation tissue.

hemostasis with no documented cases of postoperative bleeding even with 42.5% of their patients being on anticoagulation medications, and no to little postprocedural pain.[69] Although in their study they used absorbable sutures and allowed the porcine xenograft to degrade naturally with acceptable cosmetic results, we typically use a nonabsorbable suture and see the patients back in clinic 2 weeks later to assess if a new xenograft is needed or if complete removal is warranted. It is not uncommon to have the patient return with significant exudate and inflammation warranting its removal; however, this may be suggestive of poor nutritional status, vascular compromise, or tobacco use.[70] However, if the xenograft is necrotic, this is a sign that the patient may not be doing adequate wound care which would support not replacing the xenograft with a full-thickness skin graft or delayed flap due to concern for recurrence of necrosis. If the xenograft looks similar to the initial day of placement, this is suggestive of adequate wound care by the patient and viable wound bed with adequate blood supply. The surgeon can decide to either allow the wound to heal by second intention or consider placing a full-thickness skin graft or flap, given the healthy granulation tissue. Additional benefits of porcine xenografts are the ease of application and reducing the need for significant wound care by the patient.[70] Yang and Ochoa found during their retrospective review of 225 porcine xenografts following MMS or excisions that larger procedural defects and those treated with bacitracin in comparison to petrolatum jelly alone experienced longer length of time needed to heal.[71] We typically advise for patients to continue standard wound care with petrolatum jelly under occlusion. Alternative options described in the literature include the use of allografts or human skin substitute to allow for improved granulation of the MMS defect either in preparation for placement of a full-thickness skin graft closure.[72,73,74,75] These biologic dressings serve as alternatives to the standard autografts and are mainly divided into three major categories: epidermal grafts, dermal grafts, or composite grafts of epidermis and dermis.[76] These various alternative biologic dressings can reduce pain and time of healing at the surgical defect; however, we do not routinely use these options due to financial cost to the patient. Based on the size of the defect, anticipated healing time, patient comorbidities, previous healing experience of the patient, and potential for pain or complications with the patient s healing process, the editor (SNT) periodically uses biologic tissue substitutes to improve second intention healing. While he has experience and has used multiple types of tissue substitutes, he typically uses cadaveric split-thickness skin graft tissue that is removed and reapplied once every 1-2 weeks until the point where a successful patient healing outcome is deemed imminent.

12.2.3 Bolster Sutures

Postoperative hematoma or seroma formation, infection, and poor apposition of wound edges can lead to a poor surgical cosmetic outcome.[77] An ideal pressure would be approximately 30 mmHg to ensure venous compression while partially reducing arterial flow at the repair site.[78] Bolster sutures are often utilized during the repair for surgical cases to reduce bleeding and manipulation of the surgical defect by the patient.[79] Placement of a bolster suture typically entails placing multiple interrupted 4–0 Silk sutures at the periphery of a surgical defect and then crossing the suture tails over petrolatum-coated nonstick gauze or dressing to secure the bolster. An absorbent dressing is typically then applied over the tied-down bolster suture with planned suture removal 1 week later. Bolster suture placement is useful for cases in which second-intention wound healing or full-thickness skin graft closure types are used to reduce bleeding and manipulation of the surgical defect (as seen in ▶ Fig. 12.5; see also ▶ Video 12.1). Alternative approaches also include using a sponge bolster instead of the traditional bolster tie-over suture with impregnated gauze or cotton balls as the sponge allows the surgeon to visualize the status of the full-thickness skin graft and does not require additional suturing.[80] Meads et al has also described the use of Aquaplast thermoplastic bolster dressing (WFR/Aquaplast Corp., Wyckoff, NJ) which allows the surgeon to heat the perforated plastic dressing to mold the bolster over the full-thickness skin graft, thereby increasing contact between the full-thickness skin graft and the recipient

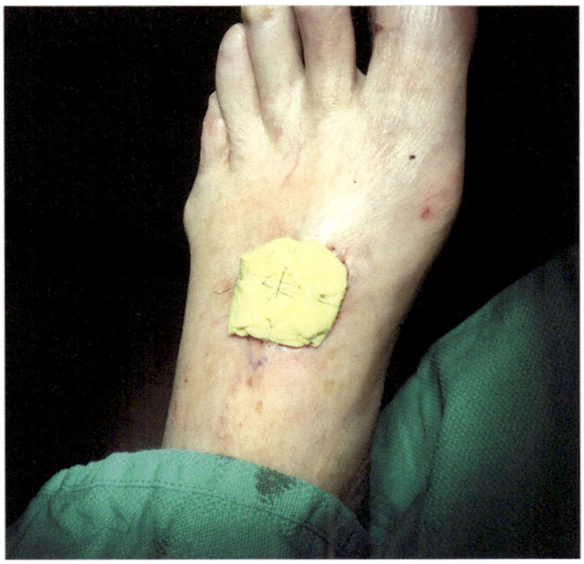

Fig. 12.5 Bolster suture placement to reduce bleeding following repair during Mohs micrographic surgery.

bed, reducing risk of hematoma formation, and allowing the patient to have the ability to shower.[81] The cost of the thermoplast dressing and risk of contact dermatitis are downsides highlighted by the authors.[81] The decision to utilize a bolster suture is patient specific and may not be required with smaller full-thickness skin grafts where an adequate pressure bandage or tie-over dressings can be used to achieve adequate hemostasis.[82,83]

12.2.4 Postdermabrasion Care

Stanislav N. Tolkachjov

Immediately following dermabrasion the abraded surface is soaked with gauze saturated with lidocaine and epinephrine (usually whatever local anesthesia is remaining in the syringe for that given case) for a period of 3 to 5 minutes to achieve hemostasis of the abraded area. Occasionally, micropoint electrocautery is used if a larger vessel on the nose continues to bleed. Do not apply Monsel's Solution or Aluminum Chloride to the abraded surface as they will stain or permanently discolor the skin. Once hemostasis is achieved, a semipermeable dressing (brand names: Vigilon or Second Skin) is applied to maintain a critical plane of humidity for reepithelialization which occurs from the skin appendages and the wound periphery. A bolster of gauze is then taped securely in place as a pressure dressing to prevent bleeding which is common during the first 24 hours postoperatively because the abraded surface is a broad open wound. This dressing is reapplied daily for 7 to 10 days until reepithelialization is complete. Hydrogen peroxide and gentle debridement is used with each dressing change in order to prevent scab or crust formation. After postoperative day 2 the pressure dressing can be reduced or eliminated because the tendency for bleeding also reduces greatly after the first 24 to 36 hours—even in anticoagulated patients. Following reepithelialization the new skin will be red or pink in color for 4 to 6 weeks. During this time patients should strictly avoid sun exposure to prevent brown hyperpigmentation which frequently occurs with UV exposure.

12.2.5 Postprimary Closure on the Lower Extremity

For our MMS cases below the knee, we often recommend the use of dilute vinegar soaks to reduce the risk of SSI. We advise the patient to mix one teaspoon of white vinegar with one 8-ounce cup of warm tap water. Following removal of the dressing, they are instructed to clean the surgical defect with normal saline or warm soap water. The patient is then advised to soak gauze in the dilute white vinegar solution and ring out any excessive liquid followed by application of the damp to leave on for 20 minutes. Following removal of the gauze the patient is advised to rinse the area with normal saline or soap water and repeat the aforementioned steps three to four times a day.[84] Compression is commonly used in distal defects on the lower extremities, given the increased venous hydrostatic pressure resulting in edema. Stebbins et al found the use of weekly Unna boots in 10 patients who underwent MMS on the distal extremity closed with either partial primary or second intention had a patient reported reduction in pain, less wound care, and no occurrence of complication of infection due to the occlusion, compression on the surgical defect site and antimicrobial and anti-inflammatory nature of zinc oxide.[85] Furthermore, Thompson et al found in their 80-patient cohort, who underwent excisions closed primary on the lower extremity, a decreased time to reepithelization with fewer complications in patients who had zinc oxide compression bandaging (Unna boot) left on for 1 week in comparison to those that had a standard pressure dressing for 48 hours.[86] The zinc oxide is thought to be both anti-inflammatory and antimicrobial to help further promote wound healing. The editors frequently use Vaseline-impregnated gauze (Xeroform) to promote healing by second intent for sites on lower extremities as well as scalp and digits. Patients are also advised standard stasis measures with elevation of the legs while at rest and graduated compression as tolerated to reduce edema of the distal lower extremity.

12.2.6 Postflap Care

Our approach to interpolation flaps is outlined in ▶ Fig. 12.6a–d. To reduce risk of postoperative bleeding, we perform pinpoint cautery to the lateral edges of the pedicle. Following adequate hemostasis, we wrap the pedicle loosely with Surgicel (Ethicon, Somerville, NJ) to reduce the risk of bleeding followed by our standard pressure dressing. Some surgeons also use a running, locked suture along the dermal edge of the pedicle to reduce postop bleeding. If there is concern for nasal valve collapse, we often secure a nose cone on the affected side prior to completion of the pressure bandage as seen in ▶ Fig. 12.7. We typically recommend a dressing change at 48 hours by the patient with standard takedown at 3 weeks. Rare postprocedural complications include venous congestion of the flap due to too tight of dressing surrounding the pedicle, hematomas due to bleeding at the distal flap, dehiscence, hypertrophic scarring, infection, and contact dermatitis to the dressings and/or ointments.[87] Newlove and Cook found in a retrospective chart review of 653 patients who underwent an interpolation flap repair following MMS that no major complications occurred.[88] Minor complications included 55 patients with bleeding for which 33 patients required electrocoagulation of bleeding venules on the flap pedicle within the first 24 hours, 4 patients with hematoma formation, 33 patients with postoperative infections either after the

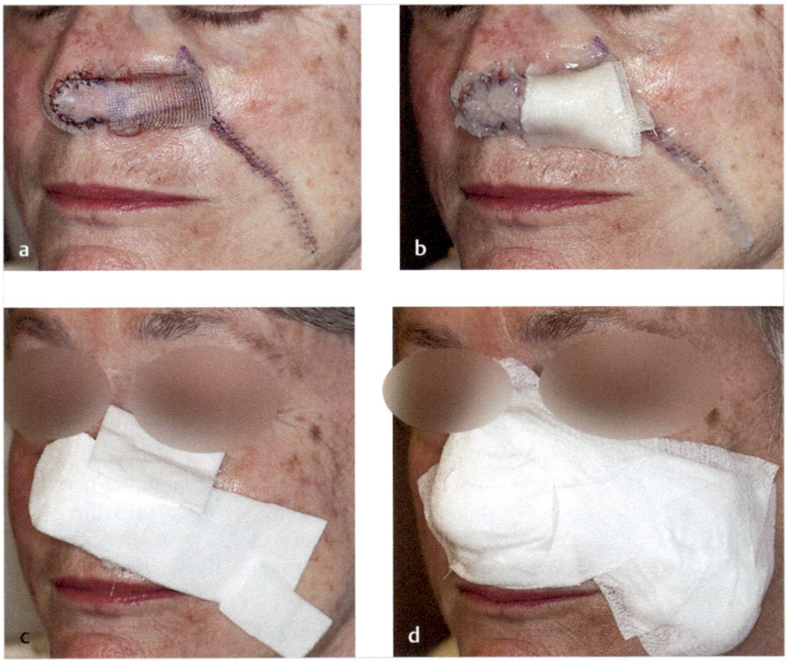

Fig. 12.6 (a) Placement of Surgicel (Ethicon, Somerville, NJ) loosely around the pedicle to aid hemostasis. (b) Placement of petrolatum jelly around pedicle and secondary defect. (c) Placement of nonadherent dressing around pedicle and secondary defect. (d) Placement of gauze with standard pressure dressing around pedicle and secondary defect.

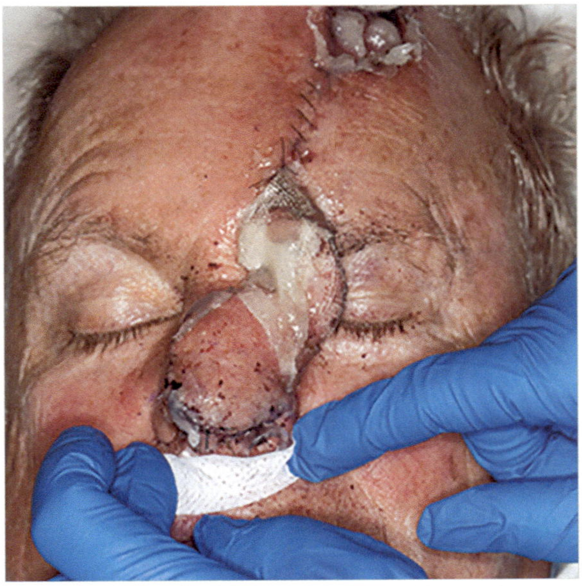

Fig. 12.7 Placement of nasal cone to help support the nasal valve.

first or second stage of the repair while on a 5-day course of either prophylactic cephalexin or ciprofloxacin, 15 patients with partial flap necrosis, and only 4 patients with total flap necrosis.[88] As described in previous chapters, dermabrasion, intralesional triamcinolone, and lasers can help to reduce the appearance of the scarring or pigmentary changes if desired.

12.3 Hematoma Management

Serious complications in MMS are rare; however, the dermatologic surgeon must be comfortable identifying and managing them when they occur. We will focus our attention to management of hematomas, infection, spitting sutures, and dehiscence for the remainder of the chapter. There are varied approaches among Mohs micrographic surgeons when managing warfarin, aspirin, and NSAID use prior to surgery. The 2002 survey results of 168 Mohs surgeons in the American College of Mohs Surgery (ACMS) highlight that 80% of providers discontinue warfarin in the perioperative time period, 26% discontinue aspirin, and 53% discontinue NSAIDs while over 90% of responders stated that they did not bridge to heparin if the patient is taken off of warfarin prior to Mohs.[89] Whereas, the 2005 survey results of 271 Mohs surgeons in the ACMS support that 44% discontinue warfarin, 37% discontinue medically necessary aspirin, 87% discontinue prophylactic aspirin, 77% discontinue NSAIDs, and 77% discontinue vitamin E.[27] As can be seen when comparing the survey results, dermatologic surgeons sampled appear to be continuing more medically necessary anticoagulation medication during dermatologic surgery. Among a meta-analysis of 1,373 patients, it was found that the risk of patients on warfarin, aspirin, and NSAIDs had a low but higher risk of bleeding than baseline.[90] Per a retrospective chart review by Kimyai-Asadi et al, out of 3,937 cases of MMS performed at two institutions, there was only one serious postprocedural complication due to naproxen use leading to gastrointestinal hemorrhage.[91] Among 2,418 patients who underwent dermatologic surgery while on anticoagulation, O'Neill et al had no patients who experienced life-threatening postprocedural bleeding.[92] Similarly, Billingsley and Maloney found that of 322 patients treated with Mohs, in comparison to the control group, patients on warfarin, aspirin, or NSAIDs had no statistically significant difference in postprocedural bleeding.[29] Although the approaches are varied, the risk of discontinuing the anticoagulant typically outweighs the benefit of reducing postprocedural bleeding in dermatologic surgery. Otley et al found that among 653 patients, severe complications occurred in 1.6% of cases in which patients were on warfarin or platelet inhibitors and there was no statistically significant reduction in severe complications for patients who had their anticoagulation medication held preoperatively.[30] Severe complications included significant hemorrhage, wound bleeding over 1 hour in duration, acute hematoma formation, necrosis of repair, or dehiscence greater than 2 mm.[30] The American College of Chest Physicians recommended that in minor dermatologic surgery (included excisions of both nonmelanoma skin cancers and melanomas) to continue vitamin K antagonists and achieve adequate local hemostasis instead of withholding anticoagulation.[93] Meticulous hemostasis with electrocautery, tying off of larger caliber bleeding vessels intraoperatively, and a well-structured pressure dressing are ways to reduce the risk of hematoma formation for patients on blood thinners during MMS.

With the aging patient population demographic, newer oral anticoagulant agents (NOACs) are commonly encountered during dermatologic surgery. Unlike vitamin K antagonists (i.e., warfarin) that can be closely monitored with INR and reversed, the NOACs until recently did not have available reversing agents and cannot be monitored as readily.[94] Given the rapid onset of NOACs and fewer drug-drug interactions, it is imperative that dermatologic surgeons are comfortable managing postprocedure bleeding if encountered. Chang et al found that among 27 patients on dabigatran undergoing 41 dermatologic surgeries, 1 patient experienced mild bleeding controlled with a pressure dressing and 4 patients on rivaroxaban undergoing 5 surgeries experienced no postprocedural bleeding complications.[40] If serious postprocedural hemorrhage occurs, NOAC effect may be lessened by use of oral-activated charcoal, antibody fragments such as Idarucizumab (Boehringer Ingelheim Pharmaceuticals, Inc., Germany), fresh frozen plasma (FFP), and hemodialysis (for dabigatran).[95] In addition to screening for NOACs during the perioperative time period, dermatologic surgeons should screen for the use of various herbal supplements that contribute to blood thinning and disrupt the clotting cascade.

Furthermore, blood pressure is part of the initial preoperative evaluation and based on current guideline it is proposed that it is acceptable to proceed with dermatologic surgery if systolic blood pressure (SBP) is less than 180 or diastolic blood pressure (DBP) is less than 100; however, it is preferred to have hypertension optimized by the primary care provider for SBP over 200 or DBP greater than 110, given increased risk of postprocedural bleeding and hematoma formation.[96] Following MMS, if the blood pressure remains elevated, the patient should have close follow-up with their primary care provider to reduce the risk of poor healing and cosmetic outcome due to bleeding or tissue ischemia related to poorly controlled hypertension.

To reduce the risk of postoperative bleeding for facial flaps we combine the use of plication sutures in the deep subcutaneous tissue along with modest undermining followed by meticulous hemostasis. If postprocedural bleeding does occur, it is advisable to have the patient hold firm pressure over the bandage for at least 30 minutes. Prolonged bleeding following dermatologic surgery places the patient at higher risk for hematoma formation and subsequent infection. Warning signs of hematoma formation following inset of facial flaps include tense flaps or closures changing in color and increasing pain.[97]

Hematomas can be divided into two types: active and passive. An active hematoma forms rapidly within 24 hours of surgery, is tense, and has active bright red blood draining from the margins and is indicative of an active arterial bleed. Active hematoma requires emergent surgical intervention to identify and coagulate or suture the arterial bleed. A passive hematoma forms slowly, up to a week after surgery, may or may not be tense but is typically dark red or blue with modest, if any, drainage at the margins. This is indicative of a mixture of venous blood in the edema that may not require active surgical intervention. Sometimes prophylactic antibiotics are used because clotted blood in the subcutaneous tissue can be a focus for infection.

As can be seen in ▸ Fig. 12.8, the tense nature underlying the large cheek rotational flap and the maroon hue to the skin are hallmark features of a rapidly expanding hematoma that should be addressed in the postoperative period. In this patient's case, he was on multiple anticoagulants, had limited social support, and due to a traumatic brain injury had removed the pressure bandage prematurely to more comfortably wear his helmet. The cheek flap was taken down within 24 hours and following careful identification and tying off of the bleeding vessels, the flap was re-sutured with no long-term complications or negative cosmetic outcome. If a hematoma is encountered, it is imperative to bring the patient back for evaluation to determine if evacuation of the hematoma is warranted. In addition, in our experience, if a patient has large repairs following MMS with little social support, it may be warranted to admit a patient for observation. Although this is not standard for the majority of our cases, this should be considered on a case-by-case basis. If a patient does have a rapidly expanding hematoma with active bleeding, the surrounding skin should be infiltrated with local

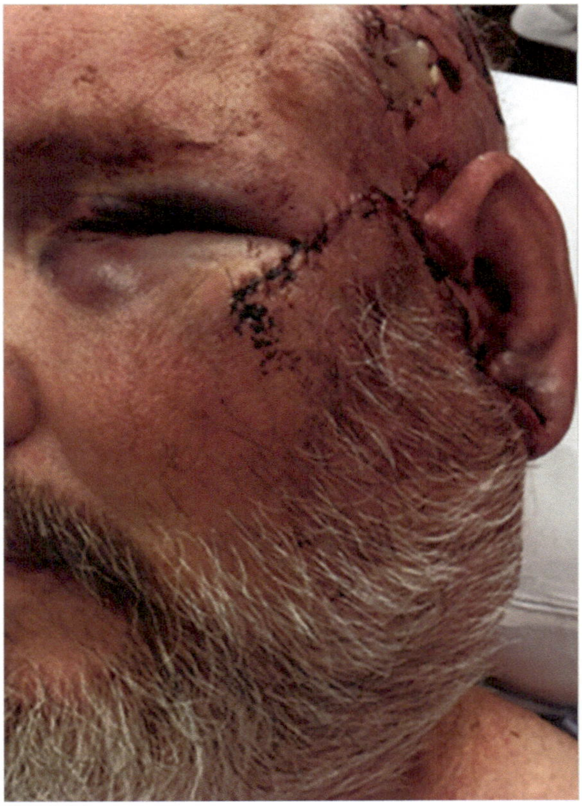

Fig. 12.8 Note the large expansive hematoma following a cheek rotational flap.

anesthesia without epinephrine. Epinephrine is not advised as this may lead to temporary vasoconstriction of the bleeding vessel, making pinpoint hemostasis more challenging. Following adequate anesthesia, the epidermal and subcutaneous sutures should be carefully removed to allow for reflection of the tissue to achieve adequate hemostasis with electrocautery or tying off of bleeding vessels. If identified early, following adequate evacuation of the hematoma, the wound can be resutured. Although rare in our practice, a Jackson-Pratt drain (JP drain) can be sutured into place at the time of repair to reduce the risk of hematoma collection as seen in ▶ Fig. 12.9. Cook found that only four hematomas developed in 1,343 cases with no significant long-term complications or poor cosmetic outcome.[98] Alternatively for an established, stable hematoma, the hematoma can be aspirated with a large-bore 18-gauge needle following surgery at which time the hematoma will have liquified.[99]

12.4 Infection Management

12.4.1 Infection

SSIs require prompt and aggressive treatment to prevent IE, prosthetic joint infection, and other adverse outcomes.

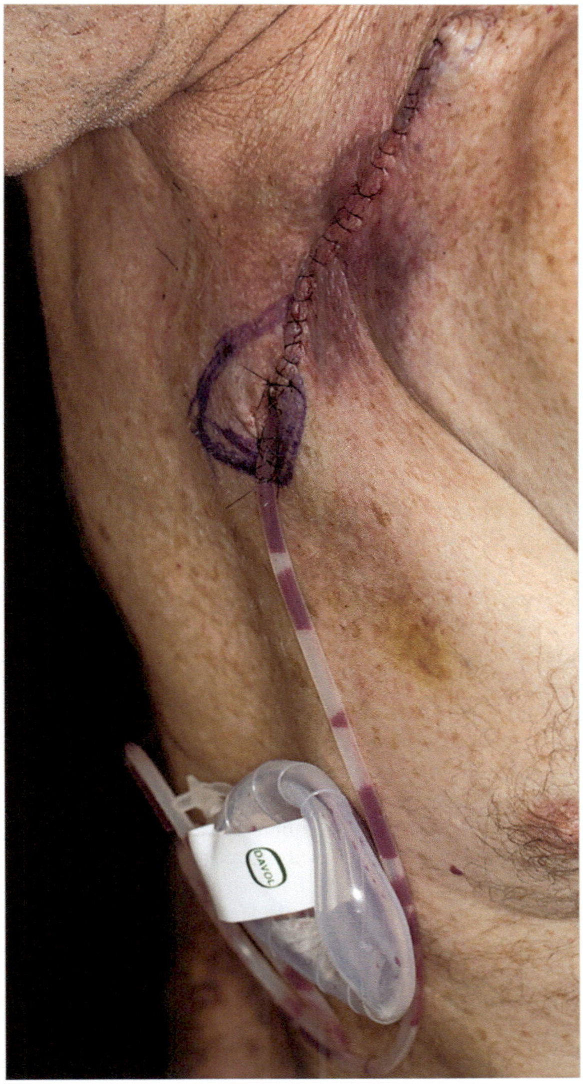

Fig. 12.9 Placement of a JP drain given depth of repair and concern for postprocedural hematoma development.

Operative locations and techniques which have been found to have a high risk for SSI are shown in ▶ Table 12.2.[2,6,7] If a surgical site is infected, cultures should be obtained prior to empiric treatment to evaluate for the causative organism and sensitivities, with the antibiotic regimen subsequently tailored according to culture results.

SSIs are caused by a multitude of factors from both endogenous and exogenous sources. Age, anatomic site, diabetes, smoking, and anticoagulant therapy have been studied as endogenous causes of SSI. The incidence of SSI has been found to be directly proportional to the patient's age,[10]with a mean age of 70.8 years among those with SSI.[100] Although smoking has been associated with higher rates of SSI in general surgery, limited studies evaluating smoking and postoperative infection in dermatology have shown no statistically significant increase in infection rates between smokers and nonsmokers[9,101]; however, one study showed smokers had an overall increased risk for postoperative complications.[102] While hematoma formation has been associated with SSI and the use of anticoagulants is associated with bleeding, there is no association seen with anticoagulant use and SSI.[9,35]

Exogenous factors contributing to SSI include personnel and environmental factors. Experienced surgeons have a lower SSI rate, thought to be secondary to decreased procedure duration and increased tissue-sparing technique.[19,103] Preoperative hair removal is thought to decrease SSIs and prevent irritation to the surgical site and potential impaired wound healing from ingrown hairs. Hair clipping has a lower rate of SSI when compared to shaving. The use of clean, nonsterile gloves, especially during tumor removal, was not associated with a higher risk of infection when compared to the use of sterile gloves, and nonsterile gloves led to significant cost savings.[104] At Mayo Clinic during MMS, layers are taken with clean, nonsterile gloves with sterile gloves utilized for the closure.

12.4.2 Antimicrobial Selection

Antibiotic selection should be guided by the most likely pathogens to cause infection at the surgical site. In dermatologic surgery, the organisms most likely to cause skin and soft tissue infection include *S. aureus* and B-hemolytic streptococci. *Streptococcus viridans*, a component of normal oral flora, is the major pathogen responsive for IE during perforating procedures involving the oral mucosa.[2] When selecting an antibiotic for surgical sites involving the groin, perineum, or in moist or macerated areas such as the axilla, and in diabetic patients, coverage should include gram-negative bacteria. Antibiotic prophylaxis for sites on the ear should take into consideration infection with pseudomonas, a frequent colonizer of the ear canal. Fluoroquinolones can be given if there is concern for pseudomonas; however, cephalexin is preferred, given infection rates with pseudomonas are low.[4,105] For patients with MRSA, doxycycline, clindamycin, or trimethoprim-sulfamethoxazole are typically utilized at Mayo Clinic. Management of abscesses includes incision and drainage and consideration of administration of antibiotics that cover MRSA.[2] The recommended evaluation of postoperative infection and antibiotic selection is shown in ▶ Fig. 12.10.[106]

12.5 Pain Management

With the overuse of opiate-based narcotic pain medications, the dermatologic surgeon must decide the appropriate means to manage acute pain in the postprocedural setting. As discussed previously, at our institution we initially recommend acetaminophen typically dosed at 1,000 mg every 6 hours, not to exceed a total of 4,000 mg in a 24-hour time period. For patients with pre-existing liver disease, the recommended amount will be dosed according to adjustment for hepatic clearance and avoid toxicity. We typically advise to avoid NSAIDs within the first 48 to 72 hours following MMS, given the effect on platelets and concern for possible increased bleeding. However, as described in more recent literature and based on previous ACMS surveys, there are varied approaches on recommending NSAIDs in combination with acetaminophen in the immediate postprocedural time period. As highlighted by Sniezek et al, in their randomized controlled study, they found that among 210 patients who underwent MMS on the head and neck and received 1,000 mg of acetaminophen with 400 mg of ibuprofen had the lowest pain score in comparison to those who received 1,000 mg of acetaminophen alone or 325 mg acetaminophen with 30 mg of codeine.[107] If the pain is not controlled, based on protocol proposed at the authors' institution by Lopez et al[110], we typically prescribe tramadol 50 mg tablets 1 tablet every 6 hours as needed for moderate-to-severe pain with a total of six tablets. Longer acting opiate-based pain medications are avoided. The total number of tablets recommended is based upon the most common time period to experience pain. As described by Firoz et al, among 433 patients administered a postoperative pain assessment sheet (Wong-Baker pain scale) to assess the level of pain following MMS, nearly half of the patients (48%) did not require any medication; the highest pain level occurred on the day of surgery and decreased until postoperative day 4.[111] Furthermore, second-intention wound healing was associated with the lowest level of pain whereas flaps had a higher level of pain.[109] Similarly, other studies support that the majority of patients experience mild-to-moderate pain on the day of MMS and postoperative day 1.[112, 113] Patients are advised if pain continues to worsen that they should be evaluated in person to monitor for signs of infection, hematoma, or dehiscence.

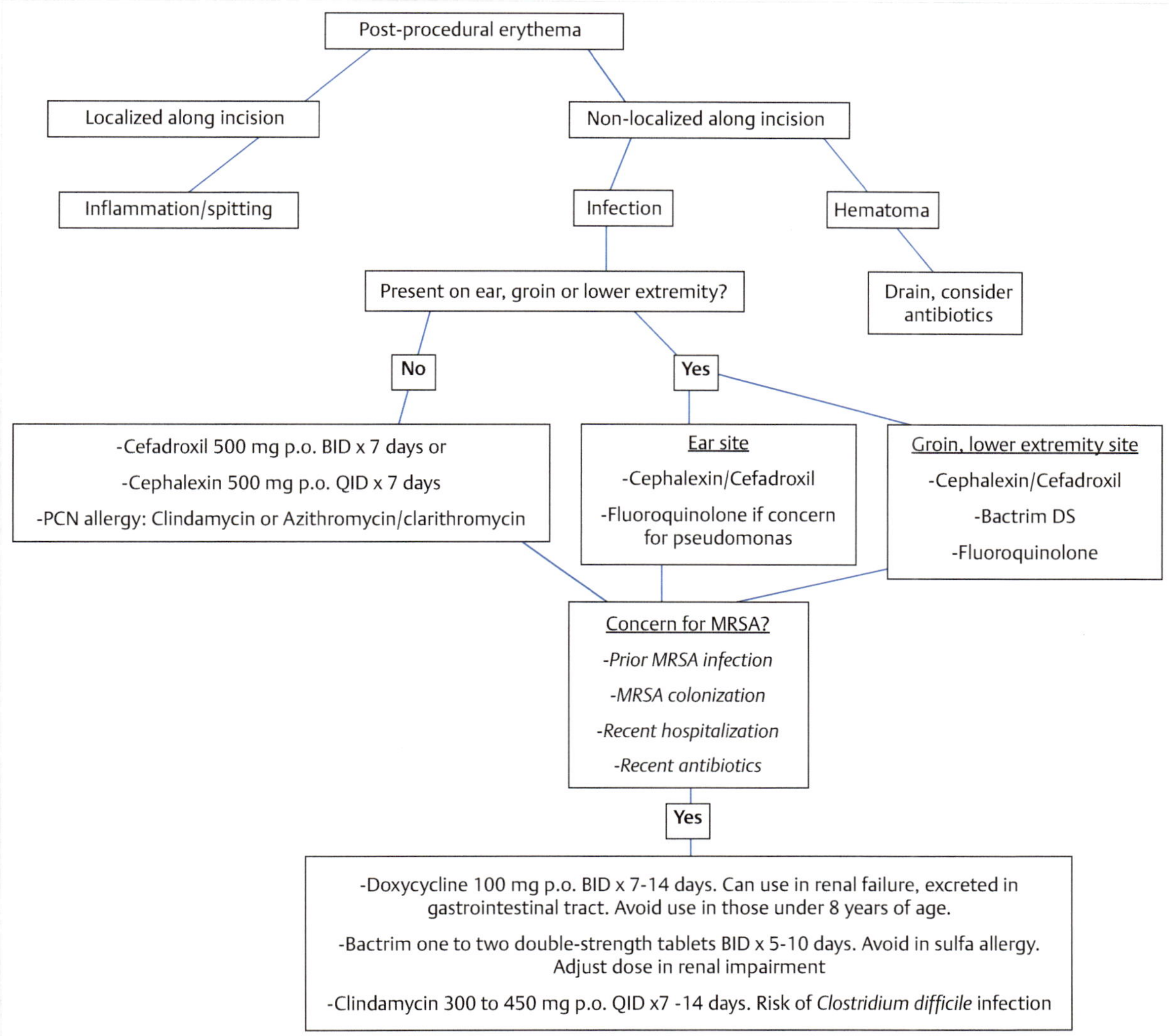

Fig. 12.10 Postoperative antibiotic recommendations. PO, by mouth; PCN, penicillin. Based on Wright et al and Stevens et al.[2,106]

References

[1] Wilson W, Taubert KA, Gewitz M, et al. American Heart Association Rheumatic Fever, Endocarditis, and Kawasaki Disease Committee, American Heart Association Council on Cardiovascular Disease in the Young, American Heart Association Council on Clinical Cardiology, American Heart Association Council on Cardiovascular Surgery and Anesthesia, Quality of Care and Outcomes Research Interdisciplinary Working Group. Prevention of infective endocarditis: guidelines from the American Heart Association: a guideline from the American Heart Association Rheumatic Fever, Endocarditis, and Kawasaki Disease Committee, Council on Cardiovascular Disease in the Young, and the Council on Clinical Cardiology, Council on Cardiovascular Surgery and Anesthesia, and the Quality of Care and Outcomes Research Interdisciplinary Working Group. Circulation. 2007; 116(15):1736–1754

[2] Wright TI, Baddour LM, Berbari EF, et al. Antibiotic prophylaxis in dermatologic surgery: advisory statement 2008. J Am Acad Dermatol. 2008; 59(3):464–473

[3] American Dental Association, American Academy of Orthopaedic Surgeons. Antibiotic prophylaxis for dental patients with total joint replacements. J Am Dent Assoc (1939). 2003; 134(7):895–899

[4] Bae-Harboe YS, Liang CA. Perioperative antibiotic use of dermatologic surgeons in 2012. Dermatol Surg. 2013; 39(11):1592–1601

[5] Messingham MJ, Arpey CJ. Update on the use of antibiotics in cutaneous surgery. Dermatol Surg. 2005; 31(8 Pt 2):1068–1078

[6] Dixon AJ, Dixon MP, Askew DA, Wilkinson D. Prospective study of wound infections in dermatologic surgery in the absence of prophylactic antibiotics. Dermatol Surg. 2006; 32(6):819–826, discussion 826–827

[7] Maragh SL, Brown MD. Prospective evaluation of surgical site infection rate among patients with Mohs micrographic surgery without the use of prophylactic antibiotics. J Am Acad Dermatol. 2008; 59 (2):275–278

[8] Wilson W, Taubert KA, Gewitz M, et al. Prevention of infective endocarditis: guidelines from the American Heart Association: a guideline from the American Heart Association Rheumatic Fever, Endocarditis and Kawasaki Disease Committee, Council on Cardiovascular Disease in the Young, and the Council on Clinical

Cardiology, Council on Cardiovascular Surgery and Anesthesia, and the Quality of Care and Outcomes Research Interdisciplinary Working Group. J Am Dent Assoc. 1939; 2008(139) Suppl:3s–24s

[9] Saleh K, Schmidtchen A. Surgical site infections in dermatologic surgery: etiology, pathogenesis, and current preventative measures. Dermatol Surg. 2015; 41(5):537–549

[10] Heal CF, Buettner PG, Drobetz H. Risk factors for surgical site infection after dermatological surgery. Int J Dermatol. 2012; 51(7):796–803

[11] Rogers HD, Desciak EB, Marcus RP, Wang S, MacKay-Wiggan J, Eliezri YD. Prospective study of wound infections in Mohs micrographic surgery using clean surgical technique in the absence of prophylactic antibiotics. J Am Acad Dermatol. 2010; 63(5):842–851

[12] Rogues AM, Lasheras A, Amici JM, et al. Infection control practices and infectious complications in dermatological surgery. J Hosp Infect. 2007; 65(3):258–263

[13] Sylaidis P, Wood S, Murray DS. Postoperative infection following clean facial surgery. Ann Plast Surg. 1997; 39(4):342–346

[14] Kaplan AL, Cook JL. The incidences of chondritis and perichondritis associated with the surgical manipulation of auricular cartilage. Dermatol Surg. 2004; 30(1):58–62, discussion 62

[15] Bari O, Eilers RE , Jr, Rubin AG, Jiang SIB. Clinical characteristics of lower extremity surgical site infections in dermatologic surgery based upon 24-month retrospective review. J Drugs Dermatol. 2018; 17(7):766–771

[16] Cherian P, Gunson T, Borchard K, Tai Y, Smith H, Vinciullo C. Oral antibiotics versus topical decolonization to prevent surgical site infection after Mohs micrographic surgery–a randomized, controlled trial. Dermatol Surg. 2013; 39(10):1486–1493

[17] Cordova KB, Grenier N, Chang KH, Dufresne R , Jr. Preoperative methicillin-resistant Staphylococcus aureus screening in Mohs surgery appears to decrease postoperative infections. Dermatol Surg. 2010; 36(10):1537–1540

[18] Tai YJ, Borchard KL, Gunson TH, Smith HR, Vinciullo C. Nasal carriage of Staphylococcus aureus in patients undergoing Mohs micrographic surgery is an important risk factor for postoperative surgical site infection: a prospective randomised study. Australas J Dermatol. 2013; 54(2):109–114

[19] Saco M, Howe N, Nathoo R, Cherpelis B. Topical antibiotic prophylaxis for prevention of surgical wound infections from dermatologic procedures: a systematic review and meta-analysis. J Dermatolog Treat. 2015; 26(2):151–158

[20] Smack DP, Harrington AC, Dunn C, et al. Infection and allergy incidence in ambulatory surgery patients using white petrolatum vs bacitracin ointment. A randomized controlled trial. JAMA. 1996; 276(12):972–977

[21] Spann CT, Tutrone WD, Weinberg JM, Scheinfeld N, Ross B. Topical antibacterial agents for wound care: a primer. Dermatol Surg. 2003; 29(6):620–626

[22] Mayo Clinic. Division of Dermatologic Surgery. Recommendations for antibiotic prophylaxis in dermatologic surgery. Rochester, MN: Mayo Clinic, Division of Dermatologic Surgery; 2008

[23] Alam M, Goldberg LH. Serious adverse vascular events associated with perioperative interruption of antiplatelet and anticoagulant therapy. Dermatol Surg. 2002; 28(11):992–998, discussion 998

[24] Eilers RE , Jr, Goldenberg A, Cowan NL, Basu P, Brian Jiang SI. A retrospective assessment of postoperative bleeding complications in anticoagulated patients following Mohs micrographic surgery. Dermatol Surg. 2018; 44(4):504–511

[25] West SW, Otley CC, Nguyen TH, et al. Cutaneous surgeons cannot predict blood-thinner status by intraoperative visual inspection. Plast Reconstr Surg. 2002; 110(1):98–103

[26] Kovich O, Otley CC. Thrombotic complications related to discontinuation of warfarin and aspirin therapy perioperatively for cutaneous operation. J Am Acad Dermatol. 2003; 48(2):233–237

[27] Kirkorian AY, Moore BL, Siskind J, Marmur ES. Perioperative management of anticoagulant therapy during cutaneous surgery: 2005 survey of Mohs surgeons. Dermatol Surg. 2007; 33(10):1189–1197

[28] Schanbacher CF, Bennett RG. Postoperative stroke after stopping warfarin for cutaneous surgery. Dermatol Surg. 2000; 26(8):785–789

[29] Billingsley EM, Maloney ME. Intraoperative and postoperative bleeding problems in patients taking warfarin, aspirin, and nonsteroidal antiinflammatory agents. A prospective study. Dermatol Surg. 1997; 23(5):381–383, discussion 384–385

[30] Otley CC, Fewkes JL, Frank W, Olbricht SM. Complications of cutaneous surgery in patients who are taking warfarin, aspirin, or nonsteroidal anti-inflammatory drugs. Arch Dermatol. 1996; 132(2):161–166

[31] Bartlett GR. Does aspirin affect the outcome of minor cutaneous surgery? Br J Plast Surg. 1999; 52(3):214–216

[32] Alcalay J. Cutaneous surgery in patients receiving warfarin therapy. Dermatol Surg. 2001; 27(8):756–758

[33] Lam J, Lim J, Clark J, Knox A, Poole MD. Warfarin and cutaneous surgery: a preliminary prospective study. Br J Plast Surg. 2001; 54 (4):372–373

[34] Ah-Weng A, Natarajan S, Velangi S, Langtry JA. Preoperative monitoring of warfarin in cutaneous surgery. Br J Dermatol. 2003; 149 (2):386–389

[35] Bordeaux JS, Martires KJ, Goldberg D, Pattee SF, Fu P, Maloney ME. Prospective evaluation of dermatologic surgery complications including patients on multiple antiplatelet and anticoagulant medications. J Am Acad Dermatol. 2011; 65(3):576–583

[36] Cook-Norris RH, Michaels JD, Weaver AL, et al. Complications of cutaneous surgery in patients taking clopidogrel-containing anticoagulation. J Am Acad Dermatol. 2011; 65(3):584–591

[37] Kargi E, Babuccu O, Hosnuter M, Babuccu B, Altinyazar C. Complications of minor cutaneous surgery in patients under anticoagulant treatment. Aesthetic Plast Surg. 2002; 26(6):483–485

[38] Shimizu I, Jellinek NJ, Dufresne RG, Li T, Devarajan K, Perlis C. Multiple antithrombotic agents increase the risk of postoperative hemorrhage in dermatologic surgery. J Am Acad Dermatol. 2008; 58 (5):810–816

[39] Khalifeh MR, Redett RJ. The management of patients on anticoagulants prior to cutaneous surgery: case report of a thromboembolic complication, review of the literature, and evidence-based recommendations. Plast Reconstr Surg. 2006; 118(5):110e–117e

[40] Chang TW, Arpey CJ, Baum CL, et al. Complications with new oral anticoagulants dabigatran and rivaroxaban in cutaneous surgery. Dermatol Surg. 2015; 41(7):784–793

[41] Spyros M Siscos, Brett C Neill, Anjali Hocker Singh, Thomas L H Hocker. Thrombotic complications with interruption of direct oral anticoagulants in dermatologic surgery. J Am Acad Dermatol. 2021; 84(2):425–431

[42] Collins SC, Dufresne RG , Jr. Dietary supplements in the setting of Mohs surgery. Dermatol Surg. 2002; 28(6):447–452

[43] Goldsmith SM, Leshin B, Owen J. Management of patients taking anticoagulants and platelet inhibitors prior to dermatologic surgery. J Dermatol Surg Oncol. 1993; 19(6):578–581

[44] Doherty JU, Gluckman TJ, Hucker WJ, et al. 2017 ACC Expert Consensus Decision Pathway for Periprocedural Management of Anticoagulation in Patients With Nonvalvular Atrial Fibrillation: A Report of the American College of Cardiology Clinical Expert Consensus Document Task Force. J Am Coll Cardiol. 2017; 69(7):871–898

[45] Siscos SM, Neill BC, Singh AH, Hocker TLH. Thrombotic complications with interruption of direct oral anticoagulants in dermatologic surgery. J Am Acad Dermatol. 2021; 84(2):425–431

[46] Lexicomp Online®, Drug Facts and Comparison, Hudson, Ohio: Wolters Kluwer Clinical Drug Information, Inc.; 2018, Apr 01, 2018

[47] Reves JG, Fragen RJ, Vinik HR, Greenblatt DJ. Midazolam: pharmacology and uses. Anesthesiology. 1985; 62(3):310–324

[48] White PF, Vasconez LO, Mathes SA, Way WL, Wender LA. Comparison of midazolam and diazepam for sedation during plastic surgery. Plast Reconstr Surg. 1988; 81(5):703–712

[49] Conway A, Rolley J, Sutherland JR. Midazolam for sedation before procedures. (Review). Cochrane Database Syst Rev. 2016(5):CD009491

[50] Kuganeswaran E, Clarkston WK, Cuddy PG, et al. A double-blind placebo controlled trial of oral midazolam as premedication before flexible sigmoidoscopy. Am J Gastroenterol. 1999; 94(11):3215–3219
[51] Beer GM, Spicher I, Seifert B, Emanuel B, Kompatscher P, Meyer VE. Oral premedication for operations on the face under local anesthesia: a placebo-controlled double-blind trial. Plast Reconstr Surg. 2001; 108(3):637–643
[52] Otley CC, Nguyen TH. Conscious sedation of pediatric patients with combination oral benzodiazepines and inhaled nitrous oxide. Dermatol Surg. 2000; 26(11):1041–1044
[53] American Society of Anesthesiologists Task Force on Sedation and Analgesia by Non-Anesthesiologists. Practice guidelines for sedation and analgesia by non-anesthesiologists. Anesthesiology. 2002; 96 (4):1004–1017
[54] Kouba DJ, LoPiccolo MC, Alam M, et al. Guidelines for the use of local anesthesia in office-based dermatologic surgery. J Am Acad Dermatol. 2016; 74(6):1201–1219
[55] Klein JA. Tumescent technique chronicles. Local anesthesia, liposuction, and beyond. Dermatol Surg. 1995; 21(5):449–457
[56] Ganz LI. Implantable cardioverter-defibrillators: Overview of indications, components, and functions. In: Piccini J, Downey BC, ed. UpToDate. Waltham, MA: UpToDate; 2017. www.uptodate.com. Accessed December 13, 2017
[57] Kumar A, Dhillon SS, Patel S, Grube M, Noheria A. Management of cardiac implantable electronic devices during interventional pulmonology procedures. J Thorac Dis. 2017; 9(10) Suppl 10:S1059–S1068
[58] Pinski SL, Trohman RG. Interference in implanted cardiac devices, Part I. Pacing Clin Electrophysiol. 2002; 25(9):1367–1381
[59] Howe N, Cherpelis B. Obtaining rapid and effective hemostasis: Part II. Electrosurgery in patients with implantable cardiac devices. J Am Acad Dermatol. 2013; 69(5):677.e1–677.e9
[60] Crossley GH, Poole JE, Rozner MA, et al. The Heart Rhythm Society (HRS)/American Society of Anesthesiologists (ASA) Expert Consensus Statement on the perioperative management of patients with implantable defibrillators, pacemakers and arrhythmia monitors: facilities and patient management this document was developed as a joint project with the American Society of Anesthesiologists (ASA), and in collaboration with the American Heart Association (AHA), and the Society of Thoracic Surgeons (STS). Heart Rhythm. 2011; 8 (7):1114–1154
[61] El-Gamal HM, Dufresne RG, Saddler K. Electrosurgery, pacemakers and ICDs: a survey of precautions and complications experienced by cutaneous surgeons. Dermatol Surg. 2001; 27(4):385–390
[62] Yerra L, Reddy PC. Effects of electromagnetic interference on implanted cardiac devices and their management. Cardiol Rev. 2007; 15(6):304–309
[63] Matzke TJ, Christenson LJ, Christenson SD, Atanashova N, Otley CC. Pacemakers and implantable cardiac defibrillators in dermatologic surgery. Dermatol Surg. 2006; 32(9):1155–1162, discussion 1162
[64] Dawes JC, Mahabir RC, Hillier K, Cassidy M, de Haas W, Gillis AM. Electrosurgery in patients with pacemakers/implanted cardioverter defibrillators. Ann Plast Surg. 2006; 57(1):33–36
[65] Machado FA, Reppold CT. The effect of deep brain stimulation on motor and cognitive symptoms of Parkinson's disease: a literature review. Dement Neuropsychol. 2015; 9(1):24–31
[66] Martinelli PT, Schulze KE, Nelson BR. Mohs micrographic surgery in a patient with a deep brain stimulator: a review of the literature on implantable electrical devices. Dermatol Surg. 2004; 30(7):1021–1030
[67] Weaver J, Kim SJ, Lee MH, Torres A. Cutaneous electrosurgery in a patient with a deep brain stimulator. Dermatol Surg. 1999; 25 (5):415–417
[68] Mayo Foundation for Medical Education and Research. Barbara Woodward Lips Patient Education Center Patient Education Care following skin surgery. Rochester, MN: Mayo Foundation for Medical Education and Research MFMER; 2006
[69] Zitelli JA. Secondary intention healing: an alternative to surgical repair. Clin Dermatol. 1984; 2(3):92–106
[70] Moreno-Arias GA, Izento-Menezes CM, Carrasco MA, Camps-Fresneda A. European Academy of Dermatology and Venereology. 2000; 14:159–165
[71] Marzolf S, Srivastava D, Nijhawan RI. Porcine xenografts for surgical defects: experience of a single center with 128 cases. J Am Acad Dermatol. 2018; 78(5):1005–1007
[72] Davis DA, Arpey CJ. Porcine heterografts in dermatologic surgery and reconstruction. Dermatol Surg. 2000; 26(1):76–80
[73] Yang YW, Ochoa SA. Use of porcine xenografts in dermatology surgery: the Mayo Clinic experience. Dermatol Surg. 2016; 42(8):985–991
[74] Kolenik SA , III, Leffell DJ. The use of cryopreserved human skin allografts in wound healing following Mohs surgery. Dermatol Surg. 1995; 21(7):615–620
[75] Gohari S, Gambla C, Healey M, et al. Evaluation of tissue-engineered skin (human skin substitute) and secondary intention healing in the treatment of full thickness wounds after Mohs micrographic or excisional surgery. Dermatol Surg. 2002; 28(12):1107–1114, discussion 1114
[76] Ahmed S, Hussein SS, Philp B, Healy C. Use of biologic dressing as a temporary wound dressing in reconstruction of a significant forehead Mohs defect. Dermatol Surg. 2006; 32(5):765–767
[77] Kontos AP, Qian Z, Urato NS, Hassanein A, Proper SA. AlloDerm grafting for large wounds after Mohs micrographic surgery. Dermatol Surg. 2009; 35(4):692–698
[78] Chern PL, Baum CL, Arpey CJ. Biologic dressings: current applications and limitations in dermatologic surgery. Dermatol Surg. 2009; 35(6):891–906
[79] Landau AG, Hudson DA, Adams K, Geldenhuys S, Pienaar C. Full-thickness skin grafts: maximizing graft take using negative pressure dressings to prepare the graft bed. Ann Plast Surg. 2008; 60(6):661–666
[80] Smith F. A rational management of skin grafts. Surg Gynecol Obstet. 1926; 42:556
[81] Sams HH, Stasko T, McDonald MA. Surgical pearl: bolster dressing for second-intention healing of Mohs micrographic surgical sites. J Am Acad Dermatol. 2004; 51(4):633–634
[82] Egan CA, Gerwels JW. Surgical pearl: use of a sponge bolster instead of a tie-over bolster as a less invasive method of securing full-thickness skin grafts. J Am Acad Dermatol. 1998; 39(6):1000–1001
[83] Meads SB, Greenway HT, Eaton JS. Surgical pearl: thermoplastic bolster dressing for full-thickness skin grafts. J Am Acad Dermatol. 2006; 54(1):152–153
[84] Langtry JAA, Kirkham P, Martin IC, Fordyce A. Tie-over bolster dressings may not be necessary to secure small full thickness skin grafts. Dermatol Surg. 1998; 24(12):1350–1353
[85] Pulvermacker B, Chaouat M, Seroussi D, Mimoun M. Tie-over dressings in full-thickness skin grafts. Dermatol Surg. 2008; 34(1):40–43, discussion 44
[86] Mayo Foundation for Medical Education and Research. Barbara Woodward Lips Patient Education Center Patient Education vinegar wound soak. Rochester, MN: Mayo Foundation for Medical Education and Research MFMER; 2008
[87] Stebbins WG, Hanke CW, Petersen J. Enhanced healing of surgical wounds of the lower leg using weekly zinc oxide compression dressings. Dermatol Surg. 2011; 37(2):158–165
[88] Thompson CB, Wiemken TL, Brown TS. Effect of postoperative dressing on excisions performed on the leg: a comparison between zinc oxide compression dressings versus standard wound care. Dermatol Surg. 2017; 43(11):1379–1384
[89] Jewett BS. Interpolated forehead and melolabial flaps. Facial Plast Surg Clin North Am. 2009; 17(3):361–377
[90] Newlove T, Cook J. Safety of staged interpolation flaps after Mohs micrographic surgery in an outpatient setting: a single-center experience. Dermatol Surg. 2013; 39(11):1671–1682
[91] Kovich O, Otley CC. Perioperative management of anticoagulants and platelet inhibitors for cutaneous surgery: a survey of current practice. Dermatol Surg. 2002; 28(6):513–517
[92] Lewis KG, Dufresne RG , Jr. A meta-analysis of complications attributed to anticoagulation among patients following cutaneous surgery. Dermatol Surg. 2008; 34(2):160–164, discussion 164–165

[93] Kimyai-Asadi A, Goldberg LH, Peterson SR, Silapint S, Jih MH. The incidence of major complications from Mohs micrographic surgery performed in office-based and hospital-based settings. J Am Acad Dermatol. 2005; 53(4):628–634
[94] O'Neill JL, Taheri A, Solomon JA, Pearce DJ. Postoperative hemorrhage risk after outpatient dermatologic surgery procedures. Dermatol Surg. 2014; 40(1):74–76
[95] Douketis JD, Spyropoulos AC, Spencer FA, et al. Perioperative management of antithrombotic therapy: Antithrombotic therapy and prevention of thrombosis. 9th ed. American College of Chest Physicians Evidence-Based Clinical Practice Guidelines. Chest. 2012; 141 (4):1129
[96] Sardar P, Chatterjee S, Lavie CJ, et al. Risk of major bleeding in different indications for new oral anticoagulants: insights from a meta-analysis of approved dosages from 50 randomized trials. Int J Cardiol. 2015; 179:279–287
[97] Fenger-Eriksen C, Münster AM, Grove EL. New oral anticoagulants: clinical indications, monitoring and treatment of acute bleeding complications. Acta Anaesthesiol Scand. 2014; 58(6):651–659
[98] Larson RJ, Aylward J. Evaluation and management of hypertension in the perioperative period of Mohs micrographic surgery: a review. Dermatol Surg. 2014; 40(6):603–609
[99] Woodard CR. Complications in facial flap surgery. Facial Plast Surg Clin North Am. 2013; 21(4):599–604
[100] Cook JL, Perone JB. A prospective evaluation of the incidence of complications associated with Mohs micrographic surgery. Arch Dermatol. 2003; 139(2):143–152
[101] Stables G, Lawrence CM. Management of patients taking anticoagulant, aspirin, non-steroidal anti-inflammatory and other antiplatelet drugs undergoing dermatological surgery. Clin Exp Dermatol. 2002; 27(6):432–435
[102] Alam M, Ibrahim O, Nodzenski M, et al. Adverse events associated with Mohs micrographic surgery: multicenter prospective cohort study of 20,821 cases at 23 centers. JAMA Dermatol. 2013; 149 (12):1378–1385
[103] Neumayer L, Hosokawa P, Itani K, El-Tamer M, Henderson WG, Khuri SF. Multivariable predictors of postoperative surgical site infection after general and vascular surgery: results from the patient safety in surgery study. J Am Coll Surg. 2007; 204(6):1178–1187
[104] Wahie S, Lawrence CM. Wound complications following diagnostic skin biopsies in dermatology inpatients. Arch Dermatol. 2007; 143 (10):1267–1271
[105] Kulichová D, Geimer T, Mühlstädt M, Ruzicka T, Kunte C. Surgical site infections in skin surgery: a single center experience. J Dermatol. 2013; 40(10):779–785
[106] Xia Y, Cho S, Greenway HT, Zelac DE, Kelley B. Infection rates of wound repairs during Mohs micrographic surgery using sterile versus nonsterile gloves: a prospective randomized pilot study. Dermatol Surg. 2011; 37(5):651–656
[107] Mailler-Savage EA, Neal KW , Jr, Godsey T, Adams BB, Gloster HM , Jr. Is levofloxacin necessary to prevent postoperative infections of auricular second-intention wounds? Dermatol Surg. 2008; 34 (1):26–30, discussion 30–31
[108] Stevens DL, Bisno AL, Chambers HF, et al. Practice guidelines for the diagnosis and management of skin and soft tissue infections: 2014 update by the infectious diseases society of America. Clin Infect Dis. 2014; 59(2):147–159
[109] Sniezek PJ, Brodland DG, Zitelli JA. A randomized controlled trial comparing acetaminophen, acetaminophen and ibuprofen, and acetaminophen and codeine for postoperative pain relief after Mohs surgery and cutaneous reconstruction. Dermatol Surg. 2011; 37 (7):1007–1013
[110] Lopez JJ, Warner NS, Arpey CJ, et al. Opioid prescribing for acute postoperative pain after cutaneous surgery. J Am Acad Dermatol. 2019; 80(3):743–748
[111] Firoz BF, Goldberg LH, Arnon O, Mamelak AJ. An analysis of pain and analgesia after Mohs micrographic surgery. J Am Acad Dermatol. 2010; 63(1):79–86
[112] Limthongkul B, Samie F, Humphreys TR. Assessment of postoperative pain after Mohs micrographic surgery. Dermatol Surg. 2013; 39 (6):857–863
[113] Chen AF, Landy DC, Kumetz E, Smith G, Weiss E, Saleeby ER. Prediction of postoperative pain after Mohs micrographic surgery with 2 validated pain anxiety scales. Dermatol Surg. 2015; 41(1):40–47

Index

Note: Page numbers set **bold** or *italic* indicate headings or figures, respectively.